CW01478593

Equine
Neonatal Medicine
A Case-Based Approach

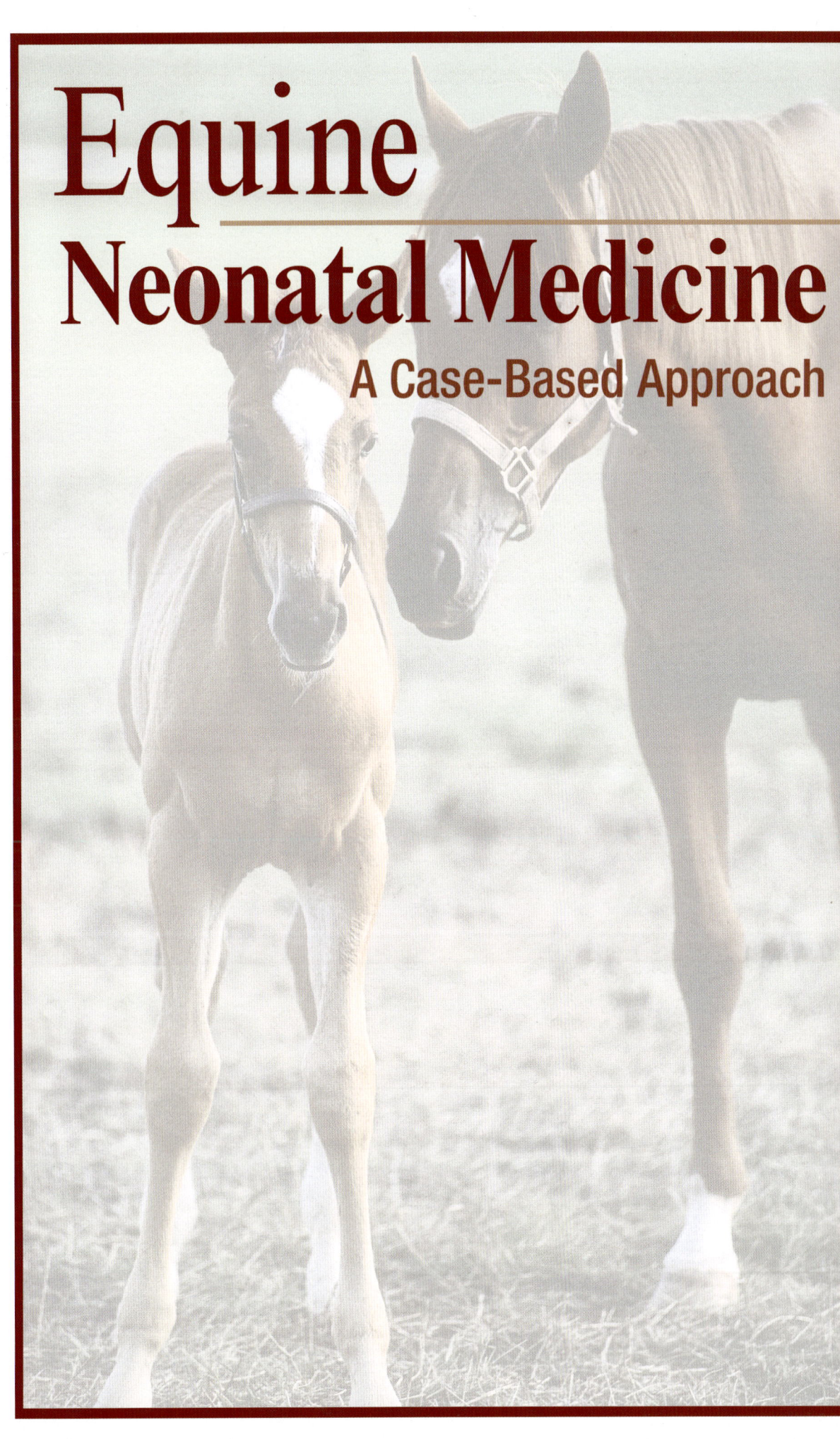

Equine
Neonatal Medicine

A Case-Based Approach

Mary Rose Paradis, DVM, MS, DACVIM(LAIM)

Tufts Cummings School of Veterinary Medicine
North Grafton, Massachusetts

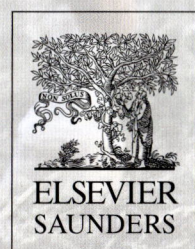

ELSEVIER
SAUNDERS

ELSEVIER
SAUNDERS

1600 John F. Kennedy Blvd.
Ste 1800
Philadelphia, PA 19103-2899

EQUINE NEONATOLOGY: A CASE-BASED APPROACH   ISBN-13: 978-1-4160-2353-1
                                                   ISBN-10: 1-4160-2353-4

Copyright © 2006 by Elsevier Inc.

Notice

Companion animal practice is an ever-changing field. Standard safety precautions must be followed, but as new research and clinical experience grow, changes in treatment and drug therapy become necessary or appropriate. The authors and editors of this work have carefully checked the generic and trade drug names and verified drug dosages to assure that dosage information is precise and in accord with standards accepted at the time of publication. Readers are advised, however, to check the product information currently provided by the manufacturer of each drug to be administered to be certain that changes have not been made in the recommended dose or in the contraindications for administration. This is of particular importance in regard to new or infrequently used drugs. Recommended dosages for animals are sometimes based on adjustments in the dosage that would be suitable for humans. Some of the drugs mentioned here have been given experimentally by the authors. Others have been used in dosages greater than those recommended by the manufacturer. In these kinds of cases, the authors have reported on their own considerable experience. It is the responsibility of those administering a drug, relying on their professional skill and experience, to determine the dosages, the best treatment for the patient, and whether the benefits of giving a drug justify the attendant risk. The editors cannot be responsible for misuse or misapplication of the material in this work.

The Publisher

ISBN-13: 978-1-4160-2353-1
ISBN-10: 1-4160-2353-4

Publishing Director: Linda Duncan
Senior Editor: Liz Fathman
Managing Editor: Jolynn Gower
Editorial Assistant: Stacy Beane
Publishing Services Manager: Julie Eddy
Project Manager: Ellen Kunkelmann
Designer: Paula Ruckenbrod

Printed in China

Last digit is the print number: 9 8 7 6 5 4 3 2 1

Dedication

This book is dedicated to the Trustees of The Dorothy Russell Havemeyer Foundation, especially Gene Pranzo, for their contribution to the acquisition and sharing of new knowledge in the field of Equine Neonatology.

Preface

Equine neonatology became a recognized area of interest in the early 1980s. In the last 25 years, research and literature on the subject of the newborn foal have flourished. The purpose of this book is two-fold: to chronicle the new developments in the field, and to write a text that presents this information in a manner that actually encourages people to read for a bigger picture.

The first goal is accomplished by assembling a team of authors who have worked intensely with the equine neonate during their careers and are willing to share their experiences and knowledge with others to continue the trend of improvement in medicine and the outcomes of our patients. Each author approaches a case in a slightly different manner, thus adding breadth to the manner in which the reader can approach a problem.

In order to accomplish the second goal, one needs to see how textbooks are currently used. As a professor teaching large animal veterinary medicine, I have found that most textbooks are only used as reference books. The only person that reads a veterinary textbook from cover to cover is the resident preparing for their specialty examination! This is certainly not a bad use of a textbook but it generally limits one's search to brief excursions into one disease and may not open one up to other possible diagnoses or treatments.

Learning a litany of facts about a certain disease without having a particular patient or story to tie those facts to is inefficient and unproductive. Telling stories or presenting examples allow the reader to use imagination to conjure up the patient and question what might be happening. The reader becomes an active participant in the case. As the case unravels and the solutions are presented, the reader receives insight into how the situation developed. This active participation is one of the most important factors in learning.

So the question becomes—How does one tell stories in a textbook? If you look at the table of contents for this book, you will see that all the normal topics will be covered. It is how they are covered that is important for this particular book. Each chapter will be made up of one or more cases. There might be a single case that the author has seen or a conglomerate of different cases that present the salient points of the particular disease. Anatomy and physiology is discussed in the context of diagnosis and treatment of the disease. Through this method, the reader will have the experience of "seeing" all of the patients, not only "experiencing" the cases but also actually beginning to understand basic mechanisms of disease and decisions behind the tests and treatments.

Of course the names of the patients have been changed to protect the confidentiality of the owners. See if you can find a connection between the foal's new name and its disease! I hope that you enjoy this format and look forward to your comments.

Acknowledgments

I would like to acknowledge all the work done by the contributors to this book—not only for this book but for the profession as a whole. I consider the contributors of this book to be not only the writers of the cases but also my colleagues who have done the research that supports the information found here. I would like to thank Andy Cunningham from the Educational Media division at Tufts Cummings School of Veterinary Medicine for the work that he did to make sure all of the pictures were clear and sharp. As the chapters started rolling in, Sue Corey was instrumental in helping me organize the drafts. My editors at Elsevier—Jolynn Gower, Andrea Campbell, and Ellen Kunkelmann—were always receptive to my ideas and vision for the book. Thank you.

As you may see I have dedicated this book to the Trustees of the Dorothy Russell Havemeyer Foundation, especially Gene Pranzo. I met Gene in 1990 when he asked me to become a primary investigator for the Foundation. The foundation has given me the freedom to investigate clinical diseases of the newborn foal, support clinical cases that may otherwise have been euthanized, and gather experts in the field to exchange the newest foal research to help develop new ideas as to what the next steps should be. I am eternally grateful for this opportunity.

A percentage of the royalties of this book will be donated to the ACVIM Foundation to support continued clinical research, and to the Travis Fund at Tufts Cummings School of Veterinary Medicine in support of patients who lack funds for treatment.

Contributors

Michelle Henry Barton, DVM, PhD, DACVIM(LAIM)
Professor, Large Animal Medicine
College of Veterinary Medicine
University of Georgia
Athens, Georgia

Daniela Bedenice, Dr. med. vet., DACVIM(LAIM)
Assistant Professor, Clinical Sciences
Tufts University School of Veterinary Medicine
North Grafton, Massachusetts

Virginia Ann Buechner-Maxwell DVM, MS, DACVIM(LAIM)
Associate Professor and Section Chief
Large Animal Clinical Sciences
Virginia-Maryland Regional College of Veterinary
  Medicine
Blacksburg, Virginia

Katherine Chope, VMD
Large Animal Ultrasound Consultant
Hospital for Large Animals
Tufts University School of Veterinary Medicine
North Grafton, Massachusetts

Brett Dolente, VMD, DACVIM(LAIM)
Staff Veterinarian
Sections of Large Animal Internal Medicine and
  Emergency, Critical Care, and Anesthesia
School of Veterinary Medicine
University of Pennsylvania
Kennett Square, Pennsylvania

Bettina Dunkel, DVM, DACVIM(LAIM)
Department of Veterinary Basic Science
Royal Veterinary College
North Mymms, Hatfield
Hertfordshire, UK

Jill R. Johnson, DVM, MS, DACVIM(LAIM), DABVP
Professor of Equine Medicine
Veterinary Clinical Sciences
School of Veterinary Medicine
Louisiana State University
Baton Rouge, Louisiana

Isabel Jurk, DVM, DACVO
Tufts Cummings School of Veterinary Medicine
Tufts University
North Grafton, Massachusetts

K. Gary Magdesian, DVM, DACVIM(LAIM), DACVECC, DACVCP
Assistant Professor, Equine Critical Care Medicine
Department of Medicine and Epidemiology
University of California, Davis
Davis, California

Melissa R. Mazan, DVM, DACVIM(LAIM)
Assistant Professor, Director of Sports Medicine
Clinical Sciences
Tufts University School of Veterinary Medicine
North Grafton, Massachusetts

Rose Nolen-Walston, DVM, DACVIM(LAIM)
Tufts Cummings School of Veterinary Medicine
Tufts University
North Grafton, Massachusetts

Jonathan Palmer, VMD, DACVIM(LAIM)
Associate Professor of Medicine
Department of Clinical Studies—New Bolton Center
School of Veterinary Medicine
University of Pennsylvania
Kennett Square, Pennsylvania

Mary Rose Paradis DVM, MS, DACVIM(LAIM)
Tufts Cummings School of Veterinary Medicine
Tufts University
North Grafton, Massachusetts

Patricia J. Provost, VMD, MS, DACVS
Department of Clinical Sciences
Tufts University Cummings School of Veterinary
    Medicine
North Grafton, Massachusetts

**Debra C. Sellon, DVM, PhD,
DACVIM(LAIM)**
Professor, Equine Medicine
Department of Veterinary Clinical Sciences
Washington State University
Pullman, Washington

**Sarah J. Stoneham, BVSc Cert, ESM,
MRCVS**
Rossdale and Partners
Newmarket, United Kingdom

**Craig D. Thatcher DVM, MS, PhD,
DACVN**
Professor
Department of Large Animal Clinical Sciences
Virginia-Maryland Regional College of Veterinary
    Medicine
Blacksburg, Virginia

**Pamela A. Wilkins, DVM, MS, PhD,
DACVIM(LAIM), DACVECC**
Chief, Section of Emergency, Critical Care and
    Anesthesia
Clinical Studies, New Bolton Center
School of Veterinary Medicine
University of Pennsylvania
Kennett Square, Pennsylvania

Contents

1 Assessing the Newborn Foal, 1

Case 1-1 '03 Labour of Love—Normal Foal (Sarah J. Stoneham), 1

2 High-Risk Pregnancy, 13

Case 2-1 '03 Vital Connection—Placentitis in the Peripartum Mare (Pamela A. Wilkins), 13

Case 2-2 Poppy—Body Wall Tear in Late Gestational Mare and Birth Resuscitation of a Compromised Foal (Pamela A. Wilkins and Brett Dolente), 22

3 Neonatal Immunology, 31

Case 3-1 '03 Vulnerable—Foal with Failure of Passive Transfer (Debra C. Sellon), 31

Case 3-2 '03 In the Red—Foal with Isoerythrolysis (Jill Johnson), 39

Case 3-3 '04 Diplomatic Immunity—Foal with Immune-mediated Thrombocytopenia (Debra C. Sellon), 46

4 Neonatal Nutrition, 51

Case 4-1 '03 Honeysuckle—Normal Foal Nutritional Needs (Virginia Ann Buechner-Maxwell and Craig D. Thatcher), 51

Case 4-2 '03 Lonely Heart—Orphan Foal (Virginia Ann Buechner-Maxwell and Craig D. Thatcher), 56

Case 4-3 '03 RunninOnEmpty—Feeding the Foal that Needs Enteral and Parenteral Nutrition (Virginia Ann Buechner-Maxwell and Craig D. Thatcher), 60

5 Septicemia, 75

Case 5-1 '02 Bugs Bunny—Septic Foal (Michelle Henry Barton), 75

6 Manifestations of Septicemia, 99

Case 6-1 '03 Hufflepuff—Foal with Septic Pneumonia (Daniela Bedenice), 99

Case 6-2 '02 Cripple Creek—Foal with Septic Arthritis (Mary Rose Paradis), 112

7 Recognition and Resuscitation of the Critically Ill Foal, 121

Case 7-1 '04 Revival—Foal in Hemodynamic Shock (Jonathan Palmer), 121

8 Non-infectious Respiratory Problems, 135

Case 8-1 '03 Surf's Up—Immature Lungs in a Foal with Maternal Stress (Melissa R. Mazan), 135

Case 8-2 '03 Last Gasp—Premature Lungs in a Foal from an Emergency C-Section (Melissa R. Mazan), 135

Case 8-3 '05 HardToSwallow—Aspiration Pneumonia Secondary to Dysphagia (Mary Rose Paradis), 148

9 Non-infectious Musculoskeletal Problems, 157

Case 9-1 '03 UpTight—Foal with Flexural Deformity (Patricia Provost), 157

Case 9-2 '04 Crooked Mile—Foal with Forelimb Valgus Deformity (Patricia Provost), 165

Case 9-3 '04 Gumby—Foal with Incomplete Ossification of Cuboidal Bones (Patricia Provost), 165

10 Neurologic Dysfunctions, 179

Case 10-1 '05 Carpe Diem—Foal with Hypoxic Encephalopathy (Mary Rose Paradis), 179

11 Gastrointestinal Problems in the Neonatal Foal, 191

Case 11-1 '03 RockN'Roll—Colic in the Newborn Foal (Michelle Henry Barton), 191

Case 11-2 '04 Belly Dancer—Gastric Ulcers and Esophageal Reflux (Endoscopy) (K. Gary Magdesian), 208

Case 11-3 '03 Liquid Assets—Diarrhea (K. Gary Magdesian), 213

CONTENTS

Case 11-4 '04 Jaundiced View—Liver Failure in the Foal (K. Gary Magdesian), 221

12 Umbilical and Urinary Disorders, 231

Case 12-1 Mutiny—Umbilical Infection/Patent Urachus (Rose Nolen-Walston), 231
Case 12-2 '04 Unzipped—Rupture of the Urinary Bladder (Pamela A. Wilkins and Bettina Dunkel), 237

13 Cardiac Disorders, 247

Case 13-1 '01 Dear John—Foal with Congenital Cardiac Defect (Katherine Chope), 247

14 Ophthalmologic Disorders, 259

Case 14-1 '04 FortyLashes—Foal with Entropion and Cataract (Isabel Jurk), 259
Case 14-2 '05 Misty—Foal with Corneal Ulceration (Isabel Jurk), 265
Case 14-3 '05 MrMagoo—Septic Foal with Hypopyon (Isabel Jurk), 268

Index, 271

1 Assessing the Newborn Foal

| Case 1-1 | Normal Foal | Sarah J. Stoneham |

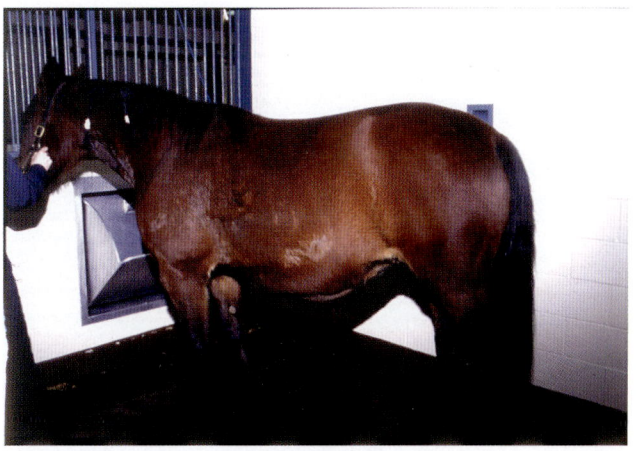

Fig. 1-1 Labour of Love, 340 days pregnant, in foaling stall.

At 340 days of pregnancy, Labour of Love, a multiparous Thoroughbred mare, had been showing signs of impending parturition over the last 5 days. She had a well-developed udder, and "wax" was beginning to form on the ends of her teats. The muscles around her hindquarters appeared to be softer, and her vulva was relaxed. As with her previous pregnancies, this pregnancy had been uneventful. (Figure 1-1)

HORMONAL SIGNALING OF PARTURITION

The fetal hypothalmo-pituitary-adrenal axis initiates fetal maturation and the cascade of hormonal events resulting in parturition and functional maturation of fetal organ systems. During the second part of pregnancy, progestagens are synthesised by the fetus and the utero-placental unit. There is a marked rise in maternal progestagen levels (principally pregnenolone:P5) during the last few weeks of pregnancy as a result of increasing stimulation of the fetal adrenal gland by ACTH. There are differences in maternal progestagens levels between horses and ponies, although the pattern of change is consistent.

This is followed by a redirection of steroidogenesis in the last few days prior to parturition. It is thought that increasing levels of cortisol induce 17α hydroxylase. This enhances metabolism of P5 to cortisol, producing a rise in fetal cortisol and a concomitant decrease in maternal progestagens. This rise in cortisol usually occurs in the last 5 days of gestation, continues for a few hours after birth,[1,2] and is essential to the viability of the foal.

Normal foals have high progestagen levels at birth, which decrease rapidly in the first few hours after birth (Figure 1-2). Progestagen levels in abnormal and premature foals remain high, and a decrease can be associated with recovery. In foals that do not survive, levels may remain elevated. It is thought that this may be due to blocking of an enzyme, which is necessary for preventing overproduction.[3,4]

Signs of impending parturition may include relaxation of the muscles of the hindquarters and lengthening of the vulvar lips. During pregnancy, the mammary glands are exposed to high levels of estrogen and progestagens. It is thought that lactation is triggered by the rise in progestagens from about 310 days gestation, then the precipitous decrease 2 to 3 days prior to parturition, combined with increasing prolactin levels during the last week of pregnancy. Udder enlargement usually begins 2 to 3 weeks before parturition. As birth becomes imminent, small amounts of beaded colostrum may form on the tips of the teats. This is called "waxing." Calcium content of

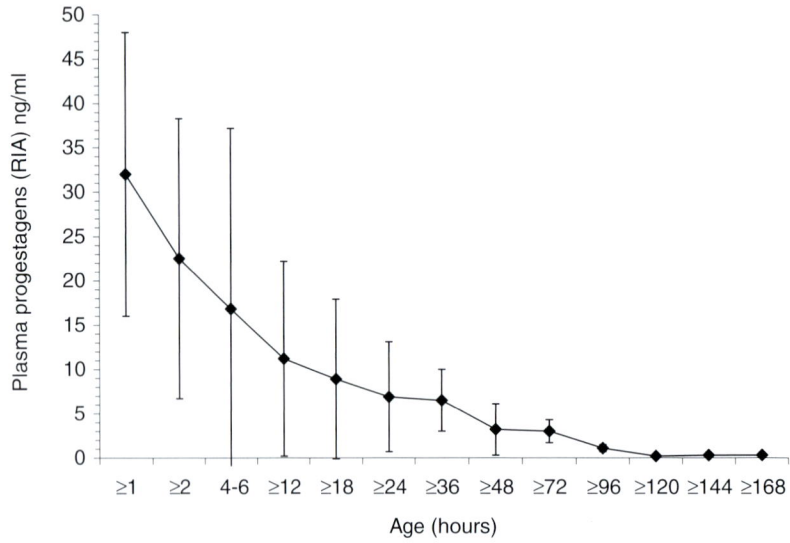

Fig. 1-2 Mean ± s.d. plasma progestagen levels in the normal foal (determined by radioimmunoassay). From Houghton E et al.: Plasma progestagen concentrations in the normal and dysmature foal, *J Reprod Fert* Suppl 44:609-617, 1991.

the mammary secretion increases over the last day of pregnancy. Field tests are available to measure calcium in the hopes of predicting when a mare will foal. These tests are not 100% reliable.[5] It is important to remember that each mare is an individual and that not all "wax up." Also, some don't enlarge the udder until days before the birth. Occasionally a mare will actually produce and leak milk 1 to 5 days before the birth. This is of grave concern because the potential loss of colostrum for the foal and failure of passive immunoglobulins.

The production of colostrum is a unique event. It is a vital component that enhances the efficacy of the foal's naïve immune system. Maternal immunoglobulins are concentrated in a nonspecific way in the mammary gland. Colostrum provides immunoglobulins, complement, lysozyme, and lactoferrin and large numbers of B-lymphocytes. It also contains growth factors important in maturation of the gastrointestinal tract. A Thoroughbred mare typically produces 1 to 2 liters of colostrum. (See Chapter 4.)

Because of her increasing restlessness, Labour of Love was placed in the foaling stall, where she appeared uninterested in hay and grain. By 10 PM, she started to sweat and pace the stall. Her tail was bandaged, and her udder and perineum were cleaned. Just after 10:30 PM, Labour of Love "broke her water," and she went down in lateral recumbency and started to strain. Gentle vaginal examination revealed the foal to be presented normally with the nose palpable between the extended forelimbs. The mare was observed and left to foal unassisted.

Ten minutes after the beginning of second-stage labor, a filly was born and rapidly attained a sternal position

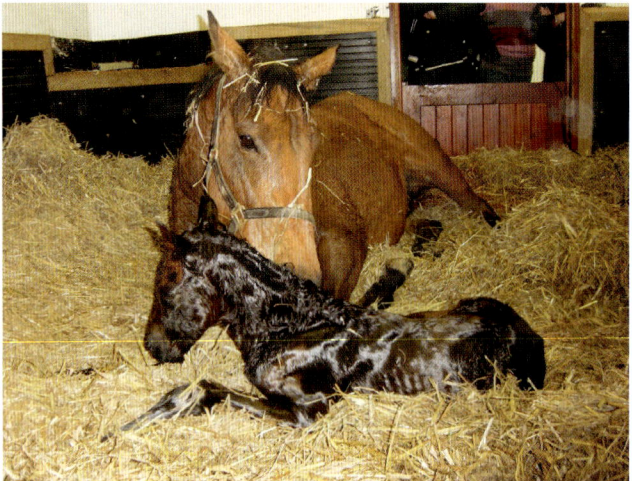

Fig. 1-3 '03 Labour of Love with mare sitting in sternal recumbency 10 minutes after birth.

(see Figure 1-3). A few minutes later the umbilical cord broke with the filly's first attempts to stand. The filly was moved in front of the mare, and the umbilical remnants were treated with a 0.5% chlorhexidine and surgical alcohol mix. The foal had a suckle reflex present, and the foal made attempts to stand as the mare licked it. Forty-five minutes after birth, the foal was able to stand with a base-wide stance and started typical udder-seeking behavior (Figure 1-4).

The mare passed an intact placenta weighing 6 kg, 1 hour after foaling. A small sample of colostrum was taken before the foal nursed and specific gravity was checked using a sugar refractometer. It measured 29%, which is considered to indicate good colostral quality. The foal suckled from the dam 65 minutes after foaling.

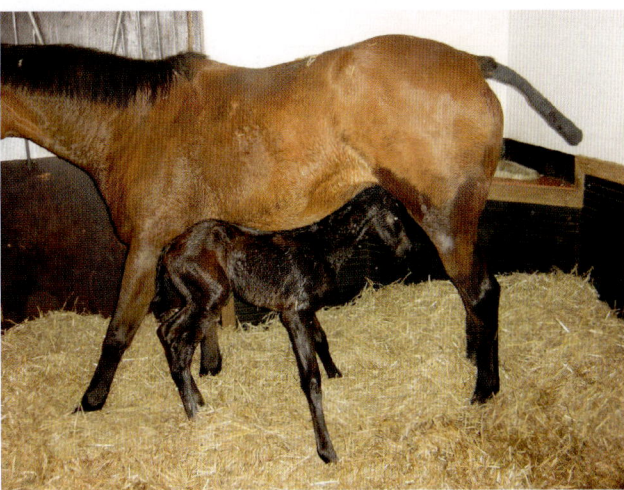

Fig. 1-4 Typical base-wide stance of newborn foal in early udder-seeking behavior.

Table 1-1	Mean (±sem) PaO₂ Values Following 100% Oxygen Administration in Foals Ages 30 Minutes to 7 Days		
Time after Birth	**Number of Foals**	**PaO₂ after 5 minutes of 100% O₂ (mm Hg)**	
30 minutes	5	238.5 ± 37.5	
2 hours	4	262.7 ± 70.4	
4 hours	4	241.8 ± 60.4	
12 hours	6	$293.8 \pm 38.3^*$	
24 hours	5	$344.1 \pm 35.6^*$	
48 hours	6	$363.8 \pm 36.0^*$	
4 days	6	$368.9 \pm 52.6^*$	
7 days	5	$483.0 \pm 43.2^{**}$	

$^*P < 0.05$.
$^{**}P < 0.01$ statistically significantly different from the value at 30 minutes after birth (from Stewart et al., 1984).

TRANSITION TO EXTRAUTERINE LIFE

At birth the foal is hypoxemic and hypercapnic; this stimulates the first gasping breaths, which start to inflate the lungs. There is also a marked decrease in pulmonary vascular resistance due to expansion of the lungs and rising PaO₂, which allows increased blood flow through the lungs. This produces increased return of blood to the left atrium and functional closure of the foramen ovale. Closure is also facilitated by the decrease in right atrial pressure, due to absence of venous return from the umbilical vein. The ductus arteriosus constricts and flow is reversed, producing physiological closure within 24 hours and anatomical closure over several days after birth.

Hypoxemia, hypothermia, and acidosis can lead to reversion to a transitional or fetal circulation with right to left shunting, as the foramen ovale and ductus arteriosus reopen and pulmonary hypertension develops. This results in a worsening of the hypoxemia and further increases in pulmonary resistance.

Stroke volume in the neonate is limited, so cardiac output is rate dependant. There are significant changes in the proportion of blood flow to the various organs at birth. In utero the kidney receives 2% of blood flow, which increases to 8% to 10% postpartum. The lungs only receive 15% in utero, which increases to 100% postpartum.[6]

The chest wall of the neonatal foal is very compliant, but the lungs are relatively inelastic, which limits tidal volume, increases work of breathing, and lowers functional reserve capacity of the lungs. High respiratory rates help to overcome this. Tidal volume increases by about 20% during the first week; there is a continued rise in PaO₂ and an increase in alveolar ventilation. The response to 100% inspired oxygen alters significantly over the first week (Table 1-1).[7,8] This results in a significant increase in respiratory reserve by day 7.

Surfactant is present in the lungs from about 300 days gestation; however, a recent study[9] has shown that at 2 days after birth, surfactant surface tension is markedly increased (tenfold) when compared with that of 5-day-old foals. Also, the sum of anionic phospholipids is decreased in normal foals when compared with that of adults. In the Thoroughbred, bronchiolar duct endings continue to increase in the foal until about 1 year of age. This continued postnatal development appears to be absent in ponies.[10]

STAGES OF LABOR

Most Thoroughbred mares foal at night, with 86% occurring between 7 PM and 7 AM, and maximal incidence between 10 PM to 11 PM.[11] During first-stage labor, coordinated uterine contractions push the allanto-chorion into the dilating cervix; at this stage, the mare starts to become restless and may begin to sweat and walk. First-stage labor ends with rupture of the membranes and release of the allantoic fluid (i.e., "breaking water"). During this first phase of parturition, the front half of the foal starts to rotate from a flexed dorsopubic position to a dorsosacral position with the forelimbs and head extending into the birth canal.[12] During second-stage labor, the caudal half of the foal rotates. Although mares can foal in a standing position, most go into lateral recumbency at the start of second-stage labor.

The passage of the foal into the birth canal stimulates oxytocin release, enhancing strong uterine and abdominal contractions that result in rapid expulsion of the foal. The white translucent amniotic sac around the

Range of parameters for foaling

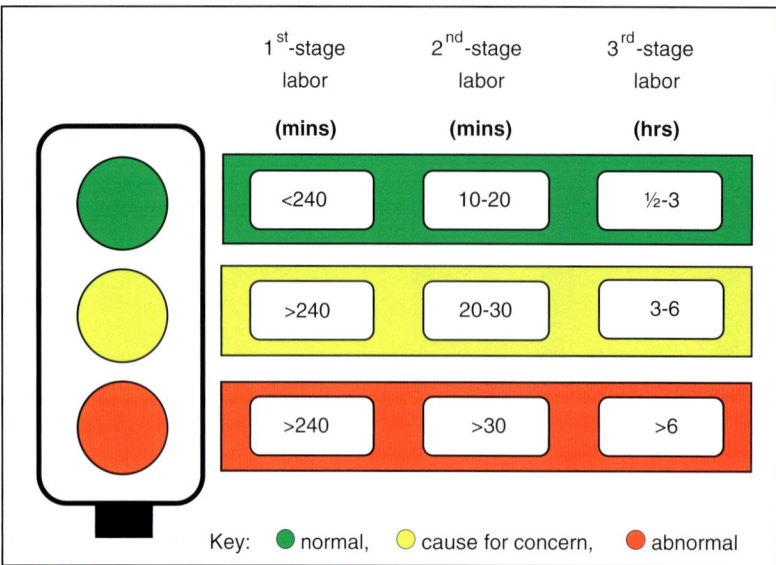

Fig. 1-5 Range of parameters for foaling. Owners should be advised to seek help if parameters fall in the yellow or red zones.

Range of parameters for newborn foal

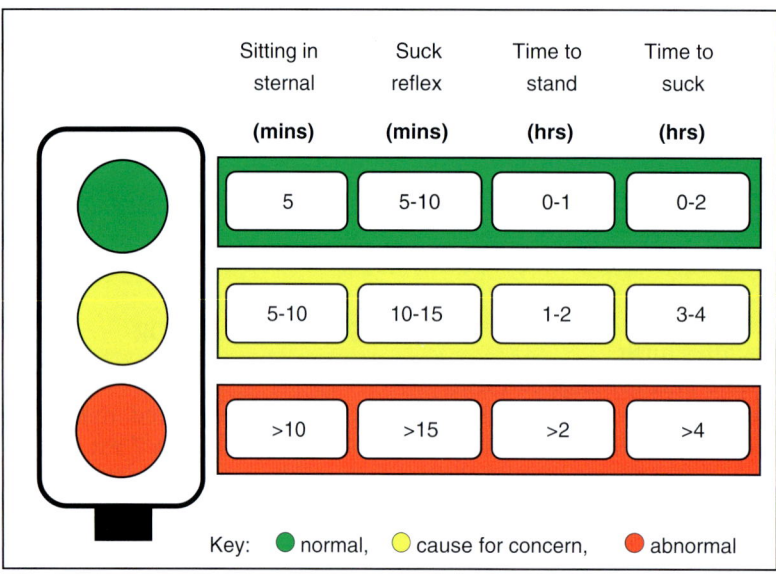

Fig. 1-6 Range of parameters for the newborn foal. Owners should be advised that they should seek veterinary intervention if the foal's parameters fall within the yellow or red zones.

foal's foot is usually visible at the vulval lips within 5 minutes of the rupture of the allantochorion. The mare often gets up and down and may roll during phase two of parturition, which may help to rotate the foal into a normal presentation.

The contractions are most forceful during delivery of the chest, and the mare usually stops straining as the hips are delivered. The foal is usually delivered within the amnion. Struggling from the foal completes delivery. Second stage labor is usually 20 to 30 minutes, and occasionally longer in primiparous mares. Expulsion of the fetal membranes constitutes third-stage labor and usually occurs within 3 hours of birth.[13]

It is important to give owners a timetable for each stage of labor and for certain foal behaviors that they can use to evaluate the progress of labor and the viability of foals (Figures 1-5 and 1-6). If labor doesn't progress as it should or if the foal fails to stand and suckle within 2 to 3 hours, then veterinary medical intervention is necessary to prevent catastrophic results.

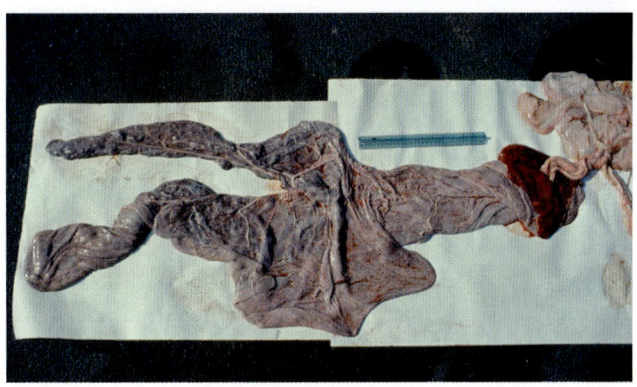

Fig. 1-7 Normal placenta laid out for evaluation. Allantoic side outermost.

EXAMINATION OF THE PLACENTA

The placenta should be weighed and checked for completeness and any signs of abnormality (Figure 1-7). There is a direct relationship between placental weight and fetal size in healthy foals. The placenta from a normal Thoroughbred weighs 5.6 to 6.3 kg (12.3 to 13.8 lbs), and the placenta from ponies averages 2.2 to 2.6 kg (4.8 to 5.7 lbs).[14]

The amnion should be bluish white and translucent with prominent tortuous vessels on its surface. "Cigarette burn" lesions are not considered significant. The amnion is attached to the cord, which should be of uniform diameter, and the whole cord usually measures 36 to 80 cm long. Cord lengths over 70 cm are more likely to be associated with abnormality.[15,16] The umbilical arteries, vein, and urachus comprise the amnionic portion of the umbilicus and usually have a gentle spiral appearance. Excessive twisting of the cord is seen in umbilical torsion and produces a dead or compromised foal.[16]

Both sides of the allanto-chorion should be examined. The smooth allantoic side has the blood vessels under a thin translucent membrane, giving the surface a whitish appearance. The chorionic side, which is attached to the mare's uterus, has a diffuse red velvety appearance; the pregnant horn, nonpregnant horn, and body can be readily identified. An uneven red coloration of the chorionic side of the placenta may be due to uneven blood congestion during the birth process. This is normal but must be differentiated from congestion and edema from placentitis.[17] (See Chapter 2.)

CARE OF THE UMBILICAL REMNANT

The umbilical remnant is a potential portal for entry of bacteria and should be treated to reduce bacterial contamination until it is sealed. *Staphylococcus spp.* is the most commonly isolated organism from this area.

It has been suggested that a concentration of 0.5% chlorhexidine is most effective in reducing bacterial colonization, with a sustained period of activity.[18,19] The addition of surgical alcohol will speed drying and sealing of the cord. Alternatively, an antibiotic in alcohol spray or diluted iodine can be applied. However, there is little evidence-based medicine on this subject. Even for human babies, it remains controversial as to which methods best reduce omalophlebitis and associated complications.

During the night, the foal was seen to suckle from both teats regularly and interact with the mare and explore her surroundings. She slept after feeding and rapidly became more coordinated at rising, lying down, and moving around the stable. She was seen to strain and pass meconium at 4 hours of age and to pass a long stream of pale-colored urine at 8 hours of age.

The following morning, a clinical examination was carried out when the foal was approximately 10 hours old. The foal weighed 57 kg (125 lbs). As the mare had not received a tetanus vaccination in the 4 to 6 weeks prior to foaling, the foal was given 1500 IU of tetanus antitoxin.

BEHAVIOR OF THE NEWBORN FOAL AND ITS DAM

The foal has a strong righting reflex within moments of birth, and the suck reflex is present within 5 to 10 minutes of birth. As the mare starts to lick the foal, the foal extends its forelimbs and attempts to stand. Most normal foals will stand within 1 hour of birth. Pony foals generally stand within the first 30 minutes of life, but larger-breed foals will take anywhere from 30 to 120 minutes to stand.[20,21] The foal should be considered abnormal if it takes longer than 120 minutes to stand. Initially the foal has a very base-wide stance and poor coordination, but this improves rapidly and the foal begins to bond with the mare and commences udder-seeking behavior.

Foals will exhibit suckling behavior before they even stand, by extending their tongue and suckling air. Udder seeking may include suckling on various parts of the mare, such as her ventrum or stifle. Most foals will suckle from the mare within 2 hours of birth. Again, there may be a difference in time to suckling related to breed or size of foal. Crossbred pony foals have been observed to start nursing from their dams within minutes of standing, whereas Thoroughbred or Standardbred foals may take up to 180 minutes after birth.[22,23] Foals that have not suckled within 3 hours should be considered abnormal (see Figure 1-6).

First urination for the foal usually occurs within 6 to 10 hours after birth, with colts urinating closer to the 6 hours and fillies closer to 10 hours.[20] Due to the large volume of milk ingested, large volumes of dilute urine are produced. A neonatal foal will produce approximately 148 ml/kg of urine per day; thus a 50-kg foal will produce about 7.4 liters/day.[24]

Meconium, which consists of allantoic fluid, cell debris, and gastrointestinal tract secretions, accumulates in the rectum and small colon. It is usually passed within 2 to 12 hours of birth. The gastrointestinal system is able to digest colostrum and milk within minutes of birth. The release of hormones and neuropeptides triggered by feeding stimulates gut development vital to postnatal function. Appearance of paler "milk dung" signifies that all the meconium has been voided. Retention of meconium may cause signs of colic in the newborn foal. (See Chapter 11.)

Digestion of mare's milk is very efficient. Lactase levels in the gut peak at birth and start to decline at around 4 months of age. Coprophagia of the mare's fresh feces is common in the newborn foal. Pony foals on pasture were observed to eat feces once every 4 hours.[25] This behavior usually occurs in the first 8 weeks of life. Although this behavior is not completely understood, the ingestion of feces in the young foal is thought to help establish colonic normal flora.

If bonded well, the mare and foal will spend 80% to 90% of their time within 1 to 5 meters of each other. Foals then develop a pattern of suckling the mare; during the first week, they suckle about 2 minutes, 5 to 7 times each hour.[26] This decreases during periods of rest. Foals normally initiate bouts of nursing by going directly to the udder or circling in front of the dam to signal to the mare to stop. Nursing bouts may begin with the foal "head butting" the dam's flank or udder. It is presumed that this signals to the mare and initiates milk letdown.[26] By day 2, Thoroughbred foals consume approximately 23% of their body weight in milk.[27] Newborn foals tend to rest in sternal recumbency for the first few days, which helps to maintain body temperature and improve lung function.

Rejection of the foal by its mare is most common in primiparous mares and often manifests as fear and avoidance of the foal.[28] In a more serious form of rejection, the mare actually attacks her foal. Certain mares are known to chronically reject their foals. It is important to try to prevent this behavior. Avoidable disturbances during the bonding process between the mare and foal immediately after birth should be eliminated. However, if the foal is in danger of not being able to suckle or is being attacked by the mare, intervention is necessary. If the mare is afraid of the foal, then calm restraint and perhaps tranquilization is sufficient for the mare to accept her newborn. If this does not achieve the goal of safe nursing or if the mare is chronically foal-aggressive, then the alternative of arranging for a "nurse" mare should be considered. (See Chapter 4.)

CLINICAL EXAMINATION

Normal neonatal foals are bright and inquisitive. When approached, the foal will usually move rapidly away from the handler to the far side of the mare. They are easily aroused from resting or sleeping and will usually jump up and go to suckle from the mare. If a foal does not behave in this manner, it is possible that it is showing the first signs of a serious illness. Because of the normal foal's liveliness, it can be difficult to determine its normal heart rate or respiratory rate, which can range from 60 to 100 beats/minute and 12 to 40 breaths/minute, respectively, depending on the foal's age and level of excitement when being caught (Table 1-2).

Very young foals may become quite relaxed, in an almost cataplectic state, once they are caught and securely restrained, with an arm around the chest and the other around the hindquarters, or when they are restrained in lateral recumbency. This is a normal response for the first few hours, but should be differentiated from the generally debilitated "floppy" foal.

Foals are extremely sensitive to tactile stimuli, and movements of the head may be exaggerated and jerky. Initially they have a rather base-wide stance and gaits may appear hypermetric. There are several significant

Table 1-2	Heart and Respiratory Rates and Temperature of Normal Newborn Foal		
Age	Heart Rate (beats/minute)	Respiratory Rate (breaths/min)	Temperature °C (°F)
birth	60–80	Gasping	37–39 (99–102)
0–2 hours	120–150	40–60	37–39 (99–102)
12 hours	80–120	30–40	37–39 (99–102)
24 hours	80–100	30–35	37–39 (99–102)

differences in the neurologic response of the newborn foal compared to the adult. Neurological examination of the newborn foal has been described.[29] It is important to be aware of these physiological differences, which in the adult may be associated with abnormality. Particular points to remember include:

- Until about 3 weeks of age, foals have a marked crossed extensor reflex of the forelimbs, with marked resting extensor tone when in lateral recumbency, and to a lesser extent in the hindlimbs

- Reflexes of hindlimbs are hyperflexic

- Gaits are hypermetric

- Movements of head and neck are rather jerky

- The menace response is a learned response and is incomplete until about 2 weeks of age[30]

- Foals have a biphasic papillary light response and for the first few days appear slower than in the adult

- Pupil position is ventromedial and becomes dorsomedial by about 1 month of age, however, position may change with brain dysfunction

- An assessment of the physical characteristics will help determine maturity; a mole-like coat, excessively pliant lips and ears, a domed forehead, and laxity of the tendons of the distal limbs are associated with immaturity. Low birth weight or poor body condition or muscular development may indicate immaturity or intrauterine growth restriction.

Mucous membranes should be moist to wet, pale pink, and have a rapid capillary refill of 1 to 2 seconds. Nostrils should be dry; evidence of milk at the nostrils may indicate a palate defect or pharyngeal dysfunction. (See Case 8-2)

Healthy full-term foals are able to effectively thermoregulate immediately after birth. Despite this, neonatal foals are susceptible to hypothermia as they have relatively little insulating subcutaneous fat, a large surface area to body weight ratio, and immature mechanisms for thermogenesis. Foals are frequently born into an environment with air temperatures below lower critical temperature and have a wet pelt resulting in a high rate of heat loss. This stimulates thermogenesis, which prior to ingestion of the first feed is dependant on endogenous energy sources and shivering to increase metabolic rate to near maximal. Metabolic rate then declines during the 6 hours following birth and then slowly increases again with age.[31] The normal body temperature of the equine neonate ranges from 99° to 101.5°F (37° to 39°C).

Foals are dependant on continuous ingestion of milk and high levels of activity to maintain body temperature. In the sick or anaesthetised individual, these mechanisms are frequently compromised.

Careful palpation of the chest should be performed to check for rib fractures, assessing pain, crepitus, or asymmetry. Fractures occur most frequently in the cranioventral portion of the chest; ribs 3-8 are most commonly involved. Fractures of 3 or more ribs increase the risk of fatality,[32] however, a fracture of a single rib that lacerates the heart or cardiac vessels is inevitably fatal.

Techniques for repair of rib fractures have in practice proved successful. If rib fractures are suspected, ultrasound evaluation and radiography of the chest are appropriate to confirm the diagnosis.[33]

Auscultation of the lungs is not as reliable as in the adult, therefore it is important to combine this with assessment of respiratory pattern and effort. Normal inspiration and expiration should cause only a gentle in and out motion of the chest wall. In foals with pulmonary disease, the respiratory effort will progressively increase from increased intercostal movement to increased synchronous abdominal effort to finally, a paradoxical movement of the chest and abdomen indicating respiratory failure. (See Case 6-1.)

Auscultation of the heart is important to determine rate and rhythm and to detect murmurs, which are common in the neonatal foal. A patent ductus arteriosus produces a grade 1-4 holosystolic murmur most clearly audible over the base of the heart. (See Chapter 13)

The abdomen should be assessed for distension and to check whether milk feces are being passed. Umbilical structures should be palpated with clean or gloved hand. The presences of an umbilical or inguinal hernia should be noted.[34]

Routine blood samples were taken on day 2 to screen for early signs of disease and efficacy of passive transfer of maternal antibodies. Routine screening tests may include haematology, proteins, IgG, and inflammatory markers. These results were within normal limits for a foal of this age (see Table 1-3) and she was considered to have good transfer of passive immunity.

CLINICAL PATHOLOGY

There are significant differences in reference ranges for the neonatal foal. It is important to be aware of variations in methodology between different laboratories, and variations in normal ranges for different breeds. The ranges suggested are considered normal for

Table 1-3	Hematology and Proteins for "Labour of Love" Taken at 18 Hours	
Test	Labour of Love Foal	Normal Range
RBC ($\times 10^{12}$/liter)	9.65	6.9–11.8
PCV	38	28–44
Hb (g/dl)	12.2	10.2–15.4
McV (fl)	39.0	31.7–40
McHc (g/dl)	32.4	31.7–39.4
McH (pg)	12.6	11.2–16.4
WBC ($\times 10^9$/liter)	8.42	6.0–15.0
Bands (%)	0	0
Segs ($\times 10^9$/liter)	6.65	4.1–9.5
Seg (%)	79	60–85
Lymphs ($\times 10^9$/liter)	1.43	1.0–3.1
Lymphs (%)	17	14–37
Monos ($\times 10^9$/liter)	0.34	0.1–0.5
Monos (%)	4	0.5–5.0
Eos ($\times 10^9$/liter)	0	0.1–0.2
Eos (%)	0	1–2
Platelets ($\times 10^9$/liter)	219	140–315
Total protein (mg/dl)	6.2	4.0–6.6
Albumin (mg/dl)	2.9	2.5–3.5
Globulin (mg/dl)	3.3	1.5–3.6
Plasma fibrinogen (mg/dl)	230	50–390
SAA (mg/l)	0.0	0–25
IgG (mg/dl)	13,500	>800

Table 1-4	Normal Range Serum Biochemistry for the Neonatal Thoroughbred Foal
Test	Normal Range
AST (IU/liter)	111–206
CK (IU/liter)	165–300
LD (IU/liter)	615–800
GGT (IU/liter)	10–32
GLDH (IU/liter)	8–45
SAP (IU/liter)	2400–4500
IAP (IU/liter)	528–1200
Urea (mg/dl)	18–22
Creatinine (mg/dl)	1.5–2.9
Calcium (mg/dl)	10–13.8
Phosphate (mg/dl)	4.2–5.85
Magnesium (mg/dl)	2–2.5
Sodium (mEq/liter)	130–140
Potassium (mEq/liter)	3.8–4.5
Glucose (mg/dl)	96–176
Chloride (mEq/liter)	95–105
SDH (IU/liter)	0.2–4.8

Thoroughbred foals (Tables 1-3 and 1-4).[35,36] It is also important to remember that even if a value falls outside the normal range, it must be considered in context with the clinical signs exhibited by the foal and other laboratory parameters.

Hematology

Packed cell volume (PCV) and red blood cell count (RBC) are generally interdependent. Erythrocyte count decreases during the first week. In the newborn foal, PCV and RBC will be influenced by the transfer of placental blood flow, catecholamine secretion, and adjustment of fluid balance as a result of osmotic effect of absorption of colostral immunoglobulins. A low PCV may be associated with premature rupture of the cord or neonatal isoerythrolysis. Mean corpuscular volume (MCV) decreases during the second half of gestation, and consequently provides an indication of maturity. It continues to decrease during the first 4 months of life when there is some degree of microcytosis, and then it gradually increases to adult values.[35]

Leukocytes

There is considerable variation in total white blood cell count (WBC) between normal foals. In general, leukopenia may be associated with bacterial infection, viral infection or immaturity, leukocytosis associated with infection, "stress," or administration of corticosteroids.

Neutrophil numbers rise in the first few hours after birth in response to the cortisol surge and tend to remain elevated. The wide neutrophil to lymphocyte ratio (>2:1) is indicative of normal adrenocortical function in the newborn foal. Neutropenia with the presence of band cells and degenerative/toxic changes are highly suggestive of systemic inflammatory response in the neonatal foal.[37]

Lymphocyte numbers increase over the last half of gestation and continue to rise for the first few months of age due to continued development of the lymphoid system.[35,38] Lymphopenia, <1 × 10^3/ml at less than 12 hours of age, has been associated with EHV or EAV infection. Severe lymphopenia is also seen in Arabian foals with the genetic severe combined immunodeficiency syndrome.

Platelet numbers are similar to adults.[39] Thrombocytopenia in the newborn foal may be associated with immune mediated disease, thought to be due to absorption of colostral antibodies to the foal's platelets. (See Case 3-3.) Routine blood samples may detect a profound thrombocytopenia.

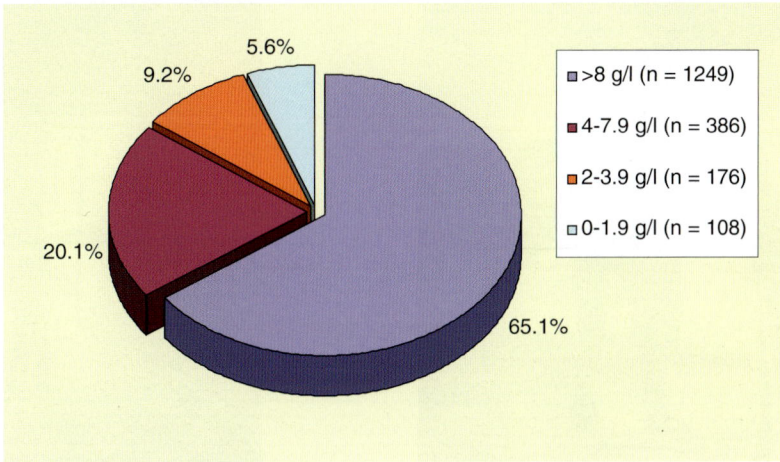

Fig. 1-8 IgG (g/liter) distribution for foals older than 24 hours (1988-1990).

Inflammatory Proteins

Due to the kinetics of fibrinogen, elevated levels in foals <48 hours of age indicate *in utero* pathology. The normal range increases significantly over the first couple of months (increasing from 2g/liter to 4g/liter).[35] An explanation that has been postulated is that it is an inflammatory response to subclinical respiratory disease.

Serum amyloid A (SAA) is an acute-phase inflammatory protein present at low levels in the normal foal. It increases rapidly in response to infection. With acute bacterial infection, levels may increase from <27mg/liter to >200mg/liter. Levels rise to a lesser extent in response to inflammation. Levels decrease rapidly in response to appropriate treatment, making this a useful test in the newborn.[40]

Serum Chemistry

Protein levels in the newborn foal before the ingestion of colostrum are generally low. The foal is virtually agammaglobulinemic at birth. A small amount of IgM can be found in a presuckle serum sample. The efficacy of absorption of colostral IgG directly correlates to globulin levels in the healthy foal in the first few days postpartum.[41] Albumin levels in the newborn tend to decrease in several diseases, therefore, it is important to consider the treatment of the sick neonate in relation to dosage of highly protein-bound drugs.

Routine measurement of IgG in foals >12 hours of age provides an indication of the efficacy of passive transfer of colostrally derived immunity. A survey of IgG levels of routine blood samples taken from clinically healthy Thoroughbred foals on well-managed stud farms indicates that the prevalence of complete or partial failure of passive transfer is as high as 35%[4] (Figure 1-8). (See Case 3-1).

Creatine kinase, an enzyme released due to muscle damage, is within the adult range in the foal. It may be increased with prolonged recumbency, convulsions, and white muscle disease.

Serum alkaline phosphatase is an enzyme that is found in bone, gastrointestinal cells, and liver. It is markedly elevated in foals at birth due to high isoenzymes associated with bone metabolism. It gradually declines over the first few weeks of life, making it less useful in assessing liver function in the neonate.[36]

Evaluation of liver pathology in foals may include aspartate amino transferase (AST), bile acids, and bilirubin. AST is frequently lower in the newborn, rising to adult levels over the first few weeks. Bile acids are elevated in foals aged 1 to 7 days, when compared to adult values, so caution must be used when evaluating this parameter in this period. Mean bile acid concentration of 54.2 ± 12.6 micromoles/liter on day 1, 27.6 ± 5.6 micromoles/liter on day 2, decreasing to 15.6 ± 3.9 micromoles/liter by day 7 have been reported.[39] Bilirubin is sometimes elevated in foals and should be monitored with awareness that it may be secondary to hemolysis of neonatal isoerythrolysis or placental dysfunction. (See Case 3-2.)

Renal function in the foal can be assessed by levels of creatinine, urea, and urine analysis. In the first few days of life, creatinine levels are in the upper end of the normal range of the adult. Elevations in the first 48 hours *postpartum* may reflect placental pathology from the mare rather than disease in the foal. Urea levels lie within the adult range. The neonatal kidney is susceptible to adverse effects, in particular those associated with nephrotoxic drugs, reduced perfusion, and hypovolemia. Urea will also rise in association with a marked negative energy balance, resulting in break-

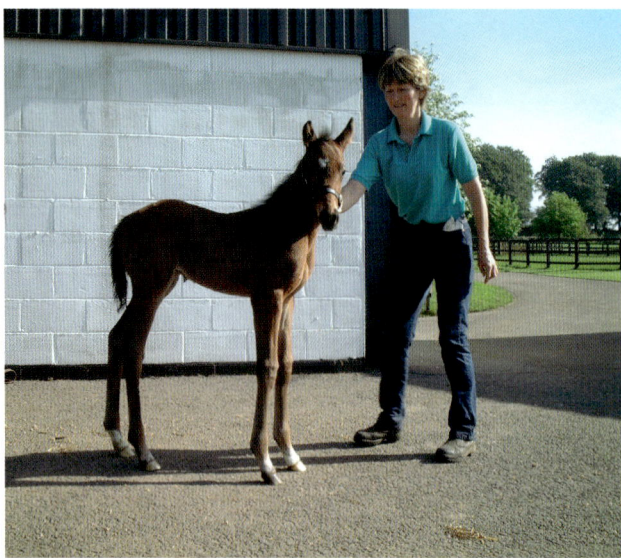

Fig. 1-9 '03 Labour of Love standing on a level hard surface to evaluate conformation.

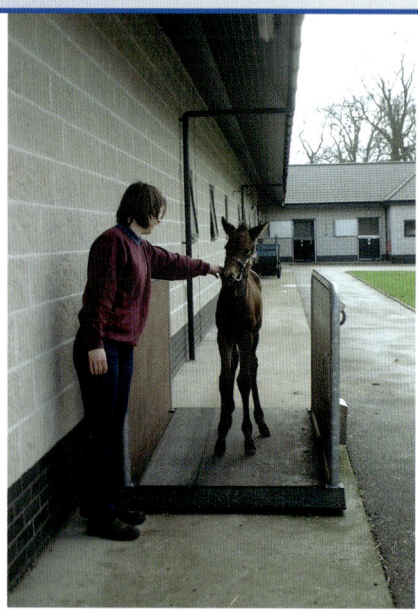

Fig. 1-10 Regular weighing of the foal is important to monitor growth.

down of the foal's body tissues to meet metabolic requirements.

Kidney function in the foal is relatively mature, with glomerular filtration rate and renal plasma flow close to adult values.[42] However, mechanism of tubular secretory function may not be as mature. There is a normal transient proteinuria for the first 24 hours postbirth due to the nonspecific absorption of low-molecular-weight proteins into the blood during this period. The specific gravity is low (1.000-1.025) and will vary in response to hydration.

Lactate measurements are useful in evaluating a sick foal. Values increase with hypoperfusion secondary to dehydration, septicaemia, or endotoxemia.

'03 Labour of Love was walked on a flat hard surface to make a preliminary assessment of conformation in order to determine an appropriate exercise regime (Figure 1-9). The filly was mildly toe out with a slight carpal valgus. There was no evidence of significant limb deformity. She was prescribed a normal exercise regime, with nursery paddock exercise for a few days followed by integration into a group of similar aged foals with their dams.

The foal was weighed the day following her birth and then weekly as she grew. Her birth weight was 57 kg. By

day 7 she was 68 kg, and by 1 month she was 92 kg (Figure 1-10).

NORMAL DEVELOPMENT

Foals have a relatively mature musculoskeletal system at birth, being able to stand and then follow their dams within a few hours of birth. Incomplete ossification of the carpal and tarsal bones is an indicator of immaturity. There is an appreciable degree of tendon and ligament laxity at birth that often produces some degree of angular limb deformity; this should improve rapidly over the first few weeks, as the foal increases its muscular mass and strength. If the abnormalities in the musculoskeletal system do not show some improvement in the first few days of life, medical intervention may be necessary. (See Chapter 9.)

Growth rates are rapid during the first month; on average Thoroughbred foals will gain 1.5-1.7 kg/day (3.3-3.7 lbs/day). Regular monitoring of weight gain can be an additional aid in determining healthy growth and development of the foal. Thoroughbred foals are approximately 68% of their mature height at birth.[43]

REFERENCES

1. Ousey JC: Peripartal endocrinology in the mare and foetus, *Reprod Dom Anim* 39:222-231, 2004.
2. Thorburn GD: A speculative review of parturition in the mare, *Equine Vet J Suppl* 14:41-49, 1993.
3. Houghton E, Holtan D, Grainger L et al: Plasma progestagen concentrations in the normal and dysmature newborn foal, *J Reprod Fert* Suppl 44:609-617, 1991.
4. Rossdale PD, Ousey JC, McGladdery AJ et al: A retrospective study of increased plasma progestagen concentrations in compromised neonatal foals, *Reprod Fertil Dev* 7(3):567-575, 1995.
5. Ousey JC: Evaluation of three strip tests for measuring electrolytes in mares' pre-partum mammary secretions and for predicting parturition, *Equine Vet J* 21:196-200, 1989.

6. Rose RJ: Cardiorespiratory adaptations in neonatal foals, *Equine Vet J* Suppl 5:11-13, 1988.
7. Stewart JH, Rose RJ, Barko AM: Respiratory studies in foals from birth to seven days, *Equine Vet J* 16:323-328, 1984.
8. Stewart JH, Rose RJ, Barko AM: Response to oxygen administration in foals: Effects of age, duration and method of administration on arterial blood gas values, *Equine Vet J* 16:329-331, 1984.
9. Christman U, Taintor J, Livesey L et al: Differences in surfactant function and composition between neonatal foals and adult horses, *JVIM* 411:100, 2004.
10. Beech DJ, Sibbons PD, Rossdale PD et al: Organogenesis of lung and kidney in thoroughbreds and ponies, 33:438-45, 2001.
11. Rossdale PD, Short RV: The time of foaling of Thoroughbred mares, *J Reprod Fert* 13:341-343, 1967.
12. Jeffcott LB, Rossdale PD: A radiographic study of the fetus in late pregnancy and during foaling *J Reprod Fert* Suppl 27:563-569, 1979.
13. Frazer GS, Perkins NR, Embertson RM: Normal parturition and evaluation of the mare in dystocia, *Equine Vet Educ* 11:41-46, 1999.
14. Whitwell K, Jeffcott LB: Morphological studies on the fetal membranes of the normal singleton foal at birth, *Res Vet Sci* 19:44-55, 1975.
15. Cottrill CM: Placental evaluation in the field, *Equine Vet Educ* 3:204-207, 1991.
16. Cottrill CM, Jeffers-Lo J, Ousey JC et al: The placenta as a determinant of fetal wellbeing in normal and abnormal pregnancies, *J Reprod Fert* Suppl 44:591-601, 1991.
17. Schlafer DH: Postmortem examination of the equine placenta, fetus, and neonate: methods and interpretation of findings, Proc 50th Ann Conv *AAEP* 144-161, 2004.
18. Lavan RP, Madigan JE, Walker R et al: Effect of disinfectant treatments on bacterial flora of the umbilicus of neonatal foals, Proc 40th Ann Conv *AAEP* 37, 1994.
19. Madigan JE: Management of the newborn foal, *AAEP* 36:99-116, 1990.
20. Jeffcott LB: Observations on parturition in crossbred pony mares, *Equine Vet J* 4:209-212, 1972.
21. Campitelli S, Carenzi C, Verga M: Factors that influence parturition in the mare and the development of the foal, *Appl Anim Ethol* 9:7-14, 1982.
22. Rossdale PD: Clinical studies on the newborn thoroughbred foal I: Perinatal behavior, *Br Vet J* 123:470-481, 1967.
23. Waring GH: Onset of behavior patterns in the newborn foal, *Equine Pract* 4:28-34, 1982.
24. Brewer BD, Clements SF, Lotz WS et al: Renal clearance: Urinary secretion of endogenous substances and urinary diagnostic indices in healthy neonatal foals, *J Vet Intern Med* 4:307, 1990.
25. Crowell-Davis SL, Houpt KA: Copraphagy by foals: Effect of age and possible functions, *Equine Vet J* 17: 17-19, 1985.
26. Carson K, Wood-Gush DGM: Behavior of Thoroughbred foals during nursing, *Equine Vet J* 15:257-262, 1983.
27. Ousey JC, McArthur AJ, Rossdale PD: How much energy do sick neonatal foals require compared to healthy ones? *Pferdeheilkunde* 12:231-237, 1996.
28. Houpt KA: Foal rejection and other behavioral problems in the postpartum period. *Compend Contin Ed Pract Vet* 6:s144-s148, 1984.
29. Adams R, Mayhew IG: Neurologic diseases, *Vet Clinics of NA Equine Pract 1:* 209-234, 1985.
30. Enzerink E: The menace response and papillary light reflex in neonatal foals, *Equine Vet J* 30:546-548, 1998.
31. Ousey JC: Thermoregulation and energy requirement of the newborn foal, with reference to prematurity, *Equine Vet J* Suppl 24:104-108, 1997.
32. Schambourg MA, Laverty S, Mullim S et al: Thoracic trauma in foals: Postmortem findings, *Equine Vet J* 35:78-81, 2003.
33. Bellezzo F, Hunt RJ, Provost P et al: Surgical repair of rib fractures in 14 neonatal foals: Case selection, surgical technique and results, *Equine Vet J* 36:557-562, 2004.
34. Acworth NRJ: The healthy neonatal foal: Routine examination and preventative medicine, *Equine Vet Edu* 15:207-211, 2004.
35. Harvey JW, Asquith RL, McNulty PK et al: Haematology of foals up to one year old, *Equine Vet J* 16(4):347-353, 1984.
36. Bauer JE, Harvey JW, Asquith RL et al: Clinical chemistry reference values of foals during the first year of life, *Equine Vet J* 16:361-363, 1984.
37. Korterba AM, Brewer BD, Tarplee FA: Clinical and clinicopathological characteristics of the septicaemic neonatal foal: Review of 38 cases, *Equine Vet J* 16:376-383, 1984.
38. Perryman LE, McGuire TC, Torbeck RL: Ontogeny of lymphocyte function in the equine fetus, *Am J Vet Res* 41(8):1197-1200, 1980.
39. Clemmons RM, Meyer DS, Dorsey-Lee MR et al: Reduced neonatal platelet function and serum bile acids, *Equine Vet J* Suppl 5:54, 1988.
40. Stoneham SJ, Palmer L, Cash R et al: Measurement of serum amyloid A in the neonatal foal using a latex agglutination immunoturbidimetric assay: Determination of the normal range, variation with age and response to disease, *Equine Vet J* 33(6):599-603, 2001.
41. Stoneham SJ, Wingfield Digby NJ, Ricketts SW: Failure of passive transfer of colostral immunity in the foal: incidence, and the effect of stud management and plasma transfusions, *Vet Record* 416-418, 1991.
42. Holdstock NB, Ousey JC, Rossdale PD: Glomerular filtration rate, effective renal plasma flow, blood pressure and pulse rate in the equine neonate during the first 10 days postpartum, *Equine Vet J* 30:335-343, 1998.
43. Jelan ZA, Jeffcott LB, Lundeheim N et al: Growth rates in Thoroughbred foals, *Pferdeheilkunde* 12:291-295, 1996.

2 High-Risk Pregnancy

| Case 2-1 | Placentitis in the Peripartum Mare | Pamela A. Wilkins |

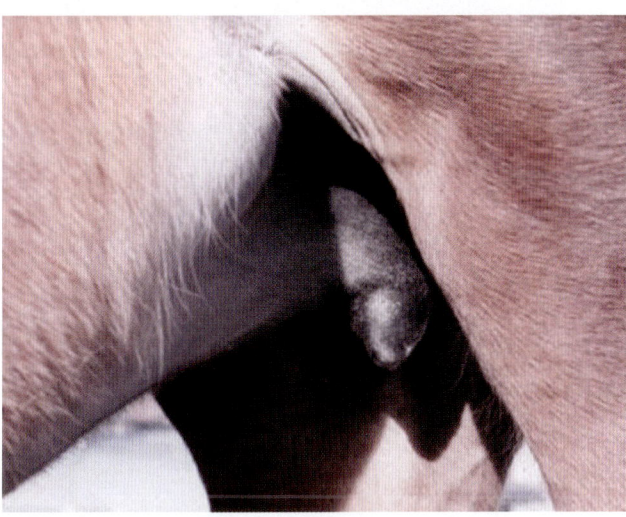

Fig. 2-1 Precocious udder development in Vital Connection at presentation on day 308 of gestation.

Vital Connection, a 13-year-old Thoroughbred mare, presented on January 29, 2004, with a primary complaint of premature-onset lactation. Her only cover for this pregnancy was March 25, 2003. Mammary development had begun two weeks prior to presentation, at which time Regumate (altrenogest, Intervet, Inc., Millsboro, DE) was administered at 10 cc twice daily by mouth (Figure 2-1). She stabilized until five days prior to presentation when her udder suddenly increased in size again. She was treated with intramuscular estrogen in addition to the oral altrenogest. She again stabilized until the day prior to presentation when she showed signs of early labor or mild colic and had wax present at both teats. Her reproductive history included five previous gestations. The first three gestations resulted in parturition occurring approximately "two weeks early" and nonsurviving foals dying at three to four days of age. No further specifics were available, although she may have been in Kentucky during the "Mare Reproductive Loss Syndrome" (MRLS) outbreak. The last two gestations produced normal healthy foals with an average gestation length of 333 days. For the last three gestations, including this one, she had received 10 cc Regumate PO daily until two weeks before her anticipated foaling date.

At presentation, Vital Connection was on day 308 of her current gestation. Initial physical examination revealed her to be bright, alert, and responsive. Her body weight was 1406 pounds, and her heart rate was 40 bpm with normal regular rhythm and synchronous pulses. No murmurs were ausculted. Her respiratory rate was 24 with mildly harsh lung sounds present cranioventrally bilaterally. Her udder was full and well-developed with wax present on both teats. There were no signs of stage-two labor. She had mild ventral edema, her vulvar lips were mild edematous, and she had evidence of mild pelvic ligament relaxation. She ambulated normally. An episiotomy had been performed prior to referral. The pregnancy was determined to be "high-risk" based on her history, gestation length and onset of premature lactation.

HISTORY AND PHYSICAL EXAMINATION

Prepartum disorders in the mare are usually readily recognized, but disorders of the fetus and placenta can be more subtle and difficult to determine. Problems resulting in premature mammary development generally fall into one of three categories: placentitis, twins, and incorrect breeding date. The first step in determining which might be the case is acquisition of a thorough history of the mare. Of particular interest is any history of previous abnormal foals. However, the history taking should also include questions regarding transportation, establishment of an accurate breeding date (sometimes more difficult than one would suspect), and any pertinent medical history (including diagnostic testing performed for the pregnancy such as culture, endometrial biopsy, and cytology, and any rectal and ultrasound examination results). Additionally, information regarding possible ingestion of endophyte-infected fescue or exposure to potential infectious causes of abortion should be obtained.[1,2] A complete vaccination and deworming history is requisite, as is a complete history of any medications and supplements administered during pregnancy.

Rectal palpation of Vital Connection demonstrated a softened cervix and decreased uterine tone. The fetus was positioned with its head near the pelvic inlet. Transrectal ultrasongraphic evaluation of the fetus and caudal reproductive tract revealed normal fetal fluid character. The fetal orbital diameter was 33 by 35 mm, consistent with the reported gestational age. The chorioallantois was edematous and appeared quite convoluted.

Transabdominal ultrasonographic evaluation of the fetus and placenta revealed no evidence of placental detachment but demonstrated generalized uteroplacental thickening and folding. The fetal fluid character was unremarkable. The fetal heart rate was 60 bpm at rest and increased to 69 to 71 bpm with activity, although the fetus was not particularly active. Breathing motions were observed, and were of a regular rhythm, and fetal tone was normal. Routine serum chemistry and hematology of the mare was within normal limits. Her PCV was 34% and her total protein was 6.7 gm/dl. Fetal ECG monitoring was performed overnight and was unremarkable with an acceptable resting heart rate and appropriate accelerations noted. A diagnosis of probable placentitis was made.

DIAGNOSTICS

Once a history is obtained and the initial physical examination complete, examination *per rectum* should be performed. When a pregnancy is identified as high risk, the fetus should be evaluated for viability. This should also encompass as thorough an evaluation as possible of the reproductive tract, placenta, and fetal fluids. The examination should include palpation of the cervix, uterus, fetus, and all palpable abdominal contents. Any abnormalities should be noted. The cervix should be tight throughout gestation; the late-gestation uterus will be large and fluid-distended and usually pulled craniad in the abdomen. Palpation of the fetus will frequently result in some fetal movement; however, lack of movement should be interpreted with caution, as some normal fetuses will not respond.

Ultrasonographic evaluation of the uterus and conceptus *per rectum* can provide valuable information, particularly regarding placental thickness if placentitis is a concern (Figure 2-2). Fetal fluids can be evaluated

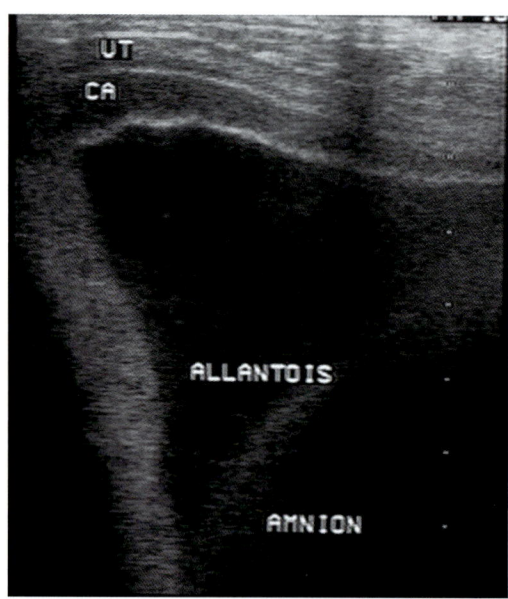

Fig. 2-2 Ultrasonographic evaluation of the uterus and conceptus per rectum. UT = uterus; CA = chorioallantois.

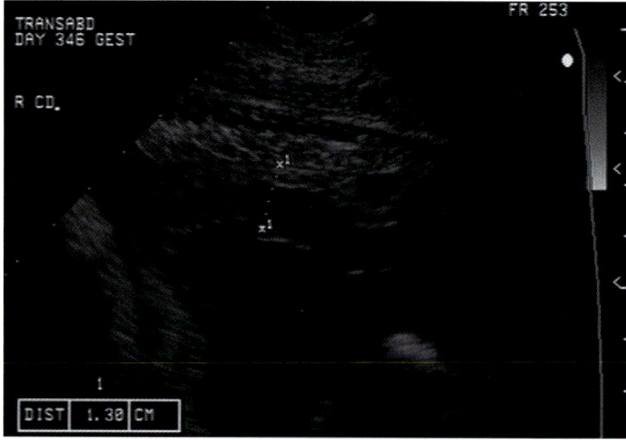

Fig. 2-3 Transabdominal ultrasonography of right caudal uterus/placenta. Note significant thickening of the placenta with evidence of edema.

and fetal size can be estimated from the size of the eye later in gestation.[3] In our hospital we choose not to perform vaginal examinations or speculum examinations as we have seen an association between these exams and the subsequent development of placentitis and, unless placentitis is recognized with ultrasonographic evaluation *per rectum* and culture is desirable, these types of examinations are generally not necessary.

Following examination *per rectum*, transabdominal ultrasonographic evaluation of the uterus and conceptus is performed[4] (Figure 2-3). The sonogram is performed through the acoustic window present from the udder to the xiphoid ventrally and laterally to the skinfolds of the flank (Figure 2-4). Imaging of the fetus usually requires a low-frequency (3.5 MHz) probe, while examination of the placenta and endometrium usually requires a higher frequency (7.5 MHz) probe (Figure

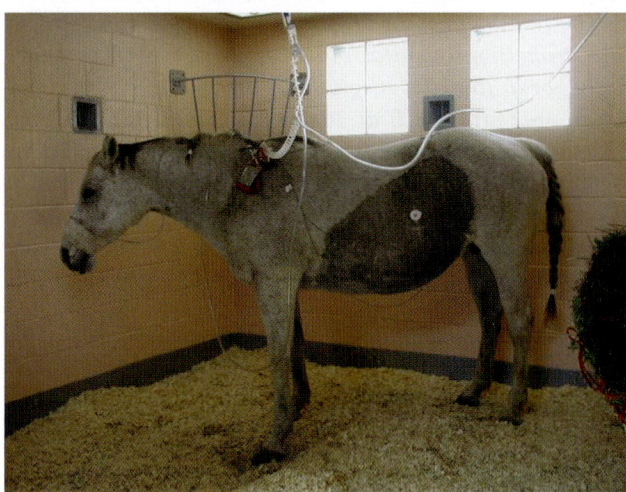

Fig. 2-4 High-risk pregnancy mare. Clipped area of her abdomen represents acoustic window for transabdominal ultrasonography of fetus and placenta. Mare is also wearing fetal ECG leads and is receiving intranasal oxygen insufflation and intravenous fluid support. Reprinted with permission from Wilkins PA: Monitoring the pregnant mare in the ICU, *Clin Tech in Equine Pract* 2:212-219, 2003.

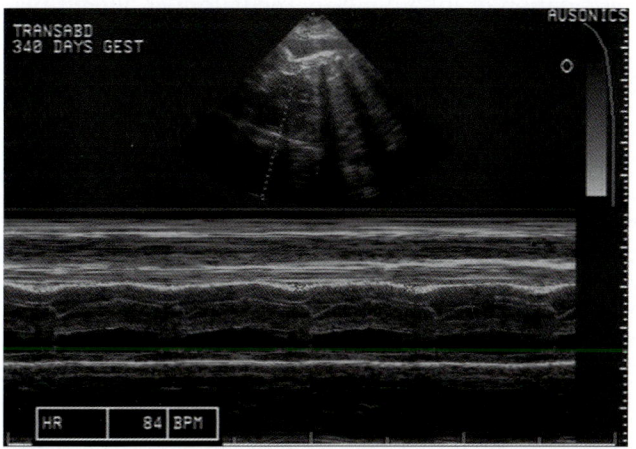

Fig. 2-5 Ultrasonographic evaluation of fetal heart and thorax and determination of fetal heart rate using M-mode echocardiography. Reprinted with permission from Wilkins PA: Monitoring the pregnant mare in the ICU, *Clin Tech in Equine Pract* 2:212-219, 2003.

Table 2-1	Late Gestation Biophysical Profile of Fetal Placental Unit Generated by Transabdominal Ultrasound Examination
Parameters	**Normal**
Fetal heart rate	70–90 beats/minute
Fetal activity	Less than 10 minutes of inactivity
Placental thickness	7–13 mm
Amniotic fluid depth	0–8 cm
Allantoic fluid depth	0–13 cm

A companion to transabdominal ultrasonography is evaluation of the fetal electrocardiogram (ECG).[4,6,7] Fetal ECGs can be measured continuously using telemetry or can be obtained using more conventional techniques several times throughout the day. Electrodes are placed on the skin of the mare in locations aimed at maximizing the magnitude of the fetal ECG but, because the fetus frequently changes position, multiple sites may be needed in any 24-hour period. We begin with an electrode placed dorsally in the area of the sacral prominence with two electrodes placed bilaterally in a transverse plane in the region of the flank (Figure 2-6). The fetal ECG maximal amplitude is low, usually 0.05 to 0.1 mV, and can be lost in artifact or background noise, so it is common to move electrodes to a new position to maximize the appearance of the fetal ECG. The normal fetal heart rate during the last months of gestation ranges from 65 to 115 bpm, a fairly wide distribution (Figure 2-7). The range of heart rate of an individual fetus can be quite narrow, however. Bradycardia in the fetus is an adaptation to *in utero* stress, and is usually thought to be hypoxia. By slowing the heart rate, the fetus prolongs exposure of fetal blood to maternal blood, increasing the time for equilibration of dissolved gas across the placenta and improving the oxygen content of the fetal blood. The fetus also alters the distribution of its cardiac output in response to hypoxia, centralizing blood distribution.[8,9] Tachycardia in the fetus can be associated with fetal movement, and brief periods of tachycardia should occur in the fetus in any 24-hour period. Persistent tachycardia is a sign of fetal distress and represents more severe fetal compromise than bradycardia.[10]

PATHOGENESIS

Placentitis is a common cause of late-term abortion in mares and perhaps the most common cause of mares presenting with clinical signs of precocious udder development, premature lactation, cervical softening, and vaginal discharge.[11] The cause is generally considered to be ascending infection that enters the uterus via the cervix, although hematogenous spread of some bac-

2-5). The utility of this type of examination lies in its repeatability and low risk to the dam and fetus. Sequential examinations over time will allow the clinician to follow the pregnancy and identify changes as they occur.

A biophysical profile of the fetus consisting of heart rate, fetal movement, placental thickening, and aminiotic/allantoic fluid volume can be generated from this examination in the late term fetus, and viability can be readily determined[4,5] (Table 2-1). The presence or absence of twins is also readily determined in the late pregnant mare in this manner. Uteroplacental thickening (>13 mm), placental separation (anechoic spaces between the chorion and uterus), and sudden increases in fetal fluid turbidity may be associated with placentitis.[4]

terial and viral agents (EHV-1 and EVA in particular) is possible. Mares with poor perineal conformation, abnormal cervical anatomy (sometimes secondary to previous birth trauma), a history of vaginal/cervical examination performed late in pregnancy, or a history of being placed in dorsal recumbency while pregnant, are at increased risk of placentitis, although for many there is no identified underlying cause.

Common bacteria that have been isolated in equine placentitis/abortions include *Streptococcus equi* (subspecies *zooepidemicu*), *Escherichia coli*, *Pseudomonas aeruginosa*, *Klebsiella pneumoniae*, and nocardioform species.[12]

Fetal loss and premature delivery secondary to placentitis are not fully understood. Recent studies, however, suggest that infection of the chorioallantois results in increased expression of inflammatory mediators that, in addition to other local effects, alters myometrial contractility.[12,13,14] Combined, these observations suggest that fetal loss can occur due to a compromised fetus, increased myometrial contractility, or both.

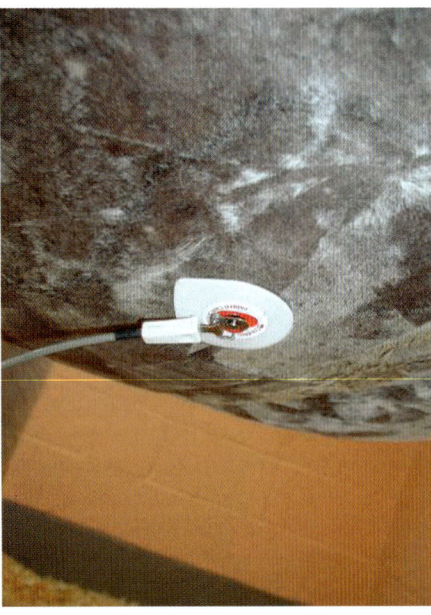

Fig. 2-6 Placement of ventral-lateral fetal ECG electrode. Reprinted with permission from Wilkins PA: Monitoring the pregnant mare in the ICU, *Clin Tech in Equine Pract* 2:212-219, 2003.

The treatment plan for Vital Connection consisted of oral trimethoprimsulfa, oral altrenogest at 14 cc twice daily, oral flunixin meglumine at 150 mg three times daily, oral vitamin E at 10,000 IU once daily, and fetal heart rate monitoring by telemetry. She was observed for signs of stage two labor by video monitoring and walk-by examinations every hour. Her vital parameters and external reproductive signs were evaluated and recorded daily. Transabdominal ultrasonographic evaluations were performed every four to seven days.

TREATMENT

The approach to management of the high-risk pregnancy is dictated to some degree by the exact cause for concern, but for many mares therapy is similar.[15,16] Many high-risk mares present with placentitis, primarily caused by ascending bacterial or fungal infections originating in the region of the cervix. These infections can cause *in utero* sepsis or compromise the fetus by local elucidation of inflammatory mediators or altered placental function. Premature udder development and vaginal discharge are common clinical signs. Treatment consists of administration of broad-spectrum antimicrobial agents and nonsteroidal anti-inflammatory drugs (Table 2-2). Trimethoprimsulfa (TMS) drugs appear to cross the placental/uterine barrier. Studies by Sertich and Vaala have demonstrated increased concentration of these agents in the fetal fluids when compared to less detectable levels of penicillin and gentamicin.[17] Other research by Murchie and colleagues using microdialysis showed that gentamicin and penicillin were found in the allantoic fluid after administration to mares. The elimination of these drugs from the allantoic fluid was slower than that from the mare's serum probably due to lack of mechanisms to eliminate drugs in this compartment.[18] If culture and sensitivity results are available, directed therapy should be instituted toward the specific organism isolated.

Nonsteroidal anti-inflammatory agents, such as flunixin meglumine, are used in an effort to combat alter-

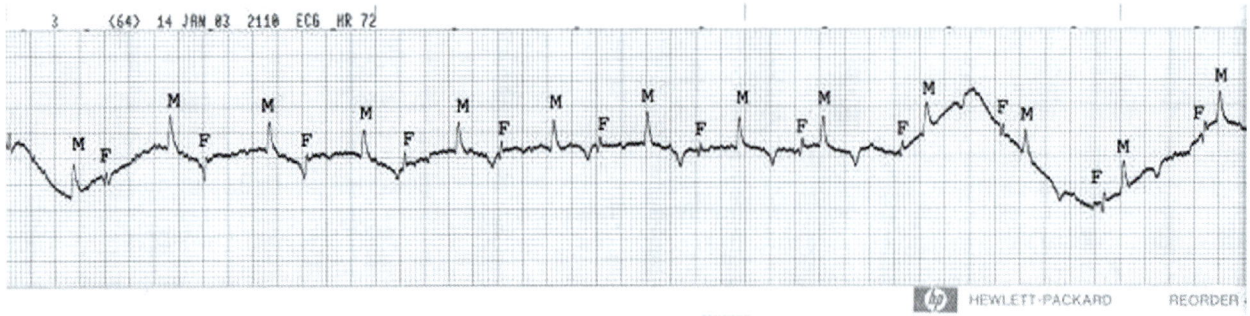

Fig. 2-7 Fetal ECG tracing. Fetal complexes *(F)* are of lower amplitude than maternal *(M)* complexes. Reprinted with permission from Wilkins PA: Monitoring the pregnant mare in the ICU, *Clin Tech in Equine Pract* 2:212-219, 2003.

Table 2-2	Drugs Used to Treat Mares with High-Risk Pregnancy	
Drug	**Dose/Frequency/Route**	**Reason**
Trimethoprim sulfonamide	25 mg/kg BID PO	Antimicrobial
Flunixin meglumine	0.25 mg/kg TID PO/IV	Anti-inflammatory
Altrenogest	0.44 mg/kg SID PO	Tocolytic
Isoxuprine	0.4–0.6 mg/kg BID PO	Tocolytic
Clenbuterol	0.8 µg/kg PRN PO	Tocolytic
Pentoxifylline	4–6 gm/500 kg BID PO	Anti-inflammatory
Vitamin E	1,000–10,000 IU/day PO	Antioxidant

SID = once daily, BID = twice daily, TID = three times daily, PRN = as needed, PO = by mouth, IV = intravenously.

ations in prostaglandin balance that may be associated with infection and inflammation. Although the efficacy of these agents is best when administered prior to the development of clinical signs, to date no detrimental effects have been reported in the fetus or dam when chronically used at low doses in well-hydrated patients. In the Murchie study, there was an attempt to measure flunixin meglumine levels in the allantoic fluid postadministration to pregnant mares. It was determined that flunixin meglumine was not measurable due to the method of microdialysis.[18] Pentoxifylline has been used for its rheologic effect, potentially improving blood flow within the placenta, and also for its general anti-inflammatory effect.[19-21]

Tocolytic agents and agents that promote uterine quiescence have been used and include altrenogest (Regumate, Intervet, Inc.) isoxuprine, and clenbuterol.[22-26] Although the use of altrenogest or progesterone in late gestation has been challenged, one study found that progestin supplementation helped to prevent prostaglandin-induced abortion in early gestation.[27] Though the mechanism of action is unclear, some feel that progestins have an anti-prostaglandin effect by interfering with prostaglandin and oxytocin receptors, thus reducing myometrial activity.[28] The efficacy of isoxuprine as a tocolytic in the horse is unproven, and bioavailability of orally administered isoxuprine appears to be highly variable. Clenbuterol may be indicated during management of dystocia in preparation for assisted delivery or caesarian section because it has been shown to decrease uterine tone for up to 120 minutes when administered intraveneously.[29] Unfortunately, the intravenous form of clenbuterol is not currently available in the United States. In a more recent study by Palmer and colleagues, 29 pregnant pony mares were treated daily in late gestation with intravenous clenbuterol; the treatment did not delay normal partuition.[30] The long-term use of clenbuterol is inadvisable due to receptor population changes associated with chronic use and its unknown effects on the fetus at this time.

Three additional strategies can be used in managing high-risk pregnancy patients. Where there is evidence of placental dysfunction, with or without signs of fetal distress, we provide intranasal oxygen supplementation to the mare in the hope of improving oxygen delivery to the fetus. Intranasal oxygen insufflation of 10 to 15 L/min has been shown to significantly increase both PaO_2 and percent oxygen saturation of hemoglobin (% O_2 sat).[31] Because of the placental vessel arrangement of the horse, improvement of these two arterial blood gas parameters should result in improved oxygen delivery to the fetus.[32,33] Blood gas transport is largely independent of diffusion distance in the equine placenta, particularly in late gestation, and is more dependent on blood flow. Information from other species cannot be extrapolated to the equine placenta because of its diffuse epitheliochorial nature and the arrangement of the maternal and fetal blood vessels within the microcotyledons.[34,35] Umbilical venous PO_2 is 50 to 54 mmHg in the horse fetus, compared to 30 to 34 mmHg in the sheep, while the maternal uterine vein to umbilical vein PO_2 difference is near zero. Also unlike the sheep, the umbilical venous PO_2 values decrease 5 to 10 mmHg in response to maternal hypoxemia and increase in response to maternal hyperoxia.[36,37]

Vitamin E (tocopherol) is administered orally to some high-risk mares as an antioxidant for both the placental/uterine inflammation and as a neuroprotectant strategy for the fetus. Administration of large doses of vitamin E prior to traumatic brain injury improves neurologic outcome in experimental models and has been examined as possible prophylaxis for human neonatal encephalopathy (NE).[38-40] Extrapolation of that information to the compromised equine fetus suggests that increased antioxidant concentrations in the fetus may mitigate some of the consequences of uterine and/or birth hypoxia, but no evidence is available to date demonstrating that protection occurs, or that vitamin E accumulates in the fetus in response to supplementation of the mare. Recent evidence suggests that large (>5,000 IU/day) vitamin E doses do not increase maternal vitamin E concentration more than smaller doses (1,000 IU/day).[41] In that study, no increase in plasma vitamin E concentration was seen in the newborn foal at any dose; however, vitamin E accumulation in tissues was not directly examined.

Finally, many high-risk mares are anorexic or held off feed because of their medical condition. These mares are at particularly large risk for fetal loss due to their lack of feed intake, which alters prostaglandin metabolism.[42] Therefore, intravenous dextrose, 2.5% to 5% dextrose in 0.45% saline or water (5% dextrose), at fluid rates providing 1 to 2 mg/kg/min dextrose, should be administered to these patients.

Few of the strategies described above are specifically aimed at the fetus, but rather in maintaining the pregnancy. Recently, evidence has appeared that prenatal ACTH administration may be beneficial in advancing the maturity of the fetus.[43] In a compromised pregnancy where clinical signs of early delivery do not regress with treatment, this therapy, or exogenous corticosteroid therapy, may be considered to increase the chances of fetal survival. However, potential risk for loss of the fetus may well outweigh any advantage provided by fetal ACTH administration.

Perhaps the most important aspect of managing high-risk pregnancy mares is frequent observation and development of a plan. Mares should be observed at least hourly for evidence of early-stage labor and should be under constant video surveillance if possible. Depending on the primary problem, the team managing the mare should develop a plan for handling the parturition once labor begins and for fetal resuscitation following delivery. Any equipment that might be needed should be readily available stallside. A call sheet, listing contact numbers for all involved, should be posted on or near the stall. The plan should include a decision as to how to handle a complicated dystocia with permission for general anesthesia and cesarian section obtained prior to the event so that time is not wasted.[44,45] It is important to ask the owner at the outset which is more important, the mare or the foal, as the answer may dictate the direction of the decision tree once labor begins.

Over the next several days, Vital Connection's signs of premature lactation and imminent parturition decreased. Improvement was noted in the degree of thickening of the uteroplacental unit on follow-up transabdominal ultrasonography. At approximately 7:00 AM on March 16, 2004, the mare entered stage two labor and delivered a filly foal on day 323 of gestation. The total duration of stage two labor was approximately 12 minutes; the fetus presented in anterior longitudinal dorsosacral position with head and both forelimbs extended. Mild assistance was provided to aid in passage of the foal's shoulders. Vital Connection experienced minimal perineal trauma. Stage three labor lasted approximately 40 minutes, with the placenta being passed with the chorionic surface outermost.

The fetal membranes were intact and malodorous despite being passed in a timely manner. There was a 15 by 30 cm well-demarcated tan area of discoloration at the

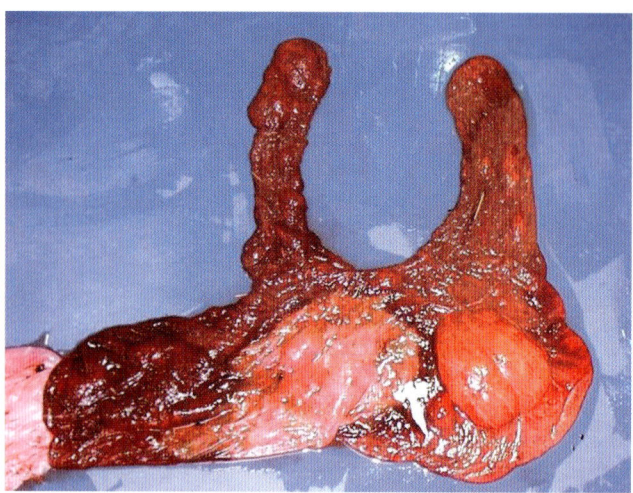

Fig. 2-8 Placenta from Vital Connection. Chorionic surface. Note large tan discolored region at the body of the uterus. This region can be very difficult to visualize with either transrectal or transabdominal ultrasonography.

base of the horns associated with a thick coffee-colored exudate. Approximately 80% of the chorion was discolored with the tip of the pregnant horn particularly discolored. Samples were obtained for culture and histopathology. The allanotoic surface was unremarkable. The amnion had prominent vasculature and was slightly edematous with opaque red-tan watery exudate present on the chorionic surface (Figure 2-8).

PLACENTAL EXAMINATION

The placenta of each pregnancy should be examined grossly to insure that the entire placenta has been expelled. There are serious complications, such as endotoxemia and laminitis, for the mare if pieces are retained. For mares with suspected placentitis, placental examination may provide clues to the cause of the inciting problem. Knowledge of the normal placental anatomy and normal artifacts that can be found in the placenta is helpful in distinguishing normal from abnormal.[46]

Structures of the placental unit include the umbilicus, the chorioallantois, the amnion, and the hippomanes. The amnionic umbilicus consists of two arteries, a vein, and the urachus. These vessels loosely spiral along the length of the umbilicus. The length of the umbilicus varies with different pregnancies but averages about 55 cm in the thoroughbred fetus.[47] Hippomanes are amorphous tan to brown oval-shaped masses that are found in the allantoic cavity of most mares. Their significance is unknown.[46]

On presentation, the chorioallantois is usually inverted from its normal orientation within the mare with the allantoic side on the outside, unlike the chorionic placental presentation seen in Vital Connection. The allantoic surface should be glistening and whitish with prominent vessels. If one orients the placenta so that the chorionic surface is on the outside, then a red velvetlike surface is apparent. The color can vary in places because of uneven expulsion of blood from the placenta during parturition.[46]

In normal parturition, the foal emerges through an avillous area called the cervical star. Examination of this area is important because it is the area first affected by an ascending placental infection.[48] Large avillous regions of the placenta, particularly when extending from the cervical region in a symmetric manner, may represent vascular abnormalities with subsequent avascular necrosis of the placental villi.[4] Other avillous areas can be found on a placenta where the placenta has folded on itself and not been exposed to the endometrial surface; lack of contact with the endometrial surface inhibits the normal formation of microcotyledonary villi. In placentas from twins, there is an avillous area where the two placentas touch.[46]

One pathological feature of placentitis may be a heavy placenta. Normal placentas are approximately 11% of the foal's weight.[46] As stated before, the area around the cervical star should be evaluated for inflammation and necrosis from an ascending infection. Placentitis secondary to *Nocardia spp* differs in that it is usually located near the cranial ventral uterine body and the attachment of the horns, as seen in this case.[49]

During normal parturition, the foal breaks through the cervical star of the placenta and is presented within the amnionic sac. The amnion is a whitish membrane that is markedly vascularized. Amnionitis denoted by diffuse inflammation may be evident in some cases of placentitis.[50]

Samples from various parts of the placenta should be placed in 10% buffered formalin for histopathic examination. Placental tissue from the cervical star and any other suspicious areas are especially important.[46]

'04 Vital Connection stood and suckled from the dam in an appropriate time frame. The foal was small and had a soft silky hair coat and somewhat lax flexure tendons. These characteristics were considered appropriate for gestational age. The colostrum was of good quality with a specific gravity of 1.065. The foal was bright and alert, although it was born with an increased fibrinogen concentration and leukocytosis. Antimicrobial therapy was administered for five days. The foal was monitored closely and experienced appropriate weight gain and demonstrated appropriate mentation. The hyperfibrinogenemia and leukocytosis rapidly resolved, with the foal showing no evidence of sepsis. A blood culture obtained from the foal at birth was negative.

INTRAUTERINE GROWTH RESTRICTION (IUGR)

The presence of placentitis or other placental abnormalities that reduce or interfere with normal placenta functions can result in a foal that is born too early (premature birth), a foal that is born at appropriate gestational age but with evidence of disparate or inappropriate growth patterns (dysmature or with IUGR), or a foal that is delivered from an abnormally prolonged gestation with evidence of growth problems (postmature). In human neonatal intensive care units (NICUs) the survival rates of low-gestation-length, low-birth-weight, infants has increased dramatically since the 1980s concurrent with improvements in obstetric and neonatal care. The now routine, well-validated use of antenatal steroid and post-parturient artificial surfactant therapies has contributed greatly to the enhanced survival of this patient population, although the use of these particular therapies is not common in the equine NICU.[51,52] However, with improved care, outcomes in the equine NICU population have also improved, with survival of premature patients in many NICUs exceeding 80%.[53]

In the equine population, gestation length is much more flexible than is observed in the human population. Therefore, the definition of the term *prematurity* should be re-examined. Traditionally prematurity is defined as a preterm birth of less than 320 days gestation in the horse. Given the variability of gestation length in the horse, ranging from 310 days to more than 370 days in some mares, it is possible for a mare whose usual gestation length is 315 days to have a term foal at 313 days, and a mare whose usual gestation length is 365 days to have a premature foal at 340 days. This underscores the importance of having very accurate breeding dates for mares with high-risk pregnancies and keeping valuable information regarding the gestation length and outcome of any previous pregnancies. This information may be significant in guiding treatment decisions made by the clinician and owner.

Foals that are born post-term but are small are termed *dysmature* (IUGR). Foals that are born post-term with a normal axial skeletal size but are thin to emaciated are termed *postmature*. Dysmature foals may have been classified in the past as *small for gestational age* (SGA) and are thought to have suffered placental insufficiency. Postmature foals are usually normal foals that have been retained too long in utero, perhaps due to an abnormal signaling of readiness for birth, and have outgrown their somewhat aged placenta. Postmature foals become more abnormal the longer they are maintained, may also suffer from placental insufficiency, and are best represented by the classic

Table 2-3	Characteristics of Premature/Dysmature and Postmature Foals	
Premature/Dysmature	**Postmature**
Low birth weight	Normal to high birth weight
Small frame; thin	Large frame; thin
Poor muscle development possible	Poor muscle development possible
Short, silky hair coat	Long hair coat
Weak suck reflex	Weak suck reflex
Poor thermoregulation	Poor thermoregulation
Delayed maturation of renal function: low urine output	Delayed maturation of renal function: low urine output
Gastrointestinal tract dysfunction	Gastrointestinal tract dysfunction
Poor glucose regulation	Poor glucose regulation
Flexor laxity common	Flexor contraction common
Hypotonia more common	Hypertonia more common
Periarticular laxity	Delayed time to standing
Floppy ears; poor cartilage development	Poor postural reflexes
High chest wall compliance	Hyperreactive
Low lung compliance	Fully erupted incisors
Domed forehead	
Entropion with secondary corneal ulcers	

Adapted from Palmer JE: Prematurity, dysmaturity, postmaturity. Proceedings of the IVECCS VI, 1998. pp 722-723.

foal born to a mare ingesting endophyte infested fescue.[1] The characteristics of premature/dysmature foals are compared and contrasted with those of postmature foals in Table 2-3.

The causes of prematurity, dysmaturity, and postmaturity include the causes of high-risk pregnancy. Additional causes include iatrogenic causes such as early elective induction of labor based on inaccurate breeding dates or misinterpretation of late-term colic or uterine bleeding as ineffective labor. The majority of causes remain in the category of idiopathic, with no discernible precipitating factor. Despite the lack of an obvious cause, premature labor and delivery does not just happen and, even if undetermined, the cause may continue to affect the foal in the postparturient period. All body systems may be affected by prematurity, dysmaturity, and postmaturity, and thorough evaluation of all body systems is necessary.

The effects of placental pathology on organ development have been studied. In one recent study, fetuses from placental pathology pregnancies had lower body weights, particularly after 320 days gestation.[54] When compared to normal controls, fetuses delivered from pregnancies with placental pathology had proportionally lower lung weights, although kidney weights were similar. Lung microstructure was compromised in some term foals with placenta pathology, implying that placental abnormalities may disrupt pulmonary development and contribute to some of the respiratory problems observed in sick newborn foals. The development of the fetal kidney was not compromised in fetuses from placental pathology pregnancies. This is in contrast to studies of sheep and infants in which glomerular numbers are reduced in IUGR.[55,56] Brain weight was unaffected by placental pathology. Adrenal weight was proportional to body weight throughout gestation in normal pregnancies, but was higher in abnormal pregnancies. This supports the clinical observation that foals born with clinical signs of IUGR (emaciation, abnormal skeletal development, and small size for gestational age) that have clearly suffered from in utero malnourishment are often viable even when born many weeks before full-term. Some require minimal veterinary care for survival and anecdotally appear to have functional maturity of many organ systems. These foals frequently have been demonstrated to have normal or even hyperadrenocortical function.

The overall prognosis for premature, dysmature, and postmature foals remains good with intensive care and good attention to detail. Many of these foals (up to 80%) will survive and become productive athletes.[53] Complications associated with sepsis and musculoskeletal abnormalities are the most significant indicators of poor athletic outcome.

Vital Connection became moderately febrile and tachycardic the day following parturition. Metritis was suspected, and treatment with flunixin meglumine (150 mg PO twice daily) and trimethoprim sulfa was initiated. Her uterus was lavaged daily, with lavage producing copious amounts of exudate. By day three, lavage fluids were clearer and Vital Connection was afebrile. An episoplasty was placed. Treatment with oral medications was discontinued five days postparturition, and Vital Connection and her foal were discharged on March 21, 2004.

Results of histopathology were consistent with a diagnosis of placentitis. A Nocardia-like organism was grown on culture of the exudate.

REFERENCES

1. Putnam MR, Bransby DI, Schumacher J et al: Effects of the fungal endophyte Acremonium coenophialum in fescue on pregnant mares and foal viability, Am J Vet Res 52:2071-2074, 1991.

2. Redmond LM, Cross DL, Strickland JR et al: Efficacy of domperidone and sulpiride as treatments for fescue toxicosis in horses, Am J Vet Res 55:722-729, 1994.

3. Kahn W, Leidl W: Ultrasonic biometry of horse fetuses in utero and sonographic representation of their organs, *Dtsch Tierarztl Wochenschr* 94:509-515, 1987.

4. Vaala WE, Sertich PL: Management strategies for mares at risk for periparturient complications, *Vet Clin North Am* (Equine Pract) 10:237-265, 1994.

5. Adams-Brendemuehl C, Pipers FS: Antepartum evaluations of the equine fetus, *J Reprod Fertil Suppl* 35:565-573, 1987.

6. LeBlanc MM: Identification and treatment of the compromised equine fetus: A clinical perspective, *Equine Vet J Suppl* (24):100-103, 1997.

7. Buss DD, Asbury AC, Chevalier L: Limitations in equine fetal electrocardiography, *Am Vet Med Assoc* 177:174-176, 1980.

8. Jensen A, Garnier Y, Berger R: Dynamics of fetal circulatory responses to hypoxia and asphyxia, *Eur J Obstet Gynecol Reprod Biol* 84:155-172, 1999.

9. Cohn HE, Piasecki GJ, Jackson BT: The effect of fetal heart rate on cardiovascular function during hypoxemia, *Am J Obstet Gynecol* 138:1190-1199, 1980.

10. Palmer JE: Fetal monitoring, *Proceedings of the Equine Symposium and Annual Conference 2000*, San Antonio, November 2000.

11. Troedsson MHT, Zent WW: Clinical ultrasonographic evaluation of the equine placenta as a method to successfully identify and treat mares with placentitis. In: Powell DG, Furry D, Hale G, eds: Proceedings of a Workshop on the Equine Placenta, Lexington KY, 2004, Kentucky Agricultural Experiment Station.

12. Giles RC, Donahue JM, Hong CB et al: Causes of abortion, stillbirth, and perinatal death in horses: 3,527 cases (1986-1991), *J Am Vet Med Assoc* 203:1170-1175, 1993.

13. Cottrill CM, Jeffers-Lo J, Ousey JC et al: The placenta as a determinant of fetal well-being in normal and abnormal equine pregnancies, *J Reprod Fertil Suppl* 44:591-601, 1991.

14. McGlothlin JA, Lester GD, Hansen PJ et al: Alteration in uterine contractility in mares with experimentally induced placentitis, *Reproduction* 127:57-66. 2004.

15. Bain FT: A clinician's approach to placentitis. In: Powell DG, Furry D, Hale G, eds: *Proceedings of a workshop on the equine placenta*, Lexington KY, 2004, Kentucky Agricultural Experiment Station.

16. Wilkins PA: Monitoring the pregnant mare in the ICU, *Clin Tech in Equine Pract* 2:212-219, 2003.

17. Sertich PL, Vaala, WE: Concentrations of antibiotics in mare, foals and fetal fluids after antibiotic administration during late pregnancy, In: *Proc 38 Ann Conv AAEP* 727-733, 1992.

18. Murchie TA, Macpherson ML, LeBlanc MM et al: A microdialysis model to detect drugs in the allantoic fluid of pregnant pony mares, In: *Proc 49 Ann Conv AAEP* 118-119, 2003.

19. Baskett A, Barton MH, Norton N et al: Effect of pentoxifylline, flunixin meglumine, and their combination on a model of endotoxemia in horses, *Am J Vet Res* 58:1291-1299, 1997.

20. Barton MH, Ferguson D, Davis PJ et al: The effects of pentoxifylline infusion on plasma 6-keto-prostaglandin F1 alpha and ex vivo endotoxin-induced tumour necrosis factor activity in horses, *J Vet Pharmacol Ther* 20:487-492, 1997.

21. Barton MH, Moore JN, Norton N: Effects of pentoxifylline infusion on response of horses to in vivo challenge exposure with endotoxin, *Am J Vet Res* 58:1300-1307, 1997.

22. Daels PF, Stabenfeldt GH, Hughes JP et al: Evaluation of progesterone deficiency as a cause of fetal death in mares with experimentally induced endotoxemia, *Am J Vet Res* 52:282-288, 1991.

23. McKinnon AO, Lescun TB, Walker JH et al: The inability of some synthetic progestagens to maintain pregnancy in the mare, *Equine Vet J* 32:83-85, 2000.

24. Gastal MO, Gastal EL, Torres CA et al: Effect of oxytocin, prostaglandin F2 alpha, and clenbuterol on uterine dynamics in mares, *Theriogenology* 50:521-534, 1998.

25. Niebyl JR, Johnson JW: Inhibition of preterm labor, *Clin Obstet Gynecol* 23:115-126, 1980.

26. Harkins JD, Mundy GD, Stanley S et al: Absence of detectable pharmacological effects after oral administration of isoxsuprine, *Equine Vet J* 30:294-299, 1998.

27. Daels PF, Besognet B, Hansen B et al: Effect of progesterone on prostaglandin F_2 secretion and outcome of pregnancy during cloprostenol induced abortion in mares, *Am J Vet Res* 57:1331-1337, 1996.

28. Garfield Re, Kannan MS, Daniel ME: Gap junction formation in the myometrium: Control by estrogens, progesterone and prostaglandins, *Am J Physiol* 238:C81-C89, 1980.

29. Card CE, Wood MR: Effects of acute administration of clenbuterol on uterine tone and equine fetal and maternal heart rates, *Biol Reprod* 1:7-11, 1995.

30. Palmer E, Chavette-Palmer P, Duchamp G et al: Lack of effect of clenbuterol for delaying parturition in late pregnant mares, *Theriogeneology* 58:797-799, 2002.

31. Wilkins PA, Seahorn TL: Intranasal oxygen therapy in adult horses, *J Vet Emerg Crit Care* 10:221, 2000.

32. Bjorkman N: Fine structure of the fetal-maternal area of exchange in the epitheliochorial and endotheliochorial types of placentation, *Acta Anat Suppl* (Basel) 61:1-22, 1973.

33. Samuel CA, Allen WR, Steven DH: Studies on the equine placenta. I. Development of the microcotyledons, *J Reprod Fertil* 41:441-445, 1974.

34. Samuel CA, Allen WR, Steven DH: Studies on the equine placenta. I. Development of the microcotyledons, *J Reprod Fertil* 41:441-445, 1974.

35. Bjorkman N: Fine structure of the fetal-maternal area of exchange in the epitheliochorial and endotheliochorial types of placentation, *Acta Anat Suppl* (Basel) 61:1-22, 1973.

36. Comline RS, Silver M: PO_2 levels in the placental circulation of the mare and ewe, *Nature* 217:76-77, 1968.

37. Fowden AL, Forhead AJ, White KL et al: Equine uteroplacental metabolism at mid- and late gestation, *Exp Physiol* 85:539-545, 2000.

38. Inci S, Ozcan OE, Kilinc K: Time-level relationship for lipid peroxidation and the protective effect of alpha-tocopherol in experimental mild and severe brain injury, *Neurosurgery* 43:330-335, 1998.

39. Clifton GL, Lyeth BG, Jenkins LW et al: Effect of D, alpha-tocopheryl succinate and polyethylene glycol on performance tests after fluid percussion brain injury, *J Neurotrauma* 6:71-81, 1989.

40. Daneyemez M, Kurt E, Cosar A et al: Methylprednisolone and vitamin E therapy in perinatal hypoxic-ischemic brain damage in rats, *Neuroscience* 92:693-697, 1999.

41. Drury EM, Whitaker TC, Palmer L: Oral water soluble vitamin E supplementation of the mare in late gestation, its effects on serum vitamin E levels in the pre- and postpartum mare and the neonate: A preliminary investigation. *Proceedings for the 2004 Equine Nutrition Conference for Feed Manufacturers*, p. 137.

42. Fowden AL, Ralph MM, Silver M: Nutritional regulation of uteroplacental prostaglandin production and metabolism in pregnant ewes and mares during late gestation, *Exp Clin Endocrinol* 102:212-21, 1994.

43. Ousey JC, Rossdale PD, Palmer L et al: Effects of maternally administered depot ACTH(1-24) on fetal maturation and the timing of parturition in the mare, *Equine Vet J* 32:489-496, 2000.

44. Freeman DE, Hungerford LL, Schaeffer D et al: Caesarean section and other methods for assisted delivery: Comparison of effects on mare mortality and complications, *Equine Vet J* 31:203-207, 1999.

45. Byron CR, Embertson RM, Bernard WV et al: Dystocia in a referral hospital setting: Approach and results, *Equine Vet J* 35:82-85, 2003.

46. Schlafer DH: Postmortem examination of the equine placenta, fetus, and neonate: Methods and interpretation of findings, In: *Proc Fiftieth Ann Conv AAEP* 144-161, 2003.

47. Whitwell KE: Morphology and pathology of the equine umbilical cord, *J Reprod Fertil Suppl* 23:599-603, 1975.
48. Whitwell KE: Equine placental pathology: The Newmarket perspective, In: Powell DG, Furry D, Hale G, eds: Proceedings of a Workshop on the Equine Placenta, Lexington KY, 2004, Kentucky Agricultural Experiment Station.
49. Donahue JM, Williams NM, Sells SF et al: *Crossiella equi sp. nov.*, isolated from equine placentas, *Int J System Evolut Microbiol* 52:2169-2173, 2002.
50. LeBlanc MM, Macpherson M, Sheerin P: Ascending placentitis: What we know about pathophysiology, diagnosis, and treatment. In: *Proc 49 Ann Conv AAEP* 118-119, 2003.
51. McEvoy C, Bowling S, Williamson K et al: Functional residual capacity and passive compliance measurements after antenatal steroid therapy in preterm infants, *Pediatr Pulmonol* 31:425-430, 2001.
52. Suresh GK, Soll RF: Current surfactant use in premature infants, *Clin Perinatol* 28:671-694, 2001.
53. Axon J, Palmer J, Wilkins PA: Short-term and long-term athletic outcome of neonatal intensive care unit survivors, *Proc Am Assoc Equine Pract* 45:224-225, 1999.
54. Ousey JC, Rossdale PD, Houghton E et al: The effects of placental pathology on equine fetal organ development and metabolism of progestagens. In: Powell DG, Furry D, Hale G, eds: *Proceedings of a workshop on the equine placenta*, Lexington KY, 2004, Kentucky Agricultural Experiment Station.
55. Hinchcliffe SA, Lynch MR, Sargent PH et al: The effect of intrauterine growth retardation on the development of renal nephrons, *Br J Obstet Gybecol* 99:296-310, 1992.
56. Bains RK, Sibbons PD, Murray RD et al: Stereological estimation of the absolute number of glomeruli in the kidneys of lambs, *Res Vet Sci* 60:122-125, 1996.

Case 2-2	Body Wall Tear in Late Gestational Mare and Birth Resuscitation of a Compromised Foal
	Pamela A. Wilkins and Brett Dolente

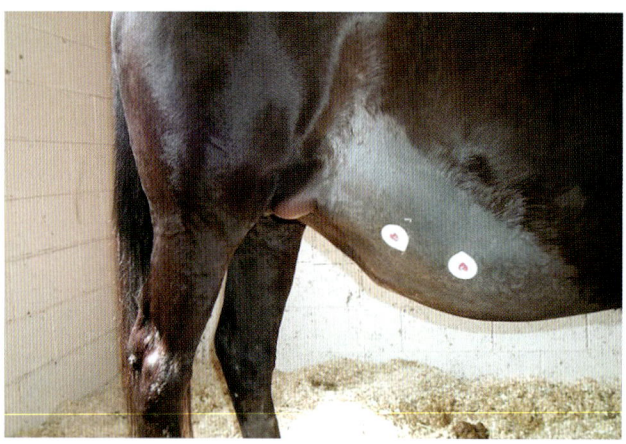

Fig. 2-9 Flank fold edema.

Poppy was presented on March 30, 2002, with a primary complaint of suspected uterine torsion. She was approximately at day 338 of gestation, which had been normal until that time. She had been leased for this pregnancy. Her owner had no detailed information regarding her reproductive history, although it was known that she had produced normal healthy foals in the past. The mare had been found sweating and colicky in the field that evening; evaluation of the uterus per rectum suggested a potential uterine torsion to the referring veterinarian. She was referred to New Bolton Center for further evaluation and treatment.

At presentation, Poppy was tachycardic and tachypneic with a slightly increased rectal temperature. She was reluctant to walk. Her abdomen was distended, primarily due to her pregnancy, but there was a plaque of ventral edema that was most prominent in her flank folds (Figure 2-9). Clear fluid was readily expressed from her teats. Her mucous membranes were pink with a normal capillary refill time, and no significant abnormalities *were present in routine clinical chemistry, hematology, and blood gas analysis. Evaluation of her uterus and pregnancy per rectum, including transrectal ultrasonography, did not reveal any significant abnormalities. Fetal ECG was unremarkable, and transabdominal ultrasonographic evaluation of the pregnancy was within normal limits. The primary differential diagnosis (based on physical examination findings of reproducible pain present in her flank fold region bilaterally and the nature and distribution of her ventral edema) was that she was developing bilateral tears in her caudal abdominal muscles. Palpation of her abdominal contents was unremarkable, and no net reflux was obtained on nasogastric intubation. No abdominal cause for her distress (colic) was uncovered.*

HISTORY AND PHYSICAL EXAMINATION

Prepartum disorders in the mare causing pain and colic-like signs can be difficult to accurately diagnose.[1] The differential diagnosis list is extensive and includes any of the usual causes of colic in addition to reproductive tract hemorrhage, uterine torsion, uterine tear, hydrops condition, body wall tears, urinary trauma/bladder rupture, and dystocia.

The first step in determining a specific cause is acquisition of a thorough history of the mare. Of particular interest is any history of previous abnormal foals or abnormal pregnancies. However, the history taking should include questions regarding transportation; establishment of an accurate breeding date; pertinent medical history, including diagnostic testing performed for the pregnancy such as culture, endometrial biopsy, and cytology results; and rectal and ultrasound examination results. A history of any episode of colic, whether or not it is associated with the pregnancy, is significant, as is any history of previous bleeding into the abdomen, uterus, or broad ligament from the middle uterine artery or other source. A complete vaccination and deworming history is requisite, as is a complete history of any medications or supplements administered during pregnancy.

A thorough physical and reproductive examination is vital to making an accurate diagnosis and therapeutic plan for the peripartum mare. Physical examination of the normal pregnant mare will often reveal mild tachycardia, secondary to the increased cardiovascular demands of pregnancy, thus a heart rate from 40-60 beats per minute may be normal for the mare in late gestation.[2,3] Mild tachypnea, secondary to reduced function residual capacity in the lung, is also not uncommon in the late-gestation pregnant mare.[3] Otherwise, examination of the cardiovascular, respiratory, and neurologic systems should be similar to findings in the nonpregnant mare. The size of the abdominal cavity should be evaluated in light of the period of gestation, and the caretakers should be inquired as to whether the abdominal size has changed significantly in a short period of time.

PATHOGENESIS

Any late-pregnant mare presenting with a rapidly enlarging abdomen and an area of painful edema along the ventral abdominal wall could be suffering from rupture of the abdominal musculature, the rectus abdominis muscle, or the prepubic tendon. These can occur together or separately in the pregnant mare. Together, these specific defects can be referred to as "ventral ruptures." Other clinical conditions include a subcutaneous or intramuscular hematoma and hydrops allantois/amnion as a primary cause leading to the above condition. There may not be an obvious predisposing cause for this condition. Some predisposing factors include pregnancies with increased uterine weight such as hydrops or twin pregnancy. Trauma in late pregnancy is another potential cause. The condition appears to be more common in older, unfit mares and, probably because of their size, in draft breeds. Affected mares are generally close to term.

Poppy was initially treated by holding her off feed overnight and providing analgesia and intravenous fluid support. She was periodically checked for gastric reflux. A large abdominal support was placed in case ventral body wall tearing was occurring (Figure 2-10). On April 1, Poppy was enrolled in a high-risk pregnancy program with the owner's consent. Bilateral body wall tearing

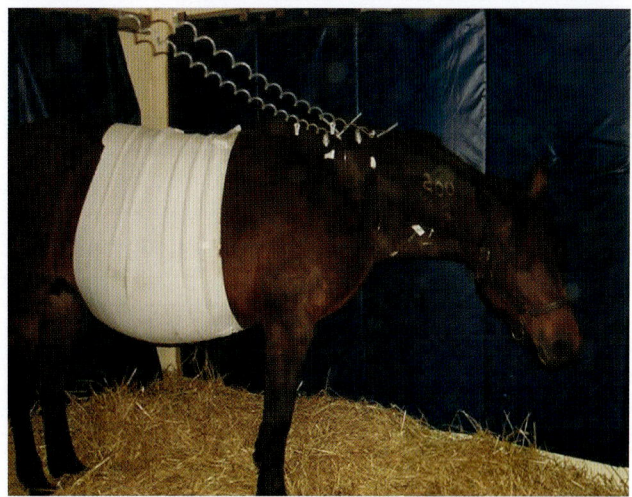

Fig. 2-10 Abdominal support wrap in place. This case was one of hydrops allantois and not ventral body wall tear; however, the abdominal support wrap is similar in both problems.

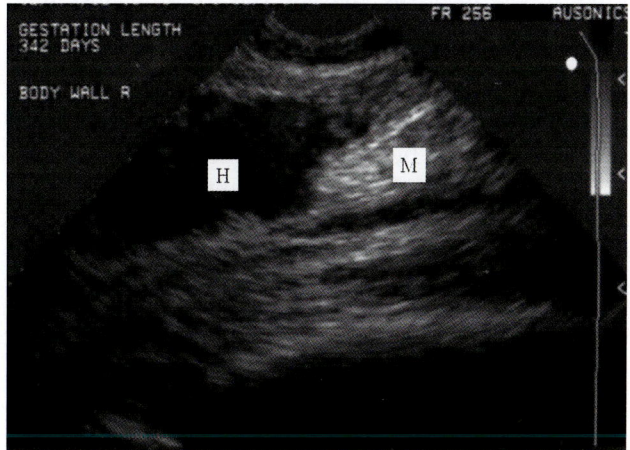

Fig. 2-11 Ultrasonographic image of body wall tear. There is large area of hematoma present *(H)* and the free edge of the torn muscle can be seen *(M)*.

was confirmed by repeat ultrasound evaluation on April 5 (Figure 2-11).

DIAGNOSTIC PLAN AND DIFFERENTIALS

Examination of the abdominal contents *per rectum* in the peripartum mare may be useful or, not unusually, very frustrating. Due to the presence of the large uterus in late gestation, rectal examination may not provide much useful information prior to parturition, particularly regarding the gastrointestinal tract. Small and large intestinal distention can be appreciated in some cases. However, rectal findings are often unremarkable despite significant disease, thus a normal rectal examination does not rule out obstructive gastrointestinal disease in the pregnant mare. Careful palpation of the reproductive tract should also be done at this time to evaluate the broad ligaments of the uterus for swellings (hematomas), or abnormal positioning or tautness (uterine torsion). Fetal activity can be assessed manually with detection of fetal movement per rectum. Sonographic examination of the reproductive tract per rectum may also provide useful information, such as abnormalities of the reproductive tract, placenta, and fetal fluids.

Clinical chemistry and hematology evaluation will aid the clinician in assessment of the peripartum mare. The presence of leukocytosis or leukopenia suggests the presence of inflammatory disease and is less common in mares with simple obstructive disease, whether gastrointestinal or reproductive in origin. The presence of anemia or hypoproteinemia with clinical signs of dehydration suggests acute blood loss, most likely from the arteries supplying the reproductive tract or from the mesenteric vessels. In the first hours after blood loss, the packed cell volume and total protein will often remain within normal limits, but will be in the low-normal range despite evidence of hypovolemia on clinical examination. Plasma fibrinogen concentration may also be inappropriately low in mares with acute hemorrhage. In acute disease, clinical chemistry values are often within normal limits. Plasma lactate concentration has been useful in identifying mares with severe postpartum hemorrhage, as they often have normal hematology and chemistry except for significant hyperlactatemia in the early stages of hemorrhagic shock. Mares that have experienced more chronic bleeding may have increased total and indirect (unconjugated) bilirubin concentrations.

Abdominocentesis can be an important tool in evaluation of the peripartum mare. If the mare is in late gestation, there is a risk of allantocentesis due to the presence of the large gravid uterus along the ventral abdomen. Abdominocentesis under sonographic guidance is indicated in these mares. Mares that have suffered uterine tears will often have evidence of septic peritonitis, as will mares that have sustained trauma to the gastrointestinal tract. If trauma to the gastrointestinal tract has led to overwhelming fecal peritonitis, nucleated cell counts may not be increased in the first 24 hours, however cytologic examination should reveal large numbers of bacteria, and plant material may also be present. Hemoperitoneum may indicate uterine artery trauma or trauma to the mesentery of the intestine. Chemical evaluation of the peritoneal fluid may aid in determination if trauma has occurred to the urinary tract. Peritoneal fluid should normally have a creatinine concentration anomalous with the peripheral blood level. If it is greater than twice the blood value, then uroperitoneum should be suspected.

Due to the difficulty of performing a thorough rectal examination in the pregnant mare, percutaneous sono-

graphic examination of the abdomen can be particularly useful in evaluating these patients.[4] Small intestinal distention may be apparent in the cranial abdomen indicating a surgical lesion. Peritoneal effusion may also be apparent. The uterus can also be evaluated via the abdominal wall. Uterine fluid quality and quantity, placental wall thickness, fetal heart rate, fetal movement, and fetal number can be determined in the pregnant mare, and will aid in future treatment decisions regarding the mare and fetus. The broad ligaments of the uterus can also be visualized, and hemorrhage within the ligament may be determined via this method.

Diagnosis of uterine torsion is most often accomplished by rectal palpation of the uterine broad ligaments. The direction of the torsion can be determined by which ligament is taut and stretched across the abdomen. Clockwise torsion is indicated if the left ligament is stretched taut across the abdomen coursing toward the right ventral abdomen (and vice versa for counterclockwise torsion). Further diagnostic information can be obtained by sonographic examination and abdominocentesis, giving the clinician additional information regarding uterine wall health, fetal fluid character, and peritoneal inflammation, suggesting more advanced uterine compromise. Fetal compromise or death may also be determined by sonographic examination.

Hydrops allantois is an emergency condition requiring attention in a short time interval to ensure the health of the mare. Secondary complications associated with intra-abdominal hypertension (IAH) may develop, potentially leading to abdominal compartment syndrome (ACS), including respiratory compromise, hypovolemic shock at delivery, and body wall hernia. In cases where IAH and/or ACS is suspected, intra-abdominal pressure may be determined by use of a bladder catheter and water manometer. Hydrop allantois is often detected by the owner as sudden onset of abdominal distention, with progressive lethargy and anorexia, and possibly dyspnea. Diagnosis is made by rectal palpation and reveals an enlarged fluid-filled uterus, and hydrops is confirmed by sonographic examination per rectum showing large amount of allantoic or amnionic fluid. The placenta from affected mares have enlarged horns and body. (Figure 2-12) Mares with hydrops conditions are more susceptible to developing ventral body wall tears.

Similar to the hydrops condition, body wall hernias and prepubic tendon rupture are usually detected by the owner as an abrupt change in the contour of the abdominal wall, and lethargy and anorexia in the mare. Mares with ventral ruptures may have ventral edema from the udder to the xiphoid cartilage of the sternum. There will be signs of distress and intermittent colic. If the pain is severe, there will be an increase

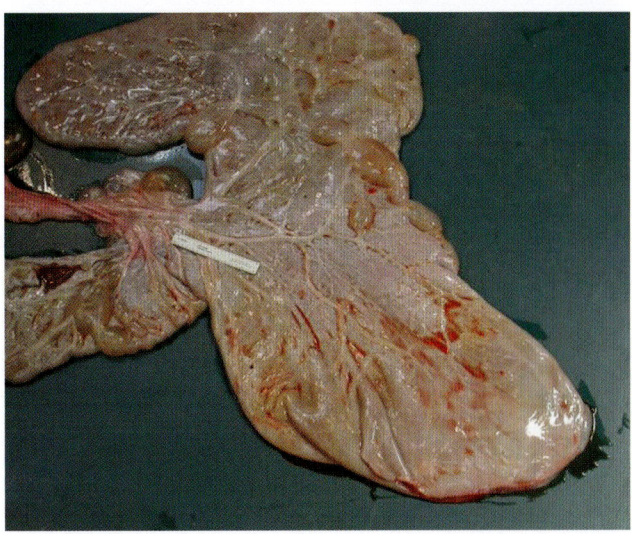

Fig. 2-12 Placenta from the mare with hydrops allantois pictured in Figure 2-10. Note the enlargement of the fetal membranes, particularly in the body and the pregnant horn. The nonpregnant horn is also larger than usual.

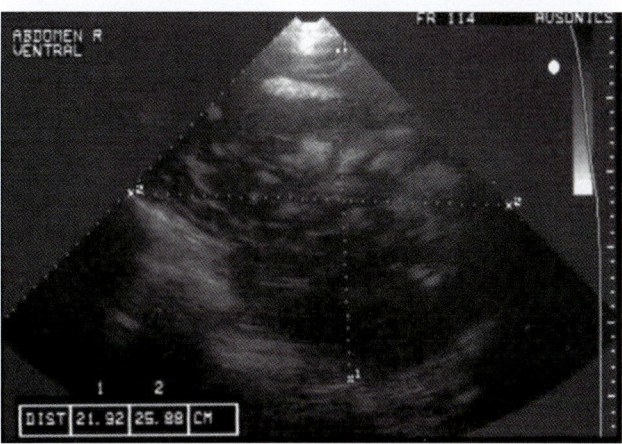

Fig. 2-13 Ultrasonographic appearance of large hematoma in uterine wall and broad ligament. Acoustic window was the right ventral flank region.

in heart rate and respiratory rate. These mares are generally reluctant to move or lie down. Ultrasonographic examination of the posterior aspect of the ventral abdomen may be useful to detect the presence of a hernia. Ultrasonography may also reveal the size of the defect and the structures involved. Any defect in the abdominal musculature may be complicated by bowel incarceration. All examinations are less than satisfactory due to the foal's presence and edema of the body wall.

Rupture of the prepubic tendon causes development of signs similar to those associated with ventral hernias. Some differences may be present, but these may not be readily noticeable. Due to loss of tension from the cranial aspect of the pelvis, the pelvis will appear tilted in cases of prepubic tendon rupture. The tail head and ischial tuberosities may be elevated. Some mares develop very obvious lordosis and adopt a "rocking horse" position because the pelvis and vertebral column cannot maintain normal alignment. The udder may be displaced cranially and ventrally because of loss of its caudal attachment to the pelvis. The plaque of edema can almost obliterate the outline of the mammary gland. Ventral body wall defects may easily lead to rupture of the blood supply to the mammary gland, disruption of its attachment to the body wall, and hemorrhage of the adjacent musculature. Blood may be detectable in the milk. Together with the reluctance to walk and lie down, these signs are strongly indicative for rupture of the ventral body wall tears.

Diagnosis of urogenital hemorrhage is often based on clinical impression. Palpation per rectum may reveal the presence of a hematoma within the uterine broad ligaments, or intralumenal uterine blood. However, rectal examination can be nondiagnostic.

Hemorrhage into the broad ligament can dissect through the fascial planes, so a discrete hematoma is not palpable despite significant blood loss. Sonographic examination via the body wall may aid in diagnosis, where the broad ligament can be visualized in some cases, or uterine or peritoneal hemorrhage may be detected (Figure 2-13).

Poppy received Regumate (Intervet, Inc.) and trimethoprim sulfa per os. Dextrose was added to her fluids to help support the pregnancy. Continuous fetal ECG monitoring was begun. Feeding was gradually reintroduced during the next several days. Poppy gradually became more comfortable during the next several days, and her pain was fairly easily controlled with phenylbutazone or flunixin meglumine in low to moderate doses. Her body support wrap was maintained. She was not allowed turn-out and was kept within a large foaling stall. A plan was developed for emergency cesarean section if dystocia should develop. Fetal heart rate monitoring by telemetry was instituted to monitor fetal well-being, and both video camera and frequent walk-by monitoring for imminent parturition was introduced.

TREATMENT

Initial treatment for ventral ruptures is aimed at stabilizing the horse by restricting activity. It is important to closely monitor for signs of blood loss (which can be significant), decreased fecal production, and development of further discomfort suggesting progression of the tear. Anti-inflammatory drugs such as phenylbutazone or flunixin meglumine may help relieve discomfort. Use of a strong bandage around the abdominal wall, acting as an abdominal sling, may provide support for the ventral abdominal wall. Any abdominal bandage must be well padded to avoid pressure necrosis along the dorsum. The possibility of bowel entrapment and strangulation should be investigated, and surgical correction may be necessary if bowel strangulation has occurred. Repeated ultrasonographic evaluation of any entrapped bowel may be necessary. In a few cases, due to rapidly changing clinical parameters, the mare gains little from supportive treatment, and induction of parturition (or termination of the pregnancy in mares earlier in gestation) must be performed. Pregnancy termination may be desirable in some mares with hydrops conditions, or twins, presenting well before their anticipated parturition date, even if ventral body wall tears have not yet occurred.

The clinician should anticipate that assistance with parturition might be necessary, as the mare may be reluctant to lie down and/or experience difficulty developing sufficient abdominal pressure during active labor. Equipment needed for assistance with parturition and resuscitation of the delivered foal should be readily at hand. It is important that clear communication has been established with the owner regarding whether the mare or the fetus is the priority, as this crucial decision may determine the decisions made as the case progresses. Edema usually resolves quickly after foaling, and the mare can suckle the foal normally. Supplementation with colostrum or plasma may be indicated when the mare has leaked colostrum prior to delivery.

On April 15, 2002, day 354 of her gestation, Poppy entered a rather prolonged Stage 1 labor. The primary concerns were that she would have difficulty moving the foal to proper position for parturition and that she would extend her body wall tears during parturition, so she was monitored closely. By late afternoon, the fetus was close to being normally positioned and she finally lay down. The fetal membranes ruptured almost immediately, and the foal was delivered at 6:03 PM with minimal assistance. The duration of stage two labor was less than 12 minutes. Poppy remained recumbent for approximately 45 minutes following delivery and received 500 mg flunixin meglumine IV during this time to ease discomfort. When she stood, a sample of her milk was obtained and appeared grossly bloody. Because she had been leaking colostrum and milk for several days prior to parturition, colostrum was provided to the foal from an alternate source. She passed her placenta within 30 minutes of standing, and the placenta was grossly normal. She demonstrated good maternal behavior and almost immediately became more comfortable. Her ventral edema improved greatly over the next several days. Ultrasonographic examination of her body wall tears postpartum revealed the presence of loops of small intestine under the

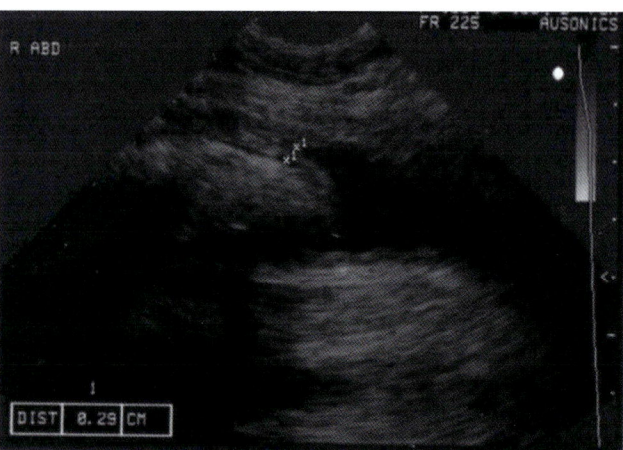

Fig. 2-14 Ultrasonographic appearance of ventral body wall tear that has become a hernia as small intestine has protruded through the defect and now lies directly under the skin. The two *x*'s associated with the 1s show a measurement of the intestinal wall. The free edge of the muscular defect can be seen on the left of the image.

skin (Figure 2-14). They appeared to move freely and were not thickened.

'02 Poppy was bradycardic at birth and was resuscitated using intranasal oxygen insufflation and intravenous epinephrine. He achieved a normal heart rate and rhythm within 10 minutes and was placed in the stall in front of his dam. The colt was standing within two hours. He received 6 ounces of high-quality banked colostrum by bottle shortly thereafter and was supplemented with additional banked colostrum by bottle during the night. He was nursing from his dam within three hours of birth. Initial bloodwork revealed an increased fibrinogen concentration at birth, although this was within the normal range on the following day. A blood culture obtained at birth was negative. On the following morning, plasma IgG concentration was >800 mg/dl. No additional treatments were instituted for the foal.

BIRTH RESUSCITATION OF FOALS FROM HIGH-RISK MARES

Most newborn foals easily make the transition to extrauterine life. Foals born from mares with high-risk pregnancies, however, may find themselves in difficulty; it is of utmost importance to recognize the condition immediately and institute appropriate resuscitation. A modified APGAR scoring system has been developed as a guide for initiating resuscitation and probable level of fetal compromise (Table 2-4).[5] This scoring system is used in foals to identify the need for medical intervention. It is useful at the moment in time that it is performed but does not alleviate the need for further monitoring. It is also important to perform at

Table 2-4	APGAR Score in the Foal		
	Assigned Value		
Parameter	1	2	3
Heart/pulse rate	Undetectable	<60 bpm; irregular	>60 bpm; regular
Respiratory rate/pattern	Undetectable	Slow; irregular	40–60 bpm; regular
Muscle tone	Limp	Lateral; some tone	Sternal
Nasal mucosal stimulation	Absent	Grimace; mild rejection	Cough or sneeze

Score at 1 and 5 minutes after birth. Scores of 7 to 8 generally indicate a normal foal, scores of 4 to 6 indicate mild to moderate asphyxia, and scores of 0 to 3 indicate severe asphyxia. For a score of 0 to 3, begin cardiopulmonary resuscitation. A score of 4 to 6 should prompt stimulation, intranasal oxygen, or mechanical ventilation.
From Martens RJ: Pediatrics. In: Mansmann RA, McAllister ES, Pratt PW, eds: *Equine medicine and surgery*, ed 3, vol 1, Santa Barbara, Calif, 1982, American Veterinary Publications.

least a cursory physical examination prior to initiating resuscitation, as there are humane issues concerning serious problems such as severe limb contracture, microophthalmia, and hydrocephalus, among others.

The initial assessment begins during presentation of the fetus. While the following applies primarily to attending the birth of a foal from a high-risk pregnancy, quiet and rapid evaluation can be performed during any attended birth. The goal in a normal birth with a normal foal is to minimally disturb the bonding process. This goal also applies to high-risk parturitions, but some disruption of normal bonding is inevitable. The lead clinician should tightly control the number of people attending the birth and the degree of activity surrounding it.

The strength and rate of any palpable peripheral pulse should be evaluated. The apical pulse should be evaluated as soon as the chest clears the birth canal. Bradycardia (pulse < 40 bpm) is expected during forceful contractions, and the pulse rate should increase rapidly once the chest clears the birth canal. Persistent bradycardia is an indication for rapid intervention.

The fetus is normally hypoxemic when compared to the newborn foal, and this hypoxemia is largely responsible for the maintenance of fetal circulation by generation of pulmonary hypertension.[6] The fetus responds to conditions producing more severe *in utero* hypoxia by strengthening the fetal circulatory pattern, and the neonate responds to hypoxia by reverting to the fetal circulatory pattern.[6] During normal parturition, mild asphyxia occurs and results in fetal responses that pave the way for a successful transition to extrauterine life. If more than mild transient asphyxia occurs, the fetus will be stimulated to breathe *in utero*. This is known as *primary asphyxia*.[7] If the initial breathing effort resulting from the primary asphyxia does not correct the asphyxia, a second gasping period, known as the *secondary asphyxia* response, will occur in several minutes. If no improvement in asphyxia occurs during this period, the foal enters *secondary apnea*, a state that is irreversible unless resuscitation is initiated.[7]

Therefore, the first priority of neonatal resuscitation is establishing an airway and breathing pattern (Figure 2-15). It should be assumed that foals not spontaneously breathing by 1 minute after delivery are in secondary apnea. Clear the airway of membranes as soon as the nose is presented. If meconium staining is present, suction the airway before delivery is completed and before the foal breathes spontaneously. Continue to the trachea if aspiration of the nasopharynx is productive. Overzealous suctioning will worsen bradycardia as it worsens hypoxia. Stop suctioning once the foal begins breathing spontaneously as hypoxia will worsen with continued suction. If the foal does not breathe or move spontaneously within several seconds of birth, begin tactile stimulation. If tactile stimulation fails to result in spontaneous breathing, the foal should be immediately intubated and manually ventilated using an Ambu-bag or equivalent with or without oxygen supplementation. Mouth to nose ventilation can be used if nasotracheal tubes and an Ambu-bag are not available. The goal of this therapy is to reverse fetal circulation ventilation and may require ventilation with 100% oxygen. This is considered the best choice for this purpose. However, recent evidence suggests that there are no apparent clinical disadvantages in using room air for ventilation of asphyxiated human neonates rather than 100% oxygen.[8,9] Room-air-resuscitated human infants recovered more quickly than those resuscitated with 100% oxygen in one study as assessed by Apgar scores, time to the first cry, and sustained pattern of breathing.[10] In addition, neonates resuscitated with 100% oxygen exhibited biochemical findings reflecting prolonged oxidative stress, present even after four weeks of postnatal life, which did not appear in the room-air resuscitated group. Thus, the current accepted recommendations for using 100% oxygen in the resuscitation of asphyxiated neonates needs further discussion and investigation.[11,12] Almost 90% of foals requiring resuscitation respond to assisted ventilation alone and require no additional therapy. Nasotracheal

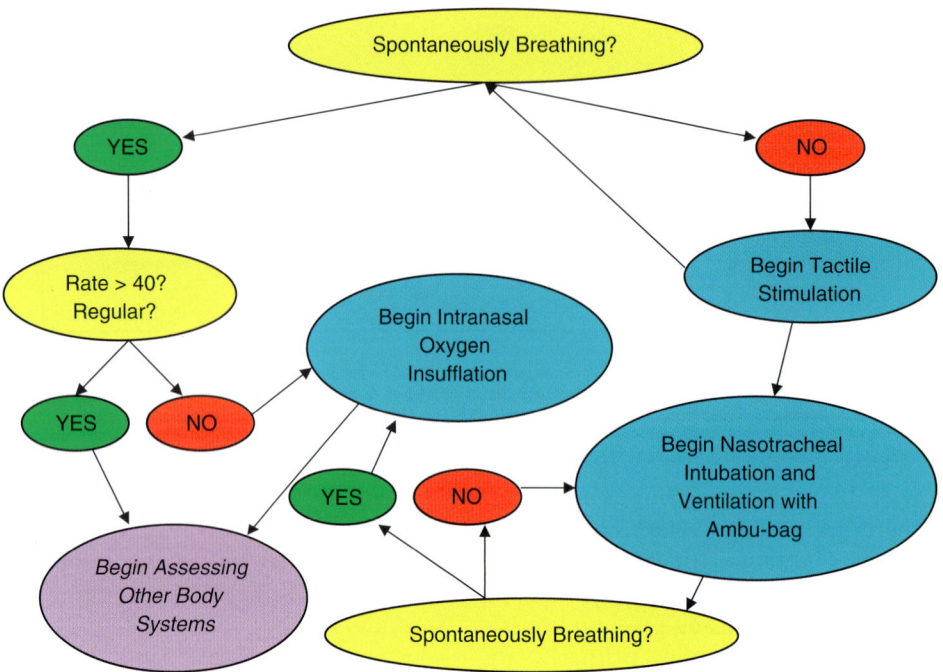

Fig. 2-15 Decision tree for respiratory resuscitation of a foal at birth.

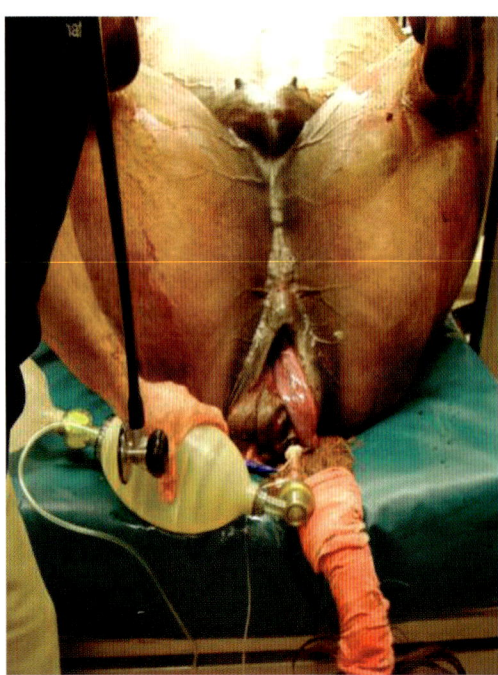

Fig. 2-16 Nasotracheal intubation can be initiated while the foal is in the birth canal if the foal will not be delivered rapidly, such as with a difficult dystocia.

intubation can be initiated while the foal is in the birth canal if the foal will not be delivered rapidly, such as with a difficult dystocia (Figure 2-16). This is a "blind" technique and requires practice, but it can be very beneficial and lifesaving. Once spontaneous breathing is

present, humidified oxygen should be provided via nasal insufflation at 8 to 10 L/min.

Cardiovascular support in the form of chest compression should be initiated if the foal remains bradycardic, despite ventilation, and a nonperfusing rhythm is present. Place the foal on a hard surface in right lateral recumbency with the topline against a wall or other support. Approximately 5% of foals are born with fractured ribs, so an assessment for the presence of rib fractures is necessary before initiating chest compressions.[13] Palpation of the ribs will identify many of these fractures. These fractures are usually multiple and consecutive on one side of the thorax. They are usually located in a relatively straight line along the part of the rib with the greatest curvature, usually 2 to 3 cm dorsal to the costochondral junction (Figure 2-17). Unfortunately, ribs 3 to 5 are frequently involved, and their location over the heart can make chest compression a potentially fatal exercise.

Initiate drug therapy if a nonperfusing rhythm persists for more than 30 to 60 seconds in the face of chest compression. Epinephrine is the first drug of choice. There are arguments regarding the best dose and the best frequency of administration for resuscitation. However, most of the data are acquired from human cardiac arrest studies and are not strictly applicable to the equine neonate, as the genesis of the cardiovascular failure is different.[14,15] Vasopressin is gaining attention as a cardiovascular resuscitation drug and, while we have used this drug in resuscitation and as a pressor, experience is limited at this time.[16] We do not

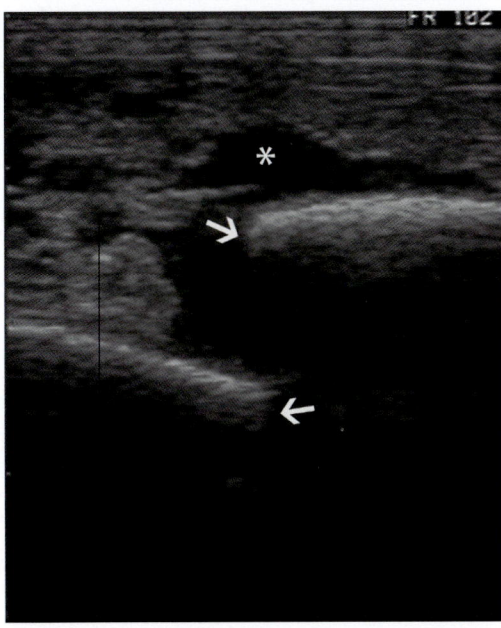

Fig. 2-17 Ultrasound of a fractured rib in a foal. Note the step-wise separation of the ends of the rib *(arrows)* and the presences of hematoma formation *(*)*.

use atropine in bradycardic newborn foals. This is because the bradycardia is usually due to hypoxia, and if the hypoxia is not corrected atropine can increase myocardial oxygen debt.[15] We also do not use doxapram as it wastes time and will not reverse secondary apnea, the most common type of apnea in newborns.

Poppy and '02 Poppy were discharged on April 20, 2002. Both mare and foal were allowed turn out in a very small turn-out area. We recommended that Poppy return in two months for follow-up ultrasound evaluation of her body wall tears, which can be done on an outpatient basis. We also recommend that she return immediately if she develops signs of abdominal discomfort due to our concerns regarding the presence of small intestine within her body wall tears, now termed hernias. We also recommended that Poppy not be bred again and that she wear her body wall support bandages until re-evaluation. Poppy never returned for follow-up.

PROGNOSIS

In situations in which the mare and foal progress well, the owner may be tempted to rebreed the mare. This must be strongly discouraged due to the likely reoccurrence or worsening of the condition. Embryo transfer is an option in mares of appropriate breeds. Surgical repair of small hernias may be possible using primary closure or mesh herniorraphy. However, this should be delayed for several months to allow for "maturation" of the damaged tissue, as edema resolves and a fibrous hernial ring develops. Spontaneous healing of partial ventral hernias can occur. In almost all cases, surgical repair of prepubic tendon rupture is not possible and euthanasia may be necessary.

REFERENCES

1. Dolente BA: Critical peripartum disease in the mare, *Vet Clin North Am Equine Pract* 20:151-165, 2004.
2. Wilson DV: Anesthesia and sedation for late-term mares, *Vet Clin North Am Equine Pract* 10:219-236, 1994.
3. Wilkins PA: Monitoring the pregnant mare in the ICU, *Clin Tech in Equine Pract* 2:212-219, 2003.
4. Reef VB: In: Reef VB, ed. *Equine diagnostic ultrasound*, Philadelphia, 1998, WB Saunders.
5. Martens RJ: Pediatrics. In: Mannsmann RA, McCallister ES, Pratt PW, eds: *Equine medicine and surgery*, ed 3, vol 1, Santa Barbara, Calif, 1982, American Veterinary Publications.
6. Soifer SJ, Kaslow D, Roman C et al: Umbilical cord compression produces pulmonary hypertension in newborn lambs: A model to study the pathophysiology of persistent pulmonary hypertension in the newborn, *J Dev Physiol* 9:239-252, 1987.
7. Gupta JM, Tizard JP: The sequence of events in neonatal apnoea, *Lancet* 2:55-59, 1967.
8. Tarnow-Mordi WO: Room air or oxygen for asphyxiated babies? *Lancet* 352:341-342, 1998.
9. Saugstad OD: Resuscitation with room-air or oxygen supplementation, *Clin Perinatol* 25:741-756, 1998.
10. Vento M, Asensi M, Sastre J et al: Resuscitation with room air instead of 100% oxygen prevents oxidative stress in moderately asphyxiated term neonates, *Pediatrics* 107:642-647, 2001.
11. Vento M, Asensi M, Sastre J et al: Six years of experience with the use of room air for the resuscitation of asphyxiated newly born term infants, *Biol Neonat* 79:261-267, 2001.
12. Saugstad OD: Resuscitation of newborn infants with room air or oxygen, *Semin Neonatol* 6:233-239, 2001.
13. Jean D, Laverty S, Halley J et al: Thoracic trauma in newborn foals, *Equine Vet J* 31:149-152, 1999.
14. Kattwinkel J, Niermeyer S, Nadkarni V et al: An advisory statement from the Pediatric Working Group of the International Liaison Committee on Resuscitation, *Middle East J Anesthesiol* 16:315-351, 2001.
15. Ushay HM, Notterman DA: Pharmacology of pediatric resuscitation, *Pediatr Clin North Am* 44:207-233, 1997.
16. Holland P, Hodge D: Vasopressin and epinephrine for cardiac arrest, *Lancet* 358:2081-2082, 2001.

3 Neonatal Immunology

Case 3-1 | Foal with Failure of Passive Transfer | Debra C. Sellon

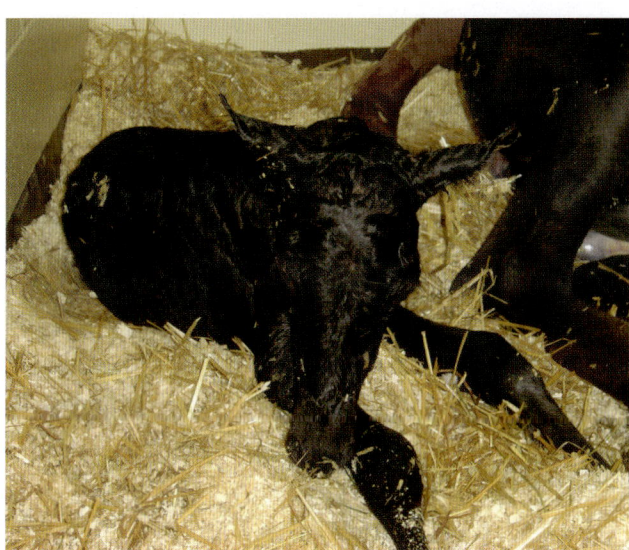

Fig. 3-1 '03 Vulnerable at birth.

*Vulnerable, a 16-year-old Standardbred mare, foaled in Kentucky in early February 2003 at 342 days gestation. The pregnancy and parturition were uneventful. This was the tenth foal from this mare. Her last foal, born in 2001, was healthy and vigorous at birth but developed **Actinobacillus equuli** septicemia and died at three days of age.*

'03 Vulnerable, a bay colt weighing approximately 50 kg, (Figure 3-1) stood within one hour of birth and nursed vigorously from his dam within two hours. The farm veterinarian examined the colt at approximately six hours of age (the morning after foaling) and found no significant abnormalities. A repeat physical examination at 36 hours of age was also within normal limits. A blood sample was collected at the time of the second examination for evaluation of serum IgG concentration.

HISTORY AND PHYSICAL EXAMINATION

The equine neonate is immune competent but immune naïve at birth. Equine lymphocytes are capable of responding to antigenic stimulation as early as 80 to 100 days of gestation and can mount a humoral response to pathogens by 200 days of gestation.[1,2] However, the fetus is protected from exposure to pathogens while in utero, and it is rare for a primary immune response to be elicited in a foal prior to birth. Maternal immunoglobulins are not transferred to the foal in utero because of the diffuse epitheliochorial placenta of the mare. The result is a foal that is born essentially agammaglobulinemic,[3-5] not yet primed to mount a rapid anamnestic response, and profoundly susceptible to infection with environmental pathogens unless the foal ingests adequate amounts of colostrum, the first milk produced by its dam.[6-9] Colostrum is widely recognized as the primary source of immunoglobulin for the equine neonate, but it also contains other immunologically important substances. Failure of the foal to ingest or absorb sufficient quantities of colostrum, primarily as defined by absorption of IgG, is termed failure of passive transfer (FPT). A foal with FPT is defined as a foal with a serum IgG concentration of <400 mg/dl at 24 hours of age. Partial FPT is defined as a foal with a serum IgG concentration of 400-800 mg/dl at 24 hours of age.

The reported incidence of complete or partial FPT in foals varies from 3% to 37.8%.[6,10-17] This wide variation is often attributed to differences in management practices on individual farms. Indeed, implementation of management factors designed to decrease the incidence of FPT in foals resulted in a significant decrease in the number of affected foals on farms in the United

Kingdom.[16] However, in one survey of 158 Standardbred mares on a single consistently managed farm, the incidence of FPT varied over a five-year period from 4% to 14%. This suggests that management may not be the only important factor.[18] Risk factors for FPT include month of foaling, adverse health events for mare and/or foal in the periparturient period, age of the dam, and colostral immunoglobulin content. A low colostral immunoglobulin concentration is associated with breed (Standardbred), age of dam (older mares) and total solar radiation.[15,18,19]

In most cases, a careful documentation of peripartum events or routine screening of all foals is critical for recognition of FPT. The most common causes of FPT in foals are loss of colostrum before parturition, failure to produce adequate quantities of good-quality colostrum, failure of the newborn foal to ingest colostrum within the first 12 hours after parturition, and insufficient absorption of ingested colostrum by the neonatal foal. Premature lactation has been associated with twin pregnancies, placentitis, and premature placental separation, but may occur without concurrent uterine, placental, or fetal pathology.

Poor-quality colostrum is difficult to identify based on appearance or available historical information; confirmation of this problem requires testing of the colostrum prior to ingestion by the foal. Increased solar radiation was associated with increased IgG concentration in colostrum and foal serum in a study by LeBlanc and colleagues,[19] perhaps explaining the observation that FPT is more common in foals born between December and March in the northern hemisphere.[18] Colostral IgG concentration was highest in mares three to ten years of age, and mean values were higher in Thoroughbred and Arabian mares than in Standardbred mares. When assessing colostral IgG concentration, it is also important to consider total quantity of colostrum produced. A mare with colostrum of lower IgG concentration may not be problematic if that mare produces a large total quantity of colostrum.

Production of colostrum with inadequate immunoglobulin content has been associated with ingestion of endophyte-contaminated fescue grass or hay. The causative agent of fescue toxicity is *Neotyphodium coenophialum* (formerly known as *Acremonium coenophialum*), a fungal endophyte that grows on stems, leaves, and seeds of tall fescue grass.[20,21] In addition to agalactia, pregnant mares consuming contaminated fescue may experience thickened fetal membranes, premature placental separation with "red bag" delivery, retained placenta, prolonged gestation, and birth of weak foals with high perinatal mortality. The ergopeptine toxins responsible for most of the reproductive manifestations of fescue toxicity act as dopamine receptor agonists that inhibit prolactin

secretion. This is compounded by decreased fetal progesterone secretion and increased serum estradiol concentrations. The net effect of decreased prolactin and progesterone and increased estradiol-17β is considered the cause of agalactia and insufficient mammary development in mares.

A foal may fail to ingest adequate quantities of colostrum if it is purposefully or inadvertently separated from the dam soon after parturition; the dam rejects the foal and does not permit it to suckle; the foal has systemic, neurologic, or orthopedic problems that cause it to be too weak to suckle or unable to stand; or the foal has neurologic problems that interfere with the development of an appropriate suckle reflex. These problems are usually readily apparent if the owner and/or farm manager are attentive during the periparturient period, and the attending veterinarian obtains a thorough history and physical examination.

Foals may develop FPT even if they are known to have ingested adequate quantities of good-quality colostrum, presumably because of a failure to absorb ingested immunoglobulins. This is most often recognized in premature or dysmature foals, possibly as a result of immature gastrointestinal function, but may also occur in otherwise healthy and vigorous full-term foals. Glucocorticoids enhance the maturation of small-intestinal epithelial cells and hence their loss of absorptive capacity[22,23] leading to speculation that endogenous corticosteroids released secondary to stress at the time of parturition may impair immunoglobulin absorption in foals.[3,24] However, administration of adrenocorticotrophic hormone to stimulate endogenous corticosteroid release failed to affect absorption in experimental foals,[25] and stress has not been a consistent historic finding in foals with FPT due to presumptive impaired immunoglobulin absorption.[13]

Foals with FPT as a sole problem do not exhibit any recognizable clinical signs. Abnormalities on physical examination are reflective of other disease processes. Therefore, unless a farm has a screening program to identify foals with FPT during the first few days of life, the problem is not recognized unless the foal becomes sick. FPT is a major risk factor for neonatal septicemia, omphalophlebitis, septic arthritis, and other infectious diseases and should be suspected in foals exhibiting clinical signs consistent with any of these disease conditions.[6-8]

PATHOGENESIS

Colostrum is produced in the mammary gland during the last weeks of gestation. As part of this process, immunoglobulin is concentrated from the mare's blood into colostrum in the mammary gland. While the predominant immunoglobulins in equine colostrum are IgG (1500-5000 mg/dl) and IgG(T) (500-2500 mg/dl), IgM (100-350 mg/dl) and IgA (500-1500 mg/dl) are also present.[26] At the time of parturition, colostral IgG concentration may exceed 9000 mg/dl in some mares.[27] The immunoglobulin concentration in milk decreases to negligible levels within 12 hours when mares are actively suckled by a healthy foal.

While immunoglobulin is the only component of colostrum that is routinely measured in veterinary medicine, colostrum also contains a wide range of other soluble and cellular substances that may have a positive impact on neonatal immunity and gastrointestinal maturity. These include cytokines,[28] growth factors,[29] hormones,[29] enzymes,[30] lymphocytes, macrophages, neutrophils, and epithelial cells.[27] The cellular components of colostrum likely play a role in local gastrointestinal immunity in the foal. Maternal cells may be found in mesenteric lymph nodes, blood, lungs, liver, and spleen of the neonate after ingestion of colostrum, suggesting they may play a role in systemic immunity as well.

Normal foals begin suckling colostrum within one to two hours of birth, and maternal antibodies are detectable in the blood of the foal within six hours. Specialized cells distributed throughout the small intestine nonselectively absorb macromolecules by pinocytosis.[5] Absorbed proteins pass through the intercellular space and lacteals into the systemic circulation via the lymph. Maximal absorptive efficiency occurs immediately after birth, declining to only 22% efficiency at 3 hours after birth and less than 1% by 20 hours.[31,32] This rapid decline in absorptive efficiency is due to rapid turnover of absorptive cells in the gastrointestinal mucosa and their replacement with more mature cells that are unable to nonselectively take up macromolecules.[5,12] The decline in absorption of colostral proteins parallels a transient proteinuria that peaks by 6-12 hours of age and declines by 24-36 hours of age.[5,33] Neonatal proteinuria most likely reflects absorption and excretion of low–molecular-weight milk proteins.

The half-life for disappearance of maternal antibodies from the foal's circulation varies between 20 and 30 days.[34-36] Antibody concentrations decline as a result of normal catabolism and gradual dilution in an increasing plasma volume as the foal grows.[5] There is also evidence for transfer of functional IgG into the gastrointestinal tract, which may account for partial clearance from the blood and enhanced gastrointestinal immunity.[37,38] Most maternal antibodies are present in only negligible concentrations by 6 months of age, although antibodies to some infectious agents have been detectable for up to 12 months after birth. The duration of detection of specific antibodies most likely depends on the quantity of specific antibodies absorbed and the sensitivity of the assay used. As passive antibody levels wane, autogenous antibody production increases with autogenous IgG first detectable at approximately two to four weeks of age.[35] The result is a nadir in serum immunoglobulin concentrations in the colostrum-fed foal at approximately one to two months of age followed by gradually increasing concentrations until adult levels are reached at approximately 5 to 10 months of age.[3,39] Serum immunoglobulin concentrations are similar in colostrum-fed and colostrum-deprived foals by three to four months of age.

Using a rapid ELISA-based screening test, it was determined that '03 Vulnerable had a serum IgG concentration of <400 mg/dl at 36 hours of age. A CBC was obtained, and results were considered within normal limits for a foal at this age. The findings were discussed with the farm manager, and it was suggested that the foal be treated. He was puzzled about the test results because the foal appeared so normal, and inquired about the pros and cons of treating the foal.

DIAGNOSIS

Ideally, all foals should be examined by a veterinarian and assessed for adequacy of passive transfer of immunoglobulin when they are 18 to 48 hours old. Foals considered to be at high risk for FPT and/or sepsis may be tested as early as 6 to 12 hours of age.[40] Serum IgG concentration should be assessed in all foals less than one month of age presenting for any type of medical problem. Foals should have a serum IgG concentration of >800 mg/dl to provide optimal passive immunity. A variety of rapid screening test kits are available for stall-side use to detect FPT in foals.[41-47] Important factors to be considered in selecting a screening test for a specific farm include overall accuracy, time necessary to perform the test, simplicity of the testing procedure, and cost. Quantitation of total serum protein by refractometry, although technically simple and cheap to perform, is relatively inaccurate as an indicator of serum IgG concentrations in foals.[47] However, there is a close correlation between serum IgG concentrations and total serum globulin concentrations in clinically healthy foals with no hematological abnormality.[16] Zinc sulfate and glutaraldehyde coagulation tests are relatively accurate, inexpensive, and results are available within an hour.[45,48] Many veterinarians and farm managers prefer to use commercial kits based on either glutaraldehyde coagulation or enzyme-linked immunosorbent assays[44,45] (Figure 3-2). In a recent comparison of the glutaraldehyde coagulation and the enzyme-linked immunosor-

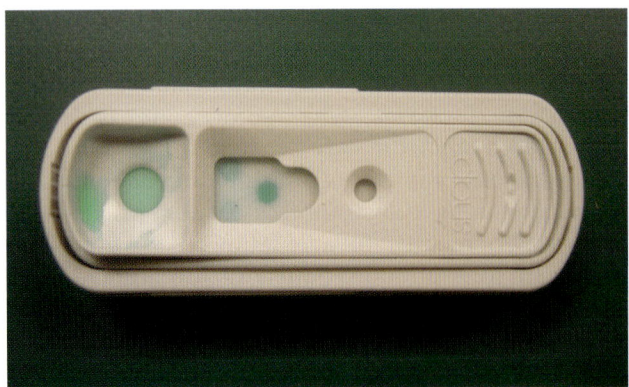

Fig. 3-2 Commercial enzyme-linked immunosorbent assay for IgG. Dark-blue spot shows the patient's sample indicating >800 mg/dl *(right)*. (SNAP, IDEXX Laboratories, Portland ME.)

bent assay (SNAP, Idexx Inc., Portland, ME), both tests were appropriate screening tests for FPT because they had high sensitivity and negative predictive value, meaning that foals with adequate IgG are identified correctly. The enzyme-linked immunosorbent assay was better than the glutaraldehyde coagulation in specificity and positive predictive value, meaning that foals with FPT were identified correctly. Immunoturbidometric testing of foal blood for serum IgG concentration is being increasingly used and appears to perform adequately in the field.[49]

False-negative and false-positive results are more common when attempting to accurately identify the foal with an IgG concentration of 400 to 800 mg/dl. When in doubt, confirmation of results can be obtained by single radial immunodiffusion (SRID) testing available through a number of commercial diagnostic laboratories. This test has the disadvantages of increased expense and a 24- to 48-hour delay in receiving results; however, it is more accurate than any of the currently available screening tests and is considered the gold standard for diagnosis of FPT in foals.

To Treat or Not to Treat

Foals that are intentionally colostrum-deprived rapidly succumb to septicemia, even when housed in a clean environment with good management practices.[9] Several field studies have confirmed that FPT is a risk factor for disease in the first few months of a foal's life.[15,18] However, Baldwin and colleagues failed to show any statistical link between serum IgG concentration and prevalence of illness, severity of illness, or survival of foals.[10,50] Hence, there is some debate regarding the significance of FPT or partial FPT in vigorous, healthy foals on well-managed farms that are known to have received some colostrum but have a serum IgG concentration of <800 mg/dl.[51] Not all foals

with FPT transfer will develop septicemia, but they are at higher risk than foals with adequate IgG. Foals from mares that have previously lost foals due to infection should also be considered high-risk foals.

The decision as to whether or not to treat a foal with partial FPT (IgG = 400 to 800 mg/dl) should be made after consultation among the owner, farm manager, and veterinarian with full consideration of the history, general physical health of the foal, farm-management practices, value of the foal, and individual tolerance for risk. If otherwise healthy foals with partial FPT are not treated, owners and farm managers should be instructed to monitor the vital parameters, appetite, attitude, gait, and respiratory rate and depth closely to facilitate early recognition of sepsis if it should occur.

Because of the mare's history of losing a previous foal to infection, the farm manager decided to pursue treatment for FPT. '03 Vulnerable was sedated, an IV catheter was placed in the left jugular vein, and 2 liters of normal equine plasma were administered IV over approximately 60 to 90 minutes. The IV catheter was removed, and the farm manager was instructed to monitor '03 Vulnerable for attitude, activity, and appetite. He was told to monitor the foal's temperature twice daily and watch for signs of lameness, diarrhea, or respiratory disease (increased rate or depth, dyspnea, cough, etc.). The farm manager was instructed to contact the farm veterinarian immediately if any abnormalities were observed.

TREATMENT

If FPT is suspected or recognized in the foal before 12 hours of age, the oral administration of good-quality colostrum is indicated. When FPT is recognized after a foal is 18 to 24 hours of age, oral administration of colostrum, colostral substitutes, or plasma is not recommended because of the relatively limited capacity of the foal's small intestine to nonselectively absorb macromolecules at that age. Healthy, vigorous foals with complete FPT (<400 mg/dl) and high-risk foals with partial or complete FPT (IgG ≤ 800 mg/dl) should be treated with intravenous normal equine plasma in sufficient quantity to increase the serum IgG concentration to >800 mg/dl. This treatment is also recommended for healthy foals with serum IgG of 400 to 800 mg/dl unless the owner and farm manager have been specifically counseled regarding the risks of not treating as described above.

Normal equine plasma with high concentrations of IgG is commercially available from several sources. The veterinarian should choose a USDA-licensed product to assure appropriate quality control in production. Donor horses should be routinely screened for equine infectious diseases and for major alloantigen or alloantibody incompatibilities. Ideally, donor horses should be negative for the Aa and Qa alloantigens to prevent sensitization of recipients to future transfusions. Donors should also be negative for all known equine alloantibodies to diminish the likelihood of adverse reaction in the recipient. For maximum benefit to the foal, donor horses should be vaccinated against common equine pathogens and contain appropriate concentrations of equine disease-specific antibodies. Some manufacturers also vaccinate their donor horses with lipid A in order to have a high level of anti-endotoxin antibodies.

An alternative to the use of commercial equine plasma is the use of plasma harvested from donor horses housed in the same environment as the foal to be treated. This approach has the advantage of increasing the likelihood that the donor plasma will contain adequate concentrations of antibodies to pathogens unique to the foal's local environment. Donor horses should have the same characteristics described above for commercial plasma donors. If blood typing or cross-matching services are not available, a previously untransfused gelding is a reasonable choice of donor horse. Donor plasma IgG concentration should minimally be 1200 mg/dl, preferably higher. Collection, processing, and storage procedures are time-consuming and must be done with strict attention to aseptic technique to prevent iatrogenic contamination of the plasma.

If the concentration of IgG in the donor plasma is known, the quantity of plasma to be transfused can be estimated. In normal foals, a dose of 200 mg IgG/kg body weight raised the serum IgG concentration by 450 mg/dl; a dose of 400 mg/kg of IgG increased the serum IgG by 575 mg/dl.[51] However, other studies suggest that there is no direct correlation between the quantity of IgG transfused and the increase in the foal's IgG concentration.[16] Septic foals often require a greater total volume of plasma to increase serum IgG concentrations by the same amount. Administering 1 liter of normal equine plasma with average quantities of IgG will typically increase the serum IgG concentration of a 45 kg foal by 200 to 300 mg/dl.[53] In order to achieve a final serum IgG concentration of >800 mg/dl in a foal with complete FPT (initial IgG <200 mg/dl), a total of 2 to 4 liters of normal equine plasma may be required.

To administer plasma, an intravenous catheter should be placed aseptically in one jugular vein. Frozen plasma should be thawed and warmed slowly to room temperature using a warm water bath. Microwave thawing or thawing with very high temperatures should be avoided because of the possibility of denaturing important plasma proteins. All blood products that are administered intravenously should

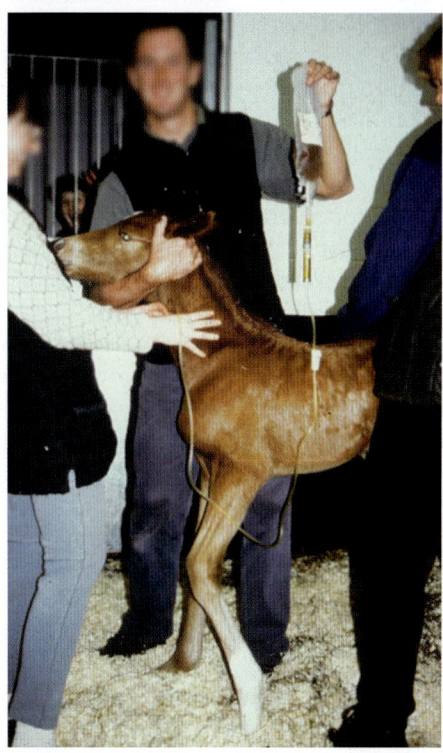

Fig. 3-3 Plasma transfusions in neonatal foals should be administered through a blood filter to remove fibrin clumps.

be administered through an appropriate in-line blood filter to remove fibrin clumps and other debris (Figure 3-3).

Even when donor and recipient are cross-matched, initial infusion rates should be slow so that the recipient foal may be closely observed for adverse reactions. Administering 0.5 ml/kg over approximately 10 to 20 minutes (approximately 20 to 30 ml to an average foal) is appropriate. Clinical signs of transfusion reactions may include muscle fasciculation, piloerection, increased heart or respiratory rates, fever, respiratory distress, abdominal pain, blanching of mucous membranes, or collapse. If no adverse reactions are observed during the initial slow infusion, the remainder of the transfusion may be administered at rates up to 40 ml/kg/hour (approximately 2 l/hour). Slower infusion rates are recommended for septic or otherwise systemically ill foals. Slower rates are also recommended if other fluids are being concurrently administered, so as to avoid iatrogenic volume overload. Vital signs and behavior of the recipient foal should be monitored throughout the transfusion and the flow rate decreased or stopped if significant changes are observed.

The foal's serum IgG concentration should be determined approximately 12 to 24 hours after administration of plasma to confirm that the desired increase has been achieved. The delay in assessing posttransfusion concentrations is necessary to allow time for distribution of the transfused immunoglobulin into vascular and extravascular spaces. In addition to redistribution into extravascular spaces, transfused immunoglobulin is rapidly catabolized or used in immune reactions. Healthy foals transfused with plasma at one day of age experienced a 30% decrease in serum IgG concentrations by seven days of age.[54] This decline might be even more precipitous in septic foals with increased vascular permeability and increased immune demands.

Equine-serum–derived products are available for intravenous use in the treatment of foals with FPT. However, these products have been associated with significant adverse reactions in some foals. Whenever possible, administration of high-quality equine plasma is preferred for treatment of foals with FPT.

PREVENTION

By the time FPT is diagnosed in many foals, it is too late to prevent exposure to potential pathogens in the environment. Therefore, the best approach to treatment begins with an aggressive program for prevention and early recognition of the problem. Owners and farm managers should be educated about the importance of ingestion of adequate colostrum within the first few hours of life. They should monitor foaling mares closely to ensure that foals stand and suckle vigorously within a few hours of birth. If this does not occur, they should contact their veterinarian to assist with oral administration of colostrum and/or colostral substitutes.

Farm managers should be encouraged to maintain a clean foaling environment during the periparturient period. Thorough cleaning and disinfection of foaling stalls between mares, replacing soiled bedding immediately after parturition, and washing the dam's perineal and mammary areas before the foal stands may decrease the ingestion of potentially pathogenic bacteria from the environment as the foal initiates environmental suckling in search of the mare's udder. Although most foals presenting for treatment of septic diseases have FPT,[6,7,16] partial FPT is not always associated with increased prevalence of illness or death.[10,16,18] Madigan has suggested that even minimal ingestion of colostrum may be associated with decreased disease because of a hastening of gut closure and prevention of absorption of bacteria,[55] however further studies suggest that feeding does not hasten gut closure.[56] Ensuring that the foal receives some colostrum immediately after birth by nasogastric tube or bottle feeding has been recommended to ensure that colostrum is present in the gastrointestinal tract prior to any exposure to bacteria.[55]

If foaling is attended, a sample of presuckle colostrum may be obtained to quantitate colostral IgG. Good colostrum tends to be sticky, yellow, and thick, but these subjective criteria are unreliable in assessing quality. Several rapid screening tests are available for stallside assessment of colostrum. One widely used method for estimating colostral quality is determination of colostral-specific gravity using a "colostrometer" (Equine Colostrometer, Lane Manufacturing Company, Denver, CO) (Figure 3-4). Specific gravity correlates directly with the IgG concentration of the colostrum. Approximately 75% of foals that ingest colostrum with a specific gravity of <1.060 will have serum IgG concentrations of <400 mg/dl; when specific gravity is >1.060, foals usually attain serum IgG concentrations of >500 mg/dl.[57] Sugar refractometry using a handheld refractometer (Brix 0-50% sugar refractometer) is also widely used for assessment of colostral quality.[58,59] A Brix % sugar reading of 20% to 30% correlates with adequate colostral quality and a reading of >30% indicates very good-quality colostrum[55] (Figure 3-5). A commercial kit based on glutaraldehyde coagulation (Gamma-Check-C, Veterinary Dynamics, Inc., San Luis Obispo, CA) is available for stallside screening of immunoglobulin concentrations in mare colostrum.[60]

Feeding foals approximately 1.5 g IgG/kg of body weight results in acceptable serum IgG concentrations. For a 45-kg foal, this requires a minimum of 1 to 2 liters of colostrum with a specific gravity of >1.060 (approximately 70 to 75 g of IgG) fed over multiple feedings in the first eight hours of life. Farm owners and managers should consider establishing a "colostrum bank" for feeding to foals that are unable to suckle colostrum from their dam. Donor colostrum should have a specific gravity of >1.060. Ideally, donor mares should be healthy, checked for blood type, negative for anti-RBC alloantibodies (especially anti-A and anti-Q), and appropriately vaccinated during the last four to six weeks of gestation. Approximately 200 to 250 ml of colostrum can be collected from a mare without depriving her own foal of IgG. Colostrum should be frozen in small aliquots (200 to 500 ml) and labeled with the name of the donor mare, blood type of the donor, level of quality, and date of collection. When frozen at −20°C and thawed slowly, colostrum should be stable for 12 to 18 months.

Studies on the induction of lactation show that normal milk production with high IgG concentration can be produced by barren mares. These results may suggest an alternative source of colostrum for freezing.[61]

If the risk for FPT is recognized during the first 8 to 12 hours of life and equine colostrum is not available, bovine colostrum[62-64] or a commercial colostrum substitute[65-69] may be administered to the foal. Bovine

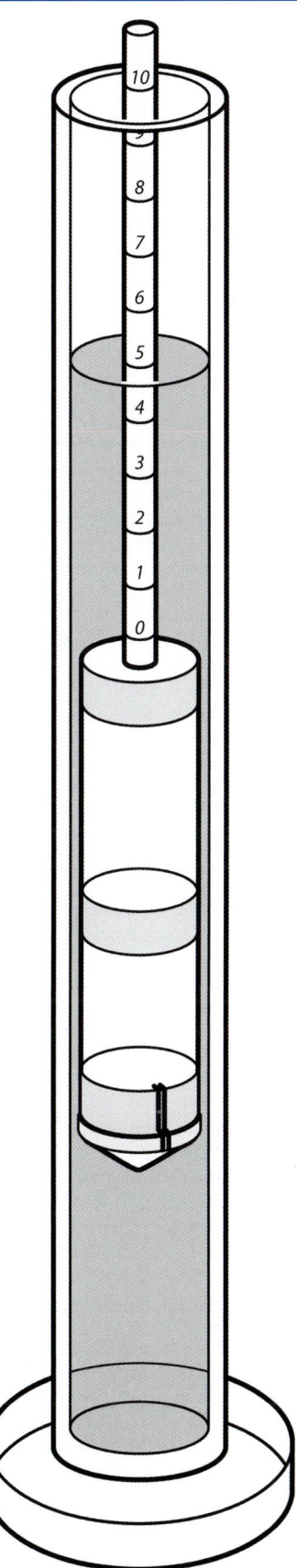

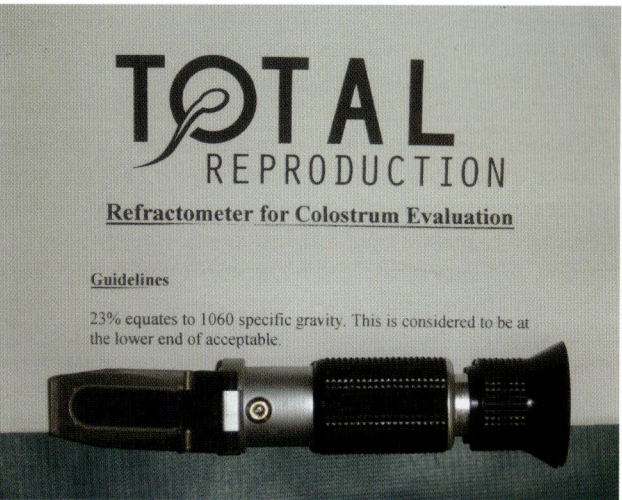

Fig. 3-5 The use of a Brix 0-50% sugar refractometer is a simple and accurate method for determining colostral quality. (Total Reproduction, Australia.)

colostral antibodies are absorbed by foals, but the half-life of these antibodies is considerably shorter than for equine antibodies. Approximately 2 to 4 liters of bovine colostrum should be administered; many foals develop transient mild diarrhea. Foals given only bovine colostrum as a source of passive antibody and raised under experimental conditions had a high incidence of respiratory disease, emphasizing the desirability of using equine colostrum whenever possible.

Lyophilized equine IgG (Lyphomune, BIOQUAL, Inc., Rockville, MD) is available as an equine colostral substitute. A minimum of 50 to 70 g of IgG is recommended for treatment of the average 45-kg foal that receives no colostrum, but in one study this dose failed to increase serum IgG concentration to >450 mg/dl in colostrum-deprived foals.[69] A concentrated equine serum product (Seramune, Sera, Inc., Shawnee Mission, KS) is available for use in foals with FPT. However, it failed to increase serum IgG concentrations in colostrum-deprived foals to adequate levels, probably because of the relatively low total IgG dose that was administered.[65] Because the product is not clearly labeled as to IgG concentration, it is difficult to formulate specific recommendations regarding the exact quantity to be administered. If the product contains 25 g of IgG per 300-ml bottle as stated by Vivrette,[65] approximately three bottles may be required to increase the serum IgG concentration of a 45-kg colostrum deprived foal to >400 mg/dl. Whereas colostrum substitutes derived from lypholized serum IgG may better used as colostrum supplements, those made from freeze-dried equine colostral IgG may have better efficacy.[70]

If there are no other available sources of immunoglobulin for a foal, oral administration of equine plasma or serum may be considered. This is

Fig. 3-4 A colostrometer can be used to determine specific gravity of colostrum, which correlates with IgG concentration. (Lane Manufacturing Company, Denver, CO 80231.)

an expensive source of oral immunoglobulin, and approximately 2 to 4 liters would be required to treat a colostrum-deprived 45-kg foal.

Because Vulnerable had a previous foal with septicemia, a condition often associated with FTP, the farm veterinarian recommended that future foals be closely monitored to ensure adequate intake of colostrum during the first 18 hours of life. Supplementation of future foals with colostrum from other mares and/or commercial colostral substitutes was discussed.

OUTCOME

Foals with uncomplicated FPT have an excellent prognosis if the condition is recognized early and treated appropriately. Prognosis for foals with FPT that is recognized only after development of sepsis or other infectious diseases is determined by the nature and severity of the infection.

REFERENCES

1. Perryman LE, Buening GM, McGuire TC et al: Fetal tissue transplantation for immunotherapy of combined immunodeficiency in horses, *Clin Immunol Immunopathol* 12:238, 1979.
2. Perryman LE, McGuire TC, Torbeck RL: Ontogeny of lymphocyte function in the equine fetus, *Am J Vet Res* 41:1197, 1980.
3. Perryman LE: Immunological management of young foals, *Comp Cont Educ Pract Vet* 3:223, 1981.
4. McGuire TC, Crawford TB: Passive immunity in the foal: Measurement of immunoglobulin classes and specific antibody, *Am J Vet Res* 34:1299, 1973.
5. Jeffcott LB: The transfer of passive immunity to the foal and its relation to immune status after birth, *J Reprod Fertil* Suppl:727, 1975.
6. McGuire TC, Crawford TB, Hallowell AL et al: Failure of colostral immunoglobulin transfer as an explanation for most infections and deaths of neonatal foals, *J Am Vet Med Assoc* 170:1302, 1977.
7. Koterba AM, Brewer BD, Tarplee FA: Clinical and clinicopathological characteristics of the septicaemic neonatal foal: Review of 38 cases, *Equine Vet J* 16:376, 1984.
8. McGuire TC, Poppie MJ, Banks KL: Hypogammaglobulinemia predisposing to infection in foals, *J Am Vet Med Assoc* 166:71, 1975.
9. Robinson JA, Allen GK, Green EM et al: A prospective study of septicaemia in colostrum-deprived foals, *Equine Vet J* 25:214, 1993.
10. Baldwin JL, Cooper WL, Vanderwall DK et al: Prevalence (treatment days) and severity of illness in hypogammaglobulinemic and normogammaglobulinemic foals, *J Am Vet Med Assoc* 198:423, 1991.
11. Clabough DL, Levine JF, Grant GL et al: Factors associated with failure of passive transfer of colostral antibodies in Standardbred foals, *J Vet Intern Med* 5:335, 1991.
12. Kohn CW, Knight D, Hueston W et al: Colostral and serum IgG, IgA, and IgM concentrations in Standardbred mares and their foals at parturition, *J Am Vet Med Assoc* 195:64, 1989.
13. Morris DD, Meirs DA, Merryman GS: Passive transfer failure in horses: Incidence and causative factors on a breeding farm, *Am J Vet Res* 46:2294, 1985.
14. Perryman LE, McGuire TC: Evaluation for immune system failures in horses and ponies, *J Am Vet Med Assoc* 176:1374, 1980.
15. Raidal SL: The incidence and consequences of failure of passive transfer of immunity on a thoroughbred breeding farm, *Aust Vet J* 73:201, 1996.
16. Stoneham SJ, Wingfield Digby NJ, Ricketts SW: Failure of passive transfer of colostral immunity in the foal: Incidence, and the effect of stud management and plasma transfusions, *Vet Rec* 128:416, 1991.
17. McClure JT, Miller J, DeLuca JL: Comparison of two ELISA screening tests and a non-commercial glutaraldehyde coagulation screening test for the detection of failure of passive transfer in neonatal foals, Proc 49th *AAEP Ann Conv* 301-305, 2003.
18. Clabough DL: Factors associated with failure of passive transfer in Standardbred foals, *Proceedings of the American College of Veterinary Internal Medicine* 8:555, 1990.
19. LeBlanc MM, Tran T, Baldwin JL et al: Factors that influence passive transfer of immunoglobulins in foals, *J Am Vet Med Assoc* 200:179, 1992.
20. Blodgett DJ: Fescue toxicosis, *Vet Clin North Am Equine Pract* 17:567, 2001.
21. Putnam MR, Bransby DI, Schumacher J et al: Effects of the fungal endophyte acremonium coenophialum in fescue on pregnant mares and foal viability, *Am J Vet Res* 52:2071, 1991.
22. Halliday R: Failure of some hill lambs to absorb maternal gammaglobulin, *Nature* 205:614, 1965.
23. Gillette DD, Filkins M: Factors affecting antibody transfer in the newborn puppy, *Am J Physiol* 210:419, 1966.
24. Jeffcott LB: Passive immunity and its transfer with special reference to the horse, *Biol Rev Camb Philos Soc* 47:439, 1972.
25. Carrick JB, Pollitt CC, Thompson HL et al: Failure of the administration of ACTH to affect the absorption of colostral immunoglobulin in neonatal foals, *Equine Vet J* 19:545, 1987.
26. Tizard I: *Veterinary immunology, an introduction*, ed 3, 1987, WB Saunders.
27. Pearson RC, Hallowell AL, Bayly WM et al: Times of appearance and disappearance of colostral IgG in the mare, *Am J Vet Res* 45:186, 1984.
28. Jan CL: Cellular components of mammary secretions and neonatal immunity: A review, *Vet Res* 27:403, 1996.
29. Grosvenor CE, Picciano MF, Baumrucker CR: Hormones and growth factors in milk, *Endocr Rev* 14:710, 1993.
30. Zou S, Brady HA, Hurley WL: Protective factors in mammary gland secretions during the periparturient period in the mare, *J Equine Vet Sci* 18:184, 1998.
31. Jeffcott LB: Duration of permeability of the intestine to macromolecules in the newly-born foal, *Vet Rec* 88:340, 1971.
32. Jeffcott LB: Studies on passive immunity in the foal. II. The absorption of 125i-labelled pvp (polyvinyl pyrrolidone) by the neonatal intestine, *J Comp Pathol* 84:279, 1974.
33. Jeffcott LB, Jeffcott TJ: Studies on passive immunity in the foal. III. The characterization and significance of neonatal proteinuria, *J Comp Pathol* 84:455, 1974.
34. Higgins WP, Gillespie JH, Robson DS: Studies of maternally-acquired antibodies in the foal to equine influenza a1 and a2, and equine rhinopneumonitis, *Equine Vet Sci* 7:207, 1987.
35. Jeffcott LB: Studies on passive immunity in the foal. I. Gammaglobulin and antibody variations associated with the maternal

transfer of immunity and the onset of active immunity, *J Comp Pathol* 84:93, 1974.

36. Reilly WJ, Macdougall DF: The metabolism of IgG in the newborn foal, *Res Vet Sci* 14:136, 1973.

37. Besser TE, Gay CC, McGuire TC et al: Passive immunity to bovine rotavirus infection associated with transfer of serum antibody into the intestinal lumen, *J Virol* 62:2238, 1988.

38. Besser TE, McGuire TC, Gay CC et al: Transfer of functional immunoglobulin G (IgG) antibody into the gastrointestinal tract accounts for IgG clearance in calves, *J Virol* 62:2234, 1988.

39. Rouse BT: The immunoglobulins of adult equine and foal sera: A quantitative study, *Br Vet J* 127:45, 1971.

40. LeBlanc MM: Update on passive transfer of immunoglobulins in the foal, *Pferdeheilkunde* 17:662-665, 2001.

41. Baird AN, Pugh DG, Rupp GP et al: Detection of immunoglobulin G in the neonate, *Equine Vet Sci* 7:124, 1987.

42. Bauer JE, Meyer DJ, Campbell M et al: Serum lipid and lipoprotein changes in ponies with experimentally induced liver disease, *Am J Vet Res* 51:1380, 1990.

43. Beetson SA, Hilbert BJ, Mills JN: The use of the glutaraldehyde coagulation test for detection of hypogammaglobulinaemia in neonatal foals, *Aust Vet J* 62:279, 1985.

44. Bertone JJ, Jones RL, Curtis CR: Evaluation of a test kit for determination of serum immunoglobulin G concentration in foals, *J Vet Intern Med* 2:181, 1988.

45. Clabough DL, Conboy HS, Roberts MC: Comparison of four screening techniques for the diagnosis of equine neonatal hypogammaglobulinemia, *J Am Vet Med Assoc* 194:1717, 1989.

46. Pugh DG, White SL: Commercially available tests for identification of the colostrum-deficient foal, *Equine Practice* 9:8, 1987.

47. Rumbaugh GE, Ardans AA, Ginno D et al: Measurement of neonatal equine immunoglobulins for assessment of colostral immunoglobulin transfer: Comparison of single radial immunodiffusion with the zinc sulfate turbidity test, serum electrophoresis, refractometry for total serum protein, and the sodium sulfite precipitation test, *J Am Vet Med Assoc* 172:321, 1978.

48. LeBlanc MM, Hurtgen JP, Lyle S: A modified zinc sulfate turbidity test for the detection of immune status in newly born foals, *Equine Vet Sci* 10:36, 1990.

49. Kent JC, Blackmore DJ: Measurement of IgG in equine blood by immunoturbidimetry and latex agglutination, *Equine Vet J* 17:125, 1985.

50. Baldwin JL, Vanderwall DK, Cooper WL et al: Immunoglobulin G and early survival of foals: A three year field study, *Proc 35th AAEP Ann Conv* 179, 1989.

51. Brewer BD, Mair TS: Failure of passive transfer: To treat or not to treat?, *Equine Vet J* 20:394, 1988.

52. White S: The use of plasma in foals with failure of passive transfer and/or sepsis, *Proc 35th AAEP Ann Conv* 215, 1989.

53. Koterba AM, Brewer B, Drummond WH: Prevention and control of infection, *Vet Clin North Am Equine Pract* 1:41, 1985.

54. White S: Exogenous IgG in the treatment of foals with failure of passive transfer and/or sepsis, *Proc ACVIM* 6:145, 1988.

55. Madigan JE: Method for preventing neonatal septicemia, the leading cause of death in the neonatal foal, *Proc 43th AAEP Ann Conv* 17, 1997.

56. Chavatte-Palmer P, Duvaux-Ponter C, Clement F: Passive transfer of immunity in horses, *Pferdeheilkunde* 17:669-672, 2001.

57. LeBlanc MM, McLaurin BI, Boswell R: Relationships among serum immunoglobulin concentration in foals, colostral specific gravity, and colostral immunoglobulin concentration, *J Am Vet Med Assoc* 189:57, 1986.

58. Cash RSG: Colostral quality determined by refractometry, *Equine Vet Educ* 11:36, 1999.

59. Chavatte P, Clement F, Cash R et al: Field determination of colostrums quality by a novel, practical method, *Proc 44th AAEP Ann Conv* 44:206-209, 1998.

60. Jones D, Brook D: Investigation of the gamma-check-C test as a means of evaluating IgG levels in equine colostrum, *Equine Vet Sci* 15:269, 1995.

61. Chavatte-Palmer P, Daels PF, Arnaud G et al: Quantitative and qualitative assessment of milk production after pharmaceutical induction of lactation in mares, *Proc Dorothy Havemeyer Neonatal Septicemia Workshop* 3, Talliores, France: 45, 2001.

62. Holmes MA, Lunn DP: A study of bovine and equine immunoglobulin levels in pony foals fed bovine colostrum, *Equine Vet J* 23:116, 1991.

63. Lavoie JP, Spensley MS, Smith BP et al: Complement activity and selected hematologic variables in newborn foals fed bovine colostrum, *Am J Vet Res* 50:1532, 1989.

64. Lavoie JP, Spensley MS, Smith BP et al: Absorption of bovine colostral immunoglobulins G and M in newborn foals, *Am J Vet Res* 50:1598, 1989.

65. Vivrette SL, Young K, Manning S: Efficacy of seramune in the treatment of failure of passive transfer in foals, *Proc 44th AAEP Ann Conv* :136, 1998.

66. Vivrette S: Colostrum and oral immunoglobulin therapy in newborn foals, *Comp Cont Educ Pract Vet* 23:286, 2001.

67. Burton SC, Hintz HF, Kemen MJ et al: Lyophilized hyperimmune equine serum as a source of antibodies for neonatal foals, *Am J Vet Res* 42:308, 1981.

68. Liu IK, Brown C, Myers RC et al: Evaluation of intravenous administration of concentrated immunoglobulin G to colostrum-deprived foals, *Am J Vet Res* 52:709, 1991.

69. Franz LC, Landon JC, Lopes LA et al: Oral and intravenous immunoglobulin therapy in neonatal foals, *Eq Vet J* 23:116, 1991.

70. Chavatte-Palmer P, Duvaux-Ponter C, Arnaud G et al: Efficacy of lyophilized colostral immunoglobulin product; effect of the 1st suckling time, *Proc Dorothy Havemeyer Neonatal Septicemia Workshop* 3, Talliores, France: 29-30, 2001.

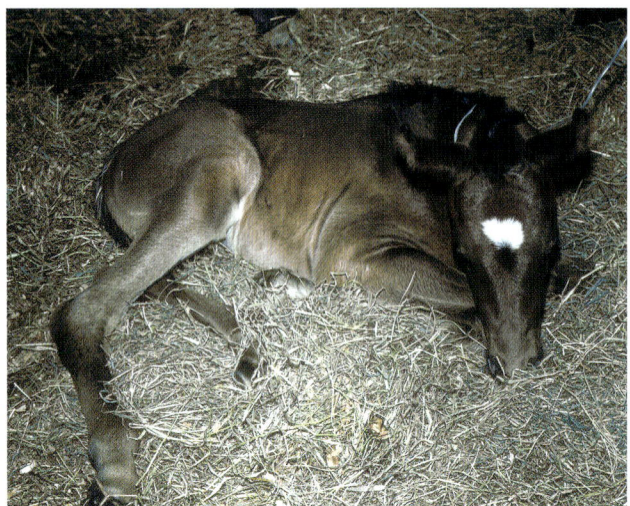

Fig. 3-6 Foal responsive but less active at two days of age.

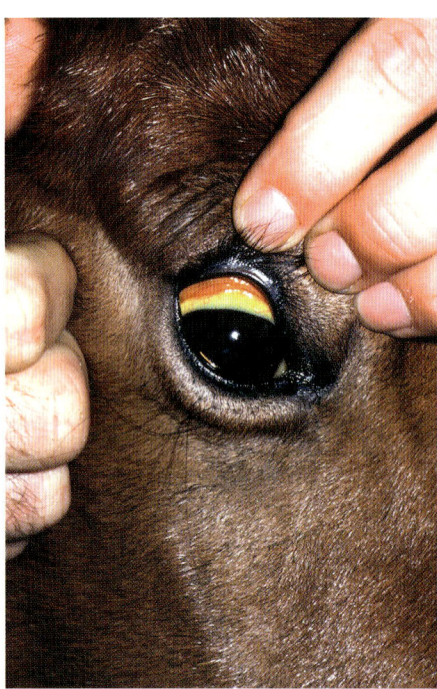

Fig. 3-7 Scleral icterus in a foal with neonatal isoerythrolysis.

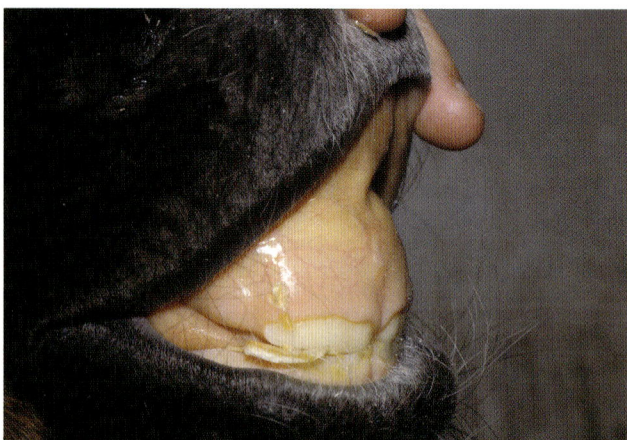

Fig. 3-8 Icteric mucous membranes in a foal with neonatal isoerythrolysis.

rate was 90 beats/minute, and respiratory rate was 40 breaths/minute. Oral mucous membranes and sclera were icteric (Figures 3-7 and 3-8). His skin tented for two seconds suggesting mild dehydration.

HISTORY AND PHYSICAL EXAMINATION

Foals affected with neonatal isoerythrolysis (NI) are normal at birth and develop disease within hours to days following ingestion of colostrum. The rapidity of onset is related to the quantity and type of offending antibody ingested in colostrum. Neonatal isoerythrolysis in the foal occurs most commonly in multiparous mares, although the diagnosis should not be excluded simply because the dam is primiparous. Often the history includes loss of a previous foal.

Pallor and icterus are the hallmark clinical signs of NI. The more rapid the onset, the more likely the foal is to exhibit pallor. In cases with slower onset, the icterus tends to be more dramatic. The severity of other clinical signs tends to relate to the rapidity of onset of anemia. Depression and neurologic signs are referable to hypoxia resulting from anemia, and occasionally kernicterus. Hemoglobinemia (evidenced by pinkish plasma) and hemoglobinuria accompany acute hemolysis (Figure 3-9). Pigment nephrosis may occur (Figure 3-10). Colic and melena may occur late in the course of the disease due to anoxia of the intestines as a result of anemia (Figure 3-11). Other considerations for icterus would include sepsis, hepatic disease, or other causes of hemolysis.

Neurologic signs in affected foals may be the result of hypoxia and ischemia or bilirubin encephalopathy.

'03 In the Red was a full-term colt with an uncomplicated birth. The foal stood and nursed within 60 minutes of delivery. The foal was bright, alert, and active. At two days of age, the foal was nursing less frequently and was less active. This was the second foal of In the Red. Her first foal is now a yearling and has had no medical problems.

On presentation, the foal was responsive but not active (Figure 3-6). His temperature was 102.6° F, heart

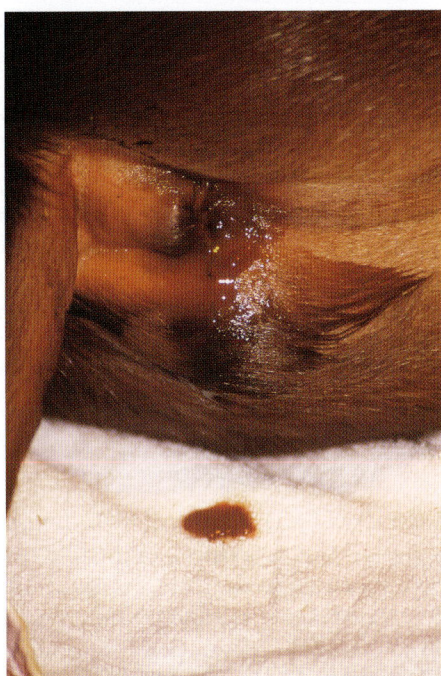

Fig. 3-9 Pigmenturia (hemoglobinuria) associated with severe hemolysis due to NI.

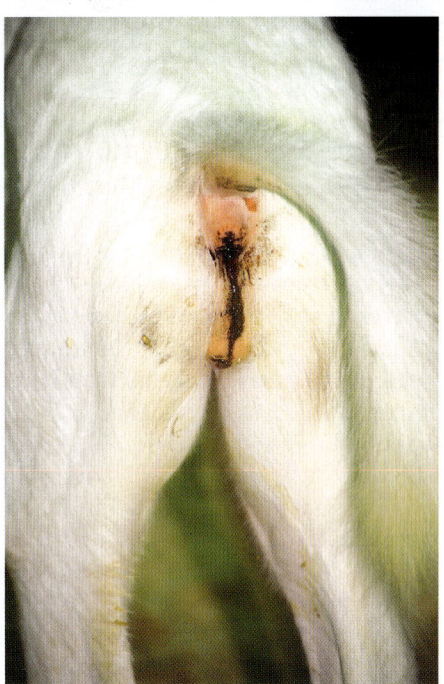

Fig. 3-11 Melena exhibited by a foal with severe NI.

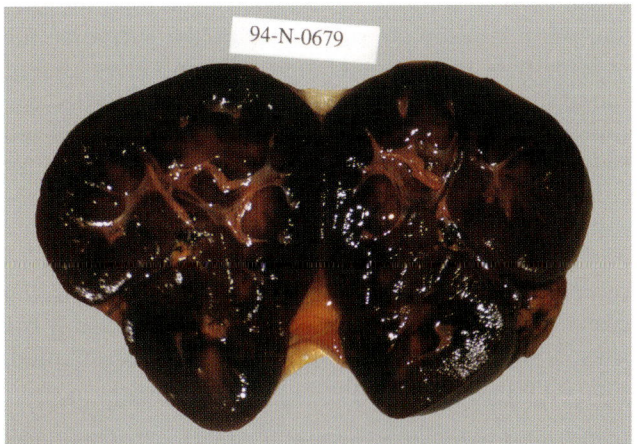

Fig. 3-10 Pigment nephropathy associated with severe hemolysis due to NI.

Kernicterus and bilirubin encephalopathy have been reported as a sequela of NI in association with markedly elevated levels of bilirubin.[1] Although free bilirubin is not toxic, toxicity develops when bilirubin is bound to cells. Multifocal yellow discoloration of the gray matter characterizes the lesion. Acidemia and septicemia are risk factors for development of kernicterus. Kernicterus is characterized by the yellow staining of the deep nuclei of the brain. Kernicterus is associated with total bilirubin levels ≥20 mg/dl, and the resulting neurologic dysfunction is characterized by abnormal muscle tone, poor suckling, opisthotonus, and deafness in children.[2]

PATHOGENESIS

NI is the immune-mediated destruction of red blood cells caused by maternal antibodies ingested in colostrum. In some ways, NI is like the "perfect storm." A large number of factors must all come together in order to produce disease. The mare must have a particular genetic makeup such that she lacks a particular red blood cell factor. The stallion must have a particular genetic makeup such that he possesses that red blood cell factor. The foal produced from this mating must inherit the gene to produce red blood cell factor from the stallion. Even when the genetic stage is set, there must be a series of other events that occur. The mare must somehow be exposed to the red blood cell factor prior to the end of gestation. This might result from an incompatible blood transfusion, a previous incompatible pregnancy/delivery, or leakage of incompatible foal red blood cells due to placentitis. Exposure to these antigens must stimulate an immune response that results in the production of antibodies. Furthermore, the mare must concentrate the antibodies to a sufficient level in her colostrum, and finally the foal must ingest and absorb sufficient colostral antibodies to cause enough red blood cell destruction to produce clinical disease.[3-5]

All red blood cell antigens (factors) stimulate the production of antibodies (that's what makes them antigens). However, certain red blood cell antigens are more antigenic under naturally occurring situations than others. Only about 25% of the recognized factors have been associated with NI, and factors Aa and Qa in the A and Q systems, respectively, have been responsible for most of the cases, however factors Ab, Qrs, Qb, Qc, Da, Db, Dc, Ka, Pa, and Ua have occasionally been associated with clinical NI.[6-9] The frequency of the various alleles that control the presence or absence of red blood cell antigens varies by breed, which in part explains the difference in prevalence of NI among breeds.[8,10] Every mule pregnancy (donkey sire/horse dam) is considered incompatible due to a factor possessed by all donkeys and lacked by all horses called donkey factor.[11]

Not all antibodies are created equal. Or perhaps it's more accurate to say that not all antigen/antibody interactions are created equal. By definition, red blood cell antigens elicit and react with anti-red blood cell antibody, but not all of these reactions produce clinical disease. Anti-Ca antibodies, for example, are very common, even in the absence of any obvious stimulatory event, yet they are not associated with the occurrence of clinical disease, and in fact, may prevent the immunization against other red blood cell antigens in "at-risk" mares by rapidly removing potentially immunizing red blood cells.[12]

The terms *sensitized* and *immunized* are equivalent with regard to NI. Immunization of a mare against red blood cell antigens usually occurs as a result of exposure to the blood of her foal (who inherited the antigens from the sire) at the time of delivery, thus making the disease more common in multiparous mares. Immunization of a mare can also occur when placentitis allows the foal's red blood cells to leak into the mare's circulation during gestation or as a result of blood transfusion. In sensitized (immunized) mares, these antibodies are concentrated in colostrum along with other antibodies. As a result of passive transfer, the foal may obtain a substantial quantity of these antibodies that then proceed to react with its red blood cells to cause intravascular hemolysis or accelerated removal by the reticuloendothelial system and extravascular hemolysis.

Incompatibilities among red blood cell antigens exist in virtually every pregnancy. Obviously not all incompatibilities result in NI. This is because many events must all converge, and sufficiently antigenic factors must be inherited by the foal for clinical disease to occur.

The initial workup on '03 In the Red included a complete blood count, chemistry profile, and immunoglobulin assessment. Anemia (PCV = 16 %, hemoglobin = 5.7 g/dl) and neutrophilic leukocytosis (16,000 WBC/μl, 14,500 segmented neutrophils/μl) was found on the CBC. Plasma was markedly icteric. Bilirubin was 12.5 mg/dl. Immunoglobulin level was >800 mg/dl. Blood urea nitrogen was 27 mg/dl. Liver enzyme activities (GGT, AST,

LDH) were within normal limits. Blood glucose was 90 mg/dl. Urine was reddish colored and tested 4+ blood on urine dipstick.

A Coombs' antiglobulin test using equine-specific reagents was submitted to assess for coating of the foal's red blood cells with immunoglobulin and complement. The test was positive at a dilution of 1:64. Serum from the mare was harvested for detection of anti-red blood cell antibodies. Anticoagulated blood samples from the mare and foal were collected for performance of red blood cell typing.

DIAGNOSTIC TESTS

The gold standard for diagnosis of NI is demonstration of antibodies (globulins) coating of the foal's red blood cells using a species-specific Coombs' test.[4,13] Presumptive evidence of NI is provided by demonstrating the presence of anti-red blood cell antibodies in the serum/plasma (or colostrum) of the dam. The presence of antibodies alone does not confirm disease because the foal must possess the corresponding antigen for disease to occur. However, if the antibodies react with the red blood cells of the foal or the sire of the foal, the presumption is quite strong. Under field conditions, the specificity of the anti-red blood cell antibodies (that is, the particular antigen to which the antibodies are directed) is seldom known, only that some anti-red blood cell antibody is present. The mare's serum (or colostrum) is the best source to test for presence of anti-red blood cell antibodies. Anti-red blood cell maternal antibodies in the foal's circulation are often attached to red blood cells and are not present in high titer in the plasma. NI and FTP are mutually exclusive, so if the presence of immunoglobulin cannot be documented, then NI is probably not the cause of the clinical signs.

Initial treatment plan for '03 In the Red included placement of an IV catheter and administration of balanced polyionic solutions to address dehydration and promote diuresis in the face of hemoglobinuria. Strict stall rest was enforced, and manipulation of the foal was kept to a minimum since stress of attempting to pass feeding tubes or other procedures may prove fatal.

Antibiotics were initiated because initially the cause of the neutrophilia and mild body temperature elevation could not be ascertained to be NI or infection. NI foals are often febrile, making it difficult to eliminate sepsis as a concern. Because the PCV was at 16% and the foal was several days old, transfusion was not immediately contemplated; however, samples were submitted for crossmatching between the mare's serum and the panel of potential available blood donors in case the PCV was found to be decreasing.

TREATMENT

Blood transfusion is indicated when PCV approaches 12%; however, due to the lengthy process of collecting and processing blood, if the PCV is at 15% and dropping, blood should be collected in anticipation of need.[14,15] Polymerized bovine hemoglobin (Oxyglobin, Biopure Corp., Cambridge, MA) has been used for short-term management of NI while awaiting a washed red blood cell transfusion.[16-18] However, this product may not be available and is very expensive. Doses used in dogs (10 to 30 ml/kg) have been extrapolated to foals. Anaphylactic reactions have been reported in adult ponies, but whether true anaphylaxis could occur in foals is unknown.[18]

The key to selection of a donor is to identify an individual whose red blood cells will not react the mare's serum (and colostral) antibody. Foals are born agammaglobulinemic, and the only antibodies present are of maternal origin; therefore, one needs to evaluate potential donors against the mare's serum. It is preferable to use the mare's serum (or colostrum) rather than the foal's serum as the source of antibodies for cross-matching because antibodies in the foal may be mostly attached to red blood cells, not freely circulating in the plasma and readily detected in agglutination or lytic assays.[19]

The odds of finding a suitable blood donor, that is, an individual that lacks the antigen to which the maternal antibody is directed, vary with the specific factor involved and the breed of donor. While there are many blood factors in numerous genetic systems, each individual factor can be thought of simply as present or absent in a potential donor. The factors are not evenly distributed among members of the population. The probability of a specific factor being present is based on the frequency of that gene in the population of a breed. As an example, over 95% of thoroughbreds have factor Aa.[8,10] That means that only about 1 in 20 thoroughbreds will be negative for the factor (and thus a suitable red blood cell donor for a foal suffering from NI associated with anti-Aa antibody). Because Aa and Qa are the antigens most commonly implicated to cause NI, horses that are Aa- and Qa-negative are frequently considered "universal donors," however, so-called universal donors have a variable complement of other red blood cell antigens that can cause transfusion reactions. Therefore, the connotation does not have the same meaning as it does for people. It is a source of confusion and should be abandoned.

The dam's red blood cells are guaranteed not to react with her own antibody; however her red blood cells must be washed free of offending antibody in order to avoid further aggravating the problem in the foal. Washing red blood cells amounts to sequential sedimentations (or centrifugations) of red blood cells with removal and discard of plasma and saline washing solutions.[20] This can be very time-consuming and may not be an option for the foal that needs an immediate transfusion.

Blood is administered at a rate of 20 ml/kg body weight initially, at a rate to avoid volume overload. Transfusion usually results in an increase in PCV for 12 to 24 hours followed by a decline.[14,15,21] This decrease may represent continued removal of the foal's own cells as well as removal of transfused red blood cells.

'03 In the Red's PCV remained stable and started to increase over the course of the next week. Antibiotics were discontinued, and the foal was discharged from the hospital with a PCV of 21. Reports from the referring veterinarian about the foal were good, as the foal experienced no further problem over the next month.

OUTCOME

In peracute cases of NI, mortality is very high and foals may die before the cause of disease is recognized. Cases with rapidly progressing anemia over one to three days can be successfully managed with more aggressive intervention, often including transfusions. In cases in which foals survive several days and do not become severely anemic, even though they may develop prominent icterus, the prognosis is generally good and these foals seldom require blood transfusions.

PREVENTION

NI is a preventable disease and one in which proactive intervention can be very rewarding. There are several strategies that can be employed to prevent the exposure of the foal to harmful antibodies.[22,23] Mares who lack an antigen (because they did not inherit the gene to produce them) are considered at risk for NI because if they are exposed to the red blood cell antigen they are likely to produce antibodies against it.[12] It is possible to identify at-risk mares by red blood cell typing. When examining a blood-typing report, of particular interest is whether factors Aa and/or Qa are present (positive). The lack of one or both factors puts the mare at risk and allows special attention to be paid to implementation of strategies to prevent NI. One exception to this is in Standardbreds, where factor Qa is not found in the breed. This would appear to leave all mares vulnerable. However, since Standardbred stallions also lack the factor, there is no mechanism for sensitization. Mates of at-risk mares can be selected based on blood type to eliminate the possibility of incompatibility (not always practical), or matings can

Box 3.1   Jaundiced Foal Agglutination Test (JFA)[25,26]

The jaundiced foal agglutination test (JFA) is used to detect the presence of agglutinating antibody in colostrum directed against red blood cell antigens. Colostrum from the mare is reacted with red blood cells from the foal. If antibody against the red blood cells is present in the colostrum, an agglutination reaction occurs and can be visualized.

The test is most useful if used presuckle, before the foal has ingested colostrums to assess the risk associated with colostral ingestion.

The test is also useful to monitor the decline in colostral antibody over time in order to determine when it will be safe to allow the foal to nurse.

If the test is performed after suckling and absorption of colostral antibody, any absorbed colostral antibody with anti–red blood cell specificity may already have attached to the red blood cells of the foal and will give a positive reaction even without the addition of colostrum. Therefore, it is important to run a saline control to check for autoagglutination.

Materials Needed:
- Centrifuge
- Test tubes (e.g., 13 × 100 ml disposable tubes or red-top blood-collection tubes)
- Pipette system capable of delivering 1.0 ml volumes
- 0.9% NaCl for preparing dilutions
- Colostrum from the mare
- Presuckle blood from the foal, preferably in EDTA anticoagulant
- Blood from the mare, preferably in EDTA anticoagulant, for use as a control sample

Testing Steps:
1. Label a set of 8 tubes as SALINE CONTROL and dilutions 1:2, 1:4, 1:8, 1:16, 1:32, 1:64, 1:128
2. Add approximately 1 ml 0.9% NaCl to each tube
3. Prepare serial dilutions of the colostrum by adding 1 ml of colostrum to the tube labeled 1:2, then transferring 1 ml of the mixture to the tube labeled 1:4, and so on until reaching the tube labeled 1:128. Discard 1 ml from the tube labeled 1:128 so that the total volume in each tube is approximately 1 ml. No colostrum is added to the saline control.
4. Add one drop of well-mixed anticoagulated whole blood from the foal to each tube of diluted colostrum and the saline control.
5. Mix the samples.
6. Centrifuge the tubes for 2 to 3 minutes at medium speed (300-500 g). The centrifugation step is important to allow cells to contact each other to promote any tendency to agglutinate. Following centrifugation, the red blood cells will be pelleted in the bottom of the tubes.
7. Invert each tube, one at a time, pouring out the liquid contents; observe the status of the button of red blood cells at the bottom of the tube.

When no agglutination exists (–), the red blood cells easily flow down the side of the tube (Unn Figure 1).

Complete agglutination (4+) causes the red blood cells to remain tightly packed in the button; strong agglutination (3+) causes the red blood cells to remain in large clumps. With weaker agglutination (1 + to 2+), the red blood cells remain in

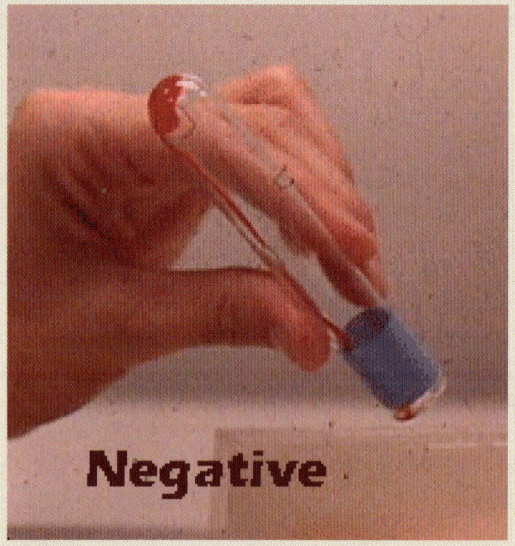

Negative

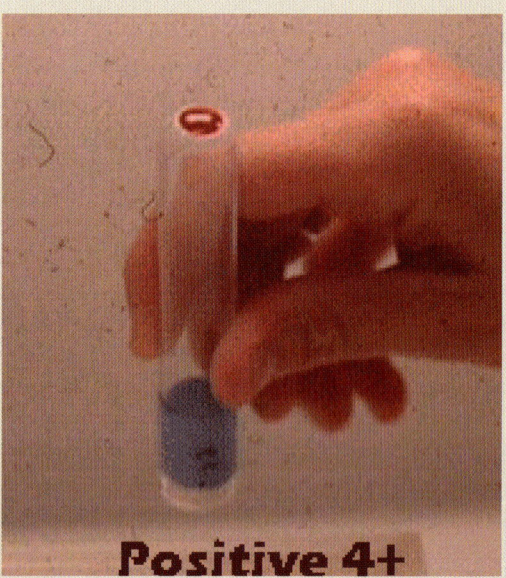

Positive 4+

small clumps as they run down the side of the tube (Unn Figure 2).

8. The titer is defined as the highest dilution that gives strong agglutination (3+ or 4+).

Interpretation:
Positive reactions at 1:16 or greater in horses and 1:64 or greater in mules are considered significant. Colostrum should be withheld until the JFA titer drops below this level.[22,25]

If the blood agglutinates in the SALINE CONTROL tube, this may indicate that the foal has already absorbed antibodies and the red blood cells are already coated with antibody. In this case, the test is not a valid assessment of the amount of antibody remaining in the colostrum.

At low dilutions, the physical characteristics of colostrum often cause clumping of the red blood cell. Colostrum can be tested using the dam's own red blood cells to be certain that it is not the viscosity of the colostrum that is causing agglutination.

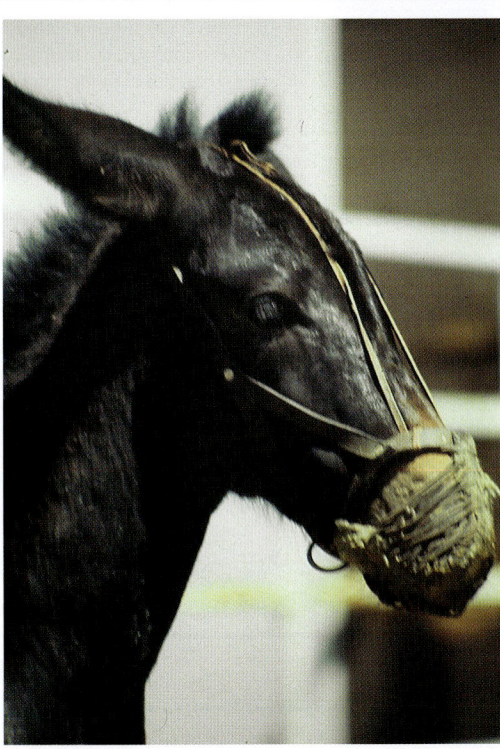

Fig. 3-12 Mule foal muzzled to prevent ingestion of colostrum and development of NI.

patibility and deal with the problems by intervening at parturition. Prevention requires attendance at birth. This can be as a result of faithful watching, or inducing parturition.[22,24] At birth, in the time between delivery and nursing, colostrum can be evaluated for the presence of offending antibodies against the foal's red blood cells prior to allowing the foal to nurse, or an alternate source of "safe" colostrums that are known to be free of anti-red blood cell antibodies can be provided.[22] Alternatively, if safe colostrum is not available, plasma transfusions can be administered and the foal managed for FTP. The jaundiced foal agglutination test (JFA), which can be completed within 10 to 20 minutes, is useful for prediction of NI (Box 3-1). If the foal has ingested colostrum, the test is less indicative of the actual situation since the foal's red blood cells are already coated with antibody and may agglutinate at all dilutions.

Colostral titers of anti-red blood cell antibody drop at a variable rate ranging from a few hours to a day. Colostrum should be withheld until the offending antibody has declined. This is best accomplished by muzzling the foal to prevent nursing (Figure 3-12). Colostrum from another mare may be given by stomach tube or bottle to ensure adequate passive transfer. Measuring titers in the dam's colostrum/milk with the JFA test (using presuckle foal blood) and withholding only until the titer drops below 1:16 (1:64 for mules)—instead of arbitrarily withholding for 36 to 72 hours—may save immense amounts of time and labor and allow the foal to bond with the mare sooner and receive the additional nutritional and health benefits of nursing (Box 3-1). The permeability of the gut to immunoglobulin also declines rapidly, so the rational for withholding longer than 24 hours is questionable. If the foal has ingested tainted colostrum, absorption takes a period of time to occur and clinical signs may progress, but will probably not be augmented by additional ingestion after about 12 to 18 hours of age.

be made without regard to blood type and strategies used to test for antibodies and/or intercept colostrum prior to ingestion. One way to prevent NI is to avoid mating a stallion that possesses the red blood cell antigen to a mare that lacks them. This is possible but not particularly practical because blood-typing information is not readily available when selecting stallions, and depending on the breed, there may be relatively small numbers of stallions that would be compatible on this basis.

Since the disease is a result of events that occur after birth, not *in utero* transfer of antibodies as with humans, it is possible to breed without regard to com-

REFERENCES

1. David JB, Byars TD, Braniecki A et al: Kernicterus in a foal with neonatal isoerythrolysis, *Comp Contin Educ Pract Vet* 20:517, 1998.
2. Shapiro SM: Definition of the clinical spectrum of kernicterus and bilirubin-induced neurologic dysfunction (BIND), *J Perinatol* 1, 2004.
3. Stormont C: Neonatal isoerythrolysis in domestic animals: A comparative review, *Adv Vet Science Comp Med* 19:23, 1975.
4. Scott AM, Jeffcott LB: Haemolytic disease of the newborn foal, *Equine Vet J* 103:71, 1978.
5. Doll ER: Observations of the clinical features and pathology of hemolytic icterus of newborn foals, *Am J Vet Res* 13:504, 1952.
6. MacLeay JM: Neonatal isoerythrolysis involving the Qc and Db antigens in a foal, *J Am Vet Med Assoc* 219:79, 2001.
7. Zaruby JF, Hearn P, Colling D: Neonatal isoerythrolysis in a foal, involving anti-Pa alloantibody, *Equine Vet J* 24:71, 1992.
8. Bailey E: Prevalence of anti–red blood cell antibodies in the serum and colostrum of mares and its relationship to neonatal isoerythrolysis, *Am J Vet Res* 43:1917, 1982.
9. Trommershausen-Smith A, Stormont C, Suzuki Y: Alloantibodies: Their role in equine neonatal isoerythrolysis, *Intl Symp Eq Hematol* 1:349, 1975.
10. Bowling AT, Clark RS: Blood group and protein polymorphism gene frequencies for seven breeds of horses in the United States, *Anim Blood Groups Biochem Genet* 16:93, 1985.
11. McClure JJ, Koch C, Traub-Dargatz J: Characterization of a red blood cell antigen in donkeys and mules associated with neonatal isoerythrolysis, *Anim Genet* 25:119, 1994.
12. Bailey E, Albright AG, Henney PJ: Equine neonatal isoerythrolysis: Evidence for prevention by maternal antibodies to the Ca blood group antigen, *Am J Vet Res* 49:1218, 1988.

13. Wilkerson MJ, Davis E, Shuman W et al: Isotype-specific anti-bodies in horses and dogs with immune-mediated hemolytic anemia, *J Vet Intern Med* 14:190, 2000.
14. McClure JJ: Neonatal isoerythrolysis. In Robinson EN, ed: *Current therapy in equine medicine*, ed 4, Philadelphia, 1997, WB Saunders.
15. Whiting JL, David JB: Neonatal isoerythrolysis, *Comp Contin Educ Pract Vet* 22:968, 2000.
16. Perkins GA, Divers TJ: Polymerized hemoglobin therapy in a foal with neonatal isoerythrolysis, *J Vet Emerg Crit Care* 11:141, 2001.
17. Polkes AC: Neonatal isoerythrolysis: Overview, management strategies, and long-term outcome, *21st Proc ACVIM Forum* 248, 2002.
18. Belgrave RL, Hines MT, Keegan RD et al: Effects of a polymer-ized ultrapurified bovine hemoglobin blood substitute adminis-tered to ponies with normovolemic anemia, *J Vet Intern Med* 16:396, 2002.
19. Swiderski CE: Hypersensitivity reactions. In Reed SM, Bayly WM, eds: *Equine internal medicine*, ed 1, Philadelphia, 1998, WB Saunders.
20. Osbaldiston GW, Coffman JR, Stowe EC: Equine isoerythroly-sis—Clinical pathological observations and transfusion of dam's red blood cells to her foal, *Can Comp Med* 33:310, 1969.
21. Smith JE, Dever M, Smith J et al: Post-transfusion survival of 50Cr-labled erythrocytes in neonatal foals, *J Vet Intern Med* 6:183, 1992.
22. Blackmer JM, Paccamonti D, Eilts B et al: Strategies for preventing neonatal isoerythrolysis, *Comp Contin Educ Pract Vet* 24:562, 2002.
23. McClure JJ: Strategies for prevention of neonatal isoerythrolysis in horses and mules, *Equine Vet Educ* 9:118, 1997.
24. Blackmer JM, Paccamonti D, Eilts B et al: Measuring calcium levels in mammary secretions, *Vet Technician* 23:590, 2002.
25. Bailey E, Conboy HS, McCarthy PF: Neonatal isoerythrolysis of foals; an update on testing, *Proc Am Assoc Equine Pract* 341, 1987.
26. Blackmer JM, Costa LRR, Koch C: The jaundiced foal agglutina-tion test, *Vet Technician* 23:577, 2002.

| Case 3-3 | Foal with Immune-Mediated Thrombocytopenia | Debra C. Sellon |

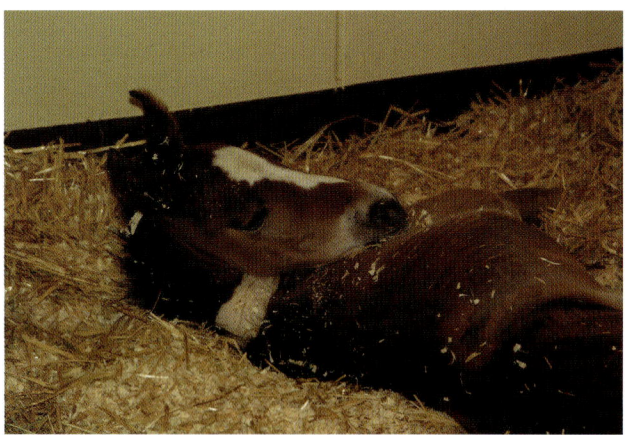

Fig. 3-13 '04 Diplomatic Immunity at three days of age.

'04 Diplomatic Immunity, a three-day-old Warmblood filly, was presented for evaluation of inadequate suck-ling, oral petechia, and ecchymoses that had developed over the previous 24 hours (Figure 3-13). Parturition was observed and uneventful. The placenta was passed rapidly after birth and appeared grossly normal. The foal's umbilicus had been treated with dilute chlorhexi-dine twice daily. The foal stood within one hour of birth and suckled vigorously. An intramuscular injection of vitamin E/selenium was administered shortly after birth. Behavior during the first 48 hours of life, including uri-nation and passage of meconium, was within normal limits. At 36 hours of age, serum IgG was >800 mg/dl. '04 Diplomatic Immunity was the fifth foal from this mare; there were no known health problems with previous foals. The preventive medicine program for the farm was excellent, and deworming and vaccinations were current.

'04 Diplomatic Immunity was in sternal recumbency at the time of presentation but was able to rise and walk. She was responsive to human interaction, but mentation was dull. She weighed 45 kg. Temperature was 100.7°F, heart rate was 72 beats/minute, and respiratory rate was 18 breaths/minute. Petechial hemorrhages were present in the inside of the foal's ear pinnae, and erosions were found on the oral mucous membranes (Figure 3-14, A and B). Capil-lary refill time was approximately two seconds. There were diffuse, small (1 to 4mm) crusting papular lesions on the skin, especially over the neck, pectoral muscles, thorax, and flanks.

HISTORY AND PHYSICAL EXAMINATION

Foals with uncomplicated alloimmune disease most commonly have a history of uneventful pregnancy and parturition. They appear healthy and vigorous at birth and ingest and absorb ample quantities of immunoglobulin from colostrum. Clinical signs become apparent at one to three days of age and owner complaints commonly include nonspecific signs of lethargy, weakness, and inability to suckle. There is no known breed or gender predilection for alloimmune thrombocytopenia in horses, however there is an apparent increased incidence in mule foals.[1,2] Findings on initial physical examination of affected foals vary depending on the duration of clinical signs, quantity, and avidity of antiplatelet antibodies consumed, and specificity of the antibodies consumed. Some foals are

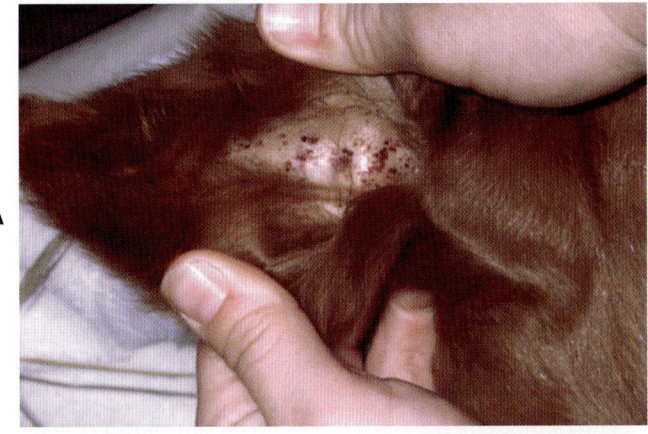

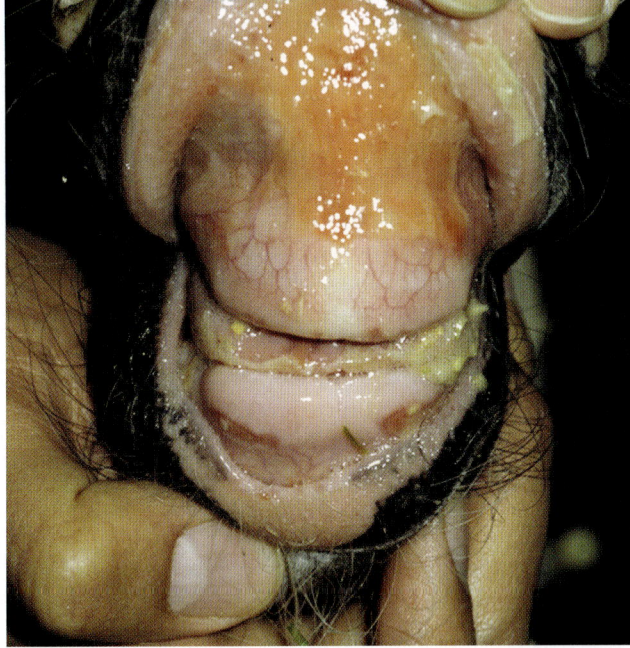

Fig. 3-14 A and **B,** Petechial and ecchymotic hemorrhages in the ear. Erosions of the oral mucous membranes of a foal. (**A,** Courtesy of Dr. Michelle Barton.)

normal and the problem is discovered on routine postfoaling bloodwork. Most clinically affected foals are in normal body condition with mild to moderate dehydration and exhibit depression, lethargy, and reluctance or inability to suckle. Petechia and ecchymoses of the mucous membranes are common.[3,4] Some affected foals have crusting miliary dermatitis, especially in the pectoral and groin regions.

PATHOGENESIS

Alloimmune disorders occur when a foal inherits antigenic determinants from the sire that are not present in the dam. If the dam is sensitized to these antigenic determinants, she will produce antibodies that are con-

centrated in colostrum. The foal ingests antibodies in colostrum that recognize epitopes on the surface of its cells. The result is destruction or damage of the targeted cells and tissues. The best described alloimmune disorder of horses is neonatal isoerythrolysis in which foals ingest colostral alloantibodies that destroy their erythrocytes (see Case 3-2).[5-7] Other alloimmune disorders documented or suggested in horses including alloimmune thrombocytopenia, neutropenia, and dermatologic disorders.[2-6,8]

Neonatal isoerythrolysis develops as a result of ingestion of alloantibodies against erythrocyte alloantigens, most commonly anti-Aa and anti-Qa. However, the specificity of antibodies causing other forms of alloimmune disease in horses has not been determined. In humans, platelet autoantibodies are most commonly directed against platelet glycoprotein (Gp) IIb-IIIa.[9] Mares have produced sequential foals with alloimmune thrombocytopenia even when bred to different stallions, suggesting that these mares lack an antigen that may be common among the horse population. When they become sensitized to the antigen, their foals are likely to experience this problem regardless of sire unless they receive colostrum from an alternative source.[3]

Foals may have isolated alloimmune thrombocytopenia, or the disorder may occur in conjunction with isoerythrolysis, neutropenia, or dermatitis.[2,3,10] '04 Diplomatic Immunity developed a common triad of clinical signs: ulcerative dermatitis, thrombocytopenia, and neutropenia.[3] Multiple alloimmune disorders may occur simultaneously because a mare has become sensitized to multiple antigens or because of sensitization to common epitopes present on multiple cell types. When antibodies attach to the surface of platelets and neutrophils, those platelets are removed from circulation by tissue mononuclear phagocytes. Skin lesions may develop because of an antibody specifically directed against epidermal or dermal antigens or secondary to immune complex deposition in the walls of small superficial blood vessels. The epidermal necrosis observed on biopsies of affected foals may be more consistent with the latter theory.[3] One report of skin lesions in a foal born to a mare with pemphigus foliatius suggests that antibodies against the mare's transmembrane proteins (desmoglein1) can also pass into the colostrum and result in similar lesions in her foal. These lesions in the foal were not present at birth and resolved without treatment in three to four weeks. This coincides with the normal fall in maternal antibodies in the foal.

The initial diagnostic evaluation of '04 Diplomatic Immunity included a CBC, serum biochemical profile, coagulation profile, arterial blood gas analysis, blood culture, and thoracic and abdominal ultrasound. The CBC revealed neutropenia (1,768/μl) with a regenerative left shift (780/μl), lymphopenia (546/μl), and profound thrombocytopenia (no platelets observed). The PCV was 31% with a total plasma protein concentration of 5.8 g/dl and a fibrinogen concentration of 100 mg/dl. The serum biochemical profile and arterial blood gas analysis were unremarkable. The prothrombin time and partial thromboplastin time were within normal limits, and fibrin degradation products (FDPs) were >40 μg/ml. Thoracic and abdominal ultrasounds were unremarkable. Serum samples for antibody titers to equine arteritis virus were submitted.

DIAGNOSTIC TESTS

The general diagnostic approach for a lethargic, depressed, inappetant neonatal foal is meant to rapidly assess the likelihood of several important differential diagnoses. The major differentials for a foal with these clinical signs at two to four days of age include sepsis, neonatal hypoxic ischemic encephalopathy, ruptured bladder, neonatal isoerythrolysis, and intestinal or abdominal disorders. Petechial and ecchymotic hemorrhages indicate a defect in primary hemostasis due to thrombocytopenia, platelet dysfunction, or vasculitis. The most important differential diagnoses to be considered for these problems are alloimmune thrombocytopenia, sepsis, and acute viral infection (equine herpesvirus or equine arteritis virus). Sepsis may result in thrombocytopenia and/or vasculitis because of widespread activation of inflammatory mediators and the coagulation cascade.[11,12] Other differential diagnoses for thrombocytopenia in foals include bone marrow disorders or pseudothrombocytopenia due to clumping of platelets that may occur when blood is analyzed using EDTA as an anticoagulant.[13] True thrombocytopenia is confirmed by determining platelet count using sodium citrate as an anticoagulant.

Initial evaluation of a depressed, lethargic, inappetant foal with petechial hemorrhages should include appropriate tests for assessment and diagnosis of sepsis (see Chapter 5) such as a CBC with plasma fibrinogen concentration, serum biochemical profile, blood electrolyte concentrations, arterial blood gas analysis, and blood culture. Determination of prothrombin time (PT) and activated partial thromboplastin time (APTT) will aid in the differentiation of foals with alloimmune thrombocytopenia and those with disseminated intravascular coagulation (DIC) secondary to sepsis.

Diagnostic tests that may aid in determining whether or not the bone marrow is increasing platelet production in response to increased destruction include mean platelet volume (MPV), flow cytometric analysis to detect thiazole orange positive (reticulated) platelets,

and bone marrow aspirate or biopsy.[14-17] MPV tends to increase during a platelet regenerative response, but the sensitivity of these results is questionable. With increased demand for replacement platelets, reticulated platelets are released from bone marrow in increased numbers and detection of reticulated platelets is probably more sensitive as an indicator of bone marrow platelet regenerative responses than MPV; however, flow cytometric assay is not readily available.[15] Bone marrow aspirates or biopsies are easy to obtain in foals and provide information regarding the ability of the bone marrow to produce platelets, but they do not indicate a specific diagnosis.[14]

The platelet factor 3 test has been recommended as an indicator of platelet surface damage that occurs commonly with immune-mediated destruction, however this test is nonspecific and is not widely available.

Flow cytometric analysis to detect immunoglobulin on the surface of platelets is probably the most specific diagnostic test available for immune-mediated thrombocytopenia in horses.[18-21] The sensitivity and specificity of this type of test has not been determined in foals with alloimmune thrombocytopenia. An immunoradiometric assay for detection of equine platelet-associated and platelet-bindable immunoglobulin has been used to confirm a diagnosis of neonatal alloimmune thrombocytopenia in a Quarter Horse foal.[4] However, this test is also not widely available. Because of the lack of availability for specific tests to detect antibody on the surface of platelets, a diagnosis of alloimmune thrombocytopenia is suggested in foals with a very low platelet count (<20,000/μl), no laboratory evidence of DIC, and bone marrow evidence of appropriate platelet production.

The initial treatment plan for '04 Diplomatic Immunity included maintenance fluid support, enteral nutrition, and broad-spectrum bactericidal antimicrobials. She began struggling and appeared somewhat disoriented and was sedated with 10 mg diazepam IV. To treat the suspected alloimmune thrombocytopenia, '04 Diplomatic Immunity received 3 mg dexamethasone IV (0.07 mg/kg). The next morning she was bright, alert, and eager to suckle. Her platelet count was 3,000/μl. Four units of platelet-rich plasma from a compatible donor were administered. Intravenous fluid therapy was discontinued, and the nasogastric tube was removed. On day two, '04 Diplomatic Immunity's platelet count was 11,000/μl and a bone marrow aspirate and skin and gingival biopsies were obtained. The platelet count decreased to 3,000/μl with a neutrophil count of 1,150/μl on day three. Four additional units of platelet-rich plasma were administered. She also received 300 μg recombinant granulocyte colony stimulating-factor subcutaneously. The next day the foal's neutrophil count was 24,000/μl, and platelet count was 6,000/μl.

The bone marrow aspirate revealed the presence of all cell lines. Blood culture results were negative. Serum titers to equine arteritis virus were 1:512 in both the mare and the foal, consistent with previous vaccination of the mare and colostral immunoglobulin absorption by the foal. Daily or every other day treatment with dexamethasone at 0.02 mg/kg was initiated; the dose was adjusted to maintain a platelet count of >10,000/μl. Gingival biopsies revealed neutrophilic ulcerative gingivitis with marked granulation tissue formation. Skin biopsies revealed multifocal, acute, neutrophilic, ulcerative epidermitis and lymphoplasmacytic perivascular dermatitis. Special stains demonstrated excessive IgG deposition in the epidermis and at the basement membranes, particularly around adnexal structures.

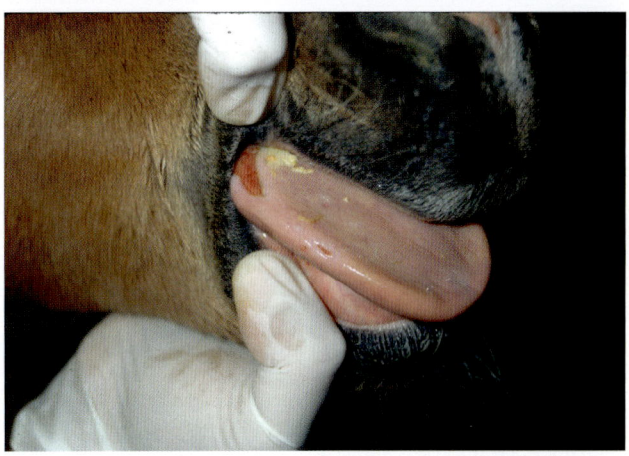

Fig. 3-15 Oral ulcer caused by candidiasis associated with suppression of the foal's immune system with corticosteroids.

TREATMENT

Treatment of foals with alloimmune thrombocytopenia is largely supportive including provision of appropriate nutritional and fluid support, antimicrobial therapy if concurrent sepsis is suspected, and nursing care. Foals should be maintained in a safe environment to minimize risk of trauma and associated hemorrhage. Platelet-rich plasma transfusions may be helpful in profoundly thrombocytopenic foals with evidence of bleeding. If platelet-rich plasma is not available, whole-blood transfusions may be administered. The therapeutic goal for transfusion is to increase the platelet count to a minimal level to provide adequate hemostasis. In most foals, this is possible if platelet count is maintained above 20,000 to 30,000/μl.[16]

Corticosteroid therapy results in rapid increases in platelet counts in foals with alloimmune thrombocytopenia,[3] presumably by inhibiting destruction of antibody-coated platelets by tissue mononuclear phagocytes. However, these drugs should be used with caution in young foals because of the immune suppression associated with prolonged or high doses. Foals are particularly susceptible to infectious diseases because of their naive immune system. Suppression of immune responses in foals with corticosteroid therapy has been associated with candidiasis, cryptosporidiosis, and other infectious complications (Figure 3-15). The therapeutic goal should be to maintain a platelet count high enough to provide adequate hemostasis rather than to increase the count to normal levels. Many affected foals will not require any corticosteroid therapy.

If concurrent profound neutropenia is present in foals with alloimmune thrombocytopenia, administration of recombinant granulocyte colony-stimulating factor (G-CSF) may be considered. In one foal in which this drug was used, the neutrophil count increased from 1800 to 20,254/μl within 24 hours.[3] There was minimal change in the platelet count during the same time period (3,000 to 6,000/μl). These results are similar to descriptions of response to G-CSF in normal foals.[22]

'04 Diplomatic Immunity was treated with corticosteroids as needed to maintain a platelet count of >10,000/μl. After two weeks, corticosteroid therapy was no longer needed. Platelet counts returned to normal by the time the foal was three to four weeks of age. No additional problems were encountered after '04 Diplomatic Immunity was discharged from the hospital. She was reported to grow and develop normally.

'04 Diplomatic Immunity's dam was bred back that spring to a different stallion. The foal born a year later in spring presented at three days of age with clinical signs identical to those of '04 Diplomatic Immunity. The diagnosis was alloimmune thrombocytopenia, neutropenia, and dermatitis. The following year, the mare's foal was not permitted to suckle her colostrum. That foal received colostrum from another mare on the farm and remained healthy.

OUTCOME AND PREVENTION

Prognosis for foals with alloimmune thrombocytopenia is good if they receive appropriate supportive care.[3,4] The dams of affected foals are at increased risk of producing subsequent foals with similar problems. Breeding to a different stallion is not sufficient to decrease risk of disease in future foals.[3] Owners should be advised to restrict the access of these foals to colostrum from this mare. Colostrum from another mare or a suitable colostrum substitute should be provided.

REFERENCES

1. Ramirez S, Gaunt SD, McClure JJ et al: Detection and effects on platelet function of anti-platelet antibody in mule foals with experimentally induced neonatal alloimmune thrombocytopenia, *J Vet Intern Med* 13:534, 1999.
2. Traub-Dargatz JL, McClure JJ, Koch C et al: Neonatal isoerythrolysis in mule foals, *J Am Vet Med Assoc* 206:67, 1995.
3. Perkins GA, Miller WH, Divers TJ et al: Ulcerative dermatitis, thrombocytopenia and neutropenia in neonatal foals, *J Vet Intern Med* 19:211, 2005.
4. Buechner-Maxwell V, Scott MA, Godber L et al: Neonatal alloimmune thrombocytopenia in a quarter horse foal, *J Vet Intern Med* 11:304, 1997.
5. McClure JJ, Koch C, Traub-Dargatz J: Characterization of a red blood cell antigen in donkeys and mules associated with neonatal isoerythrolysis, *Anim Genet* 25:119, 1994.
6. Becht JL, Semrad SD: Hematology, blood typing, and immunology of the neonatal foal, *Vet Clin North Am Equine Pract* 1:91, 1985.
7. Bailey E: Prevalence of anti–red blood cell antibodies in the serum and colostrum of mares and its relationship to neonatal isoerythrolysis, *Am J Vet Res* 43:1917, 1982.
8. Davis EG, Rush B, Bain F et al: Neonatal neutropenia in an Arabian foal, *Equine Vet J* 35:517, 2003.
9. George JN, el-Harake MA, Raskob GE: Chronic idiopathic thrombocytopenic purpura, *N Engl J Med* 331:1207, 1994.
10. Sockett DC, Traub-Dargatz J, Weiser MG: Immune-mediated hemolytic anemia and thrombocytopenia in a foal, *J Am Vet Med Assoc* 190:308, 1987.
11. Bentz AI, Wilkins PA, MacGillivray KC et al: Severe thrombocytopenia in 2 thoroughbred foals with sepsis and neonatal encephalopathy, *J Vet Intern Med* 16:494, 2002.
12. Barton MH, Morris DD, Crowe N et al: Hemostatic indices in healthy foals from birth to one month of age, *J Vet Diagn Invest* 7:380, 1995.
13. Hinchcliff KW, Kociba GJ, Mitten LA: Diagnosis of EDTA-dependent pseudothrombocytopenia in a horse, *J Am Vet Med Assoc* 203:1715, 1993.
14. Russell KE, Sellon DC, Grindem CB: Bone marrow in horses: Indications, sample handling, and complications, *Comp Cont Educ Pract Vet* 16:1359, 1994.
15. Russell KE, Perkins PC, Grindem CB et al: Flow cytometric method for detecting thiazole orange-positive (reticulated) platelets in thrombocytopenic horses, *Am J Vet Res* 58:1092, 1997.
16. Sellon DC, Grindem CB: Quantitative platelet abnormalities in horses, *Comp Cont Educ Pract Vet* 16:1335, 1994.
17. Sullivan PS, Manning KL, McDonald TP: Association of mean platelet volume and bone marrow megakaryocytopoiesis in thrombocytopenic dogs: 60 cases (1984-1993), *J Am Vet Med Assoc* 206:332, 1995.
18. Davis EG, Wilkerson MJ, Rush BR: Flow cytometry: Clinical applications in equine medicine, *J Vet Intern Med* 16:404, 2002.
19. McGurrin MK, Arroyo LG, Bienzle D: Flow cytometric detection of platelet-bound antibody in three horses with immune-mediated thrombocytopenia, *J Am Vet Med Assoc* 224:83, 2004.
20. Clabough DL, Gebhard D, Flaherty MT et al: Immune-mediated thrombocytopenia in horses infected with equine infectious anemia virus, *J Virol* 65:6242, 1991.
21. Nunez R, Gomes-Keller MA, Schwarzwald C et al: Assessment of equine autoimmune thrombocytopenia (EAT) by flow cytometry, *BMC Blood Disord* 1:1, 2001.
22. Zinkl JG, Madigan JE, Fridmann DM et al: Haematological, bone marrow and clinical chemical changes in neonatal foals given canine recombinant granulocyte-colony stimulating factor, *Equine Vet J* 26:313, 1994.

4 Neonatal Nutrition

| Case 4-1 | Normal Foal Nutritional Needs | Virginia Ann Buechner-Maxwell and Craig D. Thatcher |

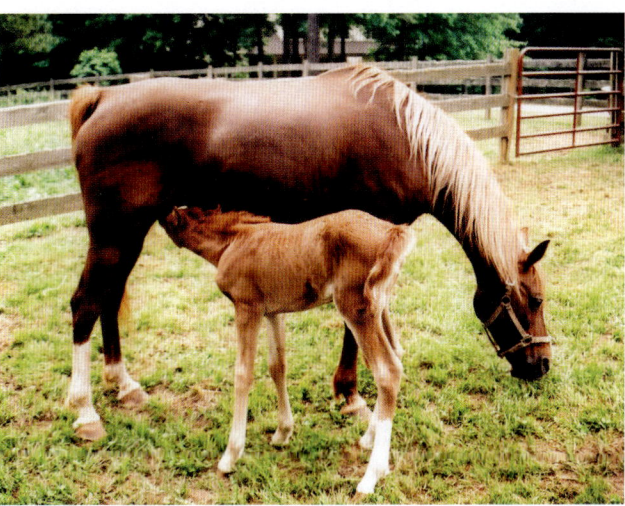

Fig. 4-1 Honeysuckle and newborn foal.

Honeysuckle, an 18-year-old Arabian mare, gave birth to a filly foal, which was now 19 hours old. The mare had been hospitalized 18 months earlier and treated for malacic keritoconjunctivitis, acute tubular necrosis, gastric ulceration, and protein-loosing enteropathy secondary to right dorsal colitis. The mare had required hospitalization for two weeks, and continued treatment and monitoring as an outpatient for an additional three months. During this period, the mare's problems resolved and, by the owner's assessment, her body weight returned to normal (body condition score of 5 out of 9). Because of the owner's attachment to Honeysuckle and the near loss of the mare due to her previous condition, the owner elected to breed her. While the mare had produced foals in the past, she had not been used as a brood mare since the time of purchase by the present owner. Honeysuckle's owner had raised weanlings in the past, but had no experience raising a foal from birth to weaning.

The foaling was attended, and no complications were observed. At the time of her examination, '03 Honeysuckle was standing, active, and had a bright attitude (Figure 4-1). The owner observed the foal initiated suckling when she was approximately $1\frac{1}{2}$ hours old, and since then, she nursed several times per hour. The owner also observed her pass feces within the last hour and urinate at least once since birth.

On physical examination, the foal's heart rate was 120 beats per minute, respiratory rate was 24 breaths per minute, and a body temperature was 100.4°F. All other examination parameters were within normal limits. The mare was also examined and no problems were identified. Her udder was well developed, and contained milk. The foal was observed while suckling the udder and had no difficulty acquiring and swallowing milk. After finishing, the udder was noticeably smaller and less distended, and the foal's appetite appeared sated.

Since the owner's experience with young horses did not include neonatal and nursing foals, she requested advice on the feeding behavior and diet of foals in this age group.

NUTRITIONAL REQUIREMENTS OF THE NORMAL FOAL

The National Research Council's *Nutrient Requirements of Horses* does not provide specific advice on feeding foals less than three months of age, and information for this age group is sparse.[1] Some indication of a young foal's requirements has been derived by observation of the normal feeding behavior, determination of milk consumption, and evaluation of milk composition.

The high metabolic needs of the foal are met through frequent feedings. Carson and Wood-Gush reported

Table 4-1	Mean Number of Attempted and Successful Nursing Bouts, and Duration of Bouts[2]		
Foal Age	**Attempted Bouts/Hour**	**Successful Bouts/Hour**	**Duration of Bouts (Seconds)**
1–7 days	7	5	140
8–14 days barn	4	3	131
8–14 days pasture	4	4	83

observations of stabled and pastured mares and foals, and measured the number of successful nursing bouts demonstrated by foals at various ages.[2] They defined a nursing "bout" as "a period of nursing activity delimited by intervals of non-nursing activity lasting for 27 seconds or longer." Within nursing bouts, activity was divided into suckling, nosing, and interval behavior, which indicated periods of less than 27 seconds when foals were neither suckling nor nosing. Their findings regarding foal nursing behavior are summarized in Table 4-1.

This study also indicated that normal foals successfully suckled each teat an equal number of times. Observations of mare-foal interaction indicated that during the first week of the foal's life the mares assisted the foals in finding the teat by shifting to positions that increased accessibly. For the following one to two weeks, the mares demonstrated more resistant behavior resulting in early termination of foal nursing. After this period, the mares became more cooperative until approximately 16 weeks postpartum. From 16 to 24 weeks, termination of the nursing sessions again became increasingly frequent.[2]

Light-breed mares produce approximately 3% of their body weight in milk/day for the first 3 months of lactations (12 to 13 liters for a 450-kg mare).[3] Using a double isotope dilution or radio-labeled water $(3H_2O)$ technique, studies have shown that 11-day-old foals consume as much as 27% of their body weight in the form of milk (12 liters for a 45-kg foal).[3,4] Mare's milk contains a caloric value of approximately 480-600 kcal/l. This amount of milk provides a mean of 159 kcal/kg/day gross energy and 7.2 g crude protein/kg/day.[4] The volume decreases to 19.3% (98 kcal/kg/day gross energy and 3.7 grams crude protein/kg/day) by the time the foal reaches 39 days of age.[3] This information demonstrates the significant energy requirements of the growing foal, and the rapid rate at which nutritional requirements change over the foal's first six weeks of life.

Detailed information regarding the composition of mare's milk has been reported elsewhere.[3,4] Equine milk is low in energy and high in water content as compared to cow's and goat's milk, and contains less fat, protein, and total solids, and more lactose.[5] The composition of mare's milk also changes over time. Initially, there is a decrease in milk total solids and protein composition from days 11 to 25.[3,6-14] Some studies also report a decline in fat content during this period, although this has not been a consistent finding.[3,6,7,10-12] The change in milk during the first three weeks postpartum is attributed a gradual change from colostrum to mature milk. Once mares reach mid-lactation (day 20 to 65 postpartum), milk composition is less changeable.[3] A comparison of published results suggests that, as fed, total solids (10.4% to 11.2%) and sugar content (6.0% to 6.9%) of milk do not change significantly between 21 and 60 days after birth.[15] Crude protein content declines minimally, and crude fat content does not follow a trend.[3] A significant animal effect (variation from animal to animal) in all contents of milk is also observed, with the exception of crude protein (whole-milk basis) and sugar (dry-matter basis).[3] These findings complicate efforts to describe the nutritional needs of the neonatal foal based upon the diet that they normally consume, since the diets of the normal foal change rapidly throughout pre-weaning life and vary significantly from individual to individual.

Management of neonatal nutrition begins before birth. Feeding management of the broodmare has been described elsewhere, and major points will be briefly highlighted here.[1,16-19] The mare's nutritional needs increase during the last three months of pregnancy and continue to increase during the first three months of lactation.[1] While supplementing adequately fed mares does not significantly improve foal growth, restricting mare's feed during lactation compromises foal growth.[20]

Indirect evidence from epidemiological and animal studies indicates that failure to meet nutritional requirements for the pregnant woman results in prenatal growth retardation and an increased risk of the child developing coronary heart disease, hypertension, and type 2 diabetes later in life.[21-24] This outcome is due to interruptions in the immediate growth pattern of tissue, resulting in a long-term effect on somatic cell programming, growth, and development.

The nutrient composition of milk may also be affected by the mare's diet. Mares fed a calcium-deficient diet before parturition and during lactation produced foals that were born with thinner and mechanically weaker bones as compared to foals from mares fed an adequate diet. This difference persisted for 40 weeks after parturition.[25] In contrast, neonatal goiter has been associated with excessive supplementation of pregnant mares with dietary iodine.[26,27] These examples support the need to pay close attention to the broodmare's diet during pregnancy and lactation to ensure the foal is receiving optimal nutrition *in utero* as well as after birth.

GASTROINTESTINAL DEVELOPMENT IN THE FOAL

At birth, lactase is the primary disaccharidase in the equine small intestine. This makes sense as the primary energy source in mare's milk will be lactose. As the foal matures, maltase activity increases until it is equal to the lactose activity at three to four months of age. Maltase is the predominant disaccharidase in the mature small intestine.[28] Also, during the first few months of life there is a significant increase in length and diameter of the foal's small intestine. By five to six months of age, the foal begins to mimic the adult feeding pattern of grazing, and it will begin to develop the large colon and cecum.[29]

Several days later, the owner observed the foal eating the mare's feces. The foal was also observed eating her dam's hay. The owner was concerned that this behavior was a sign that the foal was not getting enough to eat. She asked for methods of assessing the adequacy of the foal's diet.

COPROPHAGY

Coprophagy by foals is considered normal behavior and does not indicate inadequate nutrient availability (Figure 4-2). This behavior was initially described in the literature in 1954.[30]

More recent studies indicate that foals engage in coprophagy as early as the first week of life, and that this behavior is most frequently observed during the first two months.[31] The most common source of the feces is the mare, although feces from other adult horses may also be consumed.

While it is not known why foals participate in this behavior, several theories have been proposed. Crowell-Davis and Houpt predicted that pheromones in the feces signaled consumption by the foal, while Francis-Smith and Wood-Gush suggested that coprophagy provided gut flora and vitamins to the foal.[31,32] Foals are

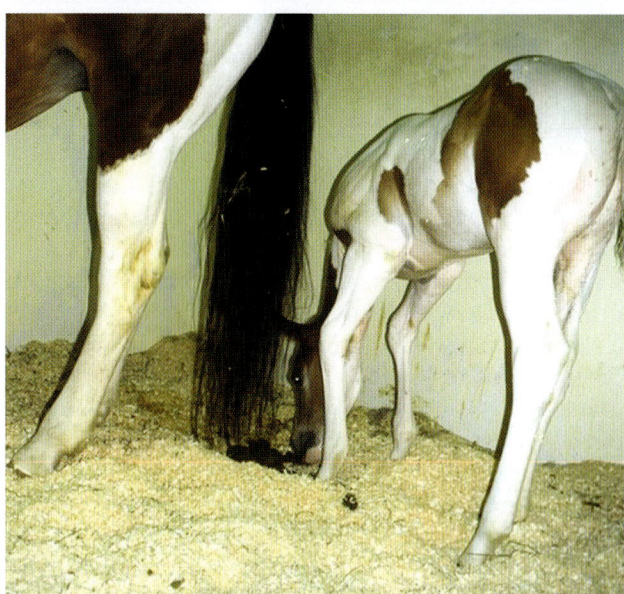

Fig. 4-2 Coprophagy is normal in young foals and is not considered an indicator of inadequate nutrition.

reported to be deficient in deoxycholic acid, and these researchers further hypothesized that the mare's feces served as a source of this nutrient. Deoxycholic acid contributes to gut immunocompetence and myelination of the nervous system, and may protect foals from developing gastrointestinal diseases like necrotizing enterocolitis. Consequently, coprophagy should not be discouraged in the neonatal foal.

ADEQUACY OF THE FOAL'S DIET

In the normal situation, the mare's milk provides all the necessary components of adequate nutrition. The foal that does not have access to milk is readily identifiable because of the rapid deterioration in its clinical status over the first 12 to 24 hours of life. Foals that are receiving less than adequate amounts of milk can be more difficult to identify. On a day-to-day basis, determining the amount of nutrition that foals receive is based upon indirect evidence that includes foal behavior, frequency of defecation and urination, weight gain, and body condition.

Foals that receive adequate nutrition typically display distinct periods of nursing and rest. Based upon the results previously discussed, one-week-old foals should latch on and suckle for about $1\frac{1}{2}$ minutes, five to seven times per hour. Foals that are not receiving adequate nutrition may attempt to suckle more frequently, and will often display agitation in between attempts. Foals may also be more aggressive toward the mare, with frequent bouts of bunting the udder, stamping, and tail flagging. The mare may respond by interrupting the foal's attempts to suckle and maneuvering in such a way to keep the foal away from the udder. These signs alone do not support inadequate nutrition, but signal the need for further investigation.

Normal foals are reported to produce 148 ml/kg/day of urine, which is approximately 10 times that of the adult horse on a per-body weight basis.[33,34] As a result, foals urinate nearly every hour. Less-frequent urination may be an indication that milk intake is restricted, especially if the foal does not have free choice access to water.

Foals begin to pass meconium within six hours of birth, and complete passage by 24 hours. Meconium evacuation is stimulated by ingestion of colostrum.[35] After meconium is passed, defecation occurs several times per day. Normal foal feces is tan in color, formed, and somewhat pasty. Although there are many reasons for foals to decrease their fecal production and/or demonstrate a change in fecal consistency, inadequate milk ingestion should be considered as a possible cause.

At birth, foals should be about 11% of their mature body weight.[36] Young, healthy foals experience rapid weight gain and growth when receiving appropriate nutrition. Neonatal foals are reported to gain 1.3 to 1.5 kg/day during the first 30 days of life.[4,37] Thoroughbred foals attain about 83% of their total body height and approximately 46% of their body weight by six months of age, doubling their weight in the first month. Restricting mare's feed during lactation diminishes milk production and compromises foals growth.[20] To detect subclinical malnutrition, the foal's height and weight should be measured every week and compared to published normal growth charts for foals of similar size and breed.[15]

BODY CONDITION SCORING

Methods for evaluating the foal's body condition have been reported. Evaluation on a weekly basis permits identification of foals that may be receiving less than adequate nutrition.[38] Foals are rarely born fat, so one can use the lower 1-5 body scores of the 1-9 Henneke Body Condition Scoring System[39] (Table 4-2, Figures 4-3, 4-4, and 4-5). Reasons for poor body condition in a foal can be divided into prepartum and postpartum causes (Table 4-3). Prepartum causes include prematurity, placental insufficiency (IRGR), twinning, and poor maternal body condition. Postpartum causes may include catabolism from a systemic illness, malabsorption/maldigestion secondary to lactase deficiency or diarrhea, agalactia in the mare, compromised ability to suckle or chew, and foal rejection.

Table 4-2	Assigning a Body Condition Score to a Young Foal[39]
Score	**Description**
1	Extremely emaciated: spinous processes, ribs, tuber coxae, tailhead, and tuber ischii very prominent; shoulder and neck structures evident (Figure 4-3)
2	Emaciated: Slight fat covering the base of the spinous processes; slightly rounded feel to traverse processes and ribs; shoulder and neck structures barely noticeable
3	Thin: Fat buildup midway down traverse processes; slight fat over ribs; individual vertebrae not discernible (Figure 4-4)
4	Moderately thin: Slight ridge along back; faint outline to ribs; fat can be felt over tailhead and withers; shoulder and neck structures not thin
5	Moderate or normal: Back flat; ribs not visible but easily palpated; fat around tailhead feels spongy, withers rounded over the spinous process; shoulder and neck structures blend well into body (Figure 4-5)

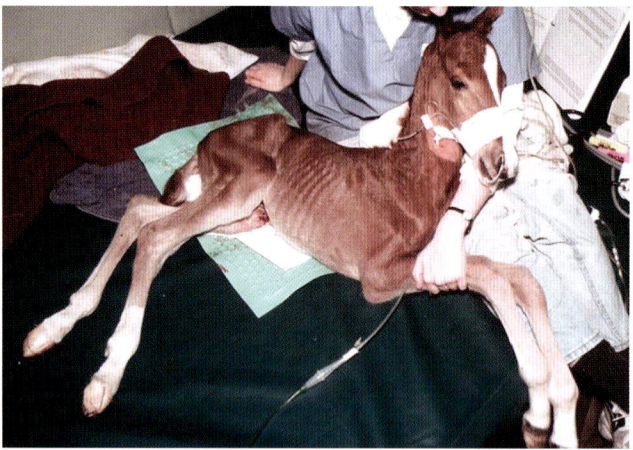

Fig. 4-3 Body score of 1.

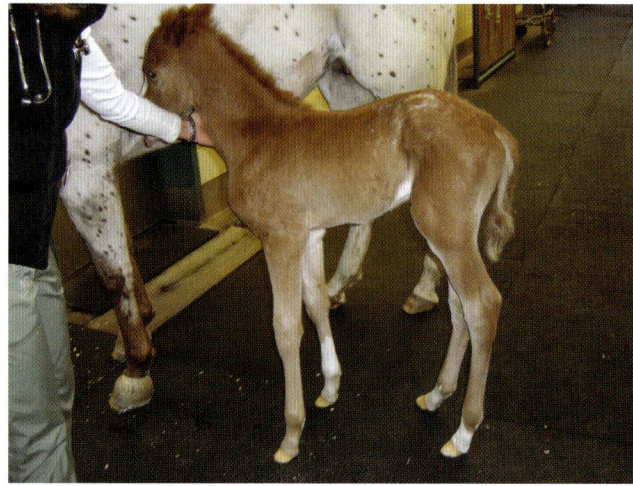

Fig. 4-4 Body score of 3.

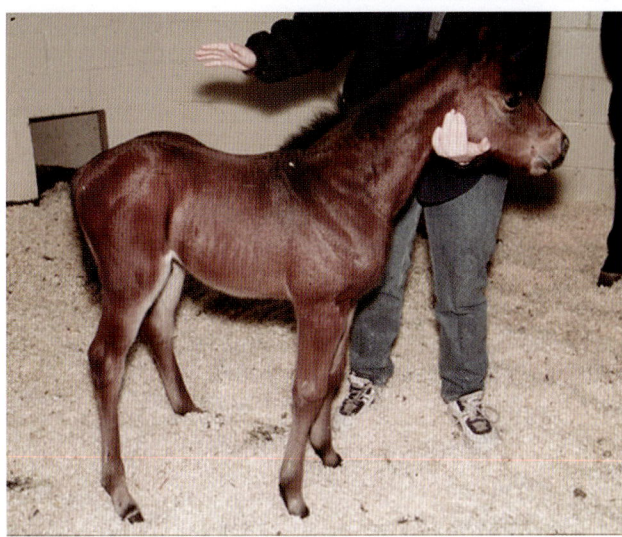

Fig. 4-5 Body score of 5.

Table 4-3	Reasons for Poor Body Score in Foals	
Prepartum Causes	**Postpartum Causes**	
Prematurity	Agalactia in the mare	
Twinning	Foal rejection by the mare	
Placental insufficiency (IUGR)	Anorexia secondary to disease	
	Malabsorption/maldigestion	
	Compromised ability to suckle or chew	

Several days later, '03 Honeysuckle's owner called to report that both the mare and foal were thriving. The foal continued to nurse vigorously and gained weight daily.

REFERENCES

1. National Research Council: *Nutrient requirements of horses,* ed 5, Washington DC, 1989, National Academy of Sciences.
2. Carson K, Wood-Gush DG: Behaviour of thoroughbred foals during nursing, *Equine Vet J* 15:257, 1983.
3. Oftedal OT, Hintz HF, Schryver HF: Lactation in the horse: Milk composition and intake by foals, *J Nutr* 113:2096, 1983.
4. Martin RG, McMeniman NP, Dowsett KF: Milk and water intakes of foals sucking grazing mares, *Equine Vet J* 24:295, 1992.
5. Koterba AM: Chapter 34: Nutritional support: Enteral feeding. In Koterba AM, Drummond WH, Kosch PC, eds: *Equine Clinical Neonatology,* Philadelphia, 1990, Lea & Febiger.
6. Linton R: The composition of mare's milk, *J Agric Sci* 21:669, 1931.
7. Linton R: The composition of mare's milk II, *J Dairy Res* 8:143, 1937.
8. Holmes A, McKey B, Wertz A et al: The vitamin content of mare's milk, *J Dairy Sci* 29:163, 1946.
9. Holmes A, Spelman A, Smith C et al: Composition of mare's milk as compared with that of other species, *J Dairy Sci* 30:385, 1947.
10. Flade E: Milchleistung und Milchqualitat bei Stuten, *Arch Tierz* 9:381, 1955.
11. Ullrey DE, Struthers RD, Hendricks DG et al: Composition of mare's milk, *J Anim Sci* 25:217, 1966.
12. Johnston RH, Kamstra LD, Kohler PH: Mares' milk composition as related to "foal heat" scours, *J Anim Sci* 31:549, 1970.
13. Balbierz H, Nikolajczuk M, Poliwoda A et al: Studies on colostrum whey and milk proteins in mares during suckling period, *Pol Arch Weter* 18:455, 1975.
14. Bouwman H, van der Schee W: Composition and production of milk from Dutch warmblood saddle horse mares, *Z Tierphysiol Tierernaehr Futtermittelkd* 40:39, 1978.
15. Lewis LD: *Growing horse feeding and care,* Media, PA, 1995, Williams & Wilkins.
16. Donoghue S, Meacham TN, Kronfeld DS: A conceptual approach to optimal nutrition of brood mares, *Vet Clin North Am Equine Pract* 6:373, 1990.
17. Pugh D, Williams W: Feeding foals from birth to weaning, *Compend Contin Educ Pract Vet* 14:526, 1992.
18. Pugh DG, Schumacher J: Feeding and nutrition of brood mares, *Compend Contin Educ Pract Vet* 15:106, 1993.
19. Lewis LD: *Broodmare feeding and care,* Media, PA, 1995, Williams & Wilkins.
20. Banach MA, Evans JW, Blacksburg, VA, 1981, Virginia Polytechnic Institute.
21. Barker DJ: Fetal origins of coronary heart disease, *BMJ* 311:171, 1995.
22. Osmond C, Barker DJ: Fetal, infant, and childhood growth are predictors of coronary heart disease, diabetes, and hypertension in adult men and women, *Environ Health Perspect* 108 Suppl 3:545, 2000.
23. Schwarzenberg SJ, Kovacs A: Metabolic effects of infection and postnatal steroids, *Clin Perinatol* 29:295, 2002.
24. Dusick AM, Poindexter BB, Ehrenkranz RA et al: Growth failure in the preterm infant: Can we catch up? *Semin Perinatol* 27:302, 2003.
25. Glade MJ: Effects of gestation, lactation, and maternal calcium intake on mechanical strength of equine bone, *J Am Coll Nutr* 12:372, 1993.
26. Drew B, Barber WP, Williams DG: The effect of excess dietary iodine on pregnant mares and foals, *Vet Rec* 97:93, 1975.
27. Eroksuz H, Eroksuz Y, Ozer H et al: Equine goiter associated with excess dietary iodine, *Vet Hum Toxicol* 46:147, 2004.
28. Roberts MC: The development and distribution of mucosal enzymes in the small intestine of the fetus and young foals, *J Reprod Fertil* (Suppl) 23:717-723, 1975.
29. Smyth GB: Effects of age, sex, and post mortem interval on intestinal lengths of horses during development, *Equine Vet J* 20:104-108, 1988.
30. Taylor EL: Grazing behavior and helmenthic disease, *Br J Anim Behav* 2:61, 1954.
31. Crowell-Davis SL, Houpt KA: Coprophagy by foals: Effect of age and possible functions, *Equine Vet J* 17:17, 1985.
32. Francis-Smith K, Wood-Gush DG: Coprophagia as seen in thoroughbred foals, *Equine Vet J* 9:155, 1977.
33. Brewer BD, Clement SF, Lotz WS et al: A comparison of inulin, para-aminohippuric acid, and endogenous creatinine clearances as measures of renal function in neonatal foals, *J Vet Intern Med* 4:301, 1990.
34. Brewer BD, Clement SF, Lotz WS et al: Renal clearance, urinary excretion of endogenous substances, and urinary diagnostic indices in healthy neonatal foals, *J Vet Intern Med* 5:28, 1991.
35. Koterba AM: Chapter 6: Physical Examination. In Koterba AM, ed: *Equine clinical neonatology,* Philadelphia, 1990, Lea & Febiger.
36. Wilson JH: Feeding considerations for neonatal foals, *Proc 24th Annu Conv AAEP* 33:823, 1987.
37. Hintz HF: Growth rate of horses, *Proc 24th Annu Conv AAEP* 455, 1978.
38. Paradis MR: Nutrition and indirect calorimetry in neonatal foals, *Proc. 19th ACVIM,* Denver, CO 19:245, 2001.
39. Henneke DR: A condition score pyslen for horses, *Equine Pract* 7:13-15, 1985.

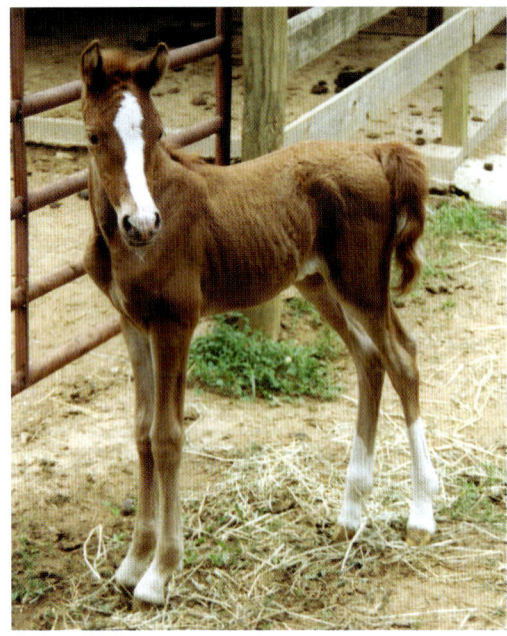

Fig. 4-6 '03 Lonely Heart, four-day-old orphan foal.

Mrs. Smith called to report that her mare, Lonely Heart, was found dead in the pasture next to her four-day-old foal. She wants to know how to provide nutrition to her now orphaned foal.

'03 Lonely Heart is a Quarter Horse filly that appears to be in good health (Figure 4-6). She has a body condition score of 5 on the Heneke system (1-9). She appears hungry and is attempting to suckle on any part of your body that she can. You discuss options of providing nutrition to this healthy foal with Mrs. Smith. These include the lease of a "nurse" mare; the use of another species, such as a goat, to rear the foal; and the use of mare's milk

replacers. You put forth the pros and cons associated with each choice (Table 4-4).

Foals may be orphaned if the mare dies, fails to lactate, or rejects the foal. There are several approaches to raising an orphaned foal. As stated, they include the use of nurse mares, nurse goats, and mare's milk replacers.

NURSE MARES

Nurse mares serve as foster dams and significantly decrease the work of raising orphaned foals. Nurse mares may be obtained from a commercial provider. A mare that has lost her foal may be used for this purpose. Most lactating mares will accept a foal, but the pair must be watched closely during the introductory phase of their interaction to avoid injury to the foal. Initially, the mare may require hobbles and a soft muzzle to prevent her from harming the foal. The least stressful method should be selected to introduce the foal to the mare. It is important that the mare not associate the foal's nursing with stress or pain.

Nurse mare chutes have been designed and are described elsewhere.[1] These chutes provide the advantage of permitting the foal to nurse with minimal restraint of the mare. Feeding the mare while the foal is nursing is also recommended. Mares accept foals by becoming familiar with their associated smell, sights, and sounds.[2] Most mares accept foals within 12 hours to 3 days, although rarely it may take as long as 10 days.[1]

Besides providing the most natural nutrition, nurse mares also provide psychological support for the

Table 4-4	Cost and Labor Comparison of Types of Feeding for the Orphan Foal		
Type of Feeding	"Nurse" Mare	"Nurse" Goat	Bucket Feeding with Milk Replacer
Labor intensity	Minimal	Moderate	Moderate to high depending upon product selected
Availability	May be limited in certain areas of the country	May be limited in availability	Available at most feed stores
Cost	$2000–$4000 for 3–4 months, plus feeding mare during that time period; lessee may be responsible for rebreeding the mare before return to lesser*	Variable; $75–$250	Approximately $850 for 90 days

*Prices reflect cost in northeast United States in 2005. Prices will vary as to location.

foal. Foals learn how to behave like horses from their dams.

NURSE GOAT

Nurse goats have also been used to assist in raising orphan foals. Larger-breed dairy goats (such as Nubians) provide the best candidates for this purpose.

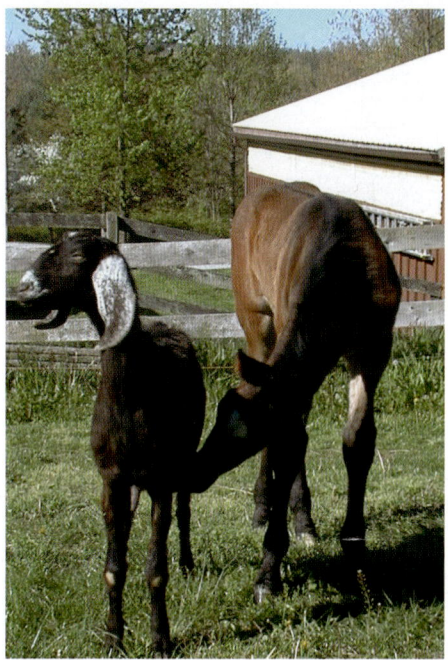

Fig. 4-7 A nurse goat can be used to raise foals. They provide milk and are often good companions.

Goats may be taught to stand on hay bales to provide better udder access to the foal.[3,4] However, even large foals can learn to position themselves to facilitate suckling. Orphan foals that are grafted on to goats should be introduced to creep feed (with milk pellets or grain mix, as described later) by two weeks of age or earlier, and should be provided access to free-choice water and hay. Alternatively, more than one goat may be provided to meet the foal's nutritional requirements.[3] Goat's milk is not a perfect match for mare's milk; it is higher in most nutrients such as fat, protein, and lactose and lower in water content. Poor weight gain and metabolic acidosis have been reported in neonatal foals that were fed 135 kcal/kg/day of goat's milk.[5] The goat's weight and the foal's growth (weight and height) should monitored closely to prevent development of poor body condition in either animal.

MILK REPLACERS

When a maternal substitute is unavailable, foals may be hand-reared. A number of commercial mare's milk replacers are available (Table 4-5). When selecting a milk replacer, it is important to obtain a product analysis sheet from the manufacturer. The milk replacer should closely match mare's milk in energy density (0.5 kcal/kg as feed), crude protein (22% dry matter), crude fat (15% dry matter), crude fiber (less than 0.2% dry matter), and total solids (11% as feed).[6,7] Replacers should also match the mineral and vitamin content of mare's milk as described by the National Research Council's *Nutrient Requirements of Horses.*[8]

	Milk			**Milk Replacers**		
Nutrient	Mare[b]	Cow	Goat	Mare's Match[c]	Foal-Lac[d]	Mare's Milk Plus[e]
Total solids[a] (DM): %	10.7	12.5	13.5	11–13	16	12.5
Crude protein: %	25	27	25	24	min 19.5	min 21
Crude fat: %	17	38	31	16	min 14	min 14
Crude fiber: %	0	0	0	0.15	max 0.1	max 0.15
Calcium: %	1.1	1.1	1.0	0.65–1.15	0.9–1.2	0.7–1.10
Phosphorus: %	0.7	0.7	0.8	0.6	min 0.75	min 0.65
Zinc: ppm	23	40	30	40	min 50	min 110
Copper: ppm	4	3	2	10	min 18	min 35
Selenium: ppm	0.04	0.024	—	0.3	0.10	min 0.3

Table 4-5 Comparison of Milk from Different Large Animal Species and Selected Milk Replacers

Buechner-Maxwell, VA, Nutritional Support for Neonatal Foals, Vet Clin Equine 21 (2005) 487-510.

[a]Values for total solids or dry matter are for the milk as fed or milk replacers diluted as recommended by the manufacturer. All other values are given for the amount in total solids or dry matter

[b]During the first four weeks of lactation

[c]Land O'Lakes, Arden Hills, MN

[d]Pet-Ag, Inc, Hampshire, IL

[e]Acidified Mare's Milk Replacer, Buckeye Nutrition, Dalton, OH

The carbohydrate source in the replacer milk should be checked. Some products use maltodextrins and corn syrup in addition to lactose. Because maltase levels are not high in the first month of life in the foal, these forms of carbohydrate may be undigestible. Undigested sugars may result in fermentation in the colon, increasing gas production and osmotic diarrhea.[9]

In a comparison of element concentrations in mare's milk versus commercial mare's milk replacement products by Rook and colleagues, most milk-replacement products meet or exceed the concentrations of calcium, iron, sulfur, potassium, sodium, copper, phosphorus, zinc, and magnesium.[10] The differences in these elements between the milk substitutes and mare's milk were not thought to be a problem except in a few medical conditions. In particular, high levels of potassium may be a problem in foals with hyperkalemic periodic paralysis or renal compromise. A scientific evaluation of the relationship between replacer formulation and foal performance has not been reported. Consequently, the effect of variations in milk replacer formula on the general health of the foal is not known.[10]

Milk replacers for lambs, kids, and calves are less expensive than those made for foals, but they are not designed to mimic the nutrition in mare's milk. Some of these products also contain antibiotics and should not be used for foals.

You discuss with Mrs. Smith the pros and cons of bottle feeding versus bucket feeding. She decides to train the foal to drink from a bucket. You leave a bag of mare's milk substitute with her and discuss how to mix it. You advise her to monitor the foal's intake and to be observant of the foal's manure production. A sudden change in diet for the foal and improper dilution of the milk substitute can result in diarrhea or constipation. You also advise her about beginning to introduce the foal to solid feed.

FEEDING METHODS AND SCHEDULE

Replacer can be provided in a bucket or bottle. Foals usually adjust to bottle feeding more rapidly than bucket feeding, but the latter is a more convenient method, and diminishes behavioral problems that may result from excessive interaction between orphaned foals and human caretakers.

Foals that have been nursing a mare or suckling from a bottle will need to be trained to drink from a bucket. To train a foal, allow it to become hungry by waiting to feed it for several hours. Place a damp finger in the foal's mouth and gently rub it between the tongue and the palate to stimulate a suckle response. Once the foal is suckling, gently guide its muzzle down to the milk. This process may need to be repeated multiple times

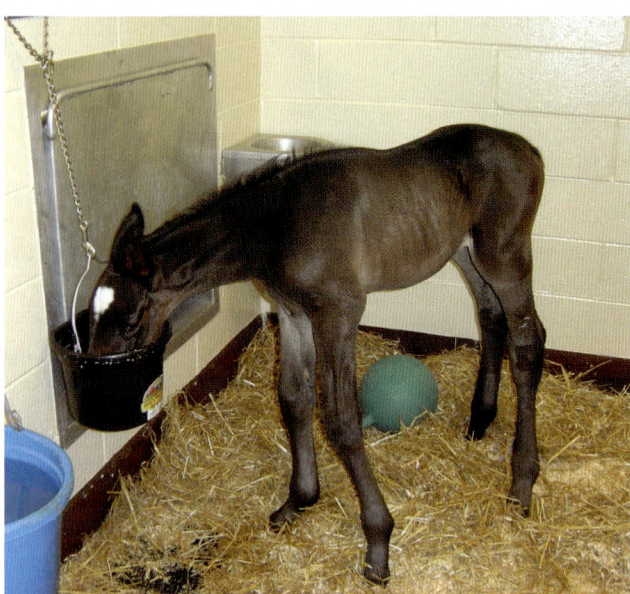

Fig. 4-8 Orphan foals readily adapt to bucket feeding.

to educate the foal to drink from the bucket. Teaching foals to drink from a bucket requires patience, and excessive force should not be used to position the foal's muzzle in the milk (Figure 4-8).

Turner reported that foals in their study took 10 to 120 minutes to learn how to bucket feed.[11] To facilitate the young foal's ability to identify the feed, light-colored buckets, preferably yellow (personal communication with Dr. Sarah Stoneham) should be used for the milk. Milk does not need to be warmed before feeding, and can be provided at room temperature.[12]

The healthy foal will consume 25% to 30% of its body weight in kilograms in mare's milk. The foal should be offered similar volumes of milk replacer if the product contains a caloric density (0.48 kcal digestible energy/ml) and nutritional composition (see Table 4-5) that closely mimics mare's milk. The amount of liters of milk that a foal ingests on a daily basis can be estimated by multiplying its body weight in kilograms by 0.25 to 0.30 to arrive at the number of liters/day that the foal needs to eat. This number is then divided by the number of feedings per day to arrive at the amount of milk needed per feeding.

The frequency that you offer milk to the orphan foal depends upon its age; the younger the foal, the more frequent the number of feedings. Normally, the foal will nurse from the dam five to seven times per hour during the first week of life. It becomes obvious that one can't meet this frequency by bucket feeding. Most normal foals do well with being fed every two to four hours by this method for the first week. As the foal becomes older, feedings can be spread to every six hours, then every eight hours.

Most manufactured products (excluding acidified milk replacer) must be made fresh and fed frequently.

The most convenient product for hand raising foals is acidified milk replacer (Buckeye Nutrition, Dalton, Ohio) and is especially useful when raising more than one orphan at a time. Acidified milk remains fresh for up to three days, but the manufacturer recommends discarding old milk, cleaning the feeding bucket, and providing fresh milk at least twice a day. This practice ensures that the milk and bucket remain sanitary, and allows the caretaker to access the foal's appetite on a regular basis.

A foal may be reluctant to consume acidified milk when it is first introduced, and foal's milk ingestion should be carefully monitored when the product is initially fed. When switching from one milk replacer to another, the change should be achieved gradually by initially mixing the old product with the new. If the foal is housed with other animals, the milk replacer should be placed in an area where access is limited to the foal, since adult horses and other animals may consume it. In addition to milk replacer, foals should have access to good-quality free-choice water.

Change in fecal consistency may occur when foals are fed milk replacers. If the product contains sugars other than lactose, the foal may develop diarrhea.[13] In addition, some milk replacers are more concentrated than mare's milk when mixed as per the manufacturer's recommendations, resulting in an increase in the percentage of total solids in the diet. The volume of water with which the replacer is reconstituted should be adjusted so that the final concentration of total solids is approximately 11% (similar to mare's milk). Making this adjustment will often resolve changes in fecal consistency associated with feeding milk replacer, but foals that experience these problems should be carefully monitored until their manure returns to a normal consistency and volume.

CREEP FEEDING

Creep feeding is the supplementation of a foal's diet with milk pellets and/or grain mix while they are receiving milk or milk replacer. Foals that are coupled with normal mares begin sampling the mare's feed as early as 10 days, but do not require creep feed until they approach four weeks of age because the amount of milk made by a normal mare is adequate to meet the foal's requirements for the first month of life.[4,12] In contrast, if the mare's milk production is inadequate or the foal is coupled with a single nurse goat, then creep feeding should be encouraged starting several days after birth.

Foals consuming milk replacer or requiring early weaning for other reasons should also be introduced to creep feed shortly after birth. Milk pellets are the feed of choice when introducing young foals (two to three days old) to creep feed. To stimulate the foal's interest in these pellets, a few should be placed in its mouth several times a day until the foal begins to eat unassisted. To facilitate the foal's acceptance, pellets should also be made available for free-choice consumption. Regardless of the amount the foal eats, the feeder should be emptied twice a day of any residual feed, cleaned, and refilled with fresh milk pellets. Once the foal is consuming 2 to 3 pounds of milk pellets per day, a good quality grain mix can be introduced.[12]

If the foal is not already familiar with eating creep feeds, grain mix must be introduced to the foal by placing small quantities in the foal's mouth several times per day. Grain mixes for pre-weaning foals should contain 16% crude protein, 0.9% calcium, and 0.6% phosphorus. Feeds for preweaning foals should also contain 60 ppm zinc, 50 ppm copper, 1365 IU/lb vitamin A, and 45 IU/lb vitamin E.[12] If the foal is already consuming milk pellets, small portions of the grain mix should be mixed with the pellets initially. Over four to six weeks, the proportion of milk pellets should be reduced while the quantity of grain mix is increased, until the pellets can be eliminated from the diet.

High-quality hay should also be made available for the foal. However, foals that consume large quantities of legume hay may develop diarrhea. This hay alone is not recommended, because the high protein and calcium content may contribute to problems such as developmental bone disease. Problems associated with feeding high-quality alfalfa hay alone can usually be avoided by mixing the alfalfa with high-quality grass hay. By eight weeks of age, the average foal should be consuming 4 to 6 lbs (1.8-2.7 kg) of creep feed per day, and can be gradually weaned off the milk replacer.[12]

'03 Lonely Heart learned to bucket feed quickly. She developed a bout of watery diarrhea that lasted for 48 hours after beginning the mare's milk replacement. Her owner decreased the concentration of the replacement by one half for a few days, and the diarrhea cleared up. The foal was seen to nibble on hay and milk pellets occasionally. Her owner was thrilled that the foal was thriving. She mentioned how cute the filly was when she was waiting for her food. The filly was charging her and bucking and kicking at her to hurry up the process!

Hand-raised orphan foals may bond to humans and actually express fear of other horses. Owners of these foals will often forget to discipline the foal for bad behavior. Bad behavior in a 50-kg foal may be cute, but it is dangerous in a 500-kg adult. Owners should be warned of this problem and encouraged to obtain an equine companion for the foal. A quiet pony or gelding may be a good choice. A slow introduction over a fence line is a good way to judge the suitability of the companion.

REFERENCES

1. O'Grady SE, Roberts L: A safe, simple way of bringing foals and "nurse mares" together, *Vet Med* 719, 1989.
2. Houpt KA: Equine maternal behavior and its aberrations, *Equine Pract* 1:7, 1979.
3. Wilson JH: Feeding considerations for neonatal foals, *Proc 24th Annu Conv AAEP* 33:823, 1987.
4. Pugh DG, Williams MA: Feeding foals from birth to weaning, *Compend Contin Educ Pract Vet* 14:526, 1992.
5. Wilson JH, Schneider CJ, Drummond WH et al: Metabolic acidosis in neonatal foals fed goat's milk, *Proceedings in the Second International Conference on Veterinary Perinatalogy* 62, 1990.
6. Koterba AM: Chapter 34: Nutritional support: Enteral feeding. In Koterba AM, Drummond WH, Kosch PC, eds: *Equine clinical neonatology*, Philadelphia, 1990, Lea & Febiger.
7. Vaala WE: Nutritional management of the critically ill neonate. In Robertson E, ed: *Current therapy in equine medicine*, ed 3, Philadelphia, 1992, WB Saunders.
8. National Research Council: *Nutrient requirements of horses*, ed 5, Washington DC, 1989, National Academy of Sciences.
9. Rooney DK: Clinical nutrition. In Reed SM, Bayly WM, eds: *Equine internal medicine*, ed 1, Philadelphia, 1998, WB Saunders.
10. Rook JS, Braselton WE, Lloyd JW et al: Comparison of element concentrations in Arabian mare's milk and commercial mare's milk replacement products, *Vet Clin Nutr* 6:17-21, 1999.
11. Turner AF: Managing mares and neonatal foals, *Vet Med* 83:502, 1988.
12. Lewis LD: *Growing horse feeding and care*, Media, PA, 1995, Williams & Wilkins.
13. Roberts MC: The development and distribution of mucosal enzymes in the small intestine of the fetus and young foals, *J Reprod Fertil* Suppl 23:717, 1975.

Case 4-3	Feeding the Foal That Needs Enteral and Parenteral Nutrition
	Virginia Ann Buechner-Maxwell and Craig D. Thatcher

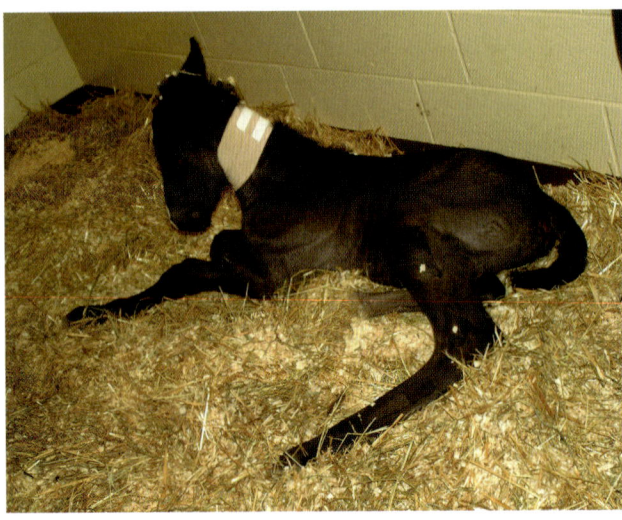

Fig. 4-9 '03 RunninOnEmpty presented to the emergency care unit at approximately 5 hours of age.

Approximately two weeks prior to her anticipated foaling date, RunninOnEmpty, a maiden five-year-old Thoroughbred mare, gave birth to a filly foal after 321 days gestation. The foaling was attended by the owners and was uncomplicated. The placenta passed within two hours and was also normal by the owner's assessment, but was not available for examination by the referring veterinarian. The foal was unable to rise after several hours. The foal had a weak suckle reflex, and her body temperature began to decrease (99°F at birth, 98°F two hours postbirth). Based upon the foal's weakness, inability to suckle, and hypothermia, a decision was made to refer her to a full-care facility.

At the time of presentation, '03 RunninOnEmpty was depressed, weak, and unable to rise. She had not ingested any colostrum or milk since birth. She displayed physical characteristics consistent with prematurity, which included a slightly dome-shaped head with curly soft crown hair, soft ear cartilage, and lax tendons (Figure 4-9). She weighed 87 lbs (40 kg). The foal's temperature was 97.5°F, heart rate was 115 beats per minute, respiratory rate was 38 breaths per minute, and she was clinically hypovolemic. Auscultation of the thorax and abdomen were within normal limits, as was palpation of all joints and the umbilicus.

Blood was obtained by jugular venipuncture and submitted for a complete blood count (CBC), blood chemistry analysis, and blood culture. The results of these tests indicated that the foal was likely septic (leukopenia with a neutropenia), hypoproteinemic, hypoglobulinemic, and hypoglycemic. The hypoglycemia (40 mg/dl, reference range of 80 to 120 mg/dl) was a clear indicator of the need for immediate nutritional support, while the hypoglobulinemia and hypoproteinemia were presumed due to failure of passive transfer. Direct evaluation of IgG concentration (190 mg/dl) in the foal's serum supported this diagnosis.

The foal was initially provided 5% dextrose at a 1.5 maintenance fluid rate (225 ml/kg/day). Other treatment modalities were started, including warming the foal with a warm air blanket and administering intravenous plasma, crystalloid fluids, and broad-spectrum antibiotics.

Two hours after initiating dextrose infusion, the foal's blood glucose increased to 185 mg/dl. The rate of infusion of 5% dextrose was decreased to one half the maintenance requirements (75 ml/kg/day), and supplemental crystalloid fluid therapy was continued.

EMERGENCY NUTRITION AND POTENTIAL COMPLICATIONS

Correction of hypoglycemia requires immediate attention. Failure to recognize and correct this problem in a foal that has not ingested colostrum/milk will result in death. In fact, this should be addressed before the foal is sent to a referral center. Administration of colostrum or milk on the farm through nasogastric intubation or 5% dextrose intravenously can be life-saving. If neither option is available to the owner, then instructions to administer sugar orally may help to support the foal's blood glucose until the foal can be presented to a hospital. Caution should be used in administering oral fluids to a depressed or obtunded foal because of the risk of aspiration.

The rate of fetal uptake of dextrose ranges between 5 and 9 mg/kg/minute in utero, with a mean average of 6.6 mg/kg/minute.[1-4] Five percent dextrose was selected to provide the foal a source of energy while a more complete diet could be formulated. At the infusion rate of 225 ml/kg/day, the foal received 7.8 mg of dextrose/kg/minute. Even though the rate of infusion for the foal was within the range of fetal uptake, she became hyperglycemic. This emphasizes the need to closely monitor the response of sick neonates to glucose infusion and adjust accordingly.

Holdstock and colleagues tested the glucoregulatory response of normal foals between 1 and 10 days of age. The beta cell of the endocrine pancreas responds to glucose by releasing both proinsulin and insulin during the neonatal period, but glucose clearance was significantly slower on day one of life suggesting a transient insulin resistance.[5] Glucose intolerance is a common problem encountered in preterm human infants.[6] Reports suggest that hyperglycemia occurs in 45% to 80% of very low birth weight infants.[7,8] The response may be due to decreased receptors in the peripheral tissue of preterm and septic neonates.[7,9] This theory is supported by the findings of Pollak and associates, who measured the insulin/glucose (I/G) ratio in normal and hyperglycemic infants. Their results demonstrated normal I/G ratios of 0.99 to 1.7 in healthy infants, while hyperglycemic infants had ratios of 0.23 or less.[10] Exceeding the ability of the foal to utilize glucose may also contribute to hypertriglyceridemia and hepatic steatosis.[11]

Lipid intolerance occurs in foals with pre-existing liver or lipid disorders (hyperlipemia, hypertriglyceridemia) and may be associated with septicemia, endotoxemia, or pancreatic disease. Endotoxemia causes the release of inflammatory mediators such as tumor necrosis factor that modulate the activity of lipoprotein lipase and lipid metabolism, increasing the risk of developing hypertriglyceridemia.[12-14]

NUTRITIONAL REQUIREMENTS OF THE NEONATAL FOAL

The newborn foal is born with limited energy stores. The hepatic glycogen stores of the neonatal foal are minimal compared to the lamb, piglet, or rat pup, and will sustain body temperature for less than one hour.[15,16] Nonstructural fat may sustain body temperature for an additional 24 hours.[16] Premature foals have lower glycogen stores, reduced fat stores, and are less insulated than full-term foals, so the need for nutritional support is more crucial in these patients.[17] Foals with failure of passive transfer also do not receive the nutritional benefits of colostrum ingestion. Colostrum contains nearly six times the protein and twice the digestible energy (DE) as early lactation milk.[18] Thus, foals that have not been fed, are premature, and have failure of passive transfer may present with severe energy and protein deficits.

Based upon the amount of milk foals ingest and the composition of mare's milk, it is estimated that the normal neonatal foal requires as much as 159 kcal of gross energy per kilogram of body weight per day.[19,20] The nutritional requirements of sick foals have been minimally studied, and the human literature provides conflicting theories regarding the energy requirements of the sick human infant.[21,22] It is often challenging to meet the patient's nutritional requirements, because the sick foal may be anorexic and/or the environment in which the foal is managed may not be conducive to some types of nutrient administration. The consequence of underfeeding include decreased lean body mass, decreased strength, impaired immune function and wound healing, and increased morbidity and mortality.

In contrast, overfeeding patients may result in metabolic derangements such as hyperglycemia, hyperlipemia, azotemia, and major organ dysfunction.[11] In formulating a diet for the sick neonate, the challenge is to provide adequate support while avoiding side effects of underfeeding or overfeeding. This goal is achieved, in part, by designing a diet that is individually tailored to the requirements of each patient. Of equal importance is careful monitoring of the patient's response to the nutritional support.

A few hours after '03 RunninOnEmpty arrived at the clinic, the foal's mentation and cardiovascular status improved, and mild gastrointestinal boborygmi were heard upon auscultation. Her blood glucose had decreased to 140 mg/dl. Because the foal presented with several problems (possible septicemia, hypovolemia) that could contribute to compromised gastrointestinal function, a decision to initiate enteral nutrition (EN) with small frequent feedings was made. A nasogastric feeding tube was placed in the left nostril and secured in place by attaching a tape butterfly around the tube and suturing the butterfly to the nares. To encourage continued lactation in the mare, 10 IU of oxytocin were given in the muscle every other time the mare was milked out (every eight hours) during the first two days. EN was initiated by providing an amount of milk equal to no more than 3% of her body weight, divided over 24 hourly feedings. '03 RunninOnEmpty weighed 40 kg, so 3% of her body weight was equivalent to 1.2 L of milk. This was divided into hourly feedings of 50 ml. Mare's milk contains 0.48 kcal of digestible energy (DE)/ml, so she was provided 576 kcal/day using EN.

CREATING A PLAN FOR NUTRITIONAL SUPPORT

Sick foals require nutritional support, but may experience problems such as metabolic derangements, organ injury, or mechanical obstructions that limit their ability to tolerate nutrients. When formulating a nutrition plan for the sick neonate, pre-existing conditions should be considered to avoid potentially harmful complications. For example, azotemia and hyperglycemia have been associated with an increase risk in the development of septicemia.[23] On an individual basis, the clinician must consider the route of nutritional support that is least likely to harm the patient, as well as the nutrient composition that the patient is most likely to tolerate.

Gut motility may be abnormal in foals that are premature, hypovolemic, dehydrated, hypoxic, or have poor gut perfusion for other reasons. Intestinal infections can also contribute to alterations in gut motility. A foal that presents with these problems may not be able to tolerate enteral feeding, or may tolerate amounts that are far less than what it requires. Foals with obstructive gastrointestinal lesions are also unable to receive nutritional support by the enteral route.

Hypercapnea may be caused or exacerbated by feeding high-carbohydrate diets to foals with severe respiratory disease.[23,24] Providing diets that are proportionally high in protein to foals with pre-existing or concurrent renal dysfunction may contribute to azotemia.[23]

SELECTING A ROUTE OF DELIVERY: ENTERAL NUTRITION VERSUS PARENTERAL NUTRITION

Enteral nutrition is delivered to the gastrointestinal tract either by suckling or by nasogastric intubation, while parenteral nutrition (PN) is given intravenously through dedicated catheters. In the treatment of sick and preterm human infants, early enteral feeding is recommended. Delayed feeding is associated with several deleterious effects. These include:

- Reduction in intestinal villi height
- Decreased weight of the stomach, pancreas, and intestine
- Decreased intestinal enzyme production
- Increased mucosal permeability, permitting translocation of bacteria
- Increased risk of necrotizing entercolitis
- Decreased secretion of gut hormones that stimulate GI development[25-28]

Enteral nutritional support is also less expensive and often easier to manage than feeding by the parenteral route. However, some sick foals cannot tolerate enteral feeding, or have conditions that require complete bowel rest. For these foals, nutrition should bypass the gut and be delivered directly to the blood.

When foals cannot tolerate enteral feeding, nutrients can be delivered directly to the blood in the form of parenteral nutrition. Formulas for parenteral support are calculated to meet part (partial PN) or all (total PN) of the patient's requirements. Evidence-based information regarding parenteral support for foals is sparse and predominantly adapted from recommendations for human infants.

Most commonly, foals are provided partial PN, which is designed to meet energy and protein requirements. Multivitamin and electrolyte supplements are usually added. Total PN is infrequently provided. Negative factors for PN include expense, complications of thrombophebitis, labor, and inadequate facilities to mix and administer. Generally, PN serves as a bridge to enteral support by allowing more time for the transition to occur.

Foals that cannot tolerate adequate amounts of enteral nutrition are often provided a combination of enteral and parenteral support. Even small amounts of oral nutrition supply the trophic benefits to the gut wall. Success with preterm and full-term sick human infants is greatest if small-volume, frequent enteral feedings are coupled with parenteral support.[29] In very compromised foals, as little as 25 ml of milk every four to six hours may benefit the gastrointestinal tract.

Enteral Nutrition

The amount of EN support that is provided to a sick neonatal foal is based upon the foal's status at the time of presentation and its response to initial therapy. In human medicine, a conservative approach to EN is recommended since many sick infants experience gut ischemia secondary to hypoxia, septic shock, and dehydration.[30] The frequency with which foals experience similar complications is not known, and a conservative approach to EN is recommended to avoid problems that result in gastrointestinal distention and bacterial overgrowth.

For moderately sick full-term foals that are unable to suckle, initial daily support is aimed at providing the amount of milk equal to 5% to 10% of the foal's body weight, in multiple small feedings. Feedings are as frequent as every hour, but may be decreased to every two hours (with double the volume) once the foal's condition stabilizes. As the foal's clinical status improves, the volume of enteral nutrition can be gradually increased over several days until the foal tolerates a volume of milk or milk replacer that is equivalent to 20% to 25% of its body weight. If the foal does not tolerate this rapid increase in enteral support, supplemental PN should be considered. Further, foals receiving less than 20% to 25% of their body weight as milk do not obtain adequate water, and should be provided additional fluid therapy by the oral (if tolerated) or IV route.

Much smaller amounts of EN (1% to 3% of body weight in milk) are used to introduce a premature or critically ill neonate to food. For these foals, EN is combined with PN support, to permit delivery of adequate nutrition without causing serious complications such as bloating, gastric distention, and enteritis. Unless a foal has an obstructive lesion, most will tolerate this amount of nutrition, but close monitoring is required (see "Monitoring" section in this chapter). Once the foal consistently tolerates ingestion of at least 15% of its body weight in milk on a daily basis, it can be weaned off of PN. Again, supplemental fluid therapy should be provided until the foal's consumption of milk approaches a normal volume (20% to 25% of body weight).

Enteral Products

Milk is described as a complex species-specific biologic fluid adapted to perfectly satisfy the nutritional and immunologic needs of the offspring.[31-33] The preferred source of enteral nutrition for the neonatal foal is the mare's milk. This is the most likely source of an inexpensive, balanced diet for the foal. Human milk has been shown to contain protectants such as secretory IgA, lactoferrin, lysozyme, lactadherin, numerous cytokines, and oligosaccharide analogues for microbial receptors on mucosal membranes.[34] Milk fat is a primary source of energy for the human infant, and the fatty acid composition supports optimal neural and

visual development.[35,36] Human breastfeeding is also considered protective against necrotizing enterocolitis, chronic lung disease of prematurity, otitis media, and general infections in infants.[30,34,37,38-42] Cymbaluk and Laarveld demonstrated that mare's milk is a significant source of insulin-like growth factor-1, which stimulates gut and somatic development.[43]

Stripping milk from the foal's dam promotes continued lactation, increasing the chance of reuniting the foal with the mare once it has recovered. Every attempt should be made to reunite the foal with the mare, since rearing an orphan foal often requires a considerable amount of labor and may produce an animal with behavioral problems.

If mare's milk is not available, goat's and cow's milk may be used as an alternative source of fresh milk products. Fresh milk products may contain nonpathogenic bacteria that assist in populating the gut. Evidence of cross-species protection from ingestion of immunoglobulins indicates that fresh milk from other species may supply some of the immunoprotective benefits.[44] While fresh milk products offer some advantages, goat's and cow's milk are not nutritionally similar to mare's milk and may be expensive if purchased from a commercial source.[45] Methods for modifying cow's milk have been described, but are recommended only for short-term use.[45,46] The source of fresh milk should also be carefully selected to avoid introducing infectious agents, such as *Salmonella*, into the foal.

A number of commercial mare's milk replacers are available, and some are listed on Table 4-5.[47] The milk replacer should closely match mare's milk in energy density (0.5 kcal/kg as feed), crude protein (22% dry matter), crude fat (15% dry matter), crude fiber (less than 0.2% dry matter), and total solids (11% as feed).[45,47] See previous orphan foal case for more discussion of selection.

Human products have also been used for short-term enteral support. Foals fed a low-residue, human liquid diet for seven days tolerated the diet.[48] These products are not suitable for long-term support, because they are expensive and are not formulated to meet the foal's nutritional requirements.

Method of EN Delivery

Foals that can suckle should be allowed to nurse the mare unless they have a specific disease in which milk ingestion is counterindicated. In cases in which foals have a weak suckle, a feeding tube should be placed to minimize the possibility of aspiration. Enteral feeding should not be attempted in foals that present with evidence of bloating or colic until a diagnosis is obtained. Distention of the small intestine is particu-

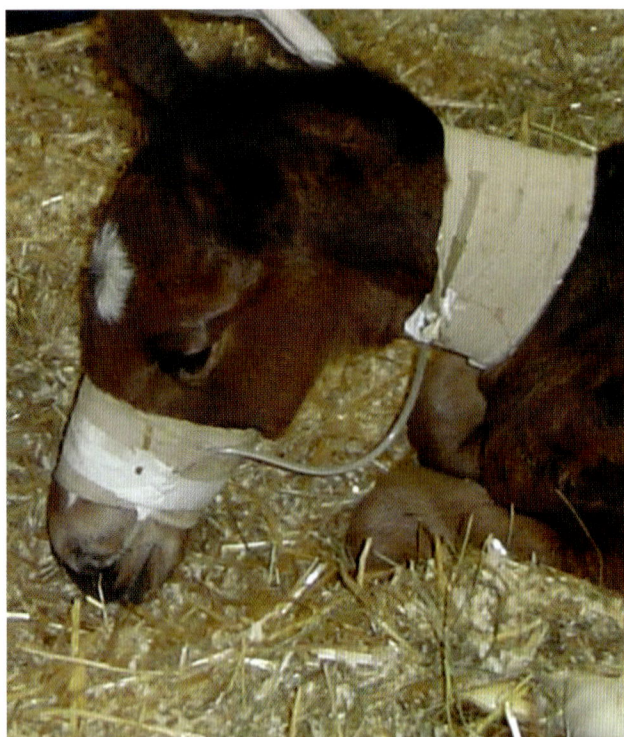

Fig. 4-10 Nasogastric feeding tubes are easily placed and maintained over long periods of time in the foal.

larly detrimental to young foals. Increased intraluminal pressures that exceed 25 cm H_2O cause collapse of the capillary beds in the wall of the gut, resulting in poor tissue perfusion and reperfusion injury.[49]

Some foals tolerate EN but have a poor suckle reflex. A feeding tube can be placed that will allow for the delivery of nutrients to the gut. A stallion catheter (1 cm or less external diameter) can be easily placed and sutured or taped into the nares. Milk will readily flow through these catheters, but their rigid nature may cause trauma to the foal's larynx if left in place for more than a few days. Feeding tubes made of polyurethane are less traumatic and may be kept in place for several weeks (Figure 4-10). Because of their smaller diameter and softer nature, polyurethane tubes are more difficult to place. Storing them in a freezer for 15 minutes prior to placement will make them more rigid and easier to pass. Some feeding tubes contain a wire stylet inside that adds to the tube's rigidity but must be removed after the tube is in place.

Rigid tubes, such as the stallion catheter, should be placed in the esophagus rather than the stomach to avoid gastric reflux between feedings. Smaller-diameter tubes of softer material may be placed in the stomach to permit the feeder to check for reflux between feedings. Generally reflux can be aspirated through small-bore soft tubes. However, in cases of obvious gastrointestinal distention, if reflux is not

obtained, the small bore tube should be replaced with a large-bore tube and attempts to obtain reflux should be repeated.

When using milk or milk replacer (excluding acidified products), the foal's diet should be fresh, or if premade, stored in a refrigerator for no longer than 24 hours. For sick foals, only the exact amount of milk/milk replacer to be fed should be warmed to room temperature before each feeding. Residual warmed milk or milk replacer should be discarded and should not be stored for future use. Human enteral feeding bags are convenient containers for the foal's diet and allow delivery by gravity flow. To minimize complications associated with EN, the following steps should be followed each time a foal is fed a meal.

1. Position the foal in sternal recumbency with the head elevated above the level of the stomach, or standing to avoid reflux and aspiration.

2. Measure the circumference of the foal's abdomen to be certain that it is not becoming distended.

3. Inject 30 ml of warm water into the feeding tube to check that the tube is patent. If the foal coughs or demonstrates discomfort, stop the feeding process and confirm proper tube position.

4. If the tube is placed in the foal's stomach, attempt to aspirate reflux. If more than 50 cc of reflux are obtained, and/or the fluid has a putrid smell, discontinue feeding for several hours.

5. Deliver the foal's diet by gravity as a slow bolus. Formula may also be delivered by a continuous rate infusion. However, human infants receiving bolus feeding, rather than continuous feeding, tolerate their diet better and require less time to reach full enteral support.[50]

6. Once the diet has been delivered, flush the line with a small amount of water, followed by air to be certain that the tube is fully evacuated.

7. Cap the tube between feedings to prevent aerophagia, and thoroughly clean all equipment used to prepare and deliver the diet.

Because '03 RunninOnEmpty's enteral intake was limited to 3% of her body weight, her remaining nutritional requirements were provided through the parenteral route. A double-bore catheter was placed in the foal's left jugular vein at the time of the foal's arrival, using sterile technique. One port of the catheter was dedicated to delivery of the PN.

'03 RunninOnEmpty was premature, likely septic, and already demonstrating evidence of glucose intolerance, so her diet was formulated to include a high percentage of lipid. Specifically, she received 40% of her nonprotein kilocalories as dextrose and 60% as lipid. The foal also

Box 4.1   Calculations for '03 RunninOnEmpty's Parenteral Nutrition

Formulating a PN Admixture

Formulating a PN admixture for '03 RunninOnEmpty will be used to demonstrate steps needed to calculate the final diet.

Step 1: Consider the patient's specific nutrient requirements and potential intolerances.
'03 RunninOnEmpty is hyperglycemic and hypoproteinemic. She also did not ingest colostrum prior to presentation.

Step 2: Calculate the foal's nonprotein energy requirements.
'03 RunninOnEmpty weighs 40 kg
40 kg × 30 kcal/kg/day = 1200 kcal/day

Step 3: Calculate the amount of protein the foal requires and the energy she will receive from that protein.
The recommended range of protein for foals is 4 to 6 grams per 100 nonprotein kilocalories. The following equation is used to calculate the protein requirements.
(1200 kcal/day × 6 g protein) ÷ 100 kcal nonprotein kcal = 72 g protein

To calculate the energy available from this amount of protein, recall that each gram of protein provides 4 kcal of digestible energy (DE).
72 g protein × 4 kcal/g = 288 kcal

Step 4: Calculate the amount of nonprotein calories that will be provided by dextrose and the amount provided by lipids.
Remember that the total nonprotein DE required by the foal = 1200 kcal, and 40% of her nonprotein calories will be derived from dextrose.
1200 kcal × 0.4 = 480 kcal in the form of dextrose
Each ml of 50% dextrose provides 1.7 kcal.
480 kcal ÷ 1.7 kcal/ml = 282 ml of 50% dextrose
60% of her nonprotein calories will be derived from lipids.
200 kcal × 0.6 = 720 kcal
Each ml of 20% lipid emulsion provides 2 kcal.
720 kcal ÷ 2 kcal/ml = 360 ml of 20% lipid emulsion

Step 5: Determine the volume of the amino acid solution required to provide 72 g of protein using the following calculation.
Each ml of 8.5% amino acid solution provides 0.085 g of protein (amino acids).
72 g ÷ 0.085 g protein/ml = 850 ml

Step 6: Check the concentration of dextrose in the solution.
Total volume of solution = dextrose (282 ml) + lipids (360 ml) + amino acids (850 ml) = 1492 ml

Grams of dextrose = 282 ml × 0.5 g/ml = 141 g

Concentration of dextrose = grams of dextrose ÷ total volume of solution
141 g ÷ 1492 ml = 9.5%

Because the final concentration of dextrose is less than 10%, this formula does not require further dilution. For formulations in which the dextrose concentration exceeds 10%, the total volume of the solution can be increased using isotonic crystalloid fluids.

Summary of PN Admixture for '03 RunninOnEmpty

50% Dextrose Solution	282 ml
20% Lipid Emulsion	360 ml
8.5% Amino Acid Solution	850 ml
Total Volume	1492 ml

Final Dextrose Concentration = 9.5%
Provides 6 g protein/100 nonprotein kcal
Provides 30 nonprotein kcal/kg/day
Provides 7.2 protein kcal/kg/day
Provides 37 total kcal/kg/day
Provides 37 ml fluid/kg/day, so foal will need supplemental fluid therapy of 113 ml/kg/day, using crystalloid fluids, to meet maintenance requirements.

---

failed to consume colostrum and was hypoproteinemic, so her diet was formulated to provide the maximum amount of protein within accepted guidelines (6 g protein/100 kcal nonprotein energy). Providing the foal a higher proportion of protein was intended to minimize catabolism of immunoglobulins provided by the plasma transfusion. Box 4-1 shows the specific calculations for '03 RunninOnEmpty.

PARENTERAL NUTRITION

Parenteral nutrition is an effective way to supply the energy and protein required for the critically ill foal that is unable to tolerate enteral nutrition. The parenteral diet is predominately formulated by mixing dextrose and lipids (to provide adequate energy to the foal) and amino acids as a protein source, combined in quantities and combinations that are tolerated. Table 4-6 describes these components. Table 4-7 provides a summary of information about each component. There are several sources for parenteral solutions listed in Table 4-8. Obtaining all of the parenteral solutions from the same source minimizes compatibility problems.

The first step in calculating a PN formula for a sick neonate is to determine the amount of energy in the form of kilocalories that the foal requires.

Calculating Energy Requirements

The requirement of the normal growing equine neonate is approximately 120 kcal/kg/day.[18,51] Using

Table 4-6	Components of Parenteral Nutrition*
Dextrose solutions	The primary nonprotein energy sources in parenteral nutrition include dextrose solutions and lipid emulsions. One gram of dextrose provides 3.4 kcal of energy. Parenteral diets are formulated using 50% solutions of dextrose, which means each ml provides 1.7 kcal of energy. Fifty percent solutions are hypertonic and should not be delivered without being first diluted to a 10% solution or less solution.
Lipid emulsions	One gram of lipids provides approximately 10 kcal of energy (based upon the specific composition of fats). Parenteral products are 10% or 20% emulsions, which provide 1 or 2 kcal/ml, respectively. When formulating parenteral diets for foals, previous recommendations suggest that lipids can provide up to 60% of energy needs, with the remainder derived from dextrose solutions.[55] Lipids are the most expensive component of parenteral nutrition, and cost can limit their use in some animals.
Protein (amino acid) solutions	Amino acids provide approximately 4 kcal/g protein. Amino acid solutions come in a variety of concentrations, ranging from 3.5% to 15% and may or may not contain electrolytes. Solutions containing 8.5% amino acids are most commonly used in veterinary medicine and provide 85 mg/ml of protein or 0.34 kcal/ml.

Dextrose solutions provide simple carbohydrates, lipid emulsions provide fat, and amino acid solutions are the source of protein.

Table 4-7	Summary of Key Information Required to Calculate a Parenteral Nutrition Admixture		
Nutrient	Commonly Used Concentration	Grams of Nutrient/ml	kcal/ml
Dextrose	50 %	0.5	1.7
Lipid emulsion	20%	0.2	2
Protein (amino acids)	8.5%	0.085	0.34

From Clinics of North America, *Equine Practice*, Buechner-Maxwell, VA, Nutritional Support for Neonatal Foals, *Vet Clin Equine* 21 (2005) 487-510.

Table 4-8	Sources for Parenteral Solutions*
Company Name	**Location**
Abbott Laboratories, Animal Health	North Chicago, IL
Baxter Health Care Corporation	Deerfield, IL
B. Braun Medical Inc.	Bethlehem, PA

Buechner-Maxwell, VA, Nutritional Support for Neonatal Foals, *Vet Clin Equine* 21 (2005) 487-510.
*Obtaining all parenteral solutions from the same source minimizes compatibility problems.

methods of indirect calorimetry, it has been recently demonstrated that sick foals require significantly less energy (44.36 kcal/kg/day) than healthy foals.[52] The nonprotein energy needed to meet the requirements of a sick foal can be estimated by providing 30 kcal/kg/day. This estimate is more applicable to sick full-term or tranquilized foals, and may not apply to premature foals since this group was not included in the previously measured study.[52] Sick human infants also have lower total energy requirements due to inhibited growth, reduced insensible losses, and decreased activity.[53] In an effort to avoid the complications associated with overfeeding, parenteral formulation is conservative, and designed to meet either basal or resting energy requirements of the sick neonate. The final calculation of total energy also includes kilocalories derived from protein added to the PN admixture.

Calculating Protein Requirements

Protein is provided in the form of amino acid solutions. While there are several ways to calculate crude protein requirements, providing 4 to 6 grams per 100 kcal of nonprotein energy is a simple method for estimating the amount that the foal requires. Protein is calculated in addition to nonprotein calories to prevent catabolism and negative nitrogen balance in critically ill patients. However, recent examination of energy balance in human patients indicate that neither a positive nonprotein energy balance nor total energy balance prevents protein catabolism in the critically ill.[54] The stressed or ill animal appears to lose the normal adaptive response to starvation of conserving lean body mass. This approach of calculating protein needs continues to be used because the protein requirements of the sick neonatal foal are not known. It is also not known how well foals tolerate formulas that contain larger proportions of protein. Azotemia is a consequence of overfeeding protein, and in the absence of better information, a conservative approach is recommended.

Each gram of protein provides 4 kcal. Using these calculations, 16 to 24 protein-derived kcal are added to every 100 kcal of nonprotein energy. The total number (protein and nonprotein) of kcal/kg delivered on a daily basis using this formulation is 37 kcal/kg/day (30 from nonprotein sources and 7 from protein). This number approaches the energy requirements of the sick foal.[52]

A similar method for determining the amount of protein in the diet is to calculate the ratio of nitrogen to non-nitrogen (nonprotein) kilocalories. One gram of nitrogen is contained in 6.25 g protein, so the conversion from nitrogen to protein is achieved by multiplying the grams of nitrogen by 6.25. For foals, the recommended ratio of nitrogen to nonnitrogen kilocalories is between 100 and 200 kcal of non-nitrogen energy per gram of nitrogen.[55-57] A similar ratio is achieved by providing 4 to 6 grams of protein/100 kcal of nonprotein.

Some additional examples of PN admixtures are provided in Box 4-2.

Preparation of Parenteral Nutrition

In preparing a parenteral diet, the components should be mixed in a very clean environment, preferably under a laminar flow hood. Solutions are usually mixed by transferring the calculated amount into a sterile PN bag (Figure 4-11). Dextrose and amino acids should be mixed first, with lipids added after the amino acids. This procedure prevents lipids from becoming unstable and coming out of the emulsion. While many PN products are available, products from the same source should be selected for formulation to minimize incompatibility.

Vitamin B complex can be added to the parenteral nutrition formula, and the amount is based upon the manufacturer recommendations. Electrolytes such as potassium can be also added, but some amino acid solutions contain electrolytes, and their concentration should be considered when determining additional electrolyte supplementation.

Foals also require maintenance fluids of 100 to 150 ml/kg body weight daily. Usually, PN is not formulated to meet the patient's fluid requirements, and these must be provided by supplementing with isotonic crystalloid fluids. If the final concentration of dextrose in the PN solution is greater than 10%, then increasing the final PN volume with isotonic crystalloid solutions is recommended. In horses, PN is usually delivered into a large-flow vessel such as the jugular vein. Therefore, it has been observed that complications such as phlebitis and thrombosis that occur with delivery of hypertonic solutions to small peripheral veins are not as common. However, solutions should be diluted to 10% dextrose concentration when prepared for sick foals that have evidence of vascular injury (such as petechia).

To deliver the diet, an intravenous catheter is placed aseptically in the jugular or peripheral vein. Catheters made of polyurethane or silastic are recommended because they are minimally thrombogenic, and are readily available for veterinary use (Mila International, Inc, Florence, KY). A double-bore catheter is preferred, and one bore is dedicated to the delivery of PN. This minimizes contamination and eliminates the need to stop and start the solution when delivering additional medications such as antibiotics. Nutrition should be delivered at a constant rate, using an infusion pump to avoid fluctuations in glucose delivery. The actual volume of parenteral nutrition should be carefully monitored and recorded.

Initiating the Diet

Between the time that the foal presents to the clinic and a nutritional plan can be formulated, every effort should be made to correct hydration, acid-base, and electrolyte abnormalities. This goal is often not fully achieved before nutritional support is instituted because foals do not have adequate energy stores to survive over the time period required to safely correct all of their deficiencies. Initiating nutritional support to critically ill foals requires a slow introduction and careful monitoring.

Once the parenteral nutrition is compounded, the maximal hourly flow rate is determined by dividing the total volume by 24. In our example, the final volume of PN is 1492 ml. To deliver this volume, 62 ml/hour must be infused. Typically, PN is initiated at 25% (15 ml/hour) to 50% (31 ml/hour) of this infusion rate for four hours, and the foal is evaluated to be certain that it tolerates the PN. If there is no evidence of complications, then the infusion rate is increased by increments of 25% every four to eight hours, until the foal reaches the desired rate of 62 ml/hour. Each time, prior to increasing the rate, the foal is assessed for evidence of complications such as hyperglycemia. If complications exist, then the infusion rate is decreased by 25% to 50% increments and the foal is re-examined in two to four hours, depending upon the severity of the intolerance.

The EN component of the diet is also best tolerated once the foal's clinical status has been stabilized. When this has not been accomplished, EN should be initiated at a very conservative rate.

Box 4.2   Additional Examples of Parenteral Diet Formulation

Example 1: Calculating PN for a Two-Day-Old 50 kg Septic Foal

Step 1: Consider the patient's specific nutritional requirements and potential intolerances.

The foal is not hyperglycemic, hypoproteinemic, or hyperlipidemic.

Step 2: Calculate the foal's nonprotein energy requirements.

DE = 30 kcal/kg/day × 50 kg = 1500 kcal/day

Step 3: Calculate the amount of protein that the foal requires and the energy provided by the protein.

Since the foal is not hypoproteinemic, 4 g of protein for every 100 kcal nonprotein energy will be provided.

(1500 kcal/day × 4 g protein) ÷ 100 kcal nonprotein kcal = 60 g protein

Calculate the energy provided by this protein.

60 g protein × 4 kcal/g = 240 kcal

Step 4: Calculate the amount of nonprotein calories that will be provided by dextrose and the amount provided by lipids.

The foal has no metabolic complications, so a formulation of using 60% dextrose and 40% lipid is appropriate. Lipid emulsions are the most expensive component when formulating PN, so less is used when it appears that the foal is capable of tolerating greater proportions of dextrose.

Remember that the total nonprotein calories required by the foal = 1500 kcal/day

60% of the nonprotein calories will be provided as dextrose
1500 kcal × 0.6 = 900 kcal in the form of dextrose

Each ml of 50% dextrose provides 1.7 kcal.
900 kcal ÷ 1.7 kcal/ml = 530 ml of 50% dextrose

40% of nonprotein calories will be derived from lipids.
1500 kcal × 0.4 = 600 kcal

Each ml of 20% lipid emulsion provides 2 kcal.
600 kcal ÷ 2 kcal/ml = 300 ml of 20% lipid emulsion

Step 5: Determine the volume of the amino acid solution required to provide 72 g of protein using the following calculation.

Each ml of 8.5% amino acid solution provides 0.085 g of protein (amino acids)
60 g ÷ 0.085 g protein/ml = 705 ml

Step 6: Check the concentration of dextrose in this solution.

Total volume of parenteral admixture =
dextrose (530 ml) + lipids (300 ml) + amino acids (705 ml) = 1535 ml

Grams of dextrose = 530 ml × 0.5 grams/ml = 265 grams

Concentration of dextrose = number of grams of dextrose ÷ total volume of solution

265 grams ÷ 1535 ml = 17% dextrose

The final concentration of dextrose solution is greater than 10%. In horses, PN is usually delivered into a large-flow vessel such as the jugular vein. Therefore, complications such as phlebitis and thrombosis that occur with delivery of hypertonic solutions to small peripheral veins are not commonly observed. However, solutions should be diluted to 10% dextrose concentration when prepared for sick foals that have evidence of vascular injury (such as petechia). This can easily be achieved by increasing the final PN volume with isotonic crystalloid solutions.

Step 7: Adjusting the dextrose concentration by adding crystalloid fluids to the admixture.

Calculation of additional crystalloid fluid volume
265 g ÷ 0.1 = 2650 ml (the total volume required to make a 10% solution)
2650 ml (total volume) − 1535 ml (PN volume) = 1115 ml isotonic fluid

Summary of PN Admixture for Example 1

50% Dextrose Solution	530 ml
20% Lipid Emulsion	300 ml
8.5% Amino Acid Solution	705 ml
Isotonic, Crystalloid Fluids	1115 ml
Total Volume	2650 ml

Final Dextrose concentration = 10%
Provides 4 g protein/100 nonprotein kcal
Provides 30 nonprotein kcal/kg/day
Provides 5 protein kcal/kg/day
Provides 35 total kcal/kg/day
Provides 53 ml of fluid/kg/day
To provide maintenance fluid therapy, the foal will need 97 ml/kg/day of crystalloid fluids.

Example 2: Calculating PN without Lipids for a Two-Day-Old 50 kg Septic Foal

When owners have limited financial resources, PN can be formulated using dextrose and amino acids, since lipid is the most expensive component of the admixture. However, this modification has a small impact on the cost of PN for sick foals in our clinic, as shown in this example. The following is a reformulation of PN for the foal described in the previous example, however, lipids are not used in the admixture.

Step 1: Consider the patient's specific nutritional requirements and potential intolerances.

The foal is not hyperglycemic, hypoproteinemic, or hyperlipidemic.

Step 2: Calculate the foal's nonprotein energy requirements.

The foal weighs 50 kg
50 kg × 30 kcal/kg/day = 1500 kcal/day

Step 3: Calculate the amount of protein that the foal requires and the energy she will receive from that protein.

Since the foal is not hypoproteinemic, 4 g of protein for every 100 kcal nonprotein energy will be provided.

(1500 kcal/day × 4 g protein) ÷ 100 kcal nonprotein kcal = 60 g protein

Calculate the energy provided by this protein.

60 g protein × 4 kcal/g = 240 kcal

Box 4.2   Additional Examples of Parenteral Diet Formulation—cont'd

Step 4: Calculate the amount of nonprotein calories that will be provided by dextrose, and the amount provided by lipids.

Remember that the total nonprotein calories required by the foal = 1500 kcal/day

100% of the nonprotein kcal will be provided as dextrose.
1500 kcal × 1 = 1500 kcal in the form of dextrose

Each ml of 50% dextrose provides 1.7 kcal
1500 kcal ÷ 1.7 kcal/ml = 882 ml of 50% dextrose

None of her nonprotein calories will be derived from lipids.

Step 5: Determine the volume of the amino acid solution required to provide 72 g of protein using the following calculation.

Each ml of 8.5% amino acid solution provides 0.085 g of protein (amino acids).
60 g ÷ 0.085 g protein/ml = 705 ml

Step 6: Check the concentration of dextrose in this solution.

Total volume of parenteral admixture is equal to
dextrose (880 ml) + lipids (0 ml) + amino acids (705 ml) = 1535 ml

Grams of dextrose = 880 ml × 0.5 grams/ml = 440 grams

Concentration of dextrose = grams of dextrose ÷ total volume of the solution
440 g ÷ 1535 ml = 28% dextrose

If the dextrose concentration exceeds 20%, regardless of the foal's condition, isotonic crystalloid fluids should be added to dilute the solution. Again, for sick foals, a solution of 10% or less is recommended.

Step 7: Adjusting the dextrose concentration by adding crystalloid fluids to the admixture

Calculation of additional isotonic crystalloid fluid volume
440 g ÷ 0.1 = 4400 ml (total volume required to make a 10% solution)

4400 ml (total volume) − 1585 ml (PN volume) = 2815 ml of isotonic fluid

Summary of PN Admixture using only 50% Dextrose (Example 2)

50% Dextrose Solution	880 ml
8.5% Amino Acid Solution	705 ml
Isotonic, Crystalloid Fluids	2816 ml
Total Volume	4400 ml

Final Dextrose concentration = 10%
Provides 4 grams protein/100 nonprotein kcal
Provides 30 nonprotein kcal/kg/day
Provides 5 protein kcal/kg/day
Provides 35 total kcal/kg/day
Provides 88 ml of fluid/kg/day
To provide maintenance fluid therapy, the foal will need 62 ml/kg/day of crystalloid fluids.

By excluding the lipids in this formulation, the cost is reduced by approximately 10% in our hospital ($4.00). This difference is minimal because none of the components are used in large volume. Cost may vary based upon the source of PN, and the savings will increase proportionally as larger volumes of PN are used. However, for foals that demonstrate glucose intolerance, the risk of inducing hyperglycemia outweighs the cost of adding lipids to the admixture. When using PN formulated without lipids, the diet should be introduced more gradually and the foal's response should be monitored closely for evidence of hyperglycemia. To avoid excessive venipuncture, urine glucose can be measured every two hours. If glucose is present in the urine, blood glucose should be immediately measured and PN infusion rate adjusted accordingly. When PN infusion rate is significantly decreased, remember to increase infusion rate of crystalloid fluids so that the total volume meets the foal's maintenance fluid requirements.

The parenteral diet for '03 RunninOn Empty was formulated as previously described. The final volume of the admixtures was 1492 ml. While the foal's clinical status had improved, her blood glucose concentration was still above normal (140 mg/dl) at the time that PN was initiated (five hours after presentation). Therefore, the initial infusion rate was 31 ml/hour (50% of the calculated volume required to deliver 100% of the formulated PN).

PN was delivered through an infusion pump to avoid fluctuations in the rate of nutrient delivery. The foal's urine glucose remained negative, and blood glucose values were less than 150 mg/dl after four hours (Figure 4-12). The foal was evaluated again after eight hours, and continued to tolerate the diet. The hourly EN feeding volume was increased to 100 ml/hour (estimated to provide 6% of the foal's body weight in kilograms). Three hours after the increase, the foal became restless and appeared more distended. Because 60 ml of putrid milk was retrieved through the nasogastric tube, enteral support was discontinued for four hours. Oral metronidazole therapy was instituted at a dose of 10 mg/kg qid PO to minimize anaerobic bacterial overgrowth in the foal's gut. Attempts to retrieve reflux were made twice, at two-hour intervals, and only small amounts of fluid were obtained. Enteral support was reinstituted at 50 ml/hour, and the foal again tolerated this volume.

Monitoring

The key to successful nutritional support is careful monitoring of the patient's response to the diet. In general, foals need to be evaluated for evidence of complications associated with the mode of delivery (catheter site reactions, nasogastric tube misplacement), and metabolic derangements associated with intolerance of the diet they receive. Patients must also be monitored more intensely when nutritional modalities are being introduced, modified, or withdrawn. Foals that are critically ill or whose condition acutely worsens warrant more frequent and careful monitoring than foals whose condition has stabilized. Recommendations for monitoring the critically ill and stable foal are summarized in Table 4-9.

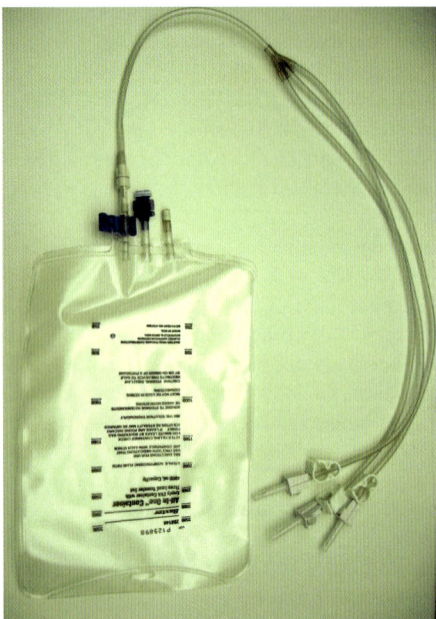

Fig. 4-11 Parenteral nutrition bag with multi access. Parenteral solutions can be delivered through one of the three tubes. Amino acid and dextrose solutions can be delivered simultaneously, while lipid emulsions must be added last.

Complications

Complications associated with EN are most commonly due to mismanagement of the tube or feeding a larger volume than the foal can tolerate. Aspiration may occur even when the tube is properly placed. Large-bore tubes, such as a stallion urinary catheter, placed into the stomach, permit dilation of the distal esophageal sphincter and regurgitation of stomach contents. Tubes may also become dislodged between feedings, especially as foals become more active. Careful evaluation of tube placement and the foal's initial response to a water bolus can minimize these problems. Also, placement of large-bore tubes in the esophagus, or use of small-bore tubes, can minimize regurgitation from the stomach and decrease the risk of aspiration.

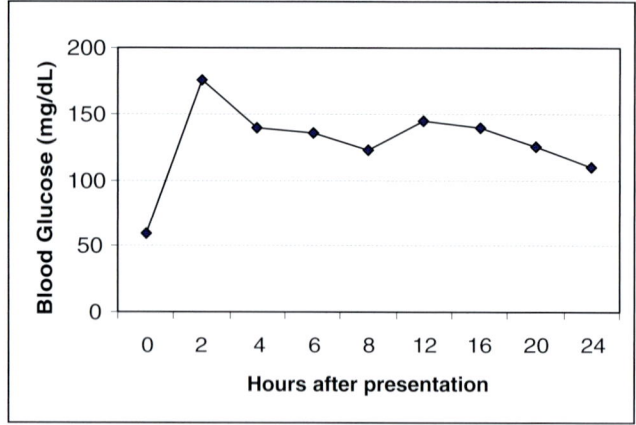

Fig. 4-12 '03 RunninOnEmpty's blood glucose concentration during the first 24 hours after presentation.

Table 4-9	Recommendations for Monitoring a Foal's Response to Nutritional Support	
	Critical Foal **Change in Diet** **Sudden Fever**	**Foal in Stable** **Condition** **Diet Unchanged**
Body weight	Daily	Daily
Urine glucose	Every 2 hours	Every 6 hours
Blood glucose	Every 2 to 4 hours or immediately if urine glucose positive	Every 6 to 8 hours
Serum creatinine	Daily	Daily or every other day
Serum protein	Every 4 to 8 hours	Daily or every other day
Serum electrolytes	Every 12 hours if abnormal	Daily or every other day
Serum triglycerides	Daily	If lipemia is noted
Lipemia	Every 4 to 8 hours	Daily
PvCO2	Every 4 hours if respiratory compromise is diagnosed	Daily or every other day if respiratory function is normal

Buechner-Maxwell, VA, Nutritional Support for Neonatal Foals, *Vet Clin Equine* 21 (2005) 487-510.

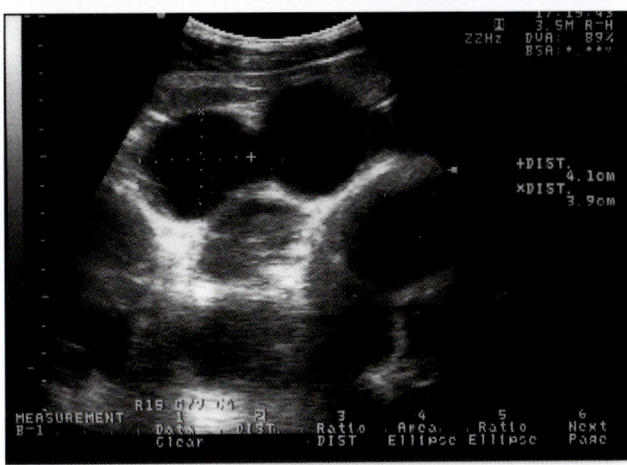

Fig. 4-13 Ultrasound evaluation of a foal with abdominal distention. Note the multiple loops of distended small intestine.

As previously discussed, foals do not tolerate intestinal distention, and monitoring for abdominal bloating must be done on a regular basis. This can be achieved by marking an area on the foal's abdomen and measuring the diameter using a tape or string before each feeding. If diameter size increases over several consecutive feedings, further evaluation is warranted. Ultrasound examination of the foal's gastrointestinal tract permits a better estimate of small-intestinal and gastrointestinal distention (Figure 4-13). If gastrointestinal distention is suspected, an attempt should be made to reflux the foal. Enteral feeding should be discontinued for four to six hours, or until the distention resolves. Feeding should then be reinstituted at a smaller initial volume.

Sick foals may also develop necrotizing enterocolitis (NEC), a life-threatening gastrointestinal infection. The likely bacterial agents associated with this disease are *Escherichia coli, Klebsiella spp,* or *Clostridia spp.*[45] Early enteral feeding and feeding of breast milk have been shown to decrease the risk of sick human infants developing NEC.[27,30,42,58] Enteral support may provide the same benefit to neonatal foals, but patients should be monitored carefully for evidence of intolerance and bloating.

Common complications associated with PN in human infants include catheter dysfunction, thrombosis, perivascular leakage, contamination, sepsis, hyperglycemia, hyperlipidemia, azotemia, and major organ failure. Similar complications have been observed in neonatal foals and can be minimized with proper monitoring and managing of the catheter site, cautious handling of the PN solutions, and diligent monitoring of the patient's response to nutritional support.

The catheter site and jugular vein should be carefully examined several times per day for evidence of infection, thrombosis, and perivascular leakage. If the catheter site is bandaged, the wrap should be removed daily to permit close visualization of the site. Prior to replacing the bandage, the site should be gently cleaned with a nonirritating antiseptic scrub and rinsed with sterile normal saline or water. If it is not bandaged, the site should be cleaned several times per day to minimize infection at the point where the catheter penetrates the skin.

As previously described, parenteral solutions should be mixed under a laminar flow hood and, once prepared, should be immediately refrigerated or used. Parenteral formulas can be stored for up to 24 hours in a refrigerator before use. Once in use, any residual PN should be discarded after 24 hours. In sick neonates, all fluid-transfer lines should be changed every 24 hours, and all injection ports should be cleaned with alcohol and allowed to dry before any substance is injected through them.

In the past, human patients receiving PN were thought to be at greater risk for developing sepsis. This was in part due to gut atrophy and increased risk of bacterial translocation across the gut wall. However, significant alterations in gut morphology were not observed in samples taken from human patients restricted to PN for one month.[59] Further, the incidence of bacterial translocation occurred with equal frequency in human subjects with intestinal obstruction whether they received PN or EN support.[60]

Hyperglycemia, hyperlipidemia, hypercapnea, azotemia, and major organ injury are side effects frequently associated with PN, but they can occur when patients are being provided any form of nutritional support. Recently, human researchers discovered that these side effects occur most frequently when patients are being overfed. Overfeeding occurs when patients are administered calories and/or a specific substrate that exceeds their requirements and/or their ability to maintain metabolic homeostasis.[54] The effects of overfeeding include azotemia, hypertonic dehydration, metabolic acidosis, hyperglycemia, sepsis, hypertriglyceridemia, hepatic stenosis, and hypercapnia.[11]

In an evaluation of 213 human patients on mechanical ventilators, 66.2% had measured resting energy expenditure (REE) of <25 kcal/kg/day. The majority of the patients were overfed (58.2%), while only 12.2% were underfed.[61] The degree of overfeeding impacted inversely with minute ventilation and also resulted in a significant increase in azotemia. Patients receiving PN tend to receive more energy than individuals receiving EN, suggesting that overfeeding rather than PN was the cause of the side effects so often associated with this mode of nutritional delivery.[61-64] These results provide additional support for a conservative approach to PN formulation.

Hyperglycemia occurs commonly in sick human infants and can occur in foals receiving parenteral support. In most cases, hyperglycemia can be managed by reducing the initial infusion rate of PN by 50% for 6 to 12 hours, then gradually increasing it until the desired infusion rate is reached. However, some septic animals may become persistently hyperglycemic, significantly limiting the amount of nutrition that can be delivered. The pathogenesis of this hyperglycemia is not well understood but may be a result of insufficient pancreatic insulin secretion, failure of insulin to suppress hepatic gluconeogenesis, and/or insulin resistance of peripheral tissues to insulin.[65] Stress-induced elevation in glucagon, epinephrine, and cortisol may also contribute to persistent hyperglycemia.[23]

Methods for managing hyperglycemia in sick foals are described briefly in this chapter and in greater detail elsewhere.[66] Insulin therapy is a beneficial tool for permitting adequate caloric delivery without causing persistent hyperglycemia. Insulin can be delivered as a continuous infusion, or may be provided as a single injection. Continuous infusion can be achieved by adding insulin to the PN solution or infusing it separately. Insulin is added to PN solutions by using 1 to 2 IU of regular insulin per 4 grams of glucose.[67] For separate infusion, the addition of 20 IU of regular insulin to 500 ml of normal saline produces a final solution with an insulin concentration of 0.04 IU/ml. Therapy is started with an infusion rate of approximately 0.0133 IU/kg/hour. For a 40 kg foal, this equals 13.3 ml of insulin-saline solution per hour. If the blood glucose concentration fails to decrease, the amount of insulin can be increased by small increments (0.002 IU/kg/hour) every six hours until blood glucose concentrations return to normal. The rate of glucose infusion should also be decreased initially until hyperglycemia resolves. Throughout this period, blood glucose concentration should be monitored closely (at least every two hours) to be certain hypoglycemia does not occur. Insulin may also be administered as an injection. The suggested dose is 0.1 to 0.5 IU/kg given SC or IV.[67] Again, blood glucose should be monitored to prevent hypoglycemia.

After initiation of nutritional support, the foal was evaluated for evidence of complications every four hours. Throughout the first 12 hours of PN, no metabolic complications were identified. The PN rate was increased to 62 ml per hour. The decision to increase PN was made to allow more time to introduce EN to the foal.

Twenty four hours after initiating nutritional support, the foal's EN was again increased to 100 ml/hour, which was tolerated well over the following 24 hours The volume was further increased to 150 ml/hr (9% body weight) and was tolerated well for an additional 24 hours. Thereafter, the EN volume was increased by 5% increments every 24 hours, until the foal was receiving 25% of her body weight in the form of milk. Once the foal was able to tolerate at least 10% of its BW in the form of milk, PN support was decreased to 31 ml/hr for 48 hours, then discontinued when the foal was capable of tolerating at least 15% of her body weight in the form of milk (Table 4-10).

The foal maintained her body weight over the first few days of hospitalization and demonstrated a continuous increase of $1/2$ to 1 pound per day starting on day four. By day six, she was bright enough to begin feeding on her own. Initially, the foal did not have a good suckle reflex and required significant stimulation to attempt any suckling activity. With repeated stimulation, her ability to suckle grew stronger, and it was decided to reintroduce her to the mare on day six. By day seven she was successfully suckling the mare.

Lactation in the mare was maintained throughout this period by evacuating her udder every two to four hours. Lactation was also supported by providing the mare free-choice access to quality grass-alfalfa hay, water, and 6 lbs of a 14% protein feed designed for lactating mare, split into two feedings. During hospitalization, the mare and foal were housed in the same stall, with a partition between them that permitted the mare to nuzzle and smell the foal. As the foal grew stronger, they were also allowed limited contact. Regardless of these efforts, the mare was not immediately accepting of the foal, and close monitoring of both was required when reunion was first attempted on

Table 4-10	Summary of PE and EN Delivered to RunninOnEmpty's '03 Foal during Seven Days of Hospitalization							
	Day 0	Day 1	Day 2	Day 3	Day 4	Day 5	Day 6	Day 7
EN (Volume)	1.2L	3L	4.5L	6L	8L	10L	10L	Return to mare
(% BW)	(3%)	(6–9%)	(9–15%)	(15%)	(20%)	(25%)	(25%)	
Volume/feeding (ml)	50	100–150	150–250	250	667	833	833	—
Feedings/day	24	24	24	24	12	12	12	—
EN (kcal/kg)[a,b]	14.4	36	54	75	100	125	125	—
PN rate (ml/hr)	31–62	62	31	31	—	—	—	
PN (kcal/kg)[b]	29	37	19	19	—	—	—	—
Total kcal/kg	43.4	73	73	94	100	125	125	—

[a]each ml of milk = 0.48 kcal[36].
[b]EN and PN kcal/kg are total kcal/kg (nonprotein plus those from protein) provided by each source.

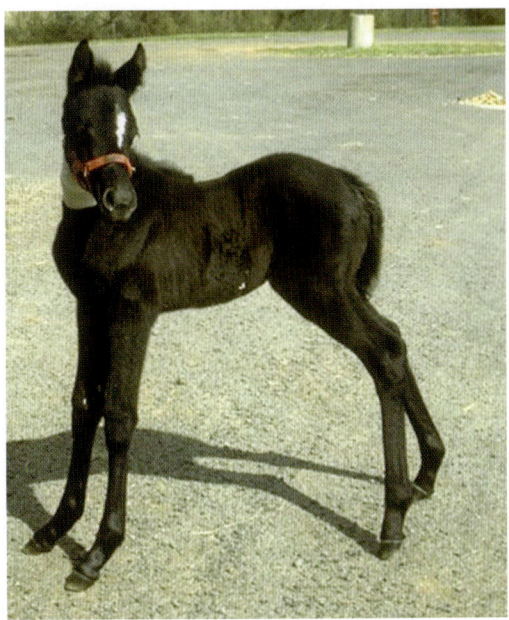

Fig. 4-14 '03 RunninOnEmpty at time of discharge.

day six of hospitalization. The mare initially required restraint and/or mild sedation. During this period, the feeding tube remained in place to permit feeding until the mare permitted the foal adequate opportunity to nurse. By day seven, the mare was more accepting of the foal, and after several successful attempts to suckle were observed, the foal's feeding tube was removed. The foal was discharged on continued therapy on day eight. One month later, the foal was reported to be normal in activity, attitude, and conformation, although she was still somewhat small for her age (Figure 4-14).

If a mare and foal have to be separated because of the care needed for the foal, then keeping them in close proximity is important to maintain some form of bond. Despite frequent hand milkings, many mares will decrease their milk production without constant stimulation from the foal. Chemical stimulation may be helpful. The frequent use of small doses of oxytocin before hand milking often will improve milk let-down. The use of domperidone, a dopamine receptor antagonist, has been helpful in milk production in agalactic mares.[68] Chavatte-Palmer describes methods of bringing nonparturient mares in to milk through the use of sulpiride, another dopamine antagonist.[69]

FINAL COMMENTS

Nutritional support is an essential therapeutic component in the treatment of sick neonatal foals. The case example described in this chapter illustrates a typical scenario encountered with moderately ill foals. RunninOnEmpty's '03 foal tolerated EN well, with the exception of bloating that occurred on the first day of treatment. Her blood glucose concentrations also remained within acceptable levels during the period that PN was being introduced and delivered. However, critically ill foals and premature foals usually require a more gradual introduction of both EN and PN. Again, monitoring is the key to determining the rate at which nutrition can be introduced. As foals recover, nutritional plans should be reassessed to provide more calories as illustrated by this case. The goal should be to attain a caloric intake that approaches that of the normal foal and supports weight gain.

REFERENCES

1. Silver M, Comline RS: Transfer of gases and metabolites in the equine placenta: A comparison with other species, *J Reprod Fertil* Suppl 589, 1975.
2. Silver M, Comline RS: Fetal and placental O₂ consumption and the uptake of different metabolites in the ruminant and horse during late gestation, *Adv Exp Med Biol* 75:731, 1976.
3. Fowden AL, Mundy L, Ousey JC et al: Tissue glycogen and glucose 6-phosphatase levels in fetal and newborn foals, *J Reprod Fertil* Suppl 44:537, 1991.
4. Fowden AL, Silver M: Glucose and oxygen metabolism in the fetal foal during late gestation, *Am J Physiol* 269:R1455, 1995.
5. Holdstock NB, Allen VL, Bloomfield MR et al: Development of insulin and proinsulin secretion in newborn pony foals, *J Endocrinology* 180:469, 2004.
6. Lopes MAF, II NAW: Parenteral nutrition for horses with gastrointestinal disease: A retrospective study of 79 cases, *Equine Vet J* 34:250, 2002.
7. Brans YW, Sumners JE, Dweck HS et al: Feeding the low birth weight infant: Orally or parenterally? Preliminary results of a comparative study, *Pediatrics* 54:15, 1974.
8. Collins JW Jr., Hoppe M, Brown K et al: A controlled trial of insulin infusion and parenteral nutrition in extremely low birth weight infants with glucose intolerance, *J Pediatr* 118:921, 1991.
9. Puukka R, Puukka M, Knip M et al: Erythrocyte insulin binding in normal infants, children and adults, *Horm Res* 17:185, 1983.
10. Pollak A, Cowett RM, Schwartz R et al: Glucose disposal in low-birth-weight infants during steady-state hyperglycemia: Effects of exogenous insulin administration, *Pediatrics* 61:546, 1978.
11. Klein CJ, Stanek GS, Wiles CE III: Overfeeding macronutrients to critically ill adults: Metabolic complications, *J Am Diet Assoc* 98:795, 1998.
12. Feingold KR, Grunfeld C: Role of cytokines in inducing hyperlipidemia, *Diabetes* 41 Suppl 2:97, 1992.
13. Feingold KR, Grunfeld C, Pang M et al: LDL subclass phenotypes and triglyceride metabolism in non-insulin-dependent diabetes, *Arterioscler Thromb* 12:1496, 1992.
14. Feingold KR, Staprans I, Memon RA et al: Endotoxin rapidly induces changes in lipid metabolism that produce hypertriglyceridemia: Low doses stimulate hepatic triglyceride production while high doses inhibit clearance, *J Lipid Res* 33:1765, 1992.
15. Fowden AL, Mundy L, Ousey JC et al: Tissue glycogen and glucose 6-phosphatase levels in fetal and newborn foals, *J Reprod Fertil* Suppl 44:537, 1991.

16. Ousey JC, McArthur AJ, Murgatroyd PR et al: Thermoregulation and total body insulation in the neonatal foal, *J Therm Biol* 17:1, 1992.

17. Ousey J: Thermoregulation and the energy requirement of the newborn foal, with reference to prematurity, *Equine Vet J Suppl* 24:104, 1997.

18. Lewis LD: *Growing horse feeding and care*, Media, PA, 1995, Williams & Wilkins.

19. Martin RG, McMeniman NP, Dowsett KF: Milk and water intakes of foals sucking grazing mares, *Equine Vet J* 24:295, 1992.

20. McMeniman NP: Nutrition of grazing brood mares and growing horses, *Aust Vet J* 74:64, 1996.

21. Scrimshaw NS: Rhoades Lecture, Effect of infection on nutrient requirements, *J Parenter Enteral Nutr* 15:589, 1991.

22. Neu J, Huang Y: Nutrition of premature and critically ill neonates, *Nestle Nutr Workshop Ser Clin Perform Programme* 171, 2003.

23. Chan S, McCowen KC, Blackburn GL: Nutrition management in the ICU, *Chest* 115:145S, 1999.

24. Mechanisms of carbohydrate-induced hypertriglyceridemia, *Nutr Rev* 32:74, 1974.

25. Lucas A, Bloom SR, Aynsley-Green A: Metabolic and endocrine consequences of depriving preterm infants of enteral nutrition, *Acta Paediatr Scand* 72:245, 1983.

26. Lucas A, Bloom SR, Aynsley-Green A: Gut hormones and "minimal enteral feeding," *Acta Paediatr Scand* 75:719, 1986.

27. Premji SS, Paes B, Jacobson K et al: Evidence-based feeding guidelines for very low-birth-weight infants, *Adv Neonatal Care* 2:5, 2002.

28. Rothman D, Udall JN, Pang KY et al: The effect of short-term starvation on mucosal barrier function in the newborn rabbit, *Pediatr Res* 19:727, 1985.

29. Evans RA, Thureen P: Early feeding strategies in preterm and critically ill neonates, *Neonat Netw* 20:7, 2001.

30. Kosloske AM: Breast milk decreases the risk of neonatal necrotizing enterocolitis, *Adv Nutr Res* 10:123, 2001.

31. Picciano MF: Human milk: nutritional aspects of a dynamic food, *Biol Neonate* 74:84, 1998.

32. Riordan J: *The biological specificity of breastmilk*, ed 2, Boston, 1998, Jones and Bartlett.

33. do Nascimento MB, Issler H: Breastfeeding: Making the difference in the development, health and nutrition of term and preterm newborns, *Rev Hosp Clin Fac Med Sao Paulo* 58:49, 2003.

34. Hanson LA, Korotkova M: The role of breastfeeding in prevention of neonatal infection, *Semin Neonatol* 7:275, 2002.

35. Morley R, Lucas A: Influence of early diet on outcome in preterm infants, *Acta Paediatr* Suppl 405:123, 1994.

36. Jewell VC, Northrop-Clewes CA, Tubman R et al: Nutritional factors and visual function in premature infants, *Proc Nutr Soc* 60:171, 2001.

37. Connor WE, Neuringer M, Reisbick S: Essential fatty acids: The importance of n-3 fatty acids in the retina and brain, *Nutr Rev* 50:21, 1992.

38. Neuringer M: Cerebral cortex docosahexaenoic acid is lower in formula-fed than in breast-fed infants, *Nutr Rev* 51:238, 1993.

39. Chandra R, Bhat BV, Puri RK: Why breast feed? *Indian Pediatr* 30:841, 1993.

40. Sheard NF: Breast-feeding protects against otitis media, *Nutr Rev* 51:275, 1993.

41. Bancalari E: Changes in the pathogenesis and prevention of chronic lung disease of prematurity, *Am J Perinatol* 18:1, 2001.

42. Pellegrini M, Lagrasta N, Garcia C et al: Neonatal necrotizing enterocolitis: A focus on, *Eur Rev Med Pharmacol Sci* 6:19, 2002.

43. Cymbaluk NF, Laarveld B: The ontogeny of serum insulin-like growth factor-I concentration in foals: Effects of dam parity, diet, and age at weaning, *Domest Anim Endocrinol* 13:197, 1996.

44. Mitra AK, Mahalanabis D, Ashraf H et al: Hyperimmune cow colostrum reduces diarrhoea due to rotavirus: A double-blind, controlled clinical trial, *Acta Paediatr* 84:996, 1995.

45. Koterba AM: Chapter 34: Nutritional support: Enteral feeding. *In* Koterba AM, Drummond WH, Kosch PC, eds: *Equine clinical neonatology*, Philadelphia, 1990, Lea & Febiger.

46. Pugh DG, Williams MA: Feeding foals from birth to weaning, *Compend Contin Educ Pract Vet* 14:526, 1992.

47. Vaala WE: *Nutritional management of the critically ill neonate*, Philadelphia, 1992, WB Saunders.

48. Kohn CW, Knight DA, Yvorchyk-St Jean KE et al: A preliminary study of the tolerance of healthy foals to a low residue enteral feeding solution, *Equine Vet J* 23:374, 1991.

49. Lundin C, Sullins KE, White NA et al: Induction of peritoneal adhesions with small intestinal ischaemia and distention in the foal, *Equine Vet J* 21:451, 1989.

50. Premji S, Chessell L: Continuous nasogastric milk feeding versus intermittent bolus milk feeding for premature infants less than 1500 grams, *Cochrane Database Syst Rev* CD001819, 2003.

51. Lewis LD: Nutrition for the broodmare and growing horse and its role in epiphysitis, *Proc 25th Annu Conv AAEP* 269, 1979.

52. Paradis MR: Nutrition and indirect calorimetry in neonatal foals, *Proc. 19th ACVIM*, Denver, CO 19:245, 2001.

53. Chwals WJ: Overfeeding the critically ill child: Fact or fantasy? *New Horiz* 2:147, 1994.

54. Plank LD, Hill GL: Energy balance in critical illness, *Proc Nutr Soc* 62:545, 2003.

55. Hansen TH: Chapter 35: Nutritional support: Parenteral feeding. *In* Koterba AM, Drummond WH, Kosch PC, eds: *Equine clinical neonatology*, Philadelphia, 1990, Lea & Febiger.

56. Koterba AM, Drummond WH: Nutritional support of the foal during intensive care, *Vet Clin North Am Equine Pract* 1:35, 1985.

57. Spurlock SL: Nutritional support of the ill equine neonate, *Equine Pract* 14:22, 1992.

58. Diehl-Jones WL, Askin DF: Nutritional modulation of neonatal outcomes, *AACN Clin Issues* 15:83, 2004.

59. Guedon C, Schmitz J, Lerebours E et al: Decreased brush border hydrolase activities without gross morphologic changes in human intestinal mucosa after prolonged total parenteral nutrition of adults, *Gastroenterology* 90:373, 1986.

60. Sedman PC, Macfie J, Sagar P et al: The prevalence of gut translocation in humans, *Gastroenterology* 107:643, 1994.

61. McClave SA, Lowen CC, Kleber MJ et al: Are patients fed appropriately according to their caloric requirements? *J Parenter Enteral Nutr* 22:375, 1998.

62. Jeejeebhoy KN: Enteral and parenteral nutrition: Evidence-based approach, *Proc Nutr Soc* 60:399, 2001.

63. Jeejeebhoy KN: Total parenteral nutrition: Potion or poison? *Am J Clin Nutr* 74:160, 2001.

64. Moore FA, Moore EE, Jones TN et al: TEN versus TPN following major abdominal trauma—reduced septic morbidity, *J Trauma* 29:916, 1989.

65. Kanarek KS, Santeiro ML, Malone JI: Continuous infusion of insulin in hyperglycemic low-birth weight infants receiving parenteral nutrition with and without lipid emulsion, *J Parenter Enteral Nutr* 15:417, 1991.

66. Buechner-Maxwell VA: Hyperglycemia in a neonatal foal: Management with continuous insulin infusion, *Equine Pract* 16:13, 1994.

67. Koterba AM: Appendix 1. In Koterba AM, Drummond WH, Kosch PC, eds: *Clinical equine neonatology*, Philadelphia, 1990, Lea & Febiger.

68. Evans TJ, Youngist RS, Loch WE, et al: A comparison of the relative efficacies of domperidone and reserpine in treating equine "fescuetoxicosis," *Proc 45th Ann Conven AAEP* 207, 1999.

69. Chavatte-Palmer P, Arnaud G, Duvaux-Ponter C, et al: Quantitative and qualitative assessment of milk production after pharmaceutical induction of lactation in the mare, *JVIM* 16:472, 2002.

5 Septicemia

Case 5-1	Septic Foal
	Michelle Henry Barton

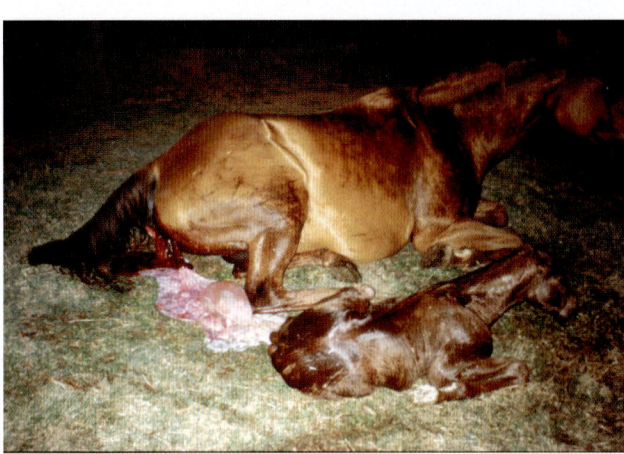

Fig. 5-1 Bugs Bunny and her 2002 foal shortly after birth. Despite prolonged gestation and an assisted delivery, the foal was able to attain sternal recumbency within minutes of birth.

Bugs Bunny, an 18-year-old Quarter Horse mare, had an uneventful fourth pregnancy, with the exception that she developed edema in the udder and the caudal dependent abdomen in the two weeks prior to parturition. All of her previous pregnancies were uncomplicated with parturition occurring between 345 and 350 days gestation. Her previous foals did well. Bugs Bunny foaled on Bermuda grass pasture in central Georgia in a gentle rain at 1 AM on March 13, 2002, at 360 days gestation. The mare was fitted with a Foal Alert™ monitor (Foal Alert, Atlanta, GA) and thus foaling was attended by the owners. Thirty minutes after presentation of both forelegs and the head, foaling had not progressed. The owners assisted delivery of the foal by traction on the forelimbs. The foal was able to attain sternal recumbency in several minutes and had a suckle reflex (Figure 5-1). The mare stood within 15 minutes of foaling. Bugs Bunny passed her placenta within one hour, and the owners reported that it appeared grossly normal and intact.

'02 Bugs Bunny stood with assistance two hours after birth and was nursing the mare within three hours of birth. The owners reported that once the foal nursed, she appeared more vigorous. The foal passed meconium within four hours. By 12 hours of age, the foal was reported to be tracking the mare and nursing several times per hour. By 24 hours of age, she appeared less interested in nursing and was seen in recumbency more frequently, but would rise when approached. By 36 hours of age, yellow diarrhea developed and the foal would only rise from recumbency if assisted. The local veterinarian was called and concurred with the owner's report of a lethargic foal. The rectal temperature was 103°F (39.4°C). The results of a SNAP™ test (IDEXX Laboratories, Westbrook, MN) revealed an IgG concentration of 400 to 800 mg/dl. Bugs Bunny and her foal were referred for further evaluation for suspicion of infection.

PATHOGENESIS OF INFECTION IN NEONATES

Infection, defined as the presence of microbes (bacteria, viruses, or fungi) inducing a host response,[1] is often cited as the most common cause of illness and/or mortality in foals in the perinatal period. However, the actual incidence of perinatal infection in the general equine population is not well-known, relative to other noninfectious causes of morbidity or mortality. "Serious" infection in the first 90 days of life was reported in 37 of 132 foals (28%) on a Standardbred farm in New York over the 1986 foaling season.[2] In contrast, in Stoneham's survey of Thoroughbred stud farms during three breeding seasons (1988 to 1990) in the United Kingdom, only 11 of 406 foals (2.7%) were reported to have infection in the first four weeks of life.[3]

In terms of neonatal mortality, the role of infection is more obvious: septicemia was the reported cause of death in 26% of 334 foals less than 10 days of age born on a large farm in 1994 in Canada.[4] In this review, sepsis was only marginally outnumbered by deaths caused from starvation or exposure (27%). In an extensive review of 3,514 pathology case reports in Kentucky from 1986 to 1991 on aborted fetuses, stillbirths, and foals that died less than 24 hours after birth, the most frequently cited cause of death was fetoplacental infection, which accounted for one third of the total cases.[5] A large-scale study of 167 farms in Texas in 1991 involving 2,468 foals revealed that septicemia was responsible for 30% of the deaths in foals less than seven days of age.[6] Geographical factors, management practices, and lack of detailed farm records likely account for the wide variation in the reported incidence of morbidity and/or mortality from perinatal infection in the general foal population.

In tertiary care centers, however, perinatal infection is consistently reported as one of the most common reasons for referral. At the University of Florida and the New Bolton Center at the University of Pennsylvania, blood is cultured from all foals that are admitted into their intensive care units. The reported incidence of positive blood cultures from these populations of foals are 26% and 28%, respectively.[7,8] At the University of Georgia, from 1986 to 2000, a review of 507 records on all foals that were less than two weeks of age revealed that 250 foals were ultimately diagnosed with infection, based on a positive blood culture, positive sepsis score, or clinical or postmortem evidence of infection in three or more tissues.[9] Considering that half of all admitted foals in the later study had evidence of significant infection, special attention needs to be focused on earlier recognition. Foal owners, care providers, and veterinarians should be familiar with historical events or prevailing conditions during the perinatal period that increase the likelihood of acquiring infection.

Colonization, or the presence of proliferating microbes without a host response, is an expected, and in many tissues, a beneficial event that prevents invasion by unwanted microbes. However, if microbial exposure or colonization leads to invasion of normally sterile tissue or evokes a response from the host, infection or sepsis has been initiated. Prevention of infection is policed by innate immunity, the branch of the host defense system that does not require previous exposure to a microbe to immediately counteract with a protective response. Simply stated, infection implies that two main events have occurred: the foal has been exposed to microbes, and the defensive response was inadequate. Whether microbial tissue invasion is contained locally or gains further widespread access depends heavily on an appropriate and competent response from the innate immune system. Microbial invasion into the bloodstream, with a concurrent systemic host response, is termed *septicemia.*

The perinatal environment is packed with microbes that may eventually gain access to the general circulation after local invasion of the skin or mucosal membranes (by inhalation or ingestion) and more directly, via the umbilical blood supply *in utero* or postpartum. Ironically, despite instinctual protective behavior, the dams themselves often serve as the direct source of potentially harmful microbes that eventually invade their offspring. The dam may inadvertently pass microbes directly to the foal *in utero* or during parturition, as a result of uterine, placental, vaginal, or intestinal (feces) infection. Bacteria that are considered "normal flora" on the mare's skin, or respiratory, vaginal, or intestinal mucosae may serve as potential contagion during normal postpartum behaviors such as the mare licking the foal and the foal udder seeking. Microbes present in the soil, feed, bedding, and feces serve as a vast reservoir of prospective invaders to which some degree of exposure is difficult, if not impossible, to avoid.

Considering the main ports of bacterial invasion, the skin, respiratory and intestinal mucosae, and umbilicus, the intestinal tract may actually serve as the most welcoming route of invasion. In the first hours of life, the cells that line the newborn foal's small intestine are uniquely poised to engulf colostral immunoglobulins. However, it appears that this process is not discriminate to immunoglobulins, as other large (synthetic) molecular weight compounds can be equally absorbed by pinocytosis during this early postpartum period.[10] Additionally, lack of tight junctions between intestinal cells during this period can freely allow large molecules to pass into the lymphatics.[11,12] Although not directly proven, this period of time during which colostral absorption occurs could hypothetically allow bacteria to cross the intestinal barrier, into the interstitium, lymphatics, and bloodstream.[11]

In light of these potential exposures, it has been suggested that the risk of microbial invasion by the oral route can be reduced if mares foal on pasture or a well-kept, clean, and disinfected stall. The mare's perineum, hindquarters, and udder should be washed and disinfected postpartum after passage of the placenta, and the foal should not be allowed to udder seek until this task has been accomplished.[11] It has also been suggested to manually strip the mare's colostrum, after disinfection of the udder, and to bottle or tube feed the foal prior to the foal contacting the mare. These practices have been shown in some situations to successfully prevent neonatal infection, even in foals with failure of passive transfer (FPT)[11] or in foals whose dams were shedding Salmonella in their feces.[13] The actual success of some of these recommendations is not entirely known. Although one large study involving 167 farms showed that the incidence of diarrhea was significantly lower in foals that were born on pasture compared to those born in stalls, the incidence of septicemia was the same despite foaling location.[6]

In consideration of the umbilical route of microbial invasion, foaling on pasture or a well-kept stall may also reduce the risk of omphalophlebitis. Allowing the cord to sever naturally allows the umbilical vessels to retract internally, and may reduce the risk of infection. If the cord must be manually severed or cut, first ligate the cord with umbilical tape and sever or cut distally. Finally, umbilical cord disinfection in the immediate postpartum period has been a long-standing recommendation as a "standard of neonatal care"; however, distinct evidence-based data on the best disinfection protocol to use in foals or if umbilical cord disinfection truly prevents infection are deficient. Allowing some degree of cord colonization may in fact be beneficial.

Avoidance of extensive wetness with disinfection of the umbilical cord is also recommended and is the premise for use of ethanol or 80% ethanol/0.5% chlorhexadine solution in human infants.[14] In foals, chlorhexadine solution (0.5%) appears to be superior to 2% iodine or Betadine solutions.[15] Harsh disinfection with tincture of iodine or Lugol's solution can cause tissue necrosis, and neither of these should be used. Often cord disinfection is repeated several times in the first day or first few days postpartum, but attention should be focused on avoiding excessive desiccation or dampness of the umbilical cord.

THE INNATE IMMUNE SYSTEM

A key player in the ultimate battle between microbial colonization and establishment of infection is the innate immune system.[16-18] Unlike adaptive immunity, which provides targeted defense against specific antigens that is magnified with each subsequent exposure, the innate immune system is comprised of components that provide unconditional defense, and therefore relies on immediate and less specific recognition of invading microbes. Neonatal foals are capable of initiating directed and specific responses against microbes, however it is the lag in the adaptive response that makes foals particularly susceptible to infection and more dependent on the innate immune system, compared to adult horses. A main feature of the innate immune system that enables immediate discrimination is pattern-recognition receptors (PRRs) that are capable of detecting a variety of microbial ligands, referred to as pathogen-associated molecular patterns (PAMPs).[17] These ligands are evolutionarily conserved molecules that are unique to microbes, are often shared by a broad range of organisms, and are usually essential for microbial survival or virulence. PRRs may be present on host cell membranes, in the circulation, or on mucosal surfaces, and they may be constitutively expressed and/or are released or secreted during the acute response to microbial invasion.

Examples of PAMPs include bacterial cell wall extracts, such as endotoxin, peptidoglycan and lipotechoic acid, and prokaryotic DNA. There is a complex and overlapping arsenal of PRRs, including the family of cationic antimicrobial peptides, such as defensins; collectins, such as mannose binding lectin; enzymes; integrins; and some of the acute-phase proteins. Ultimately, the interaction of a PRR with its PAMP can result in direct neutralization of the PAMP or microbe, or it may activate other components of the host immune system to deploy further defense mechanisms, initiate an inflammatory response, or commence tissue repair.[16,17]

A notorious PAMP in septicemia is endotoxin, with its respective mammalian host PRRs, lipopolysaccharide-binding protein (LBP), CD14, and Toll-like receptors (TLRs).[19-21] Endotoxin is released from the outer cell membrane of Gram-negative bacteria during either rapid bacterial replication or upon bacteriolysis. It is comprised of three components, a long polysaccharide outer chain, a short polysaccharide core, and lipid A, which is the toxic moiety. Once in the blood, endotoxin's amphipathic properties cause it to form aggregates that resemble micelles. LBP is a plasma constituent that serves as a PRR and efficiently extracts monomers of endotoxin from its circulating aggregates and shuttles it to various locations.[19] Through its interaction with lipid A, LBP effectively imprisons endotoxin, with its potential for toxicity determined by the complex's final destination. LBP can rapidly deliver monomers of endotoxin to the surface of host inflammatory cells to evoke an inflammatory response, or it can be transferred to other neutralizing lipoproteins, such as high-density lipoprotein, for eventual removal from the blood. Thus LBP may serve to both enhance and hinder the biologic activities of endotoxin.

Once at the cell surface, endotoxin is transferred to cluster differentiation antigen 14 (CD14), a well-conserved PRR that is attached to the cell membrane by a glycosylphosphatidylinositol anchor.[21] Mononuclear phagocytes (monocytes and macrophages) express abundant CD14, though other inflammatory cells also express minute amounts. CD14 is a 53 kDa glycoprotein that exists as both a cell membrane receptor (mCD14) and as a soluble form (sCD14) in the circulation, which is essentially identical to membrane-bound CD14 minus the glycosylphosphatidylinositol anchor. Similar to LBP's roles, sCD14 is normally present in the circulation and has dual functions. It may bind and neutralize circulating endotoxin, thereby competing with membrane CD14. However, it may also enhance endotoxin's toxic effects by transferring it to membrane CD14 or to cells that do not express membrane CD14. Another newly described source of CD14 is a smaller isoform found in extremely high concentrations in colostrum. This colostral CD14 is not present in the serum of foals prior to nursing, but it is readily detected after ingestion of colostrum.[22] The exact role of colostral CD14 has not been fully elucidated, though if its roles are similar to sCD14, it may serve to either neutralize endotoxin or to alarm the host of bacterial presence.

Because CD14 does not structurally transverse the cell membrane, it must associate with a secondary protein, TLR, which contains a transmembrane portion that is capable of communication with the intracellular domain. CD14 binds to isolated monomers of endotoxin, intact bacteria, as well as several other PAMPS of Gram-positive bacteria. The name *Toll-like receptor* was adapted because of homology with a receptor found in Drosophila, called "Toll" that is responsible for dorsal-ventral polarity and innate immunity in fruit flies.[20] Approximately a dozen TLRs have been identified, but TLR type 4 (TLR4) appears to be the isotype most important in the recognition of endotoxin, whereas TLR type 2 primarily confers recognition of Gram-positive bacterial components. Once the CD14-TLR4-endotoxin complex is complied at the cell surface, TLR4 requires a 160 amino acid helper molecule, MD2, to transmit a signal to the cytosol. Several intracellular signaling pathways have been reported to link a ligand-occupied PRR to cell activation, but the nuclear factor (NF) pathway is well characterized in its role for activating the promoter regions of inflammatory mediator genes.

Simply stated, the deleterious effects of endotoxin are the result of its interaction with host PRRs, subsequent gene activation, and synthesis of endogenous inflammatory mediators. The culmination of events in endotoxemia through the actions of these endogenous mediators is intense inflammation, immunosuppression, alterations in hemodynamics, and coagulopathy. Decreased peripheral vascular resistance, myocardial depression, hypovolemia, and microvascular thrombosis all contribute to reduction of blood flow to vital organs that may become so intense, that if left unchecked, the response to the presence of infection may be as injurious as the bacterial assault itself.

Although endotoxin and activation of its PRRs explain how the innate immune system recognizes and responds to infection, it is only a one component of host defense. The innate immune system entwines several redundant levels of protection including the macroenvironment of physiologic barriers (skin and mucosa), the microscopic protection furnished by phagocytes (principally neutrophils, monocytes, and macrophages), and molecular defense (PRRs, immunoglobulins, complement, and acute phase proteins).[17] The skin deters bacterial invasion by providing a physical barrier between the environment and deeper host tissue, in the form of host cells and normal flora. Other important components of resistance to colonization of the skin are an acidic pH, secretion of fatty acids, and the ability to "shed" cells.[23]

Like the skin, the mucosal surfaces of the gastrointestinal, respiratory, and genitourinary tracts provide a physical cell barrier that can desquamate, have normal flora, and abundant mucus that prevents colonization. The respiratory tract contains numerous "filters" that can trap bacteria that is inhaled, such as the turbinates, the long trachea, and ciliated respiratory tract lining cells. Mucosal epithelial cells in the gastrointestinal, respiratory, and genitourinary tracts secrete PRRs, such as defensins and collectins, which cause bacteriolysis and increase opsonization by phagocytes. Additional chemical defenses in the gastrointestinal tract include peroxidases, the acidic pH of the stomach, proteolytic enzymes, and lysozyme, all substances that can challenge bacterial cell wall integrity.[23] Finally, physiologic activities such as sneezing, coughing, salivation, and peristalsis can also serve to remove potential pathogens.

Phagocytes, principally neutrophils, monocytes, and tissue-fixed macrophages, play a key role in innate immunity.[17,23] In addition to engulfing and destroying bacteria via various oxidative, acidifying, and enzymatic mechanisms, neutrophils and monocytes secrete numerous substances, such as cytokines, growth factors, lactoferrin, and interferon, that can induce chemotaxis, enhance phagocytosis, cause bacteriolysis, or inhibit microbial replication.[24] Although it has been shown that equine neutrophils are functional at birth, compared to neutrophils from adult horses, phagocytosis, oxidative burst activity, and killing are reduced in the first one to two weeks of life.[25,26] These deficiencies are further exacerbated by FPT, as IgG and complement are needed for optimal phagocytosis of bacteria. Clearly these deficiencies in phagocytic activity in the newborn foal increase the susceptibility to microbial invasion in the perinatal period.

Lastly, the innate immune system is comprised of an extensive array of soluble molecules in the circulation, including PRRs, cytokines, chemokines, immunoglobulins, acute phase proteins, and other proinflammatory and anti-inflammatory mediators. Many of these molecular components are also present on cell surfaces, intracellularly, and on mucosal surfaces. Their overlapping presence in more than one tissue, the dynamic discovery of new molecules and rediscovery of new roles for previously identified molecules, confuses their classification. Although immunoglobulins are classically linked to adaptive immunity and anamnestic defense, they are a critical component for opsonization and the immediate defense against bacteria. The unique placental attachment in horses prevents placental transfer of immunoglobulins during gestation, thus foals are born agammaglobulinemic.[10] Colostrum provides an immediate source of immunoglobulins, and failure of acquisition or absorption of colostral antibodies (FPT, see Chapter 3) in the first day of life has been well recognized as a major risk for infection.[6,27-29] The fact that some foals with adequate serum IgG still acquire infection and that some foals with inadequate serum IgG do not acquire infection in the perinatal period[2] supports the notion that the likelihood of infection is a combination of the risks of exposure and colonization, counterbalanced by the ability to defend from invasion. Regardless of inadequate serum IgG concentration, if exposure to microbes is minimized, then intuitively, infection is less likely to occur. Furthermore, IgG is not the only factor available to the foal for immediate defense against microbes, thus despite FPT, other components of the immune system may provide sufficient protection.

ACUTE PHASE RESPONSE

An acute phase protein is any protein whose blood concentration significantly increases during an inflammatory response.[30] Collectively, acute phase proteins are responsible for many of the well-recognized reactions to microbial invasion, such as fever, anorexia, depression, and alterations in metabolism, hemodynamics, coagulation, and leukocyte activation. The liver is a key site of synthesis of the acute phase proteins, however some, such as ceruloplasm, complement components, and serum amyloid A, can also be produced extrahepatically.

Cytokines, principally tumor necrosis factor, interleukin 1β and interleukin 6, glucocorticoids, and growth factors stimulate and modulate gene expression and the transcription of the acute phase proteins. The serum concentrations of the major acute phase proteins—serum amyloid A (SAA) and C-reactive protein (CRP), and α-1-acid-glycoprotein (AGP)—can each increase as much as 1000-fold during the acute phase response.[30] Interestingly, despite their intense synthesis during the acute phase reaction, the roles of each of these major proteins are still not entirely clear. SAA may be involved in cholesterol regulation, chemotaxis, and mediating anti-inflammatory events, such as down-regulation of fever, phagocytosis, and prostanoid synthesis. CRP can activate complement, induce phagocytosis, and stimulate cytokine and tissue factor expression. AGP is considered an anti-inflammatory agent as it reduces both complement- and phagocyte-mediated tissue injury and inhibits platelet aggregation.[30] SAA concentrations have been determined by use of a latex agglutination assay in both healthy and ill foals.[31] The expected SAA concentration in healthy Thoroughbred foals one to three days of age is <27 mg/liter, whereas foals with focal infection or septicemia have >100 mg SAA/liter. C-reactive protein concentrations have been established in healthy foals[32] and adult horses with experimentally induced inflammation, however their utility in determining an inflammatory response in naturally-occurring diseases in foals has not be fully established.

The remaining acute phase proteins have widely diverse pathophysiologic effects. The complement system is represented by the acute phase synthesis of C3, C4, C9, Factor B, C1 inhibitor, and C4b-binding protein.[30] If a host is immunologically naïve to a pathogen, and therefore does not have specific antibody, the alternative complement pathway is evoked, activating compounds that will induce bacteriolysis, provide components that are chemotactic for neutrophils, and enhance neutrophil opsonization of both microbes and damaged host cells. The importance of complement in host defense is exemplified by the finding that opsonization of E. coli and Actinobacillus are reduced by 50% in heat-treated serum, a process that destroys complement.[33]

Balanced activation of the coagulation and fibrinolytic systems by the acute phase response of factor VIII, fibrinogen, plasminogen, tissue plasminogen activator, plasminogen activator inhibitor, fibronectin, von Willebrand factor, and tissue factor leads to formation of intravascular and extravascular "clots" that serve to capture and contain infectious organisms and inflammatory debris and to provide a scaffold for tissue repair.[34]

The release of transport and scavenger proteins, such as ceruloplasmin, haptoglobin, LBP, soluble CD14, and lactoferrin serve to bind bacterial nutrient components, such as copper and iron, and to neutralize or transport toxic bacterial components. Finally, protease inhibitors, such as α 1 protease inhibitor, serve to control tissue destruction.

SIRS, CARS, MARS, AND MODS

The ultimate goals of the innate immune system and the acute phase response are to contain infection, alarm the host to defend, and promote tissue repair. Whether these goals are achieved or defeated, the process of infection and defense against it may lead to systemic illness. In other words, even a successful campaign against microbial invasion can produce systemic disease. The host relies on a defense response from the innate immune system that is appropriate for the insult.[18,35] If the innate immune system overzealously responds, the same components that are meant to protect the host may ironically be just as detrimental as or even more harmful to the host than the initial bacterial insult. It is the intensity of the invasion and the degree of balance in the host's immune response that determine the final deposition of a microbial assault.

When the retort to infection results in an incongruous and exaggerated systemic inflammatory reaction, the clinical state is referred to as the Systemic Inflammatory Response Syndrome (SIRS).[1] It is important to note that although this discussion of SIRS focuses on an infectious stimulus, SIRS can be initiated by noninfectious insults, such as severe trauma, hypothermia, hyperthermia, or intense hypoxemia. Sepsis and septicemia are SIRS induced by local and blood infection, respectively. To counteract the pro-inflammatory response and deter the state of SIRS, the host relies on anti-inflammatory opposition that includes production of cytokines (interleukins 4, 10, 11, 13), soluble cytokine receptors, receptor antagonists, prostaglandin E_2, and corticosteroids.[36]

If there is over-recruitment of the anti-inflammatory processes, a state of anergy, increased susceptibility to infection, and inability to repair damaged tissues ensues. This scenario is referred to as Compensatory Anti-inflammatory Response Syndrome (CARS).[1] In some circumstances, a Mixed Anti-inflammatory Response Syndrome (MARS) arises in which surges of both SIRS and CARS coexist.[1] In the circle of equilibrium, if SIRS and CARS are ultimately appropriately balanced, then homeostasis resumes. Predominance of SIRS may culminate in adverse pathophysiologic events, such as disseminated intravascular coagulation (DIC), shock, organ failure, and death. In this later scenario, dissonance has occurred and the patient is defined as having Multiple Organ Dysfunction Syndrome (MODS) or the presence of organ dysfunction associated with acute illness in which homeostasis can not be restored without intervention.[1]

In summary, infection of the neonatal foal results from a combination of exposure to microbes and colonization of host tissue coupled with failure of the innate immune system to prevent microbial proliferation and invasion into deeper tissue. The outcome of infection is further determined by the appropriateness of the host's defense response. With these facts in mind, when obtaining a history on neonatal foals, careful attention should be directed toward identifying potential exposures to microbes (in magnitude and virulence), as well as identifying factors that may affect immunocompetency of the patient. Box 5-1 summarizes historical events that have been associated with increased risk of sepsis in the neonatal foal.

Box 5.1   Historical Factors Associated with Increased Risk of Acquired Infection in the Perinatal Period

Factors associated with the mare
- Advanced maternal age
- Significant stress or illness during pregnancy
- Occult carrier of pathogens, e.g., herpesvirus, Salmonella, Clostridium
- Uterine, vaginal, or placental infection
- Twinning
- Premature delivery, prolonged gestation, dystocia, induction of labor
- Premature lactation, agalactia
- Fescue toxicity
- Foaling in confinement
- Long transportation during late pregnancy
- Movement of the mare to different facilities during the last month of pregnancy
- Rejection of the foal

Factors associated with the foal
- Failure of passive transfer
- Weakness for any reason that results in delayed or inadequate nursing
  - Prematurity, dysmaturity, dystocia, twinning
  - Congenital deformities that interfere with ability to ambulate or nurse
  - Neurologic disease (Neonatal encephalopathy)
  - Neonatal isoerythrolysis
  - Perinatal asphyxia, respiratory distress, meconium aspiration
- Barrier invasion by microbes
  - Skin trauma or wounds
  - Gastrointestinal disease
  - Respiratory disease
  - Umbilicus not properly severed or disinfected, patent urachus
  - Excessive exposure to environmental microbes or normal flora of dam before ingestion of colostrum

---

In the case of Bugs Bunny, aside from normal flora, the mare did not have any additional signs of infection during pregnancy or at the time of parturition that would increase the risk of infection to the foal. By foaling on pasture, exposure to feces and soiled bedding were avoided, however the rainy weather at the time of parturition may have potentially increased exposure to soil microbes. The owners did not provide postpartum umbilical disinfection. The gestational length and delivery were prolonged. These events may have contributed to a larger birth weight foal and dystocia, which produced a weaker foal, as evidenced by a slight delay in the onset of nursing. These events were potential contributing factors for FPT. The change in nursing behavior at 24 hours of age and longer periods of time in recumbency were both early signs of illness, prompting further investigation.

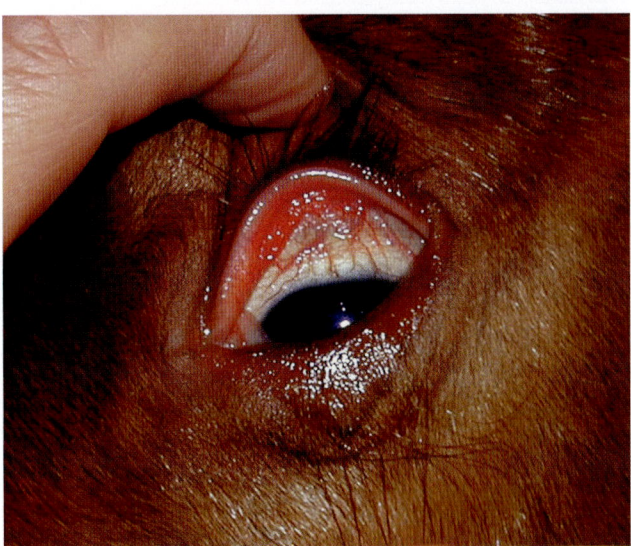

Fig. 5-2 '02 Bugs Bunny's moderately injected sclerae, an early sign of sepsis, at 36 hours of age.

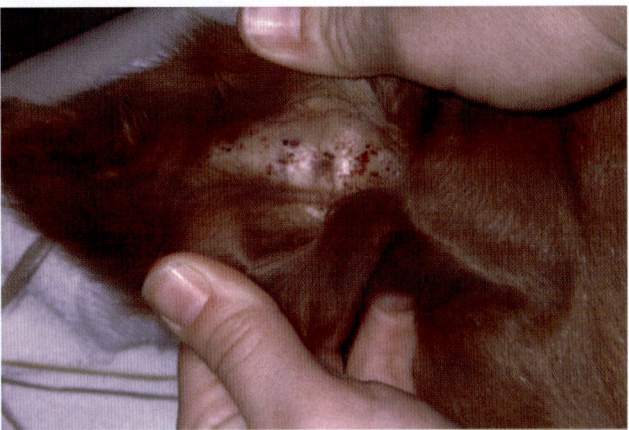

Fig. 5-3 '02 Bugs Bunny's aural petechiae, a reliable sign of sepsis, at 36 hours of age.

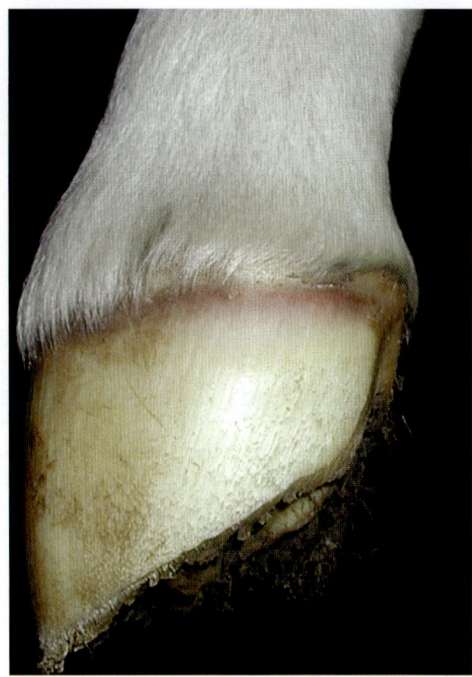

Fig. 5-4 '02 Bugs Bunny's hyperemic coronets, a sign of vasodilation, at 36 hours of age.

At the time of presentation to the Veterinary Teaching Hospital, Bugs Bunny was bright, alert, and responsive with normal vital signs. She appeared to have an adequate supply of milk. Her foal was recumbent, but able to stand with assistance. The foal's rectal temperature was 102.9°F (39.3°C), heart rate was 110 beats/minute, and respirations were 30 breaths per minute. The foal weighed 53 kg. The sclerae were moderately to severely injected (Figure 5-2), numerous petechiae were present in the pinnae (Figure 5-3), and the coronets were hyperemic (Figure 5-4). Low-volume yellow diarrhea was passed.

CLINICAL SIGNS AND PHYSICAL EXAMINATION FINDINGS ASSOCIATED WITH SEPTICEMIA

The clinical signs of sepsis depend on the duration and intensity of the microbial assault and the appropriate-

ness of the response from the host. As discussed in the last section, suitable defense should provide some degree of an effective "alarm" of infection. Typically, the prodromal signs of sepsis are subtle and often are not recognized by the caretaker. Knowledge of normal foal behavior and physical parameters (see Chapter 1) are paramount for early identification of illness. In performing the physical examination, the clinician should specifically try to identify: (1) the primary route of microbial invasion, (2) any signs of a clinical response to the presence of infection, (3) any signs of advancing microbial invasion into secondary sites, and (4) any signs of SIRS, CARS, or MODS.

FINDING THE PRIMARY SOURCE OF INFECTION

Despite thorough investigation, often the primary site or route of infection cannot be definitively identified. However, the skin; umbilicus; and digestive, respiratory, and genitourinary tracts should be carefully examined. The skin should be vigilantly examined for wounds. External evidence of omphalophlebitis may not be grossly apparent for several days to one to two weeks after initial infection. Occasionally, despite significant infection of the umbilical vessels or urachus interior to the body wall, there is no obvious evidence of disease in the external umbilical stump. Clinical signs that are consistent with infection of the umbilical remnants include heat, swelling, patency, pain of

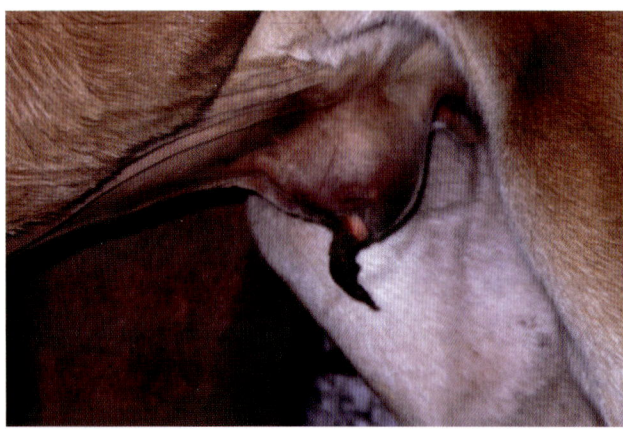

Fig. 5-5 The umbilicus should be carefully examined as a potential primary route of infection. Advanced signs of omphalophlebitis include umbilical stalk pain, heat, swelling, and discharge. Note that despite a normal appearing external umbilical stalk, significant infection may be present the internal umbilical structures.

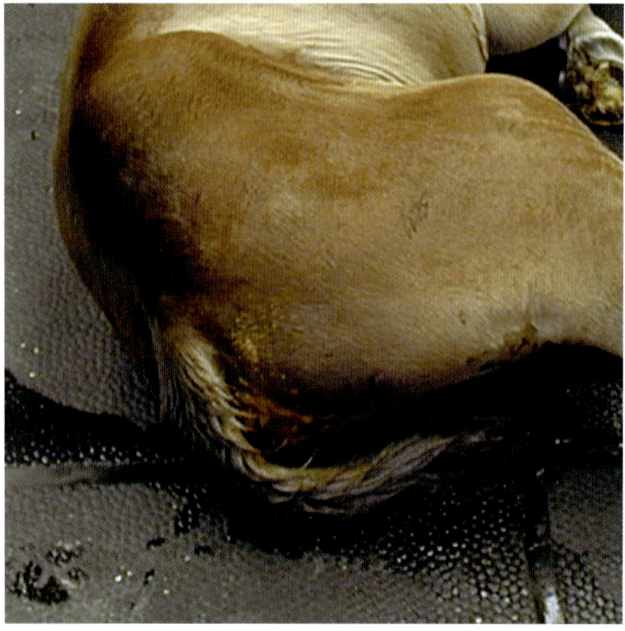

Fig. 5-6 Diarrhea in the first few days of life is not considered normal and may be a sign that the gastrointestinal tract is inflamed and a potential primary site of infection.

the umbilical stalk, or discharge or moistness from or around the stalk (Figure 5-5). Umbilical hernias are rarely associated with infection.

Diarrhea (Figure 5-6), bruxism, anorexia, and colic (see Chapter 11) may be signs that the gastrointestinal tract was the primary site of infection. Surprisingly, even severe infection of the respiratory tract may not manifest clinical signs in neonatal foals. Often the only signs of respiratory tract disease are the presence of

unexplained tachypnea, nasal flare, or dyspnea (see Case 6-1). Other localizing signs, such as nasal discharge, cough, pleurodynia, or audible abnormalities, when present, are incriminating clues.

RECOGNIZING THE FOAL'S RESPONSE TO INFECTION

The foal's response to sepsis can be highly variable, depending upon the duration and intensity of the septic insult. The acute phase response to infection should evoke signs of decreased activity, malaise, increased periods of recumbency, inability to track the mare, decreased frequency of nursing, and failure to gain weight. All of these later signs often are associated with the onset of fever triggered by synthesis of endogenous pyrogens, such as interleukin-1, tumor necrosis factor, and prostanoids. The cyclic nature of fever necessitates serial evaluation, otherwise it may be overlooked. Absence of a fever does not rule out sepsis in a foal. In fact many septic foals will present with hypothermia.

As the inflammatory response to infection intensifies, other signs of systemic disease appear including tachycardia, tachypnea, bilateral scleral injection (Figure 5-2), petechial hemorrhages of the pinnae (Figure 5-3), hyperemia of the coronary bands (Figure 5-4), unpigmented skin (Figure 5-7, *A*) and mucous membranes (Figure 5-7, *B* and *C*), and edema. Hyperemia and edema are the result of local vasodilation and increased permeability caused by the synthesis of vasoactive mediators including histamine, kinins, serotonin, eicosanoids, platelet activating factor, endothelin, and complement. Petechiae in the pinnae are an indicator of sepsis in the foal, though the exact cause is unclear. Petechiae most commonly develop as a result of either thrombocytopenia or vasculitis. As many foals with aural petechiae have normal platelet counts, it must be assumed that, in those cases, they are a sign of systemic vasculitis. Nonetheless, when petechiae are present, the platelet count should also be scrutinized.

IDENTIFICATION OF SECONDARY SITES OF INFECTION

If the innate immune system is incapable of controlling microbial invasion as septicemia progresses, secondary sites of infection may develop. With the bloodstream serving as a conduit, essentially all tissues of the body are susceptible to secondary infection (see Chapter 6). Tissues that receive a large portion of the cardiac output, and experience turbulent, slow, or unique blood supplies are targeted first and include

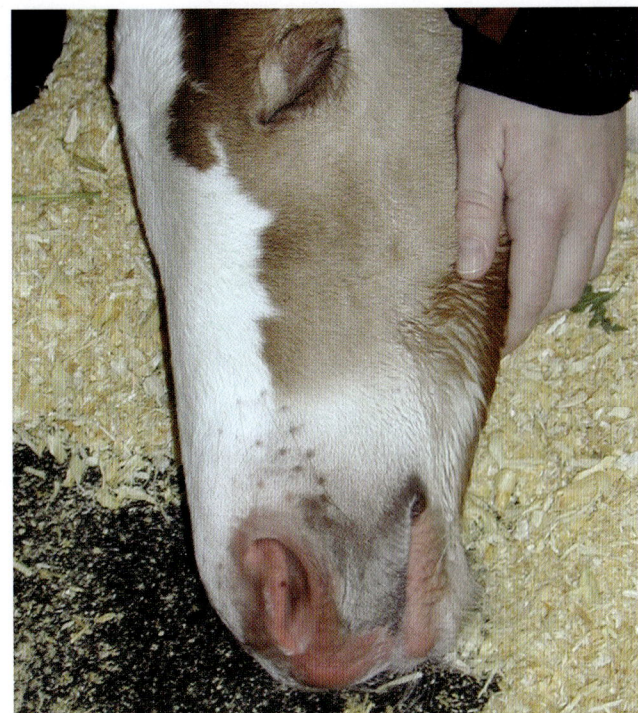

A

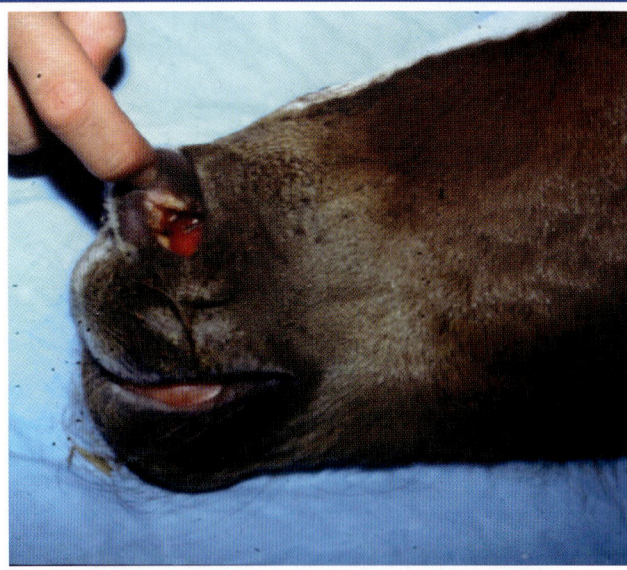

B

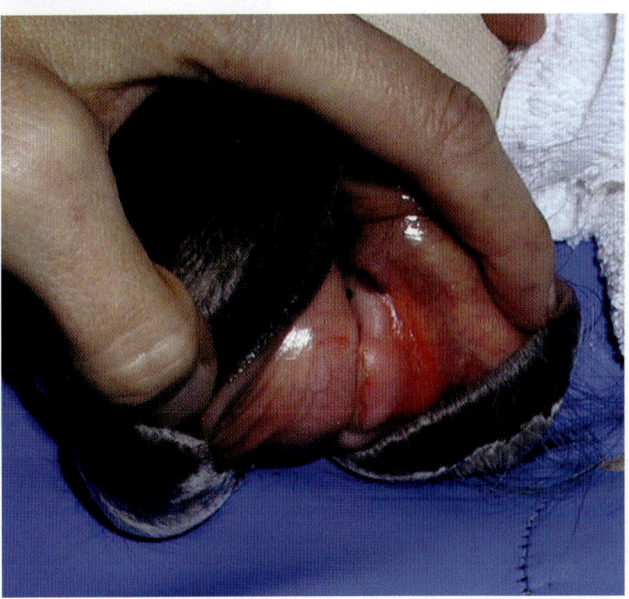

C

Fig. 5-7 Intense hyperemia is a sign of the systemic response to infection. **A,** hyperemia in the muzzle, **B,** in the nasal mucosa, and **C,** in the oral mucosa.

physes, synoviae, the uveal tract, meninges, endocardium, liver, kidney, and skin/muscle. Any neonatal foal that has joint swelling (Figure 5-8), periarticular edema, lameness, or prolonged recumbency should be carefully evaluated for sepsis (see Case 6-2). The cardinal signs of uveitis are blepharospasm, epiphora, miosis, aqueal flare, edema of the iris, and hypopyon (Figure 5-9). These signs most often manifest bilaterally in septic foals, though unilateral presentation can occur (see Chapter 14). Foals with meningitis (Figure 5-10) will often have an altered mental status, ataxia, seizures, and a stiff, "guarded" neck and gait (see Chapter 10).

Endocarditis is an infrequent complication of septicemia in foals. Tachycardia, tachyarrhythmia, lethargy, murmurs, jugular pulsation, and dependent edema may all be signs of endocarditis. Healthy neonatal foals will commonly have a low-grade systolic murmur over the semilunar valves over the left heart base. However, loud murmurs over the

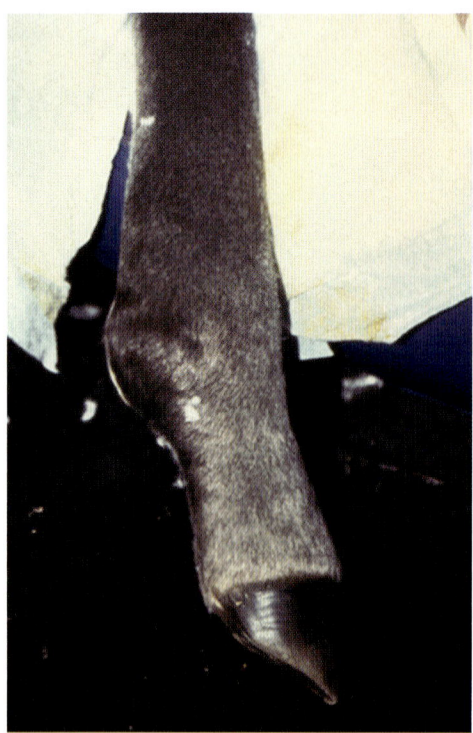

Fig. 5-8 Joint swelling, periarticular edema, and lameness are signs of secondary sites of infection and indicate advanced septicemia.

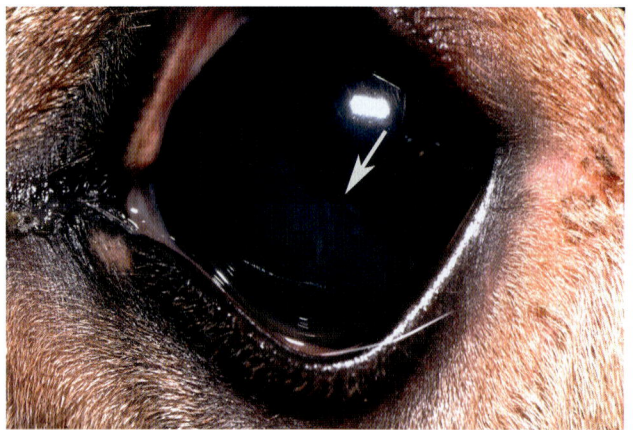

Fig. 5-9 The fibrin sheet (arrow) in the anterior chamber of this foal was present bilaterally and is a sign of uveitis and advanced septicemia.

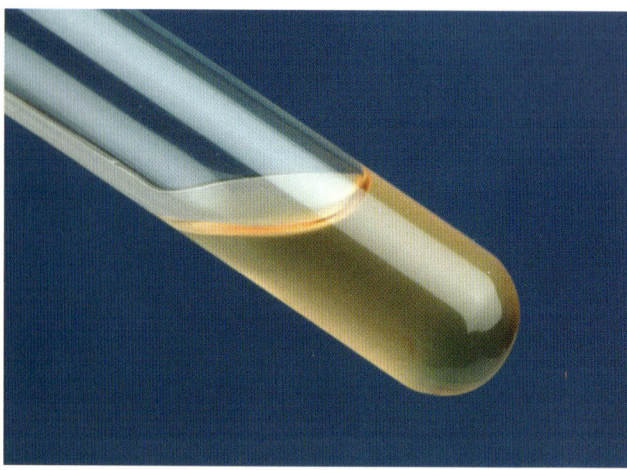

Fig. 5-10 This cerebrospinal fluid was collected from the lumbosacral site of a foal with fever, ataxia, and a stiff neck. The purulent nature of this fluid is consistent with meningitis, a sign of advanced septicemia. The nucleated cell count of this fluid was greater than 10,000/μl.

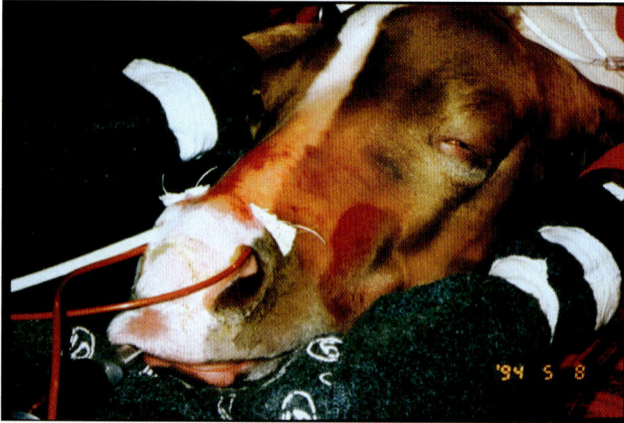

Fig. 5-11 Lack of eyelid and muzzle tone, comatose state, and large ecchymotic hemorrhages in this foal are signs of SIRS.

semilunar valves, murmurs over the mitral or tricuspid valves, or those that are accompanied by other signs of cardiac disease should be investigated further by echocardiography (see Chapter 13). Hepatic, splenic, and renal abscessation may occur secondary to septicemia, though secondary infection in these anatomic locations rarely causes significant clinical signs. *Actinobacillus equuli* is particularly known for its propensity to form secondary microabscesses in the liver and kidney.

ARE THERE SIGNS OF SHOCK OR SIRS?

When the systemic pro-inflammatory response to infection is uncontrolled and malignant, the clinical state of SIRS ensues. Any of the clinical signs of the acute phase response discussed above may be present and dynamically intensify. In addition, with loss of immunologic homeostasis, subsequent alterations in hemodynamics, the production of pro-inflammatory mediators, and unregulated coagulation, clinical signs of septic shock, DIC, and MODS arise (Figure 5-11).

Septic shock is defined as hypotension that is accompanied by signs of hypoperfusion (altered mental status, hypothermia, hypotension, shivering, cold extremities, mucous membrane pallor, bradycardia or tachycardia, poor capillary or jugular vein refill, poor pulse quality, oliguria, and ileus) that is induced by the presence of sepsis, is the result of systemic vasodilation, and persists despite adequate fluid resuscitation (see Chapter 7).

DIC is initiated by damaged endothelium, increased expression of tissue factor on monocytes and the endothelium, platelet activation and aggregation, and direct activation of the intrinsic coagulation system. Excessive consumption of components of the hemostatic and regulatory pathways (protein C, anthrombin III, fibrinolysis) transforms the process from clot formation to hemorrhage. Clinical signs of DIC are highly variable and may include thrombosis, widespread petechiae, ecchymoses, or hemorrhage into any tissue or from body orifices (Figure 5-11). The presence of an isolated cold limb with a reduced or undetectable pulse may be a sign of acute arterial thrombosis.[37,38] With the combination of endothelial damage, the release of vasoactive and proinflammatory mediators, and widespread vasodilation and microthrombi formation, tissue and organ damage ensues. The manifestations of MODS are vast, and the signs reflect the organs that are predominantly affected. These may include mental deterioration, ataxia, seizures, oliguria, dyspnea, tachypnea, tachycardia or bradycardia, colic, and/or ileus. Ultimately, identification of clinical signs or physical findings of secondary infection, SIRS, or MODS is significant. These conditions not only identify an advanced and improperly controlled disease state, but they are also associated with a more pessimistic prognosis.

Finally, when evaluating a neonatal foal for any disease entity, consider that any primary disease can induce a state of immunosuppression and/or cause loss of integrity of local protective barriers that subsequently welcomes infection. For example, other common diseases during the neonatal period, such as neonatal isoerythrolysis, neonatal encephalopathy, uroperitoneum, neonatal asphyxia syndrome, meconium impaction, diarrhea, or any cause of colic, may be complicated by concurrent infection.

While specifically examining '02 Bugs Bunny, several significant clinical findings that have been statistically associated with septicemia in foals were identified, including, depression, partial anorexia, fever, scleral injection, aural petechiae, hyperemia, and diarrhea.

*Blood was collected for immediate evaluation of glucose concentration, PCV, total solids concentration, quantification of IgG, and for submission for a complete blood count and serum chemistry profile. As detected by a glucometer (Accucheck, Roche Diagnostics, Alameda, CA), the blood glucose was 65mg/dl. The PCV was 36%, and total solids concentration was 4.5gm/dl. A SNAP™ test (IDEXX Laboratories) confirmed an IgG concentration of 400mg/dl. The complete blood count and serum chemistry results are reported in Table 5-1 and revealed neutropenia with a left shift, toxic morphology in the neutrophils, and mild hyperfibrinogenemia. The only abnormality noted on the chemistry profile was hypoproteinemia, characterized by hypoglobulinemia. The hair was clipped over the jugular vein, sterilely prepared, and 20ml of blood was aseptically collected by venipuncture for aerobic and anaerobic culture. A sample of diarrhea was collected for culture for **Salmonella** and for a **Clostridium perfringens** enterotoxin assay.*

DIAGNOSIS OF SEPTICEMIA

Blood Culture

Septicemia is defined as the systemic reaction caused by the presence of microorganisms or their toxins in the blood. Based on this definition, proof of septicemia

Table 5-1	Complete Blood Count and Serum Chemistry Evaluation of '02 Bugs Bunny						
Parameter	Admission (Two Days of Age)	Three Days of Age	Four Days of Age	Five Days of Age	Six Days of Age	Seven Days of Age	Fourteen Days of Age
White blood cell count/µl	8,920		9,345			16,137	12,101
Neutrophils/µl	2,587		3,521			12,030	7,559
Bands/µl	3,009		374			0	0
Lymphocytes/µl	3,093		5,044			3,307	4,200
Monocytes/µl	230		406			800	342
Platelets/µl	167,000						
Fibrinogen (mg/dl)	500		600			400	300
Creatinine (mg/dl)	1.7	2.9	2.8	2.2	1.7	1.1	0.9
Total protein (g/dl)	4.0	4.7				4.9	
Albumin (g/dl)	2.9	2.8				2.9	

depends upon identifying microorganisms or their toxins in the circulation or on identifying clinical signs, physical findings, or other laboratory diagnostics that are particular to the systemic response to septicemia. A positive blood culture is often considered as the "gold standard" of diagnostic proof of septicemia.

Various methods are described for obtaining blood cultures; however, controlled research determining the best method of culturing blood in foals is lacking. The hair over the site of venipuncture should be clipped and the skin surgically prepared. Use of sterile gloves and sterile handling of the venipuncture needle and syringe may reduce spurious skin contamination. The volume to be cultured varies with the collection device, but typically it is recommended to sterilely obtain 12 to 20 ml of blood. Exchanging the venipuncture needle with a new sterile needle prior to injection of the blood into the culture vials may also reduce contamination. There are several commercial blood culture vials, but most contain Columbia or trypticase soy broth, sodium polyanethol sulfonate as an anticoagulant, and are enriched with CO_2 (BBL Septi-check, Becton Dickinson, Franklin Lakes, NJ) Ideally, the blood should be split into two bottles. One bottle should be sterilely vented for aerobic culture, and the other should remain sealed for anaerobic culture.[7,8,39] Alternatively, special anaerobic bottles may be used.

The prevalence of positive blood cultures reported in foals that were ultimately diagnosed with septicemia, based on clinical signs or necropsy findings, varies from 60% to 88%.[7-9] The discrepancies in the percent of true positive blood cultures likely reflect differences in geographic location, management practices, case definition, use of antimicrobials, and culturing techniques. The results from one study suggested that it was more likely to miss a Gram-negative organism by blood culture than a Gram-positive organism.[8] Another study in foals indicated that antimicrobial use prior to blood culture did not significantly affect the culture outcome,[9] though use of cation exchange resins that remove antimicrobials from the blood sample prior to culture (Antimicrobial Removal Device [ARD], Marion Scientific, Kansas City, MO) has been shown to increase the positive blood culture rate from 72% to 95% in septicemic human patients.[40] Some clinicians prefer to obtain serial blood cultures, though this practice can be costly.

Taken collectively, although a positive blood culture is often considered a "gold standard" for proof of septicemia, its accuracy and lag time in identifying a truly septicemic foal are not ideal, and other sources of diagnostic evidence have been proposed, such as identification of pathogen-specific DNA[41] and microbial toxin analysis. Use of quantitative polymerase chain reaction (PCR) systems to detect nucleic acids of pathogens may greatly enhance the accuracy and speed of diag-

nosis, but has not been fully evaluated in septicemic foals. Lipopolysaccharide or endotoxin has been detected in the plasma of 10% to 50% of septic foals, but the assay is not commercially available and its use is currently limited to retrospective clinical studies.[34,42]

Sepsis Scoring System

To address the diagnostic limitations and the time delay inherent to blood culture analysis, one can turn to identification of historical data, clinical signs, physical findings, or routine laboratory diagnostic tests that are reliably associated with sepsis. This indeed was the premise for the development of the Sepsis Scoring System by Brewer and Koterba in the late 1980s at the University of Florida.[27] Vigorously tested, retrospectively and prospectively in foals less than 12 days of age, the Sepsis Scoring System uses a practical combination of historical, clinical, and diagnostic parameters that are statistically associated with sepsis (Table 5-2).

Historical facts and clinical findings used in this scoring system were discussed previously above in terms of how they relate to increased risk of acquiring infection or in light of the pathogenesis of septicemia. Laboratory tests that are statistically associated with sepsis include FPT, hypoglycemia, hypoxemia, acidosis, hyperfibrinogenemia, and changes in the morphology and numbers of circulating neutrophils. The role of IgG in innate immunity has been discussed previously in this chapter (also see Chapter 3).

Hypoglycemia develops as the combined result of reduced intake of milk, lack of sufficient glycogen stores in the neonate, and increased consumption by proliferating microbes. Reduced arterial oxygen content and metabolic acidosis typically reflect hypoxemia and hypovolemic shock in cases of advanced sepsis.

Fibrinogen is an acute phase protein that reliably increases with any inflammatory insult in the horse. Significant increases in plasma fibrinogen concentration may be particularly useful in determining onset. Although constitutively present in the circulation, fibrinogen is synthesized by the liver during the acute phase reaction and significant increases indicate the presence of an inflammatory response of at least 24 to 48 hours duration. Thus hyperfibrinogenemia in foals less than 24 hours of age would be consistent with the presence of infection *in utero*.

The effect of sepsis on the circulating neutrophil count is variable. With appropriate stimuli from the soluble mediators of the acute phase response, neutrophilia with or without a mild left shift are expected. Overzealous production of cytokines, prostanoids, chemokines, and chemoattractants in overwhelming or uncontrolled sepsis induces margination of neu-

| Table 5-2 | Sepsis Scoring System* |

	Score					
Parameter	4	3	2	1	0	**Score for This Case**
History:						
1. Placentitis, vulvar discharge, dystocia, long transportation of mare, sick mare, induced, prolonged gestation (>365 days)		yes			no	
2. Premature (days of gestation)		<300	300–310	311–330	>330	
Clinical signs:						
1. Petechiae, scleral injection		severe	moderate	mild	none	
2. Fever			>102°F	<100°F		
3. Hypotonia, coma, depression, seizure			marked	mild	normal	
4. Anterior uveitis, diarrhea, respiratory distress, swollen joints, open wounds		yes			none	
Laboratory data:						
1. Neutrophil count (per μl)		<2,000	2,000–4,000 or >12,000	8,000–12,000	normal	
2. Bands (per μl)		>200	50–200		none	
3. Any toxic change in neutrophils	marked	moderate	mild		none	
4. Fibrinogen (mg/dl)			>600	400–600	<400	
5. Blood glucose (mg/dl)			<50	50–80	>80	
6. IgG (mg/dl)	<200	200–400	100–800		>800	
7. Arterial oxygen (mm Hg)‡		<40	40–50	50–69	>70	
8. Metabolic acidosis‡				yes	no	
Total points for this case:						

*Each of the following parameters is evaluated and a score is assigned.[27]
A score of ≥11 predicts sepsis.
†If these two parameters are included, the positive cutoff value is 12.

trophils, extravasation into affected tissues, and/or apotosis.[36] In these scenarios, neutropenia, with or without a left shift occurs. The presence of toxic neutrophil morphology (vacuolization, basophilic cytoplasm, toxic granulation, Dohle bodies) is particularly helpful and is most intimately associated with endotoxemia or bacterial infection (Figure 5-12).[43,44] Other changes that may be found on a complete blood count or routine serum chemistry profile are not specific to septicemia, but may reflect signs of other concurrent diseases, establish organ function, and assist in determining a prognosis or therapeutic plan (i.e., fluid therapy).

A positive sepsis score (≥12) accurately identified sepsis in 94% (sensitivity) of the original cases studied, whereas scores below the cutoff value of 12 appropriately eliminated septicemia with a specificity of 86%.[27] To simplify the scoring system, a "modified" sepsis scoring system that eliminated the arterial oxygen content and bicarbonate concentration and used a cutoff score of 11 was found to have similar sensitivity and specificity in neonatal foals.[45] Although not as detailed as the sepsis scoring system for foals, sepsis in humans is defined as the systemic response to infection manifested by the presence of two or more of the following conditions: hyperthermia or hypothermia, tachycardia, tachypnea, hypocapnea, leukocytosis, leukopenia, or >10% bands.[1] Clearly this definition includes many of the same criteria identified by the neonatal foal Sepsis Scoring System.

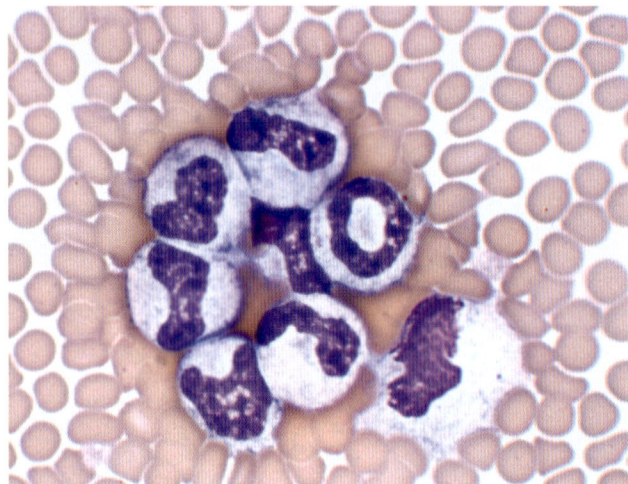

Fig. 5-12 Blood smear stained with Wright Giemsa, 100× magnification. Neutrophils clumped along the feathered edge show moderate toxic change, with Dohle bodies (amorphous clumps of blue material) and a more diffuse cytoplasmic basophilia. This and the bands present indicate inflammation. The severity of toxic change suggests a bacterial infection. (Courtesy of Dr. Joyce Knoll.)

The sepsis score is not intended to replace clinical judgment or blood culture results, but its simplicity and speed of interpretation make it a useful diagnostic aid. With the exception of a CBC to obtain information on the neutrophil and band counts and neutrophil morphology, the remaining parameters can be obtained by taking a history, doing a physical examination, and performing simple stallside tests (i.e., IgG and glucose determinations). If the sepsis score is positive without inclusion of the results of a CBC, the practitioner in the field is alerted to further investigation.

The accuracy of the sepsis score and the prognosis are directly correlated with the score: scores >23 are reported to have 100% diagnostic accuracy and are associated with mortality.[45,46] In a recent retrospective study on 250 septicemic foals at the University of Georgia, the Sepsis Scoring System remained diagnostically accurate.[46] However, another recent study at the Marion duPont Scott Equine Medical Center in Virginia found lower sensitivity and specificity than originally reported with the modified sepsis score, indicating that the scoring system's utility may vary based on the study population.[47] Although the Sepsis Scoring System in foals is easy to use and practical, lower scores or scores just below the cutoff should not be ignored. In general, the logic of "absence of proof is not proof of absence" (William Cowper, English poet, 1731–1800) and sound clinical judgment should prevail. Likewise, a positive score may not truly indicate septicemia, but does likely indicate that the foal has a systemic inflammatory reaction of some kind. Perhaps logic would dictate here to err on the side of presumed septicemia until further diagnostics are secured.

Additional Tests

Although a sign of advanced disease, the presence of multiple local sites of infection clinically or on postmortem examination is also considered a reliable indication of septicemia. With this in mind, it may be helpful to obtain additional ancillary diagnostics specifically aimed at identification of potential primary or secondary sites of infection. To this end, some clinicians prefer to routinely obtain thoracic radiographs, perform arterial blood gas analysis, and/or perform ultrasonography of the internal umbilical structures on neonatal foals with presumed septicemia. The information gained from these additional tests must be weighed against their cost.

If lameness, periarticular edema, or joint swelling is present, arthrocentesis is indicated for joint fluid analysis and culture (see Case 6-2). Radiography of joints may be helpful, but be mindful that radiographic changes of bone and articular surfaces lag behind clinical signs of septic arthritis. Occasionally lameness is present without obvious synovial distension, confounding localization of the affected joint or physis. In this situation, ultrasonography or computerized tomography may be helpful in detecting subtle changes in the synovia, articular surfaces, or physes of the affected limb. If neurologic signs are present, collection of CSF is indicated to rule out meningitis (see Chapter 10).

If sepsis is advanced and signs of shock, SIRS, or MODS are present, additional diagnostic tests to consider are blood pressure measurements, arterial blood gas analysis, determination of serum electrolyte and creatinine concentrations, and a coagulation profile. Interpretation of the former two tests is covered elsewhere (see Chapters 6 and 7). The serum creatinine and electrolyte concentrations should be periodically evaluated in septic foals, as acute renal failure is a common manifestation of sepsis.

Several hemostatic and fibrinolytic indexes are significantly different in healthy foals, compared to adult horses, and thus submission of age-matched control plasma is necessary unless neonatal references are established in the laboratory performing the analysis. Specifically, in the first month of life, platelet counts are greater; prothrombin and activated partial thromboplastin times are longer; fibrin degradation products and D-dimer concentrations and plasminogen activator inhibitor are greater; and fibrinogen and protein C antigen concentrations and antithrombin III, plasminogen, and tissue plasminogen activator activities are lower in healthy foals compared to healthy adults.[48,49] In septic foals, significant derangements in these indices have been further described, including prolongation of the prothrombin and activated partial thromboplastin times; increased fibrin degradation products concentrations and plasminogen and plasminogen activator inhibitor activities; and reduced protein C antigen and antithrombin III activity, compared to healthy age-matched foals.[34] In foals that are endotoxemic, the prothrombin and activated partial thromboplastin times were longer and plasminogen and antithrombin III activities were significantly less than foals that were not endotoxemic.[34]

Although these derangements clearly indicate that septicemic foals are at increased risk of coagulopathy, it may be difficult to predict the likelihood of hemorrhage versus thrombus formation in any given case. Interestingly, septic foals with severe coagulation abnormalities had, on average, significantly higher plasma fibrinogen concentrations, compared to healthy foals.[34] This reiterates that the fact that the equine liver is extremely capable of producing fibrinogen as an acute phase protein, even in the face of consumptive coagulopathy.

Finally, blood concentrations of several pro-inflammatory mediators, including tumor necrosis factor and interleukin-6, are significantly increased in septic neonatal foals, though their practical clinical diagnostic utility is limited at this time.[34,43]

Using the initial clinical findings and laboratory diagnostics, '02 Bugs Bunny had a sepsis score of 22. Based on this positive prediction of septicemia, an over-the-wire extended use polyurethane catheter was placed in the jugular vein and the foal was started on potassium penicillin (22,000 IU/kg IV q 6 hours) and amikacin (21 mg/kg IV q 24 hours). She was given 1 liter of LRS with 5% glucose, after which the blood glucose concentration had increased to 84 mg/dl. Two liters of plasma containing J5 anti-endotoxin antibodies was given. The foal was allowed to nurse free choice and was given 75 ml/kg body weight/day of LRS, divided into 30-minute boluses given every 6 hours. Ranitidine was given orally q 8 hours at 6.6 mg/kg, and flunixin meglumine was given at 0.5 mg/kg once. Rectal temperature, heart and respiratory rates, and blood glucose were monitored every six hours.

Treatment of Septicemia

Septicemia in neonates requires an intense combination of therapies including treatment for infection, inflammation, endotoxemia, hypotension, hypoxemia, and coagulopathy; maintenance of appropriate glucose, nutrition, and fluid and electrolyte levels; and general supportive care. Early recognition and appropriate antimicrobial therapy are paramount for successful treatment of septicemia. Until cultures from blood or local sites of infection are available, antimicrobial therapy should logically be directed against the pathogens most commonly involved in equine neonatal septicemia. Before the 1970s, *Actinobacillus equuli* and β hemolytic *Streptococcus* were reported as the primary pathogens.[7,8,50] After the 1970s, *Escherichia coli* isolates predominated. That reign has continued today. Referral center studies indicate that in the last two decades, Gram-negative bacteria account for the majority of isolates, with key players including *E. coli, Salmonella spp, Klebsiella pneumoniae, Pseudomonas aeruginosa, Enterobacter spp, Citrobacter spp, and Actinobacillus spp* (Table 5-3).[7-9,15,39,51]

Table 5-3	Most Common Pathogens Isolated from Septic Equine Neonates in the Last Fifteen Years*				
	Years isolates obtained and samples cultured				
Organisms	**1978–1987[8]** Blood and Necropsy	**1982–1987[7]** Blood and Necropsy	**1991–1998[39]** Blood	**1986–2000[9]** All Cultures	**1993–2000[51]** Blood
Escherichia coli	31	42	19	25	28
Klebsiella pneumoniae	13	9	4	8	8
Actinobacillus spp	19	6	9	6	22
Pseudomonas aeruginosa	5		5	4	1
Citrobacter spp	5	2		3	
Enterobacter spp	4	7	12	8	10
Salmonella spp		8	3	5	4
Streptococcus spp	8	8	9	12	7
Staphylococcus spp	4	3	10	6	2
Enterococcus			9	5	10

*Values are the percentage of total isolates reported within each study and represent at least 80% of the total reported isolates within each study.

Table 5-4   Antimicrobial Efficacy Against Common Bacterial Isolates from Septicemic Foals*

Organism	Amikacin	Gentamycin	Ceftiofur	Cefotaxine	Ticarcillin	TMS	CAP	TC	Amp	Pen	Cephalothin
Escherichia	90[8]	80	80		53	57			57		
coli	95[7]	95			67	71	79	3	37		
	100[9]	85	62	38		75	78	69	77		69
Klebsiella	83	67	83		0	67			0		
	100	100			10	100	100	20			
	100	92		30		92	82	83	8		50
Salmonella	100	67	100		67	67			67		
	100	100			50	100	0	50	50		
	100	77	30	50		77	62	69	77		100
Enterobacter	84	68	63		32	47			21		
	100	100			100	100	50	50			
	100	85	100	44		85	67	77	38		38
Actinobacillus	85	92	85		100	100			92		
	57	100			100	100	100	100		33	
	69	57	100	0		100	100	93	100	92	93
Pseudomonas	100	86	29		100	57			29		
Streptococcus	40	60	100		100	80			100		
	22	17	100	1		11	87	72	89	83	72
Enterococcus	0	0	0		25	33			25		
	0	0	38			0	80	50	100	100	71
Staphylococcus Coagulase neg	100	100	43		43	29			57		
Staphylococcus Coagulase pos	100	25	25		25	25			23		
Staphylococcus	94	82	100	0		70	93	76	29	35	88

*Listed number represents the percentage of total isolates that were reported to be sensitive to the listed antimicrobial agent within that study.[7-9]

†TMS = trimethoprim/sulf; CAP = chloramphenical; TC = tetracycline; Amp = ampicillin; Pen = penicillin

Information obtained on *E. coli* isolates from foals indicates that strains from healthy and diarrheic foals cannot be distinguished based on serotype or biotype; however, some of the *E. coli* isolates from foals with diarrhea possess virulence factors, such as heat-labile and heat-stable toxins and attachment factors.[52] Despite the preponderance of Gram-negative isolates, in recent years it would appear that Gram-positive bacteria are on the rise. In one report, approximately 30% of the total isolates were Gram-positive and principally consisted of *Streptococcus spp, Enterococcus,* and *Staphylococcus spp.*[39] In some cases, more than one bacterial species is isolated. Less commonly reported isolates include *Rhodococcus equi, Listeria monocytogenes, Clostridium perfringens, Bacillus, Proteus, Pasteurella, Acinetobacter, Serratia marcescens, Bacteroides,* and *Morganella morganii.*

Based on the above information, broad-spectrum antimicrobial therapy is required. Considering sensitivity data on isolates obtained at referral centers in the past 15 years, the most frequently recommended antimicrobial regimen is the combination of an aminoglycoside with a penicillin derivative. Since the 1990s, there have been increasing reports of gentamicin resistance among some *E. coli* and *Salmonella* isolates,[53] thus amikacin and penicillin or ampicillin are commonly used as the initial antimicrobial regimen for treatment of neonatal septicemia. This antimicrobial combination is projected to be effective against at least 90% of septic foal isolates (Table 5-4).[9,15,39] For single-drug therapy against the major isolates, imipenem, enrofloxacin, ceftriaxone, ceftazidime, chloramphenicol, ceftiofur, and tetracycline are reported in decreasing order of efficacy from 99% to approximately 70%.[9,15,53] The cost, mechanism of action, and side effects of each of these drugs must be carefully scrutinized before used as a first choice.

Although generalizations about antimicrobial sensitivity patterns are helpful, the decision on antimicrobial use on any given case should be driven by clinical judgment concerning the geographic location, cost of therapy, concurrent disease, and the individual's culture and sensitivity data. For foals with renal disease in which use of an aminoglycoside is a concern, third-generation cephalosporins have been recommended, but be aware that this class of drugs may also contribute to renal compromise. Table 5-5 reviews indications and dosages for antimicrobials used in *neonatal foals.*

Table 5-5 Commonly Used Antimicrobials for Treatment of Equine Neonatal Septicemia

Drug	Dose	Route	Interval	Comments
Amikacin	21 mg/kg[80] 25 mg/kg[81,82]	IV	Once daily	Trough levels should be <2 μg/ml; potentially nephrotoxic; efficacy is based on C_{max} : MIC > 10[54,82]
(Na) Ampicillin	22 mg/kg*	IV	6 hours	Prediction of efficacy is based on AUC_{0-24} : MIC
Azithromycin	10 mg/kg[83]	PO	q 24 hours; q 48 hours after 5 days	Prediction of efficacy is based on AUC_{0-24} : MIC
Ceftazidime	50 mg/kg	IV	6 hours slow over 15 minutes	Prediction of efficacy is based on T > MIC[‡]
Cefotaxime	40 mg/kg[84]	IV	4–6 hours	Higher or more frequent dosing may be needed for meningitis; prediction of efficacy is based on T > MIC[‡]
Ceftiofur	5 mg/kg[85] 10 mg/kg[86]	IV IV	12 hours 6 hours, over 30 minutes	Prediction of efficacy is based on T > MIC[‡]
Ceftriaxone	25 mg/kg[87]	IV	q 12 hour	Third generation; prediction of efficacy is based on T > MIC[‡]
Cephalothin	10–20 mg/kg*	IV	6 hours	First generation; prediction of efficacy is based on T > MIC[‡]
Cefazolin	8–16 mg/kg[15]	IV	6–8 hours	First generation; prediction of efficacy is based on T > MIC[‡]
Chloramphenicol palmitate	50 mg/kg[88]	PO	6–8 hours	Potential for aplastic anemia in humans
Cefuroxine axetil	30 mg/kg/day[86]	PO	Divided BID or TID	Second generation; prediction of efficacy is based on T > MIC[‡]
(Na) Cefuroxine	50–100 mg/kg/day[86] 200–240 mg/kg/day	IV IV	Divided TID Divided TID	Second generation; Higher dose for meningitis; prediction of efficacy is based on T > MIC[‡]
Cefpodoxime proxetil	10 mg/kg	PO	8–12 hours	Third generation; prediction of efficacy is based on T > MIC[‡]
Doxycycline	10 mg/kg*	PO	12 hours	
Clarithromycin	7.5 mg/kg[89]	PO	12 hours	
Enrofloxacin	5–10 mg/kg[81]	PO or IV	24 hours	Potential for arthropathy; prediction of efficacy is based on C_{max} : MIC > 10
Erythromycin stearate	25 mg/kg[90] 37.5 mg/kg	PO PO	8 hours 12 hours	Prediction of efficacy is based on T > MIC[‡]
Erythromycin lactobionate	5 mg/kg	IV	6 hours	
Fluconazole	4 mg/kg[56]	PO	Once daily	
Gentamicin sulfate	6.6 mg/kg 10–16 mg/kg if <7 days old[86]	IV	Once daily	Trough levels should be <2 μg/ml; potentially nephrotoxic; prediction of efficacy is based on C_{max} : MIC > 10
Imipenem	10 mg/kg†	IV	6 hours	
Metronidazole	10–15 mg/kg*	PO	6–12 hours	
Oxytetracycline	5–10 mg/kg*	IV	12 hours	
(K or Na) Penicillin	22,000 IU/kg[91]	IV	6 hours	Prediction of efficacy is based on T > MIC[‡]
Rifampin	5–10 mg/kg[92]	PO	12 hours	
Ticarcillin or Ticarcillin/ clavulanic acid	50 mg/kg[93]	IV	6 hour	
Timethoprim sulfa	20–30 mg/kg*	PO	12 hours	

*Dose established in adult horses
†Dose established in humans
‡T > MIC = plasma concentration of the drug should be one to five times the MIC for 40% to 100% of the time between dosing intervals

Antimicrobial dosing regimens can be specifically designed for the individual patient if pharmacokinetic data is available on the desired drug and the mean inhibitory concentration (MIC) has been determined for that patient's particular pathogen.[54] Time-dependent antimicrobials are those in which the time (T) the drug is in the plasma at or above the MIC is the most important factor in determining its efficacy; concentration-dependent antimicrobials are those is which the absolute concentration that the drug achieves in the plasma is the most important factor in determining its efficacy. For time-dependent drugs, such as beta-lactams and erythromycin, the plasma concentration of the drug should be one to five times the MIC for 40% to 100% of the time in between dosing intervals. Fluoroquinolones, aminoglycosides, azithromycin, and metronidazole are examples of concentration-dependent drugs for which, in general, it is recommended that the maximum plasma concentration of the drug to MIC ratio (C_{max} : MIC) be at least 10, or the area under the plasma concentration curve from 0 to 24 hours to MIC ratio (AUC_{0-24} : MIC) be greater than 125 (Table 5-5).[54]

The intravenous route is recommended for administration of antimicrobials in foals at significant risk of septicemia. Oral and intramuscular routes of administration are typically reserved for foals with less life-threatening infection or following successful control of infection with intravenous therapy. The duration of antimicrobial use will depend on the prevailing circumstances of individual cases. If culture and sensitivity results are not available, the response to treatment will be the only guide. Failure to respond to antimicrobial therapy raises the daunting question as to whether the cause is antimicrobial resistance, failure of the antimicrobial to attain adequate tissue concentrations, introduction of new pathogens, or clinician impatience.

In general, antimicrobial therapy should be continued until at least five to seven days after complete resolution of all clinical signs of infection and a normal leukogram and plasma fibrinogen concentration. For foals with a positive blood culture or localizing signs of infection, the total duration of antimicrobial therapy typically ranges between 14 and 30 days. Although this discussion on treatment has focused on bacterial isolates, it should be noted that herpesvirus and systemic candidiasis have been rarely reported in neonatal foals.[39,55,56]

Adjunctive therapy for neonatal septicemia depends upon the prevailing circumstances. Treatment of critically ill foals in septic shock with vasopressors, fluid resuscitation, glucose, and insulin is addressed elsewhere (see Chapter 7). Foals that have inadequate levels of serum IgG should receive a plasma transfusion (see Case 3-1). In cases of advanced sepsis, IgG will not only be consumed by the defense system, but it may also be catabolized as a source of energy. Thus, periodic re-evaluation of IgG concentration may be useful as a guide to the necessity of additional transfusions.

Because Gram-negative organisms predominate in neonatal septicemia, it would seem logical to direct therapy against endotoxin. Endotoxin is released during bacterial replication and during bacteriolysis incurred by host defense or antimicrobial use. In the later scenario, certain cases of antimicrobial agents, such as penicillins and cephalosporins, are more likely to generate endotoxin release, and use of such agents may in fact exacerbate clinical signs of inflammation.[57] The major commercial suppliers of equine plasma in the United States offer hyperimmune anti-endotoxin plasma (Polymune-J, Veterinary Dynamics, Templeton, CA). However, most of their plasma donor horses are immunized against endotoxin and thus even their plasma marketed for routine use or for use in foals contains anti-endotoxin antibodies to some extent (Polymune and Polymune Plus Veterinary Dynamics, Templeton, CA; and Foalimmune and HiGamm-equi, Lake Immunogenics, Ontario, NY). Although Gram-negative septicemia predominates in foals, use of plasma products that contain antibodies to endotoxin have only been shown to be beneficial in foals in controlled experimental models of sepsis or endotoxemia.[58-60]

Another drug that binds to and neutralizes endotoxin is polymyxin B sulfate, a cationic antimicrobial. The endotoxin neutralizing properties of polymyxin B have been recognized for decades, but its clinical use was hindered by the fact that the drug is neurotoxic and nephrotoxic. In recent years, it was determined that the risk of toxicity was significantly reduced, without compromising its anti-endotoxic effects, when a lower dose of the drug was used. In an experimental investigation in foals, polymyxin B was more effective in ameliorating endotoxin-induced fever and cytokine production than antiserum to endotoxin.[60] The recommended dose of polymyxin B in horses is 1000 to 5000 IU/kg IV q 8 to 12 hours.[60,61] Studies have not been conducted in neonatal foals or in clinical cases, thus polymyxin B should be used judiciously in azotemic patients.

The two main classes of drugs most commonly used to control inflammation are corticosteroids and nonsteroidal anti-inflammatory drugs. Recent meta-analysis of randomized controlled clinical trials indicates that short-term high-dose glucocorticoid therapy worsened survival of septic human patients, whereas a longer course of "physiologic doses" of hydrocortisone (200 to 300 mg q 24 hours for five days, followed by a five-day tapering dose) was beneficial in shock reversal and survival in patients with established vasopressor-dependent septic shock.[62] The positive effect of low-dose steroid therapy in septic patients may be either through augmentation of adrenal function in the stressed disease state or through anti-inflammatory properties that do not cause excessive immunosuppression. It is not clear if steroids are beneficial in septic patients without shock or those with shock that do not need vasopressor therapy. There have been no clinical studies on the use of steroids in foals with septicemia.

Although nonsteroidal anti-inflammatory therapy with flunixin meglumine has been shown to be beneficial in experimental models of endotoxemia in adult horses, such data is lacking in foals.[63] Compared to phenylbutazone, flunixin megulmine has been shown to be more effective in controlling an endotoxin-induced inflammatory response in adult horses and is associated with fewer side effects.[64,65] There is no direct data comparing the use of nonsteroidal anti-inflammatory drugs in adult horses and foals, but the anecdotal impression is that foals are more likely to develop adverse side effects, thus nonsteroid anti-inflammatory drugs should be used cautiously in the neonatal foal.

Dysregulation of the hemostatic and fibrinolytic systems is dynamic, complicated, and problematic in septic foals. In human patients with sepsis-associated coagulopathy, administration of fresh-frozen plasma and low-dose unfractionated heparin or low-molecular-weight heparin is recommended.[66,67] In adult horses with naturally-occurring proximal enteritis and DIC associated with colic, unfractionated heparin therapy reduced the incidence of laminitis and improved survival.[68,69] Although more expensive than unfractionated heparin, the low-molecular-weight heparin, dalteparin, is reported to have fewer side effects in horses.[70] The recommended dose for dalteparin in adult horses is 50 IU/kg q 24 hours subcutaneously.[70]

Recombinant human activated protein C is recommended in human patients at high risk of death from septic shock, sepsis-induced acute respiratory distress syndrome, or sepsis-induced multi-organ failure, whether or not clinical evidence of DIC exists.[71] Activated protein C therapy increases the risk of hemorrhage, and thus heparin therapy should not be given concurrently. Although protein C improves survival of septic human patients, a single dose costs approximately $8,000 to $10,000. Platelet transfusion is reserved for patients with hemorrhagic diathesis associated with thrombocytopenia.

Hypoxemic foals should receive nasal insufflation of oxygen at a rate of 2 to 6 liters/minute. The oxygen should be humidified to prevent desiccation of the respiratory mucosa. With the increased metabolic demand of infection, short-term nasal insufflation may

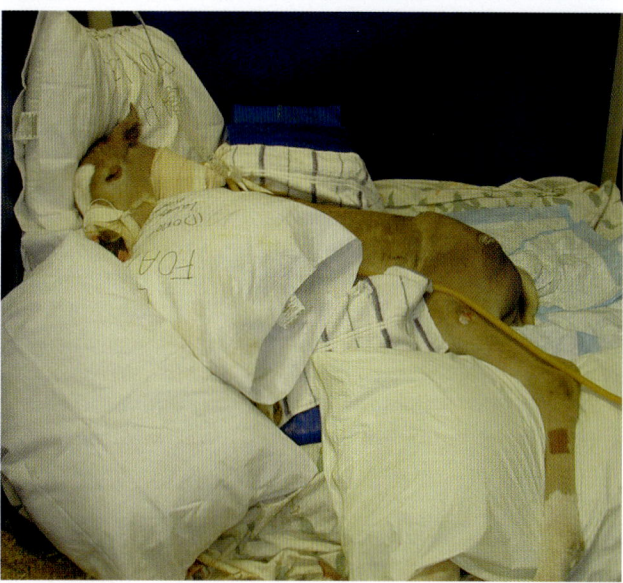

Fig. 5-13 Providing a warm, dry, clean, and quiet environment is critical in recumbent foals. Pillows and fleece pads were used on this recumbent foal to deter decubital ulcers and to maintain sternal recumbency.

benefit foals even if they do not have hypoxemia. Likewise, sepsis-induced catabolism warrants careful attention to nutritional status and assurance that the foal is gaining weight. Foals that are too weak to nurse their dams, have intense ileus, or concurrent gastrointestinal disease will require enteral or parenteral nutrition (see Case 4-3).

Perhaps the stress associated with severe illness should be controlled as best as possible to avoid further catabolism, immunosuppression, and adverse events. Gastric ulcer prophylaxis with histamine receptor antagonists is recommended in septic human patients.[67] The utility of gastric ulcer prophylaxis is questioned in critically ill foals, as the pH of their stomachs apparently is alkaline relative to healthy foals.[72] Finally, septic foals must be kept dry and warm. Recumbent foals should be maintained in sternal recumbency when possible and dependent sides frequently alternated (Figure 5-13). Diligent attention to fluid balance, urine and fecal output, catheter maintenance, and clinical progression are paramount.

After the initial fluid replacement and plasma therapy, Bugs Bunny 2002 was brighter. At three days of age (day two of hospitalization), the foal had a rectal temperature of 103.2°F (39.6°C), but was nursing more frequently and was active. The SNAP™ test (IDEXX Laboratories, Westbrook, ME) was repeated, and IgG concentration was >800 mg/dl. Blood glucose concentration remained steady at or above 80 mg/dl and thus monitoring of this param-

eter was discontinued. The serum chemistries were rechecked and revealed an unexpected increase in the serum creatinine concentration (see Table 5-1), though clinical hydration status appeared normal. Serum electrolyte concentrations were within normal limits. A transabdominal ultrasound examination was performed, and the umbilical remnants, bladder, and kidneys appeared normal. To induce diuresis, mannitol (0.25 g/kg as a CRI over 30 minutes q 12 hours) and furosemide (1 mg/kg IV q 12 hours) were given, and the daily fluid rate was increased to 100 ml/kg/day. Low-volume diarrhea continued for approximately 36 hours. Microbiology reported that the fecal culture for Salmonella and Clostridium enterotoxin tests were negative. The blood culture vial was turbid, indicative of bacterial growth.

By day four of hospitalization, the five-day-old foal's rectal temperature remained below 102°F (<38.9°C), scleral injection and petechial hemorrhages subsided, although leukocytosis and hyperfibrinogenemia were present (see Table 5-1). Serial re-evaluation of the creatinine concentration (see Table 5-1) revealed improvement, mannitol and furosemide therapy were discontinued on day four of hospitalization, and the daily IV fluid rate was decreased to 50 ml/kg/day. The foal had gained 3.5 kg of body weight since admission.

Five days after admission, microbiology reported that the blood culture yielded **Actinobacillus equuli**, sensitive to penicillin and amikacin. '02 Bugs Bunny's clinical course was "typical" for **Actinobacillus** with the exception of the unexpected increase in serum creatinine concentration on the second day of treatment. At this time, she had only received a single dose of amikacin, making aminoglycoside toxicity unlikely. Determination of the plasma amikacin level prior to the next treatment (i.e., trough level) would have assisted with this assessment, but the test was not available.

Renal ultrasonography did not reveal any significant structural changes. The exact cause of the azotemia was not definitively determined; however, possible considerations included **Actinobacillus** infection in the renal cortices or renal disease as a result of the systemic response to inflammation. A conservative diagnostic approach was taken. Amikacin therapy was continued, the foal was treated with diuretics, and the serum creatinine concentration was rechecked. Within the next 24 hours, creatinine concentration had decreased, thus amikacin therapy was continued. If the creatinine concentration had not improved, amikacin therapy would have been replaced. The foal received a total of 14 days of intravenous antimicrobial therapy, several days beyond resolution of all clinical signs and return of the leukogram and fibrinogen concentration to normal limits (see Table 5-1). She recovered fully with no long-term complications. Upon recheck by the local veterinarian seven days

later, the foal was clinically normal and had a normal CBC and creatinine concentration.

Actinobacillus equuli is a Gram-negative pleopmorphic rod that is commonly found in the tonsils and intestine of normal adult horses. Infection is reported to most commonly occur within hours to the first few days of life and accounts for as much as 30% of the organisms isolated in septic foals in some parts of the world.[51] The colloquial name of "sleepy foal disease" stems from the depression and sleeplike appearance that accompanies infection. Compared to foals with other Gram-negative bacterial infections, foals with *Actinobacillus* septicemia are more commonly reported to have diarrhea, neutropenia, a left shift, and higher sepsis scores.[51] The survival rate of foals with *Actinobacillus* septicemia is equivalent to that caused by other Gram-negative organisms.

Outcome of Septicemia

The overall survival rate of foals with septicemia is highly variable, with reported short-term survival rates of 10%,[73] 25%,[74] 44%,[9] 45%,[7,75] 54%,[51] and 70%.[76] One fact is encouragingly clear—the overall survival rate from septicemia in foals has improved over time.[46,77] The variation in survival is largely a reflection of differences in case inclusion criteria and geographic location. In general, in documented septicemia, it is probably appropriate to quote a prognosis for short-term survival of approximately 50%. Several parameters from independent retrospective studies have been statistically associated with nonsurvival, including induction of parturition, recumbency at presentation, septic arthritis, respiratory disease, hypothermia, neutropenia, hypoglycemia, acidemia, increased anion gap, hypoxemia, hyperfibrinogenemia, FPT, high sepsis score, positive blood culture, Gram-negative bacteremia, and multisystem disease.[46,73,75,78] One must be particularly cautious in using survival parameters to determine the course of treatment. Individual circumstances in each case must be carefully examined. Predictive models on survival from neonatal care units have been shown to vary by hospital, thus parameters that may be accurate in one setting may be inappropriate in another.[79]

Information on long-term survival from neonatal septicemia is scarce. In 1986, The University of Florida reported that 54% of all foals admitted to the neonatal intensive care unit survived to discharge. Of the foals that survived short-term, 18% died or were euthanized within a year after discharge from the hospital. Of the foals that did not survive after discharge, 30% died or were euthanized as sequelae suspected to be associated with their neonatal illness.[74] Recent long-term survival data is not available for foals with a general diagnosis of neonatal septicemia. However, the development of septic arthritis in a Thoroughbred foal significantly reduces the likelihood that it will successfully race.[78]

REFERENCES

1. Bone R, Balk R, Cerra F et al: Definitions of sepsis and organ failure and guidelines for the use of innovative therapies in sepsis. The ACCP/SCCM Consensus Conference Committee. American College of Chest Physicians/Society of Critical Care Medicine, *Chest* 101:1644-1655, 1992.
2. Baldwin J, Cooper W, Vanderwall D et al: Prevalence (treatment days) and severity of illness in hypogammaglobulinemic and normoglobulinemic foals, *J Am Vet Med Assoc* 198:423-428, 1991.
3. Stoneham S, Wingfield Digby N, Ricketts S: Failure of passive transfer of colostral immunity in the foal: Incidence, and the effect of stud management and plasma transfusions, *Vet Recod* 128:416-419, 1991.
4. Haas S, Bristol F, Card C: Risk factors associated with the incidence of foal mortality in an extensively managed mare herd, *Can Vet J* 37:91-95, 1996.
5. Giles R, Donahue J, Hong C et al: Causes of abortion, stillbirth, and perinatal death in horses: 3,527 cases (1986-1991), *J Am Vet Med Assoc* 203:1170-1175, 1993.
6. Cohen N: Causes of and farm management factors associated with disease and death in foals, *J Am Vet Med Assoc* 204:1644-1651, 1994.
7. Brewer B, Koterba A: Bacterial isolates and susceptibility patterns in foals in a neonatal intensive care unit, *Comp Cont Ed for Pract Vet* 12:1773-1781, 1990.
8. Wilson W, Madigan J: Comparison of bacteriologic culture of blood and necropsy specimens for determining the cause of foal septicemia: 47 cases (1978-1987), *J Am Vet Med Assoc* 195:1759-1763, 1989.
9. Henson S, Barton M: Bacterial isolates and antibiotic sensitivity patterns from septicemic neonatal foals: One 15 year retrospective study (1986-2000). Dorothy Havemeyer Foundation Third Neonatal Septicemia Workshop 2001, 50-52.
10. Jeffcott L: Studies on passive immunity in the foal II: The absorption of 125-labeled PVP (polyvinyl pyrrolidone) by the neonatal intestine, *J Comp Pathol* 84:1974.
11. Madigan J: Method for preventing neonatal septicemia, the leading cause of death in the neonatal foal. 43rd Annual American Association of Equine Practitioners Convention Proceedings 17-19, 1997.
12. Banks K, McGuire T: Neonatal immunity. In R. Halliell, N. Gorman, eds: *Veterinary clinical immunology*, Philadelphia, 1988, WB Saunders.
13. Walker R, Madigan J, DW H et al: An outbreak of equine neonatal salmonellosis, *J Vet Diag Invest* 3:223-227, 1991.
14. Oishi T, Iwata S, Nonoyama M et al: Double blind comparative study on the care of the neonatal umbilical cord using 80% ethanol with or without chlorhexidine, *J Hosp Infect* 58:34-37, 2004.
15. Madigan J: *Manual of equine neonatal medicine*, ed 3, Woodland, CA, 1997, Liveoak Publishing.
16. Giguere S, Prescott J: Equine immunity to bacteria, *Vet Clin North Am Equine Pract* 16:29-63, 2000.
17. Mackay I, Rosen F: Innate immunity, *N Engl J Med* 343:338-344, 2000.
18. Roy M: Sepsis in adults and foals, *Vet Clin North Am Equine Pract* 20:41-61, 2004.
19. Fenton M, Golenbock D: LPS-binding proteins and receptors, *J Leukocyte Biol* 64:25-32, 1998.
20. Brightbill H, Modlin R: Toll-like receptors: Molecular mechanisms of the mammalian immune response, *Immunology* 101:1-10, 2000.
21. Antal-Szalmas P: Evaluation of CD14 in host defense, *Eur J Clin Invest* 30:167-179, 2000.
22. Barton M: Colostral CD14: More than a receptor for endotoxin. Dorothy Havemeyer Foundation Neonatal Septicemia Workshop 3, 2001, 21-23.
23. Tizard I: *Veterinary immunology*, ed 7, Philadelphia, 2004, Elsevier Saunders.
24. Gershwin L, Krakowka S, Olsen R: *Innate immunity. Immunology and immunopathology of domestic animals*, St Louis, 1995, Mosby.
25. McTaggart C, Yovich J, Penhale J et al: A comparison of foal and adult horse neutrophil function using flow cytometric techniques, *Res Vet Sci* 71:73-79, 2001.
26. Demmers S, Johannisson A, Grondahl G et al: Neutrophil functions and serum IgG in growing foals, *Equine Vet J* 33:676-680, 2001.
27. Brewer B, Koterba A: Development of a scoring system for the early diagnosis of equine neonatal sepsis, *Equine Vet J* 20:18-22, 1988.
28. Brewer B, Koterba A, Rowe E: Comparison of empirically developed sepsis score with a computer generated and weighted scoring system for the identification of sepsis in the equine neonate, *Equine Vet J* 20:23-24, 1988.
29. Robinson J, Allen G, Green E et al: A prospective study of septicemia in colostrum-deprived foals, *Equine Vet J* 25:214-219, 1993.
30. Ceciliani F, Giordano A, Spagnolo V: The systemic response during inflammation: The acute phase proteins, *Protein Peptide Lett* 9:211-233, 2002.
31. Stoneham S, Palmer L, Cash R et al: Measurement of serum amyloid A in the neonatal foal using a latex agglutination immunoturbidimetric assay: Determination of the normal range, variation with age, and response to disease, *Equine Vet J* 33:599-603, 2001.
32. Yamashita K, Fujinaga T, Okumura M et al: Serum C-reactive protein (CRP) in horses: The effect of aging, sex, delivery and inflammations on its concentration, *J Vet Med Sci* 53:1019-1024, 1991.
33. Grondahl G, Sternberg S, Jensen-Waern M et al: Opsonic capacity of foal serum for the two neonatal pathogens, *Escherichia coli* and *Actinobacillus equuli*, *Equine Vet J* 33:670-675, 2001.
34. Barton M, Morris D, Norton N et al: Hemostatic and fibrinolytic indices in neonatal foals with presumed septicemia, *J Vet Intern Med* 12:26-35, 1998.
35. McKenzie H, Furr M: Equine neonatal sepsis: The pathophysiology of severe inflammatory and infection, *Comp Cont Ed for Pract Vet* 23:661-670, 2001.
36. MacKay R: Inflammation in horses, *Vet Clin North Am Equine Pract* 16:15-27, 2000.

37. Forrest L, Cooley A, Darien B: Digital arterial thrombosis in a septicemic foal, *J Vet Intern Med* 13:382-385, 1999.

38. Brianceau P, Divers T: Acute thrombosis of limb arteries in horses with sepsis: Five cases, *Equine Vet J* 33:105-109, 2001.

39. Marsh P, Palmer J: Bacterial isolates from blood and their susceptibility patterns in critically ill foals: 543 cases (1991-1998), *J Am Vet Med Assoc* 218:1608-1610, 2001.

40. Wallis C, Melnick J, RD W et al: Rapid isolation of bacteria from septicemic patients by use of an antimicrobial removal device, *J Clin Microbiol II* 462-464, 1980.

41. Madigan J: Development of real-time TaqMan PCR systems to facilitate the diagnosis and research of septicemia in foals. Neonatal septicemia workshop 3: Dorothy Havenmeyer Foundation 2001, 37-40.

42. Breuhaus B, Gegraves F: Plasma endotoxin concentration in clinically normal and potentially septic equine neonates, *J Vet Intern Med* 7:296-302, 1993.

43. Morris D, Moore J: Tumor necrosis factor activity in serum from neonatal foals with presumed septicemia, *J Am Vet Med Assoc* 199:1584-1590, 1991.

44. Lavoie J, Madigan J, Cullor J et al: Haemodynamic, pathologic, haematological, and behavioral changes during endotoxin infusion in equine neonates, *Equine Vet J* 22:23-29, 1990.

45. Brewer B: Neonatal foal evaluation: Sepsis and survival scoring in private practice. Thirty-third Annual Conference of the American Association of Equine Practitioners 1988, 817-822.

46. White S, Barton M: The sepsis score revised. Neonatal Septicemia Workshop 3: Dorothy Havenmeyer Foundation 2001, 13-15.

47. Corley K, Furr M: Evaluation of a score designed to predict sepsis in foals, *J Vet Emerg Crit Care* 13:149-155, 2003.

48. Barton M, Morris D, Crowe N et al: Hemostatic indices in healthy foals from birth to one-month of age, *J Vet Diagnostic Invest* 7:380-385, 1995.

49. Figueiredo M, Divers T, Brooks M et al: Comparisons of dimer concentration in septic and healthy foals, *J Vet Intern Med* 18:412, 2004.

50. Platt H: Septicemia in the foal: A review of 61 cases, *Br Vet J* 129:221-229, 1973.

51. Stewart A, Hinchcliff K, Saville W et al: *Actinobacillus sp* bacteremia in foals: Clinical signs and prognosis, *J Vet Intern Med* 16:464-471, 2002.

52. Holland R, Schmidt A, Sriranganathan N et al: Characterization of *Escherichia coli* isolated from foals, *Vet Microbiol* 48:243-255, 1996.

53. Sanchez L, Lester G: Equine neonatal sepsis: Microbial isolates, antimicrobial resistance, and short and long term outcomes. Eighteenth Annual Forum of the American Veterinary Medical Association 2000, 223-224.

54. McKellar Q, Sanchez Bruni S, Jone D: Pharmacokinetic/pharmacodynamic relationships of antimicrobial drugs used in veterinary medicine, *J Vet Pharm Ther* 27:503-514, 2004.

55. Perkins G, Ainsworth D, Erb H et al: Clinical, haematological and biochemical findings in foals with neonatal equine herpesvirus-1 infection compared with septic and premature foals, *Equine Vet J* 31:422-426, 1999.

56. Reilly L, Palmer J: Systemic candidiasis in four foals, *J Am Vet Med Assoc* 205:464-466, 1994.

57. Bentley A, Barton M, Lee M et al: Antimicrobial-induced endotoxin and cytokine activity in an in vitro model of septicemia in foals, *Am J Vet Res* 63:660-668, 2002.

58. Morris D, Whitlock R: Therapy of suspected septicemia in neonatal foals using plasma-containing antibodies to core lipopolysaccharide (LPS), *J Vet Intern Med* 1:175-182, 1987.

59. Ellefson D, Pierce R: Effects of an *Escherichia coli* antiserum in preventing foal diarrhea and septicemia. Annual Convention of the AAEP 1993, 515-520.

60. Durando M, Mackay R, Linda S et al: Effects of polymixin B and salmonella typimurium antiserum on horses given endotoxin intravenously, *Am J Vet Res* 55:921-927, 1994.

61. Barton M, Parviainen A, Norton N: Polymyxin B protects horses against induced endotoxaemia in vivo, *Equine Vet J* 36:397-401, 2004.

62. Keh D, Sprung C: Use of corticosteroid therapy in patients with sepsis and septic shock: An evidence-based review, *Crit Care Med* 32:S527-S533, 2004.

63. Semrad S, Hardee G, Hardee M et al: Low dose flunixin meglumine: Effects on eicosanoid production and clinical signs induced by experimental endotoxemia in horses, *Equine Vet J* 19:201-206, 1987.

64. Moore J, Hardee M, Hardee G: Modulation of arachidonic acid metabolism in endotoxic horses: Comparison of flunixin meglumine, phenylbutazone, and a selective thromboxane synthetase inhibitor, *Am J Vet Res* 47:110-113, 1986.

65. MacAllister C, Morgan S, Borne A et al: Comparison of adverse effects of phenylbutazone, flunixin meglumine, and ketoprofen in horses, *J Am Vet Med Assoc* 202:71-77, 1993.

66. Zimmerman J: Use of blood products in sepsis: An evidence based review, *Crit Care Med* 32:S542-547, 2004.

67. Treciak S, Dellinger R: Other supportive therapies in sepsis: An evidence based review, *Crit Care Med* 32:S571-577, 2004.

68. Cohen N, Parson E, Seahorn T et al: Prevalence and factors associated with development of laminitis in horses with duodenitis/proximal jejunitis: 33 cases (1985-1991), *J Am Vet Med Assoc* 204:250-254, 1994.

69. Welch R, Watkins J, Taylor T et al: Disseminated intravascular coagulation associated with colic in 23 horses (1984-1989), *J Vet Intern Med* 6:29-35, 1992.

70. Feige K, Schwarzwald C, Bombeli T: Comparison of unfractioned and low molecular weight heparin for prophylaxis of coagulopathies in 52 horses with colic: A randomized double-blind clinical trial, *Equine Vet J* 35:506-513, 2003.

71. Fourrier F: Recombinant human activated protein C in the treatment of severe sepsis: An evidence based review, *Crit Care Med* 32:S534-541, 2004.

72. Sanchez L, Lester G, Merritt A: Intragastric pH in critically ill neonatal foals and the effect of ranitidine, *J Am Vet Med Assoc* 218:907-913, 2001.

73. Hoffman A, Staempfli H, Willan A: Prognostic variables for survival of neonatal foals under intensive care, *J Vet Intern Med* 6:89-95, 1992.

74. Baker S, Drummond W, Lane T et al: Follow up evaluation of horses after neonatal intensive care, *J Am Vet Med Assoc* 189:1454-1457, 1986.

75. Gayle J, Cohen N, Chaffin M: Factors associated with survival in septicemic foals: 65 cases (1988-1995), *J Vet Intern Med* 12:140-146, 1998.

76. Raisis A, Hodgson J, Hodgson D: Equine neonatal septicemia: 24 cases, *Aust Vet J* 73:137-140, 1996.

77. Paradis M, Uri L: The effectiveness of equine neonatal care: A retrospective study. Eighth American College of Veterinary Internal Medicine Forum 543-546, 1990.

78. Smith L, Marr C, Payne R et al: What is the likelihood that Thoroughbred foals treated for septic arthritis will race?, *Equine Vet J* 36:452-456, 2004.

79. Furr M, Tinker M, Edens L: Prognosis for neonatal foals in an intensive care unit, *J Vet Intern Med* 11:183-188, 1997.

80. Madgesian K, Wilson W, Mihalyi J: Deposition pharmacokinetics and evaluation for nephrotoxicity of a high dose, once daily administration of amikacin to neonatal foals. Neonatal Septicemia Workshop 2: Dorothy Havenmeyer Foundation 1998, 36-37.

81. Vivrette S: Update on treatment of neonatal septicemia and failure of passive transfer. Neonatal Septicemia Workshop 2: Dorothy Havenmeyer Foundation 1998, 38.

82. Bucki E, Giguère S, Macpherson M et al.: Pharmacokinetics of once-daily amikacin in healthy foals and therapeutic drug

monitoring in hospitalized equine neonates, *J Vet Intern Med* 18:728-733, 2004.

83. Jacks S, Giguère S, Gronwall R et al: Pharmacokinetics of azithromycin and concentration in body fluids and bronchoalveolar cells in foals, *Am J Vet Res* 62:1870-1875, 2001.

84. Gardner S, Duvers T, Sweeney R: Pharmacokinetics of cefotaxime in neonatal pony foals, *Am J Vet Res* 54:576-579, 1993.

85. Wilson W, Mihalyi J: Comparative pharmacokinetics of ceftiofur in neonatal foals and adult horses. Neonatal Septicemia Workshop 2: Dorothy Havenmeyer Foundation 1998, 34-35.

86. Palmer J. 2004. Personal Communication.

87. Ringger N, Brown M, Kohlepp S et al: Pharmacokinetics of ceftriaxone in neonatal foals, *Equine Vet J* 30:163-165, 1998.

88. Buopane R: Serum concentrations and pharmacokinetics of chloramphenicol in foals after a single oral dose, *Equine Vet J* 20:59, 1988.

89. Jacks S, Giguère S, Gronwall R et al: Disposition of oral clarithromycin in foals, *J Vet Pharm Therap* 25:359-362, 2002.

90. Prescott J, Hoover D, Dohoo I: Pharmacokinetics of erythromycin in foals and adult horses, *J Vet Pharm Ther* 6:67, 1985.

91. Brown M, Gronwall R, Boos D et al: Aqueous procaine penicillin G in foals: Serum concentrations and pharmacokinetics after a single intravenous dose, *Equine Vet J* 16:374, 1984.

92. Burrows G, MacAllister C, Ewing P et al: Rifampin disposition in the horse: Effects of age and method of oral administration, *J Vet Pharm Ther* 15:124-132, 1992.

93. Sweeney R, Beech J, Simmons R: Pharmacokinetics of intravenously and intramuscularly administered ticarcillin and clavulanic acid in foals, *Am J Vet Res* 49:23-26, 1988.

Manifestations of Septicemia

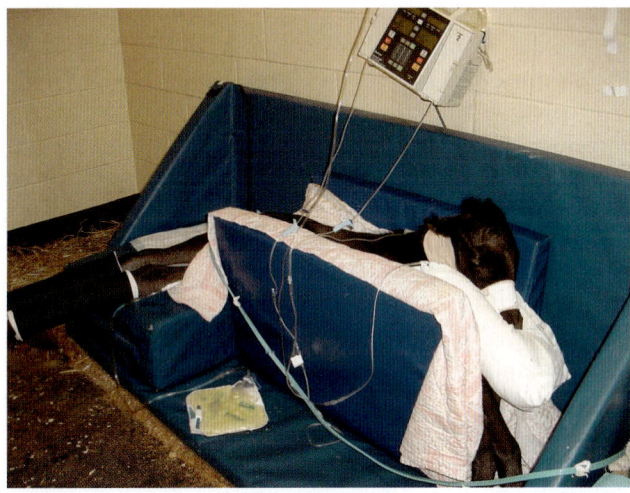

Fig. 6-1 '03 Hufflepuff was maintained in sternal recumbency to limit positional atelectasis.

'03 Hufflepuff, a 48-hour-old Thoroughbred foal, presented to a referral hospital after an uncomplicated, attended birth of 337 days of gestation. Hufflepuff, the six-year-old dam, is a primiparous mare in good general health. There was no colostrum leakage prior to parturition. Her foal stood within 110 minutes after birth and attempted to nurse the mare by 180 minutes. Hufflepuff, however, acted restless and agitated after parturition with minimal interest in the foal. The farm manager bottle fed approximately 80 ml of colostrum to the foal and subsequently assisted the foal to nurse every four hours by restraining the mare.

Eighteen hours after parturition, the foal was evaluated by the farm veterinarian. '03 Hufflepuff was reported to lie down frequently, but was readily aroused to stand for examination and nursed from the mare. Physical examination did not reveal any significant abnormalities at the time. Based on the history of delayed nursing and the possibility of inadequate colostrum intake, the farm veterinarian administered 1 liter of intravenous plasma to the foal. An IgG level >800 mg/dl was confirmed after transfusion. During the following 12 hours, the foal became increasingly lethargic, with a weak suckle reflex. The decision was made to refer the foal to a full-care facility.

On presentation, '03 Hufflepuff was markedly depressed (Figure 6-1). The foal had a poor suckle reflex and bright pink mucous membranes with a capillary refill time of two seconds. His temperature was 100.3°F, heart rate was 112 beats per minute, and respiratory rate was 48 breaths per minute with an increased respiratory effort (excessive rib excursion). Auscultation revealed harsh broncho-vesicular lung sounds, without other abnormalities. The remainder of the physical examination was considered normal.

HISTORY AND PHYSICAL EXAMINATION

The respiratory system of the neonatal foal is particularly vulnerable to injury. In one retrospective study, 50% of all foals presented to a referral hospital had some form of pulmonary involvement.[1] Foals with respiratory dysfunction also showed the highest mortality rate. This was reflected in a recent postmortem study of equine neonates, where the respiratory system was the most common system affected.[2]

Pneumonia as a clinical manifestation of sepsis shares similar historical findings as a foal with sepsis, as described in Chapter 5. Colostrum leakages prior to parturition or colostrum deprivation (poor colostrum quality or quantity or delayed intake) are risk factors of bacterial pulmonary disease in neonatal foals, as they are in sepsis.[3] In the current case, a delayed and inadequate colostrum intake was probably the result of partial rejection of the foal by an inexperienced mare. Infectious neonatal respiratory diseases are usually part of complex multiorgan systemic infections (sepsis), commonly precipitated by failure of passive transfer (FPT).[4] Administration of 1 liter of intravenous plasma at 18 hours of age resulted in adequate immunoglobulin levels upon admission of the foal, but may have only been partially protective due to the foal's exposure to facultative pathogens prior to effective immune protection.

Early in life, localizing clinical signs of respiratory disease may be absent even in the presence of extensive disease. Dyspnea may be seen in affected foals and manifest as an increase in respiratory rate and effort. After the first deep breaths taken at birth, foals should breathe with a subtle chest excursion. As respiratory disease progresses, one might notice signs of increased breathing effort by an excessive movement of the intercostal muscles and an increased abdominal component to respiration. Finally, thoraco-abdominal asynchrony (paradoxical breathing) may ensue in foals in respiratory distress, fatigue, or failure. However, the initial signs of respiratory distress and hypoxemia are frequently vague. Even some severely hypoxemic foals may only show restlessness, and considerable resistance and struggling when being handled or restrained. Abnormal respiratory sounds (crackles or wheezes) may be heard on auscultation. However, even normal foals may show crackles on the down lung after having remained in lateral recumbency for a prolonged period of time. Furthermore, foals with no auscultable abnormalities may still have extensive pulmonary disease. Cough and nasal discharge are usually absent in the early stages of neonatal pulmonary disorders.[5]

Cyanosis is a sign of severe hypoxemia (Figure 6-2). The arterial PaO_2 (partial pressure of oxygen), however, must reach very low levels (35 to 45 mm Hg) before clinical cyanosis is observed. Approximately 5 g/dl of unoxygenated hemoglobin in the capillaries generates the dark-blue color that is appreciated as cyanosis in humans.[6] Therefore, severely anemic foals may never appear cyanotic even in the face of profound hypoxemia. Weakness, depression, anorexia, weak or absent suckle reflex, dehydration, and fever may also be noted in foals with respiratory disease. In this case, evidence of depression, weakness, and injected mucous membranes should alert the clinician of possible underlying sepsis.

Respiratory disease is often related to aspiration, descending or hematogenous spread of infection, birth

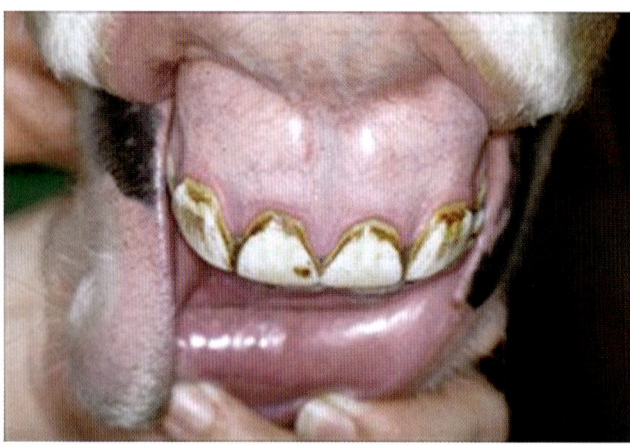
Fig. 6-2 Cyanotic mucous membranes occur when PaO_2 is <40 mm Hg. Courtesy of Dr. Michelle Barton.

asphyxia, or prematurity. In this case, underlying sepsis posed a risk factor for septic pneumonia.

PATHOGENESIS

Respiratory disease and dysfunction in neonatal foals may present as a primary condition or may occur secondary to other disease processes.[7] Equine neonatal pneumonia is generally defined as inflammation of the pulmonary parenchyma in foals less than four weeks of age. The etiologies of pneumonia in the newborn foal include systemic inflammatory response syndrome (SIRS), hematogenous spread of infection, aspiration of foreign material, and inhalation of airborne pathogens.[5] Hematogenous (ascending) infections occur in association with bacteremia or sepsis, which may be acquired in utero from a placental infection or perinatally through environmental contamination (e.g. omphalitis, omphalophlebitis).

Perinatal pulmonic infections are more common in foals that are immunocompromised due to failure of absorption of maternal antibodies (FPT). An immature ciliary apparatus and the presence of fewer alveolar macrophages in neonates in comparison to adult horses lead to decreased bacterial clearance from the lungs.[8] Reduced complement values in neonates may further contribute to decreased humoral defense against invading bacterial infections. If colostrum intake is insufficient and immunoglobulin G levels remain low, the foal is not only deprived of specific antibody protection, but neutrophil function is also seriously impaired.[9]

E. coli, Klebsiella spp, Actinobacillus equuli, Salmonella spp, and *Streptococcus spp* are some of the more common bacteria involved in neonatal foal pneumonia.[5,10] Equine viral arteritis (EVA) and herpes viral infections (EHV 1 and 4) have been implicated in in utero viral infections.[11] Although involvement of adenovirus in the pathogenesis of pneumonia has also been reported in a Thoroughbred foal, fatal adenoviral pneumonia is primarily associated with combined immunodeficiency (CID) in Arabian foals.[12,13] Additionally, a recent report documents the isolation of influenza A virus from a seven-day-old foal with bronchointerstitial pneumonia.[14] Rare opportunistic fungal pathogens may include *Pneumocystis carinii* (renamed *Pneumocystis jiroveci* in humans), *Aspergillus*, *Candida*, and *Mucor spp* in immune-deficient foals.

Descending respiratory infections may be related to inhalation pneumonia (transmission of viral, bacterial, or fungal airborne pathogens), aspiration of infected amniotic fluid due to placental infection, aspiration of gastric reflux, iatrogenic aspiration (oil, medication, oral supplements), and aspiration of milk and meconium (see Case 8-3). Aspiration of meconium occurs in utero in foals that experience fetal distress. Though the meconium is commonly sterile at this time, it creates mechanical airway obstruction, surfactant inactivation, and pulmonary inflammation (caused by vasoactive mediators, chemotactic and inflammatory cytokines, including tumor necrosis factor α, interleukin 1β, and interleukin 8).[15] The resulting edema and vasoconstriction may lead to hypoperfusion of the pulmonary parenchyma, with damage to type II pneumocytes and decreased production of surfactant.[16] This type of "secondary surfactant deficiency" may also be induced by other forms of generalized pulmonary inflammation, including diffuse bacterial pneumonia.

Neurologic dysfunction, severe inflammation, or structural abnormalities of the upper airways predispose to aspiration pneumonia postpartum (see Case 8-3). Descending infection secondary to bacterial colonization of the mucosal surfaces of the oropharynx and nasopharynx rarely occurs, except when other predisposing factors are present.

Initial laboratory analysis of '03 Hufflepuff revealed leukopenia (1.5×10³/μL) with a marked lymphopenia (0.32 × 10³/μL), neutropenia (0.62 × 10³/μL), and a band neutrophil count of 405/μL. Cytological findings were consistent with a severe degenerative left shift and associated toxic changes. The foal was hypoglycemic with a blood glucose level of 49 mg/dl. A brachial arterial blood gas analysis demonstrated a pH of 7.4, hypoxemia (58 mm Hg), and mild hypercarbia of 49.5 mm Hg. The foal's alveolar to arterial oxygen gradient (A-a gradient) was calculated to be increased at 36.5. The calculated sepsis score was also increased at 18. Blood cultures were submitted.

Because the foal exhibited signs of increased respiratory effort and evidence of hypoxemia on blood gas analysis, further diagnostic evaluation included right- and left-sided thoracic radiographs in lateral recumbency. A moderate, diffuse alveolar-interstitial lung pattern within the

caudo-dorsal lung was observed on both views. Mild to moderate diffuse interstitial infiltrates were also noted within the remaining lung quadrants.

DIAGNOSTIC TESTS

Bloodwork

As seen in the previous chapter, the effect of sepsis on the circulating neutrophil count is variable. Acute neutropenia, with or without a left shift, is commonly related to bacterial sepsis or endotoxemia when there is overzealous production of cytokines. With the appropriate stimulus, neutrophilia with or without a left shift may be present. Profound lymphopenia may be found in acute viral diseases as well as sepsis and endotoxemia.[17] Lymphocyte counts are generally higher than neutrophil counts in the fetus and may reflect the degree of immaturity in premature foals. Physiologically, neutrophil counts in neonatal foals increase to mean values of approximately 8×10^3 neutrophils/μl during the first 24 hours postparturition, due to endogenous glucocorticoid steroid release. Lymphocyte counts may physiologically decrease to mean values of 1.4×10^3 lymphocytes/μl a few hours after birth, and then gradually increase to 5×10^3 lymphocytes/μl at three months of age.[18] Neonatal respiratory disease is not consistently related to specific abnormalities in the serum biochemistry analysis, but may depend upon underlying conditions such as sepsis, SIRS, or perinatal asphyxia.

Blood Gas Analysis

Arterial blood gas analysis is preferentially used to determine oxygenation and ventilation in neonates. Although pulse oximetry provides a continuous measure of arterial oxygen saturation, this technique has not been rigorously tested in the foal, and accurate readings are often difficult to obtain in the awake foal. Technically, an arterial blood sample can be obtained from any artery where a pulse can be felt. The more common sampling sites include the dorsal metatarsal artery located between the third metatarsal (cannon) bone and the cranial ridge of the forth metatarsal (lateral splint) bone of the hind limb; the branchial artery on the medial aspect of the elbow; the femoral artery at the external inguinal ring; the carotid artery, which runs medial and deep to the jugular vein; and the transverse facial artery, which is located caudal to the lateral cantus of the eye (ventral to the zygomatic

Table 6-1	Arterial Blood Gas Interpretation	
Parameter	Rounded Mean Normal Values (mm Hg)	Age of Foal Postpartum*
PaO_2	55–60	30 minutes (lateral recumbency)
	70–80	6 hours (lateral)
	70–80	12 hours (lateral)
	70 (lateral) to 90 (standing)	24 hours
$PaCO_2$	50–55	30 minutes (lateral recumbency)
	43–47	6 hours (lateral)
	43–47	12 hours (lateral)
	42 (standing) to 50 (lateral)	24 hours

Caution
- Mild hypoxemia may be observed in foals after prolonged recumbency (especially if peripheral samples are taken).
- Changes in body temperature result in large changes in PaO_2, $PaCO_2$, and pH without affecting HCO_3. A low body temperature decreases PaO_2 and $PaCO_2$ while raising pH.
- Air contamination in the ABG sample will falsely increase measured PaO_2 and decrease $PaCO_2$ levels.
- Metabolism continues within the ABG syringe after the sample is taken (tends to decrease PaO_2 and produce CO_2). Therefore, specimens held at room temperature must be analyzed within 10 minutes of drawing; iced samples should be analyzed within two hours.

*Summarized from Harvey JW: Normal hematologic values, In Koterba AM, Drummond WH, Kosch PG, eds: *Equine clinical neonatology*, Philadelphia, 1990, Lea & Febiger.

arch). Successful arterial sampling is somewhat dependent upon the cardiovascular status of the foal. It is difficult to feel a pulse at the more distal sites in foals that are hypotensive or hypothermic. Additionally, peripheral oxygenation may not be equivalent to partial oxygen pressures obtained from central arteries.

Clipping and applying alcohol to the site of arterial puncture may help to visualize the artery. It is best to use a 22- to 25-gauge needle and a special blood gas syringe that contains an anticoagulant (e.g. sodium heparin) to obtain your sample. These syringes are usually self-filling. Once the sample has been drawn, all air bubbles should be evacuated from the syringe and the syringe should be capped to prevent exposure to room air. Room air will falsely increase the true PaO_2 and decrease the $PaCO_2$. Samples should be analyzed as soon as possible. If there is a delay (>10 minutes), then the sample can be refrigerated for two hours without significant problems. New handheld blood gas analyzers make this a practical test even in farm settings. Table 6-1 and Figure 6-3 are guidelines for the interpretation of arterial blood gas results in equine neonates.

In the absence of alterations in the inspired oxygen fraction (FiO_2), arterial hypoxemia may result from four basic processes, including hypoventilation, diffusion impairment, ventilation-perfusion inequality (VQ mismatch), and shunt (intrapulmonary and extrapulmonary shunt).[19]

Alveolar hypoventilation is defined as a reduced volume of inspired air reaching the alveoli per unit time, and is always related to an increase in $PaCO_2$ (hypercarbia). Conditions associated with alveolar hypoventilation include drug-induced respiratory depression (morphine, barbiturates), brain stem disease, abnormal respiratory muscle function (botulism, diaphragmatic hernia, dysfunction, or fatigue), thoracic cage abnormalities (rib fractures), increased airway resistance (upper and lower airway obstruction) and pleural space disease.[20] Although the mainstay of hypercarbia is hypoventilation, hypercapnic respiratory failure may also be multifactorial and can be exacerbated by severe VQ mismatch, shunt, or diffusion impairments. However, hypercarbia in foals with respiratory failure due to consolidating pneumonia, atelectasis, ARDS, etc., is more likely related to hypoxic diaphragmatic failure (secondary hypoventilation) than VQ mismatch, shunt, or diffusion impairment.

Impaired diffusion results from an increase in the blood-gas barrier. Since carbon dioxide diffuses more readily than oxygen, the $PaCO_2$ is usually not increased in conditions that only cause impaired diffusion, until the lesion is severe. Diffusion impairments may be seen in conditions such as pulmonary edema, pneumonia, atelectasis, or pulmonary contusion.[20]

The adequacy of pulmonary gas exchange is also determined by the balance between pulmonary ventilation and capillary blood flow, which is commonly expressed as the ventilation-perfusion (VQ) ratio. A VQ ratio above 1 describes conditions in which ventilation is excessive relative to capillary blood flow (dead space ventilation). In normal human subjects, dead space ventilation accounts for 20% to 30% of the

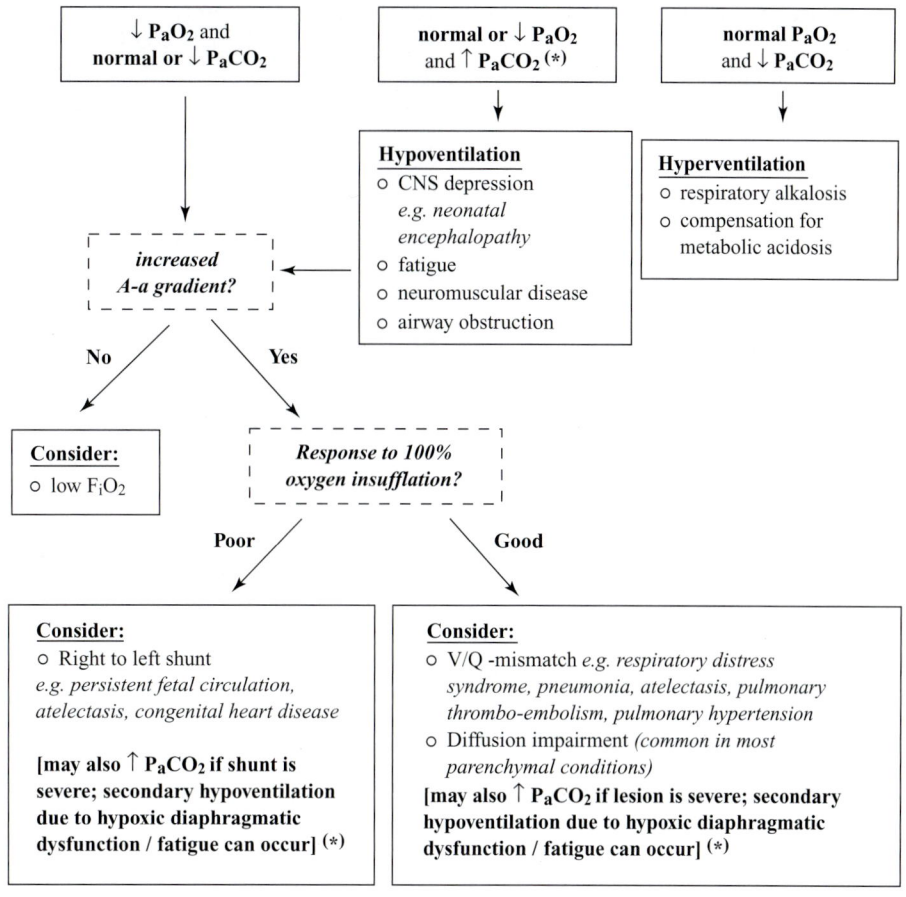

Fig. 6-3 Interpretation of arterial blood gases in neonatal foals.

total ventilation. Dead space ventilation increases when the alveolar-capillary interface is destroyed (e.g. emphysema), when blood flow is reduced (e.g. low cardiac output, pulmonary thrombo-embolism, persistent pulmonary hypertension), or when the alveoli are overdistended by positive pressure ventilation. A VQ ratio below 1 describes the condition in which capillary blood flow is excessive relative to ventilation (pulmonary edema, pneumonia, atelectasis, etc.).[21]

Shunting, on the other hand, is defined as any mechanism by which blood that has not passed through ventilated areas of the lung is added to arteries of the systemic circulation.[20] In normal human subjects, intrapulmonary shunt flow (venous admixture) represents less than 10% of the total cardiac output.[21] Rose and colleagues calculated the extent of physiologic shunt in neonatal foals and reported values of 16% to 18% in newborn term foals restrained in temporary lateral recumbency.[22] In contrast, a 15% true shunt in adult humans is generally regarded as requiring oxygen therapy and 30% as life-threatening.[23]

Increased intrapulmonary anatomical shunting can result from pulmonary artery to venous fistulas or severe lung lobe consolidation. Cardiac shunting (right to left shunt) may be related to congenital heart disease (e.g. tetralogy of Fallot, patent ductus arteriosus) or persistent fetal circulation (PFC). It is important to note that hypoxemia that is unresponsive to oxygen therapy is suggestive of shunt.[20]

Alveolar to Arterial Oxygen Gradient

The difference in partial pressure of oxygen between alveolar pressure of oxygen (PAO_2) and arterial pressure of oxygen (PaO_2) is termed *A-a gradient*. The A-a gradient can be used as an indirect measure of VQ abnormalities, severe diffusion impairment and shunt, and is determined by the alveolar gas equation.

$$A\text{-a gradient} = PAO_2 - PaO_2$$
$$= (PiO_2 - PaCO_2/RQ) - PaO_2$$

Index:
PiO_2 = inspired oxygen pressure (150 mm Hg in animals' breathing room air)
PAO_2 = alveolar pressure of oxygen
PaO_2 = arterial pressure of oxygen

PaCO$_2$ = arterial pressure of carbon dioxide

RQ = respiratory quotient (ratio of CO$_2$ production over O$_2$ consumption); is equal to 0.8 at resting conditions

A simplified formula of the A-a gradient in animals' breathing room air is

$$A\text{-a gradient} = 150 - (PaCO_2/0.8) - PaO_2$$

The normal A-a gradient is less than 15 mm Hg in healthy foals' breathing room air, and increases with VQ mismatch, shunt, and severe diffusion impairments. The normal A-a gradient increases 5 to 7 mm Hg for every 10% increase in the inspired oxygen fraction in humans (FiO$_2$ = 21% in room air). This effect is presumably caused by the loss of regional hypoxic vasoconstriction of the lungs after oxygen administration.[21] Normal A-a gradients in foals receiving supplemental oxygen have not been established.

'03 Hufflepuff's A-a gradient was more than double that of a normal foal. This was compatible with a diffusion impairment or VQ mismatch from pulmonary atelectasis, edema, consolidating pneumonia, pulmonary hypertension, or pulmonary thrombo-embolism.

Radiographic Examination

Thoracic radiography is often helpful in establishing the presence of respiratory disease and in determining the type and extent of pulmonary involvement.[7] In contrast to noninvasive and invasive pulmonary function testing (PFT, see below), thoracic radiography is used extensively in the clinical setting. Neonatal radiographic evaluation of the chest is facilitated by classifying the image appearance into radiographic patterns of pulmonary disease. Three major lung patterns (interstitial, alveolar, and bronchial patterns) are commonly used to define evidence of radiographic respiratory disease in neonatal foals. Although the vascular pattern may be helpful in assessing pulmonary perfusion, venous congestion, and cardiac anomalies, it plays a lesser role in the assessment of foal pneumonia.

Interstitial Lung Pattern

The pulmonary interstitium is composed of a connective tissue framework containing the pulmonary vasculature, lymphatics, nerves, and bronchi. Inflammatory infiltrate that affects these structures may produce radiographic changes that are referred to as the interstitial pattern. The hallmark of the interstitial

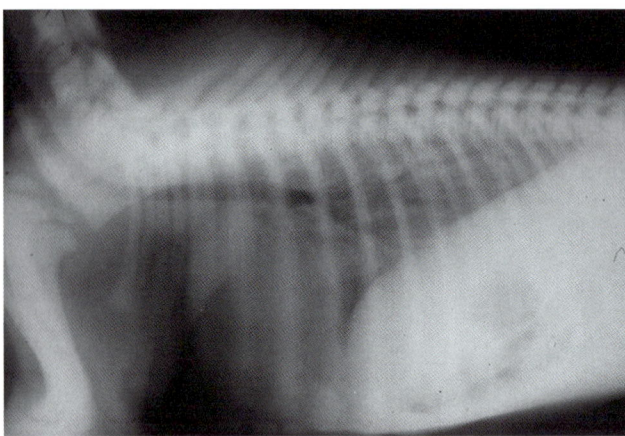

Fig. 6-4 Diffuse interstitial lung pattern, predominantly in the dorso-caudal region of the lung.

pattern is an increase in background opacity, which results in the loss of visualization of the fine vascular structure of the normal, well-aerated lung.[24]

The interstitial pattern is the most common radiographic abnormality in foals with pulmonary disease. It may be associated with bacterial or viral pneumonia, pulmonary edema, meconium aspiration, lung immaturity, acute lung injury, and prolonged recumbency due to dependent atelectasis.[25] Compression of the lung by distended abdominal viscera may also result in an apparent increase in the interstitial pattern due to decreased lung inflation (Figure 6-4).

Bronchial Lung Pattern

Although the bronchi are a component of the interstitial complex, diseases of this system are often considered separately. Radiographic signs of bronchial disease include increased thickness and density of the bronchial walls, or changes in bronchial lumen diameter (e.g. bronchiectasis). A bronchial lung pattern is more suggestive of chronic disease. However, a peribronchial pattern indicates infiltrates surrounding the bronchi and may be seen in acute and chronic inflammatory conditions.[24]

Alveolar Lung Pattern

The alveolar or air-space pattern is characterized by displacement of air from the alveoli by transudate, exudates, or blood, leading to a relatively homogenous increase in soft-tissue opacity. Air bronchograms may appear as lucent branching structures within an opaque lung field. The finding of air bronchograms is an indication of nearly complete alveolar filling.[24] Edema, aspiration, infection, hemorrhage, and pulmonary consolidation commonly produce an alveolar pattern in neonatal foals (Figure 6-5).[26] Additionally, a

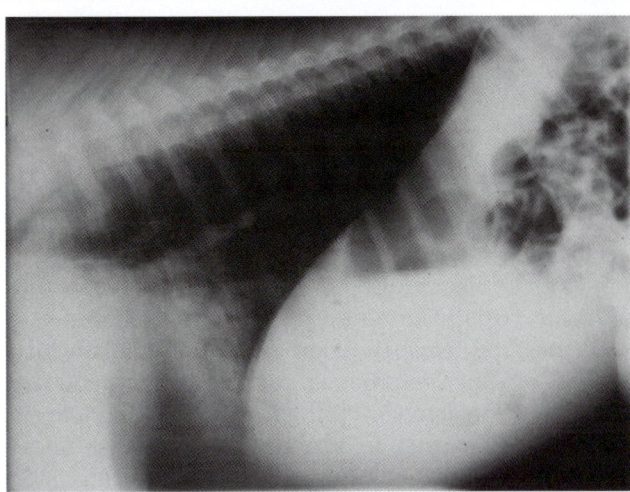

Fig. 6-5 Alveolar lung pattern in the caudo-ventral aspect of the lung field in a neonatal foal.

diffuse air-space pattern can result from respiratory distress syndrome (RDS) in the neonate, acute lung injury (ALI), and acute respiratory distress syndrome (ARDS) in the equine neonate.[27]

It is important to recognize that the clinical onset of neonatal respiratory disease may be extremely insidious and thus difficult to recognize by physical examination alone. Early thoracic radiographic imaging of compromised neonatal foals may alert the clinician and establish a prompt diagnosis of underlying respiratory disease. Since radiographic findings may precede or lag behind alteration of respiratory function, repeated diagnostic imaging is recommended. Thoracic radiography, however, should be interpreted critically. Specifically, the severity of radiographic abnormalities is significantly dependent on patient position. The most useful radiographic position to assess a foal's lung is in temporary lateral recumbency with the forelimbs extended forward. This allows for the examination of the entire lung field without interference by the tricep muscle. Because lateral recumbency can result in atelectasis of the down lung, it is recommended to maintain the foal standing or sternal prior to radiographic assessment and to obtain both right and left lateral thoracic views.

A recent study has documented that radiographic abnormalities involving the caudodorsal lung region were most common in foals admitted to a referral center.[28] Bedenice and colleagues showed that the presence of dyspnea, tachypnea, a fibrinogen concentration >400 mg/dl, SIRS, hypoxemia, or FPT in neonatal foals may be predictors of underlying respiratory disease and should prompt an early radiographic evaluation of the thorax, even in the absence of other localizing clinical signs.[3,28]

'03 Hufflepuff was tachypneic upon presentation and showed diffuse radiographic infiltrates with a predominance of caudodorsal distribution. This is consistent with previous findings that tachypnea most reliably related to diffuse (caudodorsal, caudoventral, and cranioventral) pulmonary changes.[28] The presence of underlying sepsis or SIRS in this foal may further explain the predominant caudodorsal pulmonary infiltrates. Pulmonary ventilation and perfusion is closely matched in horses, and the percent regional blood flow is increased in the caudal lung lobes.[29] Additionally, Amis and coworkers documented that ventilation and perfusion follow a vertical gradient and increase in the dorsal lung regions of horses.[30] SIRS may initiate severe vascular leakage and thus contribute directly to the pathogenesis of lung injury in regions of increased relative blood flow.[28]

Ultrasonography

Thoracic ultrasonography has become a popular diagnostic tool for the assessment of equine lung and pleural disease. Consolidation, pleural effusion, abscesses, penetrating thoracic wounds, rib fractures, and diaphragmatic hernias are some of the diseases that have been detected ultrasonographically in the lung and pleural cavity of adult horses and foals. The side(s) of the thorax affected, as well as the precise location of the lesion, can be determined in most cases.

Computed Tomography

Additionally, computed tomography (CT) may serve as an important and sensitive means of thoracic imaging in anesthetized patients. Computed tomography has played an important role in improving our knowledge of the pathophysiology, morphology, and progression of pulmonary dysfunction in humans.[31] It is not only a research tool, but an invaluable technique that allows for the quantitative and qualitative characterization of structural lung abnormalities, assessment of lung structure–pulmonary function relationships, the effect of ventilation strategies (e.g., PEEP), and therapeutic maneuvers (e.g., patient position) on lung structure and the progression of pulmonary disease (Figure 6-6). However, the use of CT in equine neonatal pulmonary disease is currently restricted to referral centers.

Diagnostic Sampling

Diagnostic sampling of the respiratory tract is less commonly performed in neonatal foals compared to

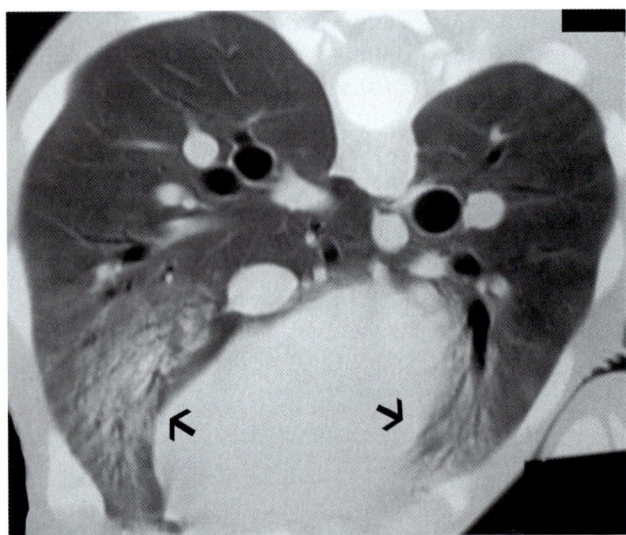

Fig. 6-6 Computed tomography of the lung in a foal with acute lung injury indicating affected lung tissue (arrows).

adult horses. Transtracheal aspirates (TTA), broncho-alveolar lavage (BAL), protected catheter brush (PCB), or protected aspiration catheter sampling (PAC) is useful in stabilized patients to direct antimicrobial therapy and evaluate therapeutic efficacy. Generally, the clinician will depend upon the blood culture results to direct antibiotic therapy in the critically ill foal with respiratory compromise. Although rare in foals, thoracocentesis may also be of diagnostic and therapeutic importance in cases of pleuropneumonia and chylothorax. Lung biopsies are rarely performed and are limited to patients with chronic disease or suspected fungal pneumonia.

'03 Hufflepuff was diagnosed with presumptive septic pneumonia based on physical, laboratory, and radiographic interpretation. Blood culture results confirmed bacteremia at the time of admission; both E. coli and Streptococcus spp were isolated with moderate growth. The initial thoracic radiographs were not consistent with postpartum aspiration based on the predominant caudodorsal distribution of radiographic infiltrates, nor did the foal's history suggest intrauterine compromise. Postpartum sepsis, facilitated by inadequate transfer of colostral antibodies and hematogenous spread of the bacteria, appeared to be the most likely cause of lung injury in this foal.

Pathophysiology

The term *lung injury* is generally used to describe the pulmonary response to a wide range of injuries occurring either directly to the lung or as a consequence of injury or inflammation at other sites in the body.[32] Lung injury is a common sequela to sepsis, aspiration, or trauma and may be clinically difficult to differentiate from primary pneumonia, ARDS or RDS in premature foals (see Case 8-1).

The pathophysiology of ALI is driven by an aggressive inflammatory reaction. In the exudative or acute phase, injury to the alveolar epithelial barrier leads to an increase in permeability to protein and extravasation of solutes and water. Pathologically, diffuse alveolar damage with neutrophils, macrophages, erythrocytes, protein-rich edema fluid in the alveolar spaces, hyaline membranes, capillary injury, and disruption of the alveolar epithelium may be evident.[33]

ALI is diagnosed in humans if acute respiratory symptoms, a PaO_2/FiO_2 ratio <300 mm Hg, and noncardiogenic diffuse radiographic infiltrates occur following direct lung injury (e.g., aspiration, lung contusion, diffuse pulmonary infection) or indirect lung injury (e.g., sepsis, severe nonthoracic trauma, hypertransfusion). ARDS represents the more severe form of lung injury and is associated with a PaO_2/FiO_2 ratio <200 mm Hg in humans.[34] Mortality rates from ARDS in humans have ranged from 40% to 60% in the past with the majority of deaths being related to sepsis or multiorgan dysfunction rather than primary respiratory causes.[33] More recent studies indicate a reduced mortality of 36% and 34%.[35]

Initial arterial blood gas analysis of '03 Hufflepuff confirmed a PaO_2/FiO_2 ratio <300 mm Hg (58/.21 = 276 mm Hg). In the face of acute respiratory symptoms and the presence of noncardiogenic diffuse radiographic infiltrates as a sequela of sepsis, '03 Hufflepuff met the human criteria of defining "acute lung injury." However, further research is required to determine the validity of these definitions in neonatal foals.

To further clarify the foal's respiratory compromise, noninvasive pulmonary function testing including functional residual capacity (FRC) via helium dilution and capnography were performed. A markedly reduced FRC of 1.05 liters was found on presentation. When this test was repeated at 48 hours postpresentation, the FRC had increased to 1.4 liters. Repeated capnography via facemask demonstrated an end-tidal CO_2 between 30 and 40 mm Hg. Dead space to tidal volume ratio was normal at 0.4. The foal further showed a normal minute ventilation of 21 liters/minute, with a peak inspiratory and expiratory flow of 0.9 and 1.27 liters/second.

Noninvasive Pulmonary Function Testing

Diagnostic imaging helps to identify structural thoracic changes, but does not quantify functional respiratory impairment in foals with pneumonia. Arterial blood gas analysis and the calculation of the A-a gradient give us further information about gas exchange. However, only novel noninvasive PFT helps clarify the true pulmonary function or dysfunction of foals with respiratory compromise. Clinical PFT is generally divided into the assessment of respiratory mechanics and gas exchange. Lung mechanics determine the static and dynamic properties of the lung—resistance, compliance, FRC, and ventilatory parameters.[36] Analysis of gas exchange investigates ventilation-perfusion (VQ) matching, shunt, diffusion capacity, and dead space to tidal volume ratios (V_D/V_T).

One potential application of noninvasive PFT in neonatal foals includes measurements of FRC via helium dilution[37] (Figure 6-7). FRC is a measure of the amount of gas that remains in the lung at end-expiration. FRC = residual volume + expiratory reserve volume (Figure 6-8). FRC is lower in patients with increased "lung stiffness" (reduced compliance of the lung) as well as airway inflammation. '03 Hufflepuff had a lower than expected FRC on presentation, which appeared to improve over time with treatment. This finding was most likely related to improving airway inflammation (resolving ALI).

Measurement of pulmonary diffusion capacity and VQ mismatch via nuclear scintigraphy may also be used to monitor pulmonary disease progression in neonatal foals, although the clinical application of this technique is limited. A lower diffusion capacity may be found in foals with pulmonary parenchymal disease (e.g., edema, pneumonia).

Capnography

Capnography measures end-tidal CO_2 concentrations ($PetCO_2$) using infrared spectroscopy (via facemask or endotracheal tube). It serves as a noninvasive approximation of $PaCO_2$ in animals without significant VQ mismatch, diffusion impairment, or shunt. The amount of CO_2 that appears in the exhaled gas is dependent upon three main components of respiration:

(1) CO_2 production due to cellular metabolism, e.g., $PetCO_2$ is increased during shivering and decreased during hypothermia

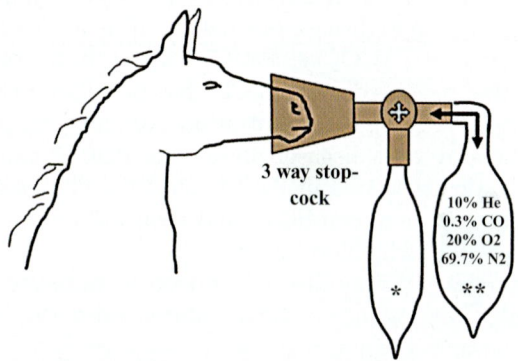

3 way stop-cock

10% He
0.3% CO
20% O2
69.7% N2

$*$ $**$

FRC = {[(initial [He] x bag volume / final [He]) x (1-[CO2])]–[bag volume + inst.d. space]} x 1.11 L

Fig. 6-7 Schematic of FRC measurement in a foal.

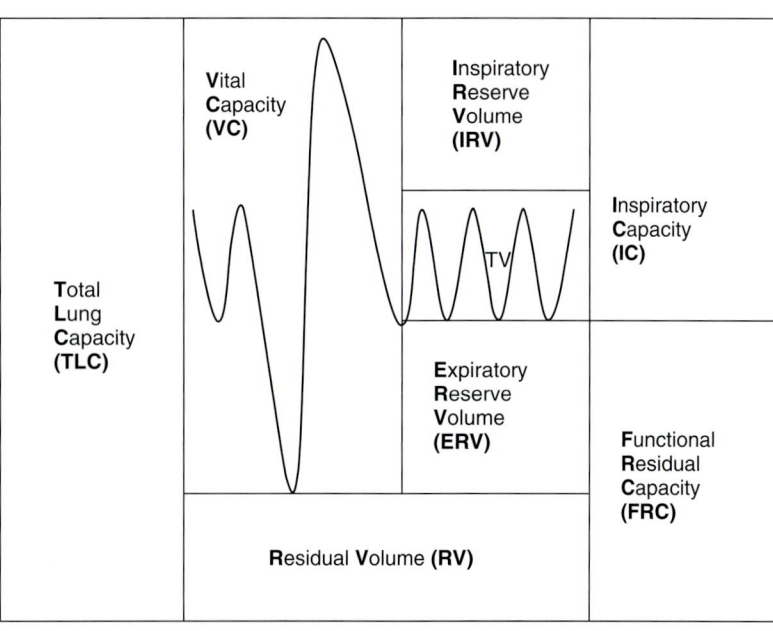

Total Lung Capacity (TLC)

Vital Capacity (VC)

Inspiratory Reserve Volume (IRV)

Inspiratory Capacity (IC)

TV

Expiratory Reserve Volume (ERV)

Functional Residual Capacity (FRC)

Residual Volume (RV)

Fig. 6-8 Schematic of differentiation of lung volumes.

(2) Transport of CO_2 between cells and pulmonary capillaries as well as diffusion of CO_2 into and from the alveoli, e.g., $PetCO_2$ is decreased in the face of hypovolemia (low cardiac output) or pulmonary embolism

(3) Pulmonary ventilation, e.g., $PetCO_2$ decreases during hyperventilation or bronchospasm

Under normal physiologic conditions, the difference between arterial PCO_2 ($PaCO_2$ from an arterial blood gas) and alveolar PCO_2 ($PetCO_2$ from a capnograph) is 2 to 5 mm Hg (capnographic values are usually slightly lower). This $PaCO_2 - PetCO_2$ difference may increase due to leaks in the sampling system or foals with diseased lungs. It is also important to remember that the $PetCO_2$ in foals with shallow breaths (e.g. shallow tachypnea due to disease or excitement) is *neither* representative of $PACO_2$ *nor* $PaCO_2$. Under these conditions, the measured expired CO_2 has not equilibrated with the alveolar gas concentration. Nonetheless, with both healthy and diseased lungs, the $PetCO_2$ can be used to detect trends in $PaCO_2$, alert the clinician to changes in patient condition, and reduce the required number of arterial blood gases.[38]

Capnography may also be utilized to measure the patient's dead space to tidal volume ratio (V_D/V_T). This variable estimates the percentage of ventilated lung where no gas exchange occurs, and is calculated according to the following formula[21]:

$$V_D/V_T = (PaCO_2 - PeCO_2)/PaCO_2$$

$PaCO_2$ = arterial pressure of carbon dioxide (can be approximated by $PetCO_2$)
$PeCO_2$ = mixed expired CO_2

For example, foals with a pulmonary thromboembolism or shunt will ventilate areas of the lung that are poorly perfused, thus leading to increased dead-space ventilation (where no gas exchange can occur) and a higher V_D/V_T ratio. Additionally, shallow breaths (low tidal volume ventilation) will increase V_D/V_T.

In summary, better clinical monitoring may improve the clinician's assessment concerning 1) aggressive management of lung disease, 2) decisions for ventilation, 3) intensity of monitoring, 4) ventilator weaning, 5) cost analyses, and 6) prognosis of foals with neonatal respiratory disease.

Initial management of '03 Hufflepuff included cardiovascular support with dextrose-containing fluids, nutritional management via an indwelling nasogastric tube, continuous nasal insufflation of oxygen at 6 liters/minute, and systemic broad-spectrum antibiotic treatment with amikacin and potassium penicillin.

Initial indirect blood pressure measurements revealed a systolic/diastolic blood pressure of 95/60, with a mean

of 75 mm Hg. Following fluid therapy, the foal's blood pressure increased to 116/58, with a normal central venous pressure (CVP) of 5 cm H_2O, which indicated adequate volume resuscitation.

TREATMENT

The treatment of equine neonatal pneumonia is multifaceted. The interim goal of therapy is to maintain adequate gas exchange to ensure patient survival, limit progressive pulmonary damage, and ultimately eradicate infection. Long-term goals should be directed at maintaining optimal pulmonary function and conserving adult athletic performance. Specific treatment strategies of septic pneumonia may include: antimicrobial therapy, treatment of inflammation independent of antimicrobial therapy, and respiratory and cardiovascular support.

Broad-spectrum antibiotic treatment of septic pneumonia should be initiated before culture results are available, and are targeted toward the most common pathogenic bacteria involved (see Chapter 5). A combination of amikacin and penicillin is a reasonable initial empirical choice in patients with adequate peripheral perfusion. Aminoglycosides penetrate lung tissue at 10% to 45% of serum levels. However, the acidic environment of infected airways may reduce the drug's activity below levels sufficient to eradicate the offending bacteria.[39,40]

Third- or fourth-generation cephalosporins (Ceftiofur and Cefepime, respectively) may be safer in markedly cardiovascular compromised patients and show good penetration into lung tissues.[41] In the human ICU, however, the routine use of third-generation cephalosporins is limited by rapid induction of resistance in the hospital setting.[42] Since equine neonatal pneumonia is frequently a result of bloodstream infection or may seed the circulation secondarily, it is essential to attain adequate plasma bloodstream concentrations of the antimicrobial agent via a parenteral route. Alveolar delivery of antibiotics typically occurs via diffusion of a free, nonprotein-bound drug and is usually satisfactory if plasma concentrations and alveolar perfusion are adequate.[43] Antibiotic therapy should not be discontinued prematurely, since pulmonary infection is commonly well established prior to its diagnosis.[44] Duration of antimicrobial treatment for established pneumonia may extend from two to five weeks. Long-term therapy should therefore be carefully monitored, especially in premature and debilitated foals. Assessment of plasma antibiotic concentrations will ensure drug adequacy and reduce the toxic potential if they are available.

Considerable speculation exists about whether bactericidal antimicrobial treatment transiently worsens inflammatory responses and host injury by releasing pro-inflammatory structural and metabolic constituents into the surrounding microenvironment. The utility and efficacy of current anti-inflammatory therapy, however, needs to be further explored.[43]

Adequate gas exchange not only depends upon alveolar ventilation, but also upon perfusion and diffusion capacity. Preservation of pulmonary and systemic perfusion is essential in the treatment of compromised foals using volume expanders, inotropes, afterload reduction, and blood products, as needed (see Chapter 7). Foals should also be maintained in sternal recumbency to limit positional atelectasis.

Maintenance of airway patency may be more challenging in foals with pneumonia, due to the presence of potentially profuse and obstructive secretions and mucopurulent exudates of variable viscosity.[43] Specific respiratory support may, therefore, include judicious suctioning, coupage, bronchodilators (albuterol inhalants), and mucolytic agents (e.g., 10% acetylcysteine; 30 ml nebulized over 30 minutes bid). Theophylline and aminophylline are commonly used as bronchodilators (theophylline: 4 to 7 mg/kg PO tid, or 6 to 10 mg/kg diluted in 100 ml administered slowly IV bid; keeping serum levels below 15 µg/ml), which may also strengthen diaphragmatic function. In calculating doses, 1 mg theophylline equals about 1.25 mg aminophylline. Aminophylline (starting dose of 2 mg/kg) should be diluted in at least 100 ml NaCl and given slowly IV, at rates not exceeding 25 mg/minute.[5]

Nasal insufflation of oxygen is a simple technique to stabilize foals with poor oxygenation due to V/Q mismatch, hypoventilation, and diffusion limitations. The goals of correct oxygen therapy are three-fold: (1) treatment of hypoxemia, (2) reduction of ventilatory work necessary to maintain a given alveolar oxygen tension (PaO_2), and (3) decrease in myocardial work necessary to maintain a given PaO_2.[23]

Previous studies in healthy neonatal foals have shown that age-dependent differences in PaO_2 were attributed to a right to left shunt and related to a closing foramen ovale, ductus arteriosus, or ventilation-perfusion inequality in the postnatal period.[45] (see Table 6-1) PaO_2 response to administered O_2 also increases from birth to seven days of age (see Table 1-1). The administration of 100% oxygen via facemask versus intranasal oxygen insufflation at 10 liters/minute to the level of the pharynx results in comparable increases in PaO_2. Peak concentrations of PaO_2 are generally obtained after two minutes of oxygen administration.

Intranasal administration of oxygen to a foal is most easily accomplished through a small tube inserted into the nostril up to the level of the pharynx. The tube can

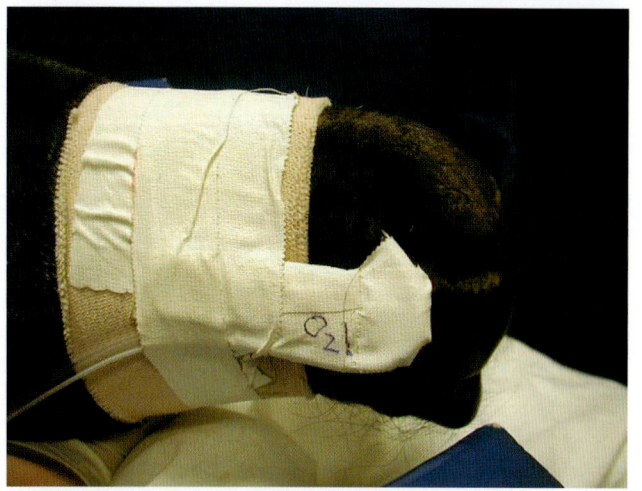

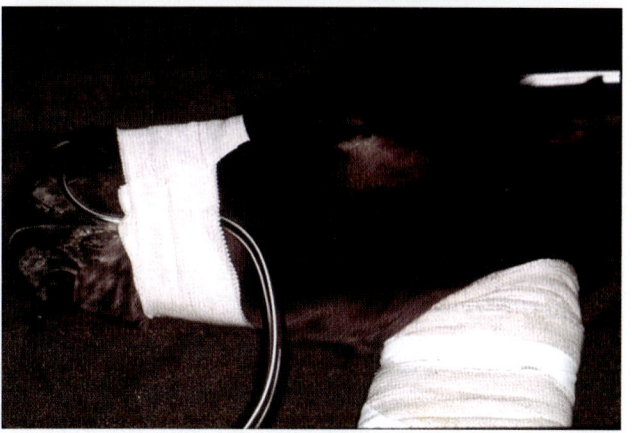

Fig. 6-9 A, Foal with nasal insufflation of oxygen with nasal tube taped to the nose. **B,** Foal with nasal tube sewn into nasal fold.

be fixed to a tongue depressor and taped to the muzzle of the foal or alternatively fixed to the nostril through the use of a Chinese finger trap suture. The flow of oxygen should be passed through a humidifier to prevent drying of the respiratory mucosa (Figure 6-9).

In cases of respiratory failure in which there is a progressive increase in $PaCO_2$, oxygen therapy alone is not sufficient. Respiratory support in the form of mechanical ventilation may be necessary (see Chapter 8).

Cardiac and intrapulmonary shunts show a limited response to oxygen therapy, in contrast to hypoxemia due to VQ mismatch, hypoventilation, and diffusion impairment. Figure 6-10 is a helpful guideline to calculate shunt fractions in humans.

'03 Hufflepuff responded favorably to nasal insufflation of oxygen at 6 liters/minute. A recheck arterial blood gas analysis revealed a pH of 7.44, $PaCO_2$ of 44 mm Hg, and PaO_2 of 184 mm Hg. Based on his favorable response to oxygen therapy alone, a pathologic shunt was consid-

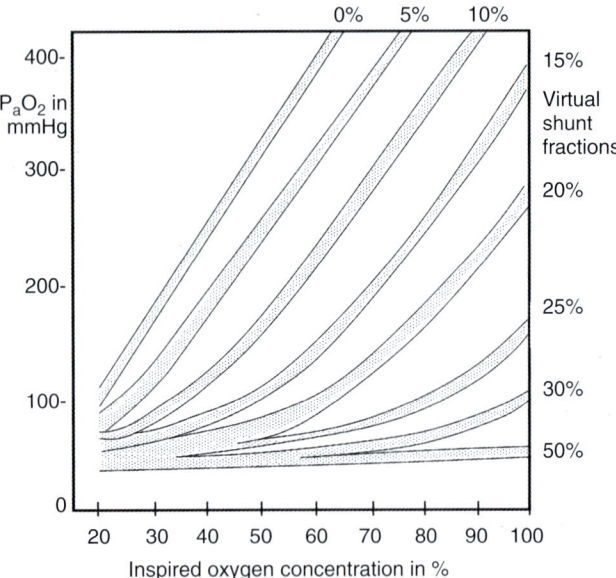

Fig. 6-10 Calculation of shunt fractions in humans. Redrawn from Lumb A: *Nunn's applied respiratory physiology*, ed 5, Oxford, 2000, Butterworth Heinemann.

ered less likely. Hypoxemia in this foal was most likely related to V/Q mismatch or diffusion impairment.

'03 Hufflepuff responded well to broad-spectrum antimicrobial treatment. His arterial blood gases and pulmonary function parameters normalized by day four of hospitalization. A recheck CBC at this time showed a resolution of his neutropenia and left shift. However, the fibrinogen level was markedly elevated at 700 mg/dl, indicative of continuing inflammation. Improvement of the thoracic radiographic appearance was observed on day five.

The foal was discharged on day seven, with a recommendation of continued antimicrobial treatment until recheck evaluation in three weeks. Chest radiographs at the time of recheck demonstrated a marked improvement in radiographic appearance. A residual mildly increased interstitial lung pattern within the caudal lung field was observed, the clinical significance of which was unclear. The foal had gained 20 kg since the previous discharge, and all laboratory data had normalized at this time. Antimicrobial treatment was discontinued after a total of four weeks of therapy.

PROGNOSIS

The survival of foals with septic pneumonia is contingent on the underlying disease conditions, a prompt diagnosis, and the etiology and severity of pulmonary dysfunction. Several studies have observed prognostic variables of survival in critically ill foals.[46-49] It is important to note, however, that many foals are euthanized before a life-threatening disease becomes terminal. Termination of treatment may be related to financial constraints or the clinician's impression of futility of treatment, which may alter the objectivity of outcome studies.

A variety of clinical variables have been correlated with outcome. Only ones that demonstrated some respiratory component will be presented here. Gayle and colleagues determined that the ability to stand at admission, a respiratory rate ≥60 breaths per minute, and normal-appearing mucous membranes were significantly associated with survival of septic foals.[47] In a separate study, Hoffman and coworkers studied prognostic factors in critically ill neonates with a variety of primary problems. He reported that a decreased PvO_2 and increased anion gap were indicators of poor prognosis.[48]

Few studies have objectively evaluated the outcome of neonatal foal pneumonia. One report documented a 50% prevalence of pulmonary disease in hospitalized neonatal foals with a 39% survival to discharge.[1] A subsequent study from the same institution demonstrated that 65% of foals with radiographic evidence of pulmonary disease were discharged alive between 1990 and 1998. In this study, the presence of diffuse radiographic infiltrates (caudodorsal, caudoventral, and cranioventral involvement) or concurrent alveolar patterns within the caudodorsal and caudoventral lung indicated lower survival rates.[3] An increase of survival from 39% to 65% over time represents an improved outcome as we learn more about the pathophysiology of lung injury. The clinician should be aware that aggressive medical management, early fluid resuscitation, and specific respiratory support may be crucial for the successful outcome of these patients.[3,28]

The long-term effect on athletic performance has thus far been only evaluated in older foals that survived rhodococcus pneumonia. *R. equi* infection in foals was associated with a decreased chance of racing as adults. However, the performance of foals that went on to race was not significantly different from that of the general U.S. racing population.[50] It still remains speculative whether severe equine neonatal pneumonia has a high propensity to limit peak athletic future performance. Human studies have shown that many hosts develop long-lasting or permanent pulmonary changes after recovery from neonatal pneumonia. The documented residual pulmonary damage in humans may significantly affect the quality of life and susceptibility to later infections.[43]

Case-based evaluations in horses have demonstrated that functional and structural pulmonary impairment may occur in survivors of severe neonatal pneumonia. However, the clinical significance of this finding currently remains unclear.

REFERENCES

1. Freeman L, Paradis MR: Evaluation the effectiveness of equine neonatal care, *Vet Med* 87:921, 1992.
2. Magee T, Bedenice D, Paradis MR: Unpublished data, MA, Tufts University School of Veterinary Medicine, 2004.
3. Bedenice D, Heuwieser W, Solano M et al: Risk factors and prognostic variables for survival of foals with radiographic evidence of pulmonary disease, *J Vet Intern Med* 17:868, 2003.
4. Paradis MR: Infectious diseases of the equine respiratory tract: From gestation to five months, *Vet Med* 84:1174, 1989.
5. Bedenice D, Paradis MR: Equine neonatal pneumonia. In Brown CM, Bertone JJ, eds: *The 5-Minute veterinary consult—equine*, Philadelphia, 2002, Lippincott Williams & Wilkins.
6. Martin L. *Cyanosis*: In emedicine.com, Inc., 2004.
7. Koterba AM: Respiratory disease: Approach to diagnosis. In Koterba AM, Drummond WH, Kosch PG, eds: *Equine clinical neonatology*, Philadelphia, 1990, Lea & Febiger.
8. Zink MC, Johnson JA: Cellular constituents of clinically normal foal bronchoalveolar lavage fluid during postnatal maturation, *Am J Vet Res* 45:893, 1984.
9. LeBlanc PH: Responses of plasma transfusion in clinically healthy and clinically ill foals, *AAEP* 755, 1988.
10. Beech J: Respiratory problems in foals, *Vet Clin North Am Equine Pract* 1:131, 1985.
11. Vaala WE: Fatal congenital acquired infection with equine arteritis virus in a neonatal thoroughbred, *Equine Vet J* 24:155, 1992.
12. Webb RF, Knight PR, Walker KH: Involvement of adenovirus in pneumonia in a Thoroughbred foal, *Aust Vet J* 57:142, 1981.
13. Thompson DB, Spradborw PB, Studdert M: Isolation of an adenovirus from an Arab foal with a combined immunodeficiency disease, *Aust Vet J* 52:435, 1976.
14. Britton AP, Robinson JH: Isolation of influenza A virus from a 7-day-old foal with bronchointerstitial pneumonia, *Can Vet J* 43:55, 2002.
15. Klingner CM, Kruse J: Meconium aspiration syndrome: Pathophysiology and prevention, *J Am Board Fam Pract* 12:450, 1999.
16. Ghidini A, Spong CY: Severe meconium aspiration syndrome is not caused by aspiration of meconium, *Am J Obstet Gynecol* 185:931, 2001.
17. Morris DD: Alterations in the leukogram. In Smith BP, ed: *Large animal internal medicine*, St Louis, 2002, Mosby.
18. Harvey JW: Normal hematologic values, In Koterba AM, Drummond WH, Kosch PG, eds: *Equine clinical neonatology*, Philadelphia, 1990, Lea & Febiger.
19. West JB: *Pulmonary pathophysiology*, Baltimore, 1982, Williams & Wilkins.
20. Wilson WD, Lofstedt J: Alterations in respiratory function. In Smith BP, ed: *Large animal internal medicine*, ed 3, St Louis, 2002, Mosby.
21. Marino PL: Hypoxemia and Hypercapnia. In Zinner SR, ed: *The ICU book*, ed 2, Philadelphia, 1998, Lippincott Williams &Wilkins.
22. Rose RJ, Hodgson DH, Leadon DP et al: The effect of intranasal oxygen administration on arterial blood gas and acid base parameters in spontaneously delivered, term-induced and induced premature foals, *Res Vet Sci* 34:159, 1983.
23. Shapiro DL, Harrison RA, Walton JR: *Clinical application of blood gases*, ed 3, Chicago, 1982, Yearbook Medical Publishers.
24. Butler et al, eds: *Clinical radiology of the horse*, 1st ed, Blackwell, 1995.
25. Lester GD, Lester NV: Abdominal and thoracic radiography in the neonate, *Vet Clin North Am Equine Pract* 17:19, 2001.
26. Lamb CR, O'Callaghan MW: *Diagnostic imaging of equine pulmonary disease, the compendium—equine* 11:1110, 1989.
27. Lamb CR, O'Callaghan MW, Paradis MR: Thoracic radiography in the neonatal foal: A preliminary report, *Vet Radiol* 31:11, 1990.
28. Bedenice D, Heuwieser W, Brawer R, et al: The clinical and prognostic significance of radiographic pattern, distribution and severity of thoracic radiographic changes in neonatal foals, *J Vet Intern Med* 17:876, 2003.
29. Stewart JH, Young IH, Rose RJ et al: The distribution of ventilation-perfusion ratios in the lungs of newborn foals, *J Dev Physiol* 9:309, 1987.
30. Amis TC, Pascoe JR, Hornof W: Topographic distribution of pulmonary ventilation and perfusion in the horse, *Am J Vet Res* 45:1597, 1984.
31. Pelosi P, Crotti S, Brazzi L, et al: Computed tomography in adult respiratory distress syndrome: What has it taught us?, *Eur Respir J* 9:1055, 1996.
32. Bellingan GJ: The pulmonary physician in critical care 6: The pathogenesis of ALI/ARDS, *Thorax* 57:540, 2002.
33. Tweardy DJ: Acute respiratory distress syndrome (ARDS): Update on pathogenesis and new therapeutic directions, *VCRS*, San Antonio, 2003.
34. Desai SR: Acute respiratory distress syndrome: Imaging of the injured lung, *Clin Radiol* 57:8, 2002.
35. Abel SJ, Finney SJ, Brett SJ, et al: Reduced mortality in association with the acute respiratory distress syndrome (ARDS), *Thorax* 53:292, 1998.
36. Hoffman AM: Clinical application of pulmonary function in the horse. In International Veterinary Information Service (IVIS), 2002.
37. Amis TC, Jones HA: Measurement of functional residual capacity and pulmonary carbon monoxide uptake in conscious greyhounds, *Am J Vet Res* 45:1447, 1984.
38. Capnography: A reference handbook, *Respironics*, 2002.
39. Pennington JE: Penetration of antibiotics into respiratory secretions, *Rev Infect Dis* 3:67, 1981.
40. Bodem CR: Endobronchial pH: Relevance to aminoglycoside activity in Gram-negative bacillary pneumonia, *Am Rev Resp Dis* 127:39, 1983.
41. Cohen SH: Entry of four cephalosporins into the ovine lung, *J Infect Dis* 149:264, 1984.
42. Bryan CS. Gentamicin vs. cefotaxime for therapy of neonatal sepsis. Relationship to drug resistance, *Am J Dis Child* 139:1086, 1985.
43. Faix R: *Congenital pneumonia*, e-medicine, 2004.
44. Koterba AM, Paradis MR: Specific respiratory conditions. In Koterba AM, Drummond WH, Kosch PG, eds: *Equine clinical neonatology*, Philadelphia, 1990, Lea & Febiger.
45. Stewart JH, Rose RJ, Barko AM: Response to oxygen administration in foals: Effect of age, duration and method of administration on arterial blood gas values, *Equine Vet J* 16:329, 1984.
46. Barton MH, Morris DD, Norton N, et al: Hemostatic and fibrinolytic indices in neonatal foals with presumed septicemia, *J Vet Intern Med* 12:26, 1998.
47. Gayle JM, Cohen ND, Chaffin MK: Factors associated with survival in septicemic foals: 65 cases (1988-1995), *J Vet Intern Med* 12:140, 1998.
48. Hoffman AM, Staempfli HR, Willan A: Prognostic variables for survival of neonatal foals under intensive care, *J Vet Intern Med* 6:89, 1992.
49. Furr M, Tinker MK, Edens L: Prognosis for neonatal foals in an intensive care unit, *J Vet Intern Med* 11:183, 1997.
50. Ainsworth DM, Eicker SW, Yeagar AE et al: Associations between physical examination, laboratory, and radiographic findings and outcome and subsequent racing performance of foals with *Rhodococcus equi* infection: 115 cases (1984-1992), *J Am Vet Med Assoc* 213:510, 1998.

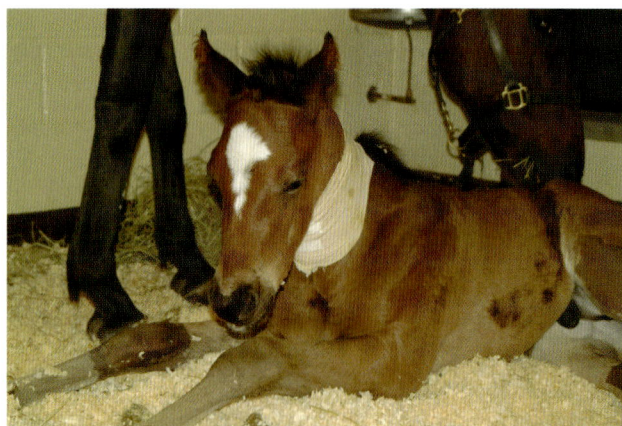

Fig. 6-11 '02 CrippleCreek, a two-day-old Thoroughbred foal, was presented with lameness and tarso-crural joint effusion.

Three days prior to parturition, CrippleCreek, an eight-year-old Thoroughbred mare, began leaking colostrum. There was evidence of caked milk on her hindlimbs. The birth of '02 CrippleCreek, a large foal, was uncomplicated (Figure 6-11). He stood within 120 minutes of birth and nursed by 180 minutes. Because of the colostral leakage and the possibility of FPT of maternal antibodies, the farm veterinarian administered 1 liter of plasma intravenously to the foal.

At two days of age, '02 CrippleCreek was found trembling. The owner found him recumbent in the morning. Though he would stand, the owner felt that he was lying down more than was normal. The decision was made to refer the foal to a full-care facility.

On presentation to the hospital, '02 CrippleCreek was bright and alert. His temperature was 102.6°F, heart rate was 104 beats per minute, and respiratory rate was 52 breathes per minute. Lameness in the left hindlimb was noted at the walk, and effusion of the left tarso-crural joint and edema of the physeal region of the lateral left hind fetlock were palpated.

HISTORY AND PHYSICAL EXAMINATION

Septic arthritis in the foal is often accompanied by a history of some incident that may have resulted in a decrease in the ingestion of adequate maternal antibodies from colostrum.[1,2] McCoy found the foals with FPT were 1.7 to 1.9 times more likely to develop septic arthritis or septic osteomyelitis, respectively, than foals that received adequate colostrum.[2] In this case, an inadequate immunoglobulin level was probably the

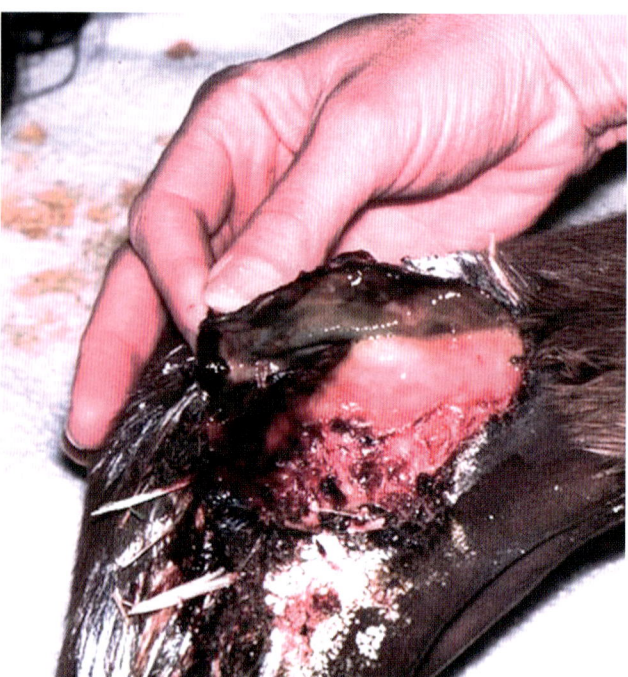

Fig. 6-12 Decubital ulcers form in areas where there is little body fat. The first signs include a sharp demarcation between healthy and affected skin. The affected skin becomes dry and less supple. In the final stages the skin sloughs, leaving a raw open wound.

result of the mare leaking colostrum before parturition. The administration of 1 liter of plasma by the referring veterinarian was enough to prevent a full-blown septic shock but not enough to provide complete protection. So over the course of two days, the foal became bacteremic.

The age range of neonatal foals presenting with septic arthritis is usually from the time of birth to 21 days of age with a mean age of presentation around eight days of age.[2] Clinically, the younger neonatal foal (birth to 36 hours) usually presents with joint effusion as a part of general signs of septicemia on the first day of life. Alternatively, the slightly older neonate (>36 hours) may appear relatively normal at first and develop lameness over a period of days or even weeks. Owners may report that the foal seems to spend more time recumbent than other foals. Evidence of thickened or leatherlike skin over boney prominences such as the elbows, hips, hocks, and carpi are signs of development of pressure decubital ulcers secondary to orthopedic pain and recumbency (Figure 6-12).

Careful palpation of all joints and physis should be done on the physical examination of the neonatal foal.

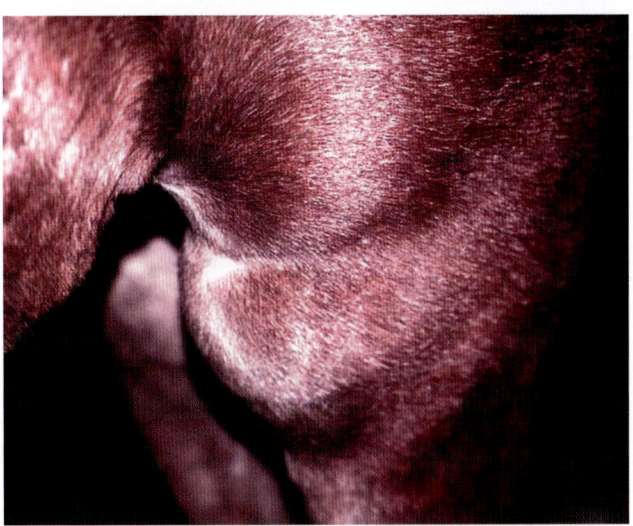

Fig. 6-13 Different joints may be affected in septic arthritis. A swollen stifle as seen in this photo may be obvious by sight, but subtle differences in size may only be detected by simultaneous palpation of the opposite joint.

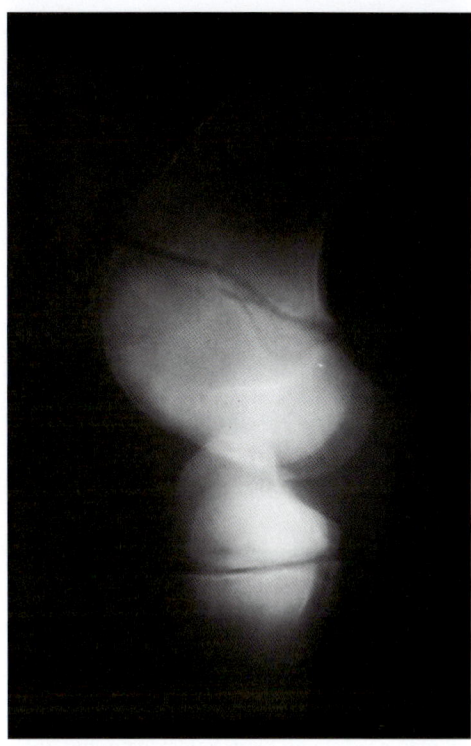

Fig. 6-14 Radiographs of *E*-type osteomyelitis in a foal. Note the lytic lesion in the epiphysis. These lesions are subchondral.

Though all joints and growth plates in the foal have the potential for hematogenous infection, the joints of the appendicular skeleton are most commonly affected. In one study of 36 foals, 89 joints were affected. The site prevalence varies in different studies, but in the McCoy study the following joints were affected in decreasing order: tarsus, stifle, fetlock, and carpus[2] (Figure 6-13). Effusion may be hard to detect in joints such as the shoulder, elbow, and hip. Subtle joint effusion may be detected by palpating the opposite joint for comparison. Septic physitis may not present with joint swelling but rather with edema over the growth plate region. Manual pressure applied at this site may illicit a painful response from the foal with an infected physis. In chronic septic physitis, the infection can erode through the bone and result in subcutaneous abcessation.[3]

Though other considerations for the cause of lameness would include trauma and congenital deformities, septic arthritis/osteomyelitis should be investigated first. Certainly any newborn foal with lameness, edema at the level of the physis, or joint effusion should be treated by the clinician as having a septic process until proven otherwise. Septic arthritis/osteomyelitis is an emergency situation. Delayed treatment can result is permanent orthopedic damage.

PATHOGENESIS

Septic arthritis/osteomyelitis is a manifestation of bacteremia in foals. Approximately one fourth of foals presented to a referral hospital with sepsis scores >11 will present with or develop evidence of septic arthritis.[4] Cohen and colleagues recognized septic arthritis as the cause of death in 12.5% of foals (8 to 31 days of age) on farms.[5] It is felt that hematogenous seeding of the synovium and the physis/epiphysis with bacteria is the cause for this problem.

Blood supply to the joint of the young foal is supplied through a main arteriole that branches into the synovial membrane and the epiphysis.[3] In the newborn foal, the blood supply of the epiphysis also supplies the metaphysis through transphyseal vessels.[6,7] Hematogenous bacteria can settle in any of these three areas creating a septic foci. Sluggish blood flow and decreased oxygen tension may encourage the proliferation of bacterial growth at the chondo-osseous junctions.[3,6,7] The types of lesions in the foal have been described by Firth according to their location in joint or bone. Synovial lesions (*S*-type) are located within the joint and involve the synovial structures only, with no bone involvement. Epiphyseal lesions (*E*-type) occur in the subchondral bone adjacent to the articular cartilage (Figure 6-14). Physeal infection (*P*-type) involves bone on the metaphyseal side of the growth plate (Figure 6-15). A fourth type of osteomyelitis in young foals involves the small tarsal bones (*T*-type).[3]

It appears that the *S*- and *E*-type infections are more prominent in younger foals, and the *P*-type infections occur in older foals. The closure of the transphyseal vessels may play a role in this finding. Closure of the

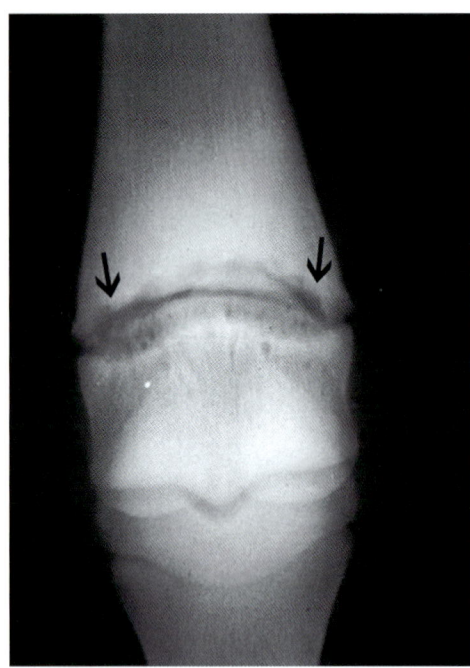

Fig. 6-15 Radiographs of *P*-type osteomyelitis in a foal. The presence of transphyseal vessels from the epiphysis in the young foal may predispose them to lesions in this region.

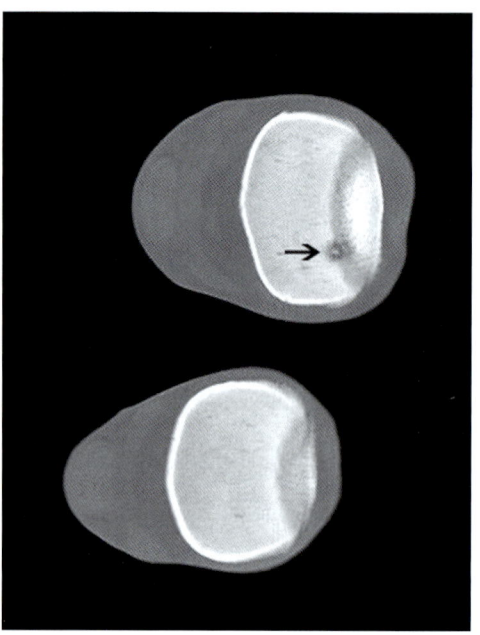

Fig. 6-16 Computed tomography of suspect joints may reveal osteomyelitis earlier than radiographs. Note small lesion in the distal metatarsal physis.

vessels is said to occur anywhere from 7 to 45 days of age.[3,7] Foals may present with one or multiple joints affected, and they may have more than one type of infection. Though foals can have an *S*-type alone with no bone involvement, most foals with *E*-type osteomyelitis have an accompanying *S*-type because of the proximity of the lesion to the synovial structures. *P*-type infections may also extend into the joints where the physis are partially intra-articular (proximal humerus, proximal, and distal femur).[3]

The initial workup on '02 CrippleCreek included a complete blood count (CBC), chemistry profile, and immunoglobulin assessment. A neutrophilic leukocytosis (11,600 WBC/μl, 10,208 segmented neutrophils/μl) with a lymphopenia (696 lymphocytes/μl) and an elevated fibrinogen of 600 mg/dl was found on the CBC. A slightly low globulin (2.1 g/dl) was the only abnormality found on the serum chemistry profile. The foal's immunoglobulin level was less than 400 mg/dl despite the previous plasma transfusion. Blood cultures were submitted.

Arthrocentesis of the affected joint yielded a cloudy, yellow flocculent fluid with poor viscosity. The fluid analysis from this joint had an elevated total nucleated cell count of TNCC = 205,000 cells/μl, and protein count of TP = 4 gm/dl. The differential for the WBC in the synovial fluid samples was 94% nondegenerate neutrophils and 6% monocytes. Two neutrophils had inclusions that could be compatible with degenerating bacteria or Dohle bodies. A diagnosis of marked suppurative inflammation was made. Cultures of this fluid were submitted. An

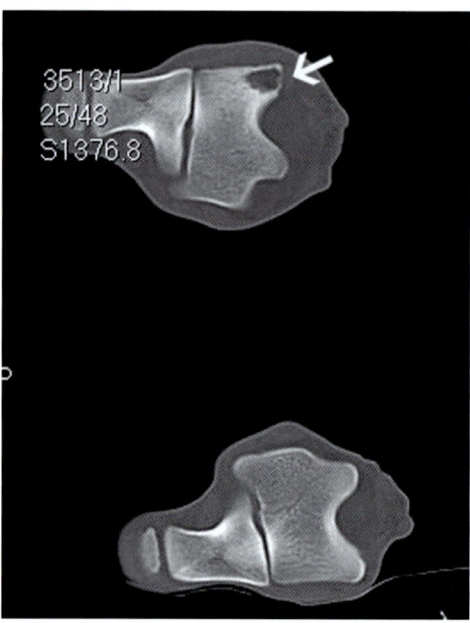

Fig. 6-17 Computed tomography of '02 CrippleCreek's tarsus. Note lytic cystlike lesion in left lateral condylar ridge of the talus.

arthrocentesis of the left hind fetlock yielded normal synovial fluid.

Radiographs of the affected joints were taken. Soft tissue swelling consistent with the increased joint effusion of the hock was seen on radiographs. A suspicious lytic lesion was also noted on the lateral trochlea of the talus. No evidence of osteomyelitis was found on radiographs of the left hind fetlock. To further investigate the possibility of early bone involvement, a CT was performed. A small lytic lesion was noted in the distal lateral physis of the left metatarsus, and a cystic lesion was confirmed in the lateral trochlea of the left talus (Figures 6-16 and 6-17).

Further diagnostics on the foal included an ultrasonic examination of the foal's umbilical structures. A slight enlargement of the umbilical stalk was the only abnormality.

DIAGNOSTIC TESTS

The clinical pathology of foals with septic arthritis/osteomyelitis can vary depending upon whether the foal has overwhelming septicemia accompanying the joint infection and the length of time the foal has been affected. In foals that present with overwhelming infection and sepsis, neutropenia is the usual finding. Foals that show mainly signs of musculoskeletal involvement may have normal or elevated WBC counts. The longer the duration, the more likely the foal will have higher than normal WBCs with increased fibrinogen. Because septic arthritis is often the consequence of low immunoglobulins, IgG levels need to be assessed. The standard should be levels ≥800 mg/dl.

Arthrocentesis of a distended joint is usually straightforward. The joint to be aspirated is aseptically prepared and an 18- or 20-gauge needle is directed through the distended joint capsule. Landmarks for the different joints are published. The clinician should aspirate enough fluid to place it in an EDTA tube for fluid analysis, in blood culture media for incubation, and on a culturette for immediate plating.

Synovial fluid is a dialysate of plasma with the addition of hyaluronan, a polymer produced by the synovial membrane.[8] Hyaluronan in synovial fluid is responsible for the viscosity of the fluid and aids in lubrication of the joint. It has been suggested that hyaluronan may be responsible for the composition of the rest of the synovial fluid components, allowing only small molecules to enter and restricting the entry of large molecules such as fibrinogen.[9]

Normal synovial fluid analysis yields a nucleated cell count of less than 200 cells/mm³. Though the differential count should have a mixture of neutrophils, lymphocytes, and mononuclear cells, neutrophils should make up less than 25% of the distribution. Protein levels in the fluid can be measured on a refractometer and should be less than 2 g/dl. Normal synovial fluid has a high level of viscosity. This can be roughly estimated by watching a fluid drop from the syringe or placing a drop of fluid between two fingers. As the fluid drops or the two fingers are separated, the synovial fluid should create a 4- to 5-cm strand (Figure 6-18).

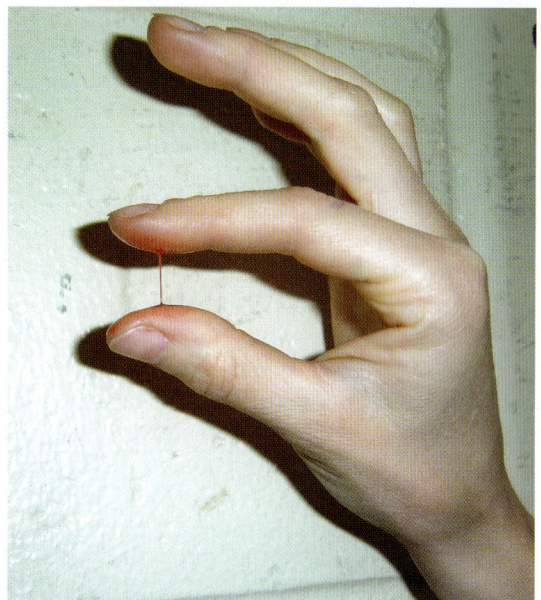

Fig. 6-18 Normal synovial fluid is clear yellow with a high level of viscosity. When placed between two fingers that are then separated, the normal synovial fluid will be "stringy."

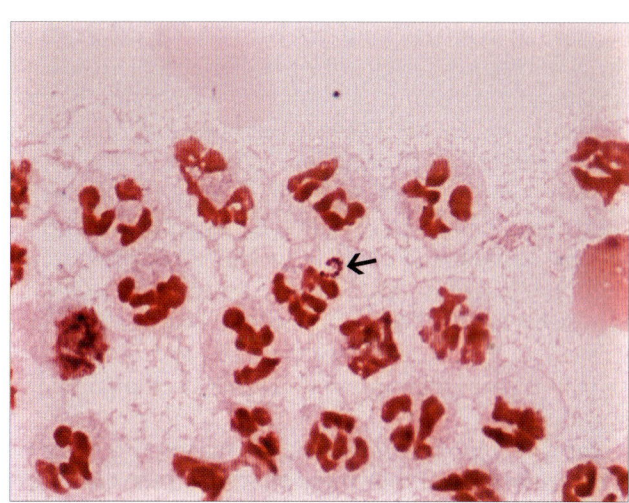

Fig. 6-19 Bacteria are not often seen on cytology of synovial fluid, but occasionally can be seen with a Gram stain or even a Wright Giemsa stain. This photo depicts Gram-negative cocci within the neutrophils of synovial fluid from a foal with septic arthritis. (Gram stain is 100×.)

Synovial fluid from infected joints has a high total nucleated cell count and an elevated total protein. Cell counts can range from several thousand to several hundred thousand. The differential of cells in the infected joint is generally >90% neutrophils; some may be degenerate. Bacteria can occasionally be seen on a Gram stain of the fluid (Figure 6-19). The joint fluid from infected joints becomes serous in nature, losing its viscosity.[10] Inflammation in the joint will cause hyaluronan to depolymerize. This depolymerization and the relationship of hyaluronan are probably responsible for the loss of viscosity in the joint fluid.[11]

Blood cultures should be taken at the time of admission when dealing with a potentially bacteremic animal. In the case of septic arthritis/osteomyelitis, joint fluid cultures should also be taken. Vatistas reported that only 50% of foals with positive blood cultures and positive synovial fluid culture were found to have the same organism(s), so having both would give a more complete microbial assessment.[12] Madison and colleagues found that culturing synovial fluid yields bacterial growth from suspected septic arthritis more often that culturing of synovial membranes.[13] Even so, there was only a 52% recovery rate of bacteria. In a canine model of bacterial arthritis, the best recovery of organism on culture came from synovial fluid placed in blood culture media and incubated for 24 hours. It is suggested that submission of synovial fluid on a culturette for immediate plating and in blood culture media for incubation would give the clinician the best chance at identifying the organism. Synovial biopsies are more invasive and less helpful in culture.[14] Cultures of needle aspirates from infected physis have also been advocated.

The use of PCR technology for early detection of bacteria in synovial fluid has been tested. Analysis of the 531 base-pair segment of bacterial DNA enabled nonspecific detection of *Salmonella enteritidis, E. coli, Actinobacillus equuli, Staphylococcus aureus, Streptococcus zooepidemicus, Bacteroides fragilis,* and *Clostridium perfringes* in previously inoculated aliquots of synovial fluid. This method may be helpful in rapidly identifying the presence of bacteria in joint fluid that is not definitively septic on fluid cell count or in joints in which bacterial cultures are not positive for bacterial growth. But because it is a nonspecific test, culture and sensitivity are still important in determining antibiotic sensitivity.[15]

Radiographic imaging is helpful in the presence of bone involvement, but there is a lag period in which bone demineralization goes unrecognized. This makes early recognition difficult or impossible. CT has been shown to demonstrate osteomyelitis in some foals before radiographic changes and, therefore, may be helpful in identifying bony involvement at an earlier stage of the disease process. If CT is not available and the foal does not respond to therapy, radiographs should be repeated every three to five days. Epiphyseal or physeal lesions, if present, will become more evident over time.

Radionuclide bone imaging has been used in identifying septic arthritis and osteomyelitis in children where it was difficult to localize the exact site of pathology.[16] This technique has also been useful in the foal.[17]

As with generalized septicemia, it is helpful to identify the point of entry or source of the infection. Several studies indicate that omphalophlebitis is a risk factor in the development of septic arthritis/osteomyelitis.[2,18]

Paradis found that in a group of foals with sepsis scores >11, 25% of the foals had surgical removal of the umbilical remnants while 50% of the foals with septic arthritis had the same surgical procedure, indicating a higher incidence of umbilical disease in foals with septic arthritis/osteomyelitis.[18] Similarly, McCoy and Paradis found that foals with omphalitis were 2.6 times more likely to have septic synovitis and 1.9 times more likely to develop osteomyelitis.[2] Ultrasonographic examination of the umbilical stalk, arteries, and veins is recommended for all sick foals.

The initial treatment plan for '02 CrippleCreek included immunologic support through an additional 1.5 liters of intravenous plasma, and antibiotic support with amikacin and penicillin. Specific therapy for the fetlock and hock lesions of the left hindlimb included regional limb perfusion (RLP) with 500 mg amikacin in 30 ml of saline, through and through joint lavage of the tarsocrural joint with 1 liter of lactated Ringer's solution and intra-articular injection 250 mg of amikacin into both joints. Joint treatment was performed after surgical preparation of the area and under a short-acting anesthesia.

Adjunct therapy included oral chondroitin sulfate, banamine (0.5 mg/kg) and oral ranididine (6 mg/kg). The foal was restricted to stall rest.

RLP of the left hindlimb and lavage of the tarsocrural joint was repeated two days later. The TNCC of the tarsus had decreased to 80,000 cells/mm³. Despite the decrease in cell count, the foal continued to have an elevated temperature (102°F). He spent increasing amounts of time in sternal recumbency. The skin over his elbows began to feel somewhat thickened.

Both blood culture and synovial fluid cultures were reported positive for **Klebsiella pneumoniae** *on the fourth day of hospitalization. A small lytic lesion was found in the lateral physis on repeat radiographs of the left hind fetlock, supporting the earlier diagnosis made through CT imaging.*

The decision was made to arthroscopically evaluate the left tarsocrural joint. During surgery, a moderate amount of fibrin was seen and removed. The lateral trochlear ridge had an area of discoloration, which was debrided to reveal a cystlike cavity. The affected joint was lavaged at surgery with a copious amount of sterile lactated Ringer's solution. The foal's temperature decreased over several days, and his activity level increased.

TREATMENT

Treatment of a septic joint is directed at providing immunologic support, antimicrobial coverage, and joint health maintenance. Immunologic support is accomplished with the use of intravenous plasma to increase immunoglobulin levels. Antimicrobial coverage is directed at the selection and administration of the most effective antibiotics both systemically and locally. Joint health maintenance is aimed at removing the proteolytic enzymes that are present in the diseased joint, which will in turn improve joint fluid viscosity.

Antimicrobial support is initiated before culture results are available, so the selection of antibiotic coverage should be based on its known effectiveness against the most common pathogenic bacteria. Bacterial organisms involved in septic arthritis/osteomyelitis mirror the same bacteria seen in other manifestations of sepsis. These include both Gram-negative organisms, such as the *E. coli, Klebsiella, Enterobacter, Salmonella, Pseudomonas*, and *Acinetobacter*, and Gram-positive organisms, such as *Streptococcus* or *Staphylococcus*.[2,19,20] Anaerobic organisms are less frequent but do occur. Broad-spectrum antibiotic coverage is best while awaiting culture results. Amikacin is the most effective first-line antibiotic against the enterobacteriaceae, coagulase-positive staphylococci, and *Pseudomonas* organisms. Gentocin is more limited in its effectiveness. Penicillin and ampicillin are highly effective against the beta-hemolytic streptococci. Cephalothin is also effective against Gram-positive bacterial infections. Trimethoprim sulphonamides have a narrow spectrum against the common pathogens and should not be used without culture and sensitivity results.[18,21-24] The best empirical selection therefore would include amikacin (20 to 25 mg/kg IV, qd) and either penicillin (22,000 IU/kg, IV, qid), ampicillin (22 mg/kg, IV tid), or cephalothin (10 to 20 mg/kg, IV, qid).

Systemic antibiotics alone are not effective in eliminating deep-seated synovitis or osteomyelitis in most cases. Foals with septic joint/osteomyelitis will also benefit from aggressive local therapy. Lloyd and colleagues found that synovial gentocin concentration in *E. coli* experimentally infected joints was 1000 times greater in joints that had received intra-articular gentocin than in joints that had received only systemic gentocin. In addition, the levels remained above MIC of most pathogenic organism for at least 24 hours.[25] Bone levels of gentocin remained above MIC for eight hours post–intra-articular administration.[26]

RLP of antibiotics is also a useful technique in achieving high local concentration of antibiotic to the infected synovial lining or bone.[26-30] RLP is best performed in the anesthetized foal. With the foal in lateral recumbency, either a venous catheter or an intraosseous catheter is placed proximal to the affected joint. An Esmarch bandage is tightly wrapped around the limb from the toe to the affected joint. A tourniquet is applied above the catheter (Figure 6-20). The Esmarch is then released around the affected joint but left on the lower part of the limb. Amikacin (500 mg) diluted with 20 to 30 ml sterile saline is then injected into the venous

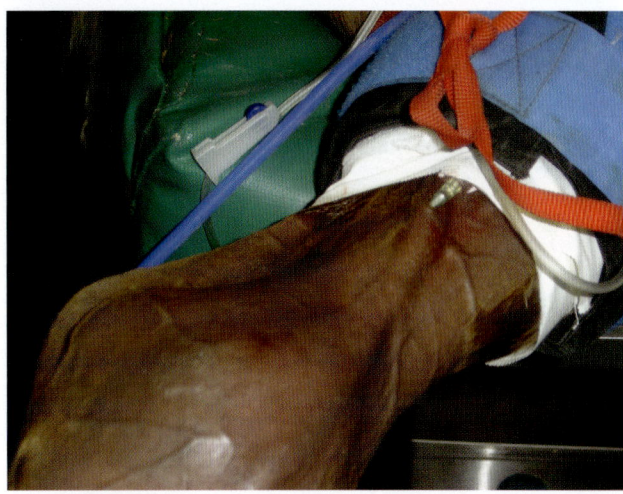

Fig. 6-20 For regional limb perfusion, a tourniquet is placed above the catheter that is placed proximal to the affected joint.

system under pressure and left for 20 to 30 minutes. This method of treatment delivers high levels of antimicrobial drugs locally by diffusion. Synovial fluid and bone concentration of gentocin post-RLP remained above MIC for 24 hours and eight hours, respectively.[26] RLP is most effective when using concentration-dependent drugs, such amikacin and gentocin, instead of time-dependent drugs, such as penicillin.

As noted previously, joint infection results in an increase in joint effusion and an influx of WBCs, particularly neutrophils. Activation of these neutrophils and of the synoviocyte by bacteria lead to the release of inflammatory mediators and proteolytic enzymes that are capable of degrading connective tissue within the joint.[31] Depolymerization of hyaluronate is evidenced in the decreased viscosity of the joint fluid. Increased cytokine production increases the vascular permeability of the joint and activates the kinin, coagulation, complement, and fibrinolytic systems. Severe distension of the joint reduces blood flow to the synovial membrane and joint capsule. Clinically, the end result of all of these processes is a joint distended with fibrin and destructive enzymes.[33]

Joint lavage is a technique for decreasing the tension within the joint capsule and diluting the inflammatory products in the joint fluid. Joint lavage is best performed in the heavily sedated or anesthetized foal. The affected joint is aseptically prepared, and a 14- to 16-gauge needle is inserted into the joint. Fluid is allowed to flow into the joint causing further distension. Once fully distended, a second needle is inserted into the joint on the opposite side and the joint is allowed to drain (Figure 6-21). For larger joints, 1 to 2 liters of sterile saline may be used to lavage the joint. Less fluid can be used for smaller joints such as the fetlock. Intermittent distention of the joint by covering the exit needle hub is helpful in achieving a thorough flush.

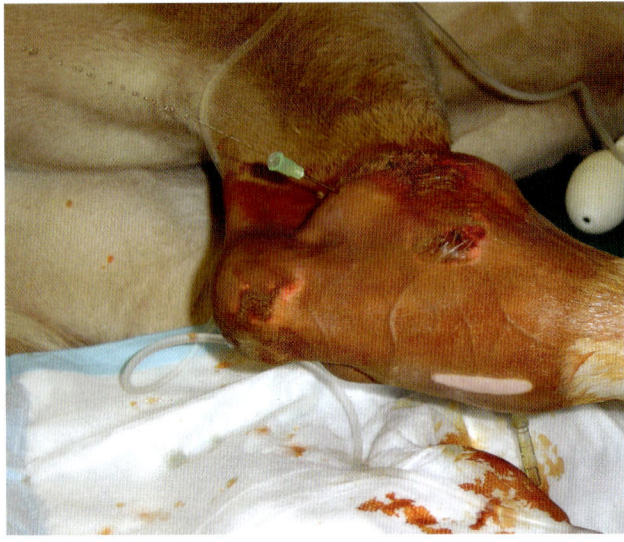

Fig. 6-21 Joint lavage is best undertaken in the heavily sedated or anesthetized foal. A through and through lavage is accomplished by inserting one needle as a flushing port and a second needle as an exit port. Copious lavage aids in decreasing detrimental enzymes in the joint fluid.

For difficult joints such as the shoulder and hip, it may be necessary to use a single needle for both ingress and egress of fluid.

The addition of povidone-iodine, chlorhexidine, or DMSO to the lavage solution are not recommended and in fact can cause further inflammation to the joint.[34] Though the addition of antibiotics to the lavage solutions is not helpful, intra-articular antibiotics should be instilled after the lavage is finished. Joint lavage should be repeated every other day until clinical signs improve.[35] If the joint is unresponsive, then more aggressive therapy, such as arthroscopy, should be undertaken.[36]

Arthroscopic evaluation is helpful when there is a large amount of fibrin in the joint (as evidenced by ultrasound or poor results obtained by joint lavage or inadequate lavage) or when epiphyseal lesions connect to the joint. Subchondral lesions can be curetted and fibrin removed. Arthroscopy facilitates large volumes of fluid lavage. In chronic nonresponsive septic arthritis, arthrotomy with open drainage has been advocated.[24] The open drainage technique requires daily sterile bandaging. Arthrotomy with closed suction drainage has also been successful in treatment of septic arthritis.

Other adjunctive therapy that may be helpful for the foal with septic arthritis includes the use of chondroprotective agents.[37] The oral administration of chondrotin sulfate and glucosamine can be easily administered to affected foals. Intra-articular injection of hyluronic acid post through and through lavage has been shown to decrease inflammation.[38] Intravenous use of hyaluronate sodium has also be advocated in affected foals. None of these products have been tested for efficacy in the foal.

Many foals that experience orthopedic pain will develop pressure sores secondary to recumbency. Skin over bony processes will begin to feel thickened and leathery. This usually progresses to large decubital ulcers. Deep bedding is not always sufficient to stop this process. Keeping the wound clean and well padded helps the healing, but it often takes several weeks before bandaging is unnecessary. Bandaging decubita of the hip area can be difficult. However, this can be accomplished by encircling the wound with preplaced stent sutures through which umbilical tape is threaded. The wound can be covered with gauze sponges and then umbilical tape can be laced over them to hold the bandage in place.

Over the next five days post surgery, '02 CrippleCreek exhibited less lameness and his left hock was only mildly distended. Joint fluid analysis was within the normal limits of protein and TNCC. Intravenous antibiotics were continued, and a final RLP of the left hock was performed. Banamine therapy was discontinued. The foal was discharged with instructions for stall rest and continued intravenous amikacin and penicillin for another 14 days.

On the two-week recheck, '02 CrippleCreek was actively moving around. There was only a mild thickening of the joint capsule of the left hock. No swelling or pain response could be elicited with palpation of the left hind distal metatarsal physis. Resolution of the previously visible radiographic lesions was seen. A repeat CT confirmed resolution of the distal metatarsal physeal lesion and the surgical defect on the lateral trochlear ridge of the left talus.

Discharge instructions included restricted exercise in a small paddock and continued close observation of the foal for any signs of recurrence of lameness or joint distension.

OUTCOME

The survival rate to discharge of foals with septic arthritis/osteomyelitis has been variably stated in different studies as ranging from 16.7% to 73%.[2,12,19,39,40] A large part of the variability in the studies is probably due to the time period of when they were studied. In the past decade, treatment of affected foals has become more aggressive and produced better results. In one study, the survival of foals with septic arthritis/ osteomyelitis (71%) was only slightly less than that of foals admitted to the hospital (75%).[2] It is felt that the death of foals with septic arthritis/osteomyelitis is equally due to other concurrent problems such as septicemia and pneumonia.

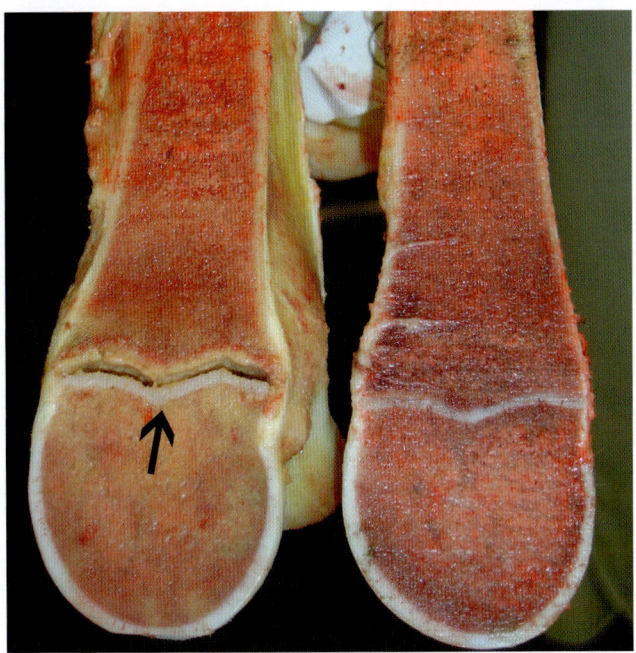

Fig. 6-22 Postmortem photo of a septic distal metatarsal physis that has fractured.

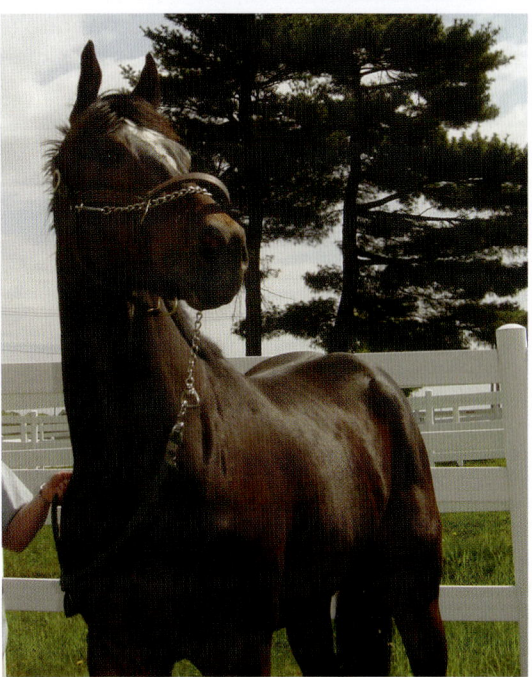

Fig. 6-23 '02 Cripple Creek as a three-year-old. He is sound at walk and trot with a slightly positive hock flexion test on the left hindlimb.

Though many factors probably influence the survivability of each foal such as the virulence of the bacterial organism, contrary to common belief, McCoy and colleagues found that the number of joints affected did not have a significant impact on foal survival.[2] Probably the most important factor for survival is the early recognition of the problem and the initiation of aggressive treatment. Steel and coworkers found that 71% of foals with septic arthritis that presented before two days survived to discharge, while only 40% of foals with a duration of >2 days survived to discharge.[10] In experimental models of septic arthritis in horses, a large influx of WBCs, proteolytic enzymes, and inflammatory cytokines occurs within the first 12 to 24 hours postinfection.[31] This leads to depletion of proteoglycans for the cartilage matrix within five days.[41] In human medicine, it is felt that chronic and sometime irreversible changes occur after seven days.

Clinically some of the foals with the worst prognosis are foals with physeal lesions. Many of these go undiagnosed because of the lack of joint swelling. By the time the treatment is started, the lesions have spread to the entire physeal surface and weaken the junction between the metaphysis and the epiphysis, resulting in a Salter fracture (Figure 6-22). Careful palpation of the physeal regions of the long bones of any lame foal may elicit pain or discover edema and in turn aid in early diagnosis.

One important factor to consider in the survival rate of foals is the expense of the therapy and how it influences decisions on euthanasia. In general, foals with septic arthritis/osteomyelitis have long hospitalization times, multiple anesthesia for joint lavage and

RLP, long-term antimicrobial therapy, and possible arthroscopic surgery. Financial constraints of the owner may limit the aggressiveness of treatment. Without the knowledge of the long-term prognosis for the foal's future soundness, it is a difficult decision for owners to financially and emotionally make or undertake.

Residual dysfunction after septic arthritis in children ranges from 13% to 27%.[42] An important question that needs to be answered is not the short-term survivability of affected foals, but the long-term athletic ability.

Steel reviewed the outcomes of 93 foals with septic arthritis. Factors that were found to be unfavorable for survival and ability to race included the isolation of *Salmonella sp.* and the presence of multisystemic disease. Approximately one third of the animals that survived went on to race at least once. Most raced fewer than five times. It is difficult to ascertain whether or not the other two thirds did not race as a direct result of damage secondary to septic arthritis.[20] Smith and colleagues found that 50% of foals with a diagnosis of septic arthritis went on to start at least one race. When compared with unaffected siblings, foals that had had septic arthritis were significantly less likely to race and those that raced took a significantly longer time to start.[43]

No one has studied the long-term effects of septic arthritis on foals that are not destined to be racehorses. Perhaps their ability to perform at a less-strenuous activity is less affected. Septic arthritis or "joint ill" was a death sentence to foals in the past. The key to success with these affected foals is early recognition and aggressive therapy. If these criteria can be met, then many of these foals survive in the long term and may go on to be useful athletes in the short term (Figure 6-23).

REFERENCES

1. Goedegebuure SA, Dik KJ, Firth EC et al: Polyarthritis and polyosteomyelitis in foals, *Vet Pathol* 17:651, 1980.
2. McCoy J, Paradis MR: An Assessment of Neonatal Septic Arthritis at Tufts University School of Veterinary Medicine, 1990-1998, Dorothy Havemeyer Neonatal Septicemia Workshop 2, 29, 1998.
3. Firth EC: Current concepts of infectious polyarthritis in foals, *Equine Vet J* 15:5, 1983.
4. Paradis MR: Septic arthritis in the equine neonate: A retrospective study, *Proc ACVIM*, 1992.
5. Cohen ND: Causes of and farm management factors associated with disease and death in foals, *J Am Vet Med Assoc* 204:1644, 1994.
6. Bennett D: Pathological feature of multiple bone infections in the foal, *Vet Rec* 103:482, 1978.
7. Firth EC, Poulos PW: Blood vessels in the developing growth plate of the equine distal radius and metacarpus, *Research Vet Sci* 33:159, 1982.
8. Cohen AS: Synovial fluid. In Cohen AS, ed: *Laboratory diagnostic procedures in the rheumatic diseases*, Boston, 1967, Little Brown.
9. Nettelbladt E, Sundblad L, Jonsson E: Permeability of the synovial membrane to proteins, *Acta Rheum Scand* 9:28, 1963.
10. Orsini JA: Strategies for treatment of bone and joint infections in large animals, *J Am Vet Med Assoc* 185:1190, 1984.
11. Holt PJ, How MJ, Long VJ, et al: Mucopolysac-chlorides in synovial fluids. Effect of aspirin and indomethacin on hyaluronic acid, *Ann Rheum Dis* 27:264, 1968.
12. Vatistas NJ, Wilson WD, Pascoe JR, et al: Septic arthritis in foals (141 cases): 1978-1992. In Proc Third International Conf on Vet Perinatology, California, 1993.
13. Madison JB, Sommer M, Spencer PA: Relations among synovial membrane histopathologic findings, and bacterial culture results in horses with suspected infectious arthritis: 64 cases (1979-1987), *J Am Vet Med Assoc* 198:1655, 1991.
14. Montgomery RD, Long IR, Milton JL: Comparison of aerobic culturette, synovial membrane biopsy, and blood culture medium in detection of canine bacterial arthritis, *Vet Surg* 18:300, 1989.
15. Crabill MR, Cohen ND, Martin LJ, et al: Detection of bacteria in equine synovial fluid by use of the polymerase chain reaction, *Vet Surg* 25:195-198, 1996.
16. Tuson CE, Hoffman EB, Mann MD: Isotope bone scanning for acute osteomyelitis and septic arthritis in children, *J Bone and Joint Surg* 76B:306, 1994.
17. Hardy J: Septic arthritis in foals, Proceedings, ACVS, San Francisco, 63, 1999.
18. Paradis MR: Equine neonatal sepsis—update, *Vet Clin North Am Equine Prac* 109, 1994.
19. Schneider RK, Bramlage LR, Moore RM, et al: A retrospective study of 192 horses affected with septic arthritis/tenosynovitis, *Equine Vet J* 24:436, 1992.
20. Steel CM, Hunt AR, Adams PLE et al: Factors associated with prognosis for survival and athletic use in foals with septic arthritis: 93 cases (1987-1994), *J Am Vet Med Assoc* 215:973, 1999.
21. Snyder JR, Pascoe JR, Hirsh DC: Antimicrobial susceptibility of microorganisms isolated from equine orthopedic patients, *Vet Surg* 16:197, 1987.
22. Hanie EA: Antibiotic therapy for infections of skeletal and synovial structures, part II, *Equine Pract* 2:7, 1989.
23. Moore RM, Schneider RK, Kowalski J et al: Antimicrobial susceptibility of bacterial isolates from 233 horses with musculoskeletal infection during 1979-1989, *Equine Vet J* 24:450, 1992.
24. Schneider RK, Bramlage LR, Mecklenburg LM et al: Open drainage, intra-articular and systemic antibiotics in the treatment of septic arthritis/tenosynovitis in horses, *Equine Vet J* 24:443, 1992.
25. Lloyd KCK, Stover SM, Pascoe JR et al: Synovial fluid pH, cytologic characteristics, and gentamicin concentration after intra-articular administration of the drug in an experimental model of infectious arthritis in horses, *Am J Vet Res* 51:1363, 1990.
26. Werner LA, Hardy J, Bertone AL: Bone Gentamicin Concentration After Intra-articular Injection or Regional Intravenous Perfusion in the Horse, *Vet Surg* 32:559, 2003.
27. Whitehair KJ, Blevins WE, Fessler JF et al: Regional Perfusion of the Equine Carpus for Antibiotic Delivery, *Vet Surg* 21:279, 1992.
28. Whitehair KJ, Bowersock TL, Blevins WE et al: Regional limb perfusion for antibiotic treatment of experimentally induced septic arthritis, *Vet Surg* 21:367, 1992.
29. Scheuch BC, Van Hoogmoed LM, Wilson WD et al: Comparison of intraosseous or intravenous infusion for delivery of amikacin sulfate to the tibiotarsal joint of horses, *AJVR* 63:374, 2002.
30. Kettner NU, Parker JE, Watrous BJ: Intraosseous regional perfusion for treatment of septic physitis in a two-week-old foal, *J Am Vet Med Assoc* 222:346, 2003.
31. Tulamo RM, Ramlage LR, Gabel AA: Sequential clinical and synovial fluid changes associated with acute infectious arthritis in the horse, *Equine Vet J* 21:325, 1989.
32. Spiers S, May SA, Harrison LJ et al: Proteolytic enzymes in equine joints with infectious arthritis, *Equine Vet J* 26:48, 1994.
33. Martens RJ, Auer JA, Carter GK: Equine pediatrics: Septic arthritis and osteomyelitis, *J Am Vet Med Assoc* 188:582, 1986.
34. Bertone AL, McIlwraith CW, Powers BE et al: Effect of four antimicrobial lavage solutions on the tarsocrural joint of horses, *Vet Surg* 15:305, 1986.
35. Meijer MC, Van Weeren PR, Rijkenhuizen AB: Clinical experiences of treating septic arthritis in the equine by repeated joint lavage: A series of 39 cases, *J Vet Med* 47:351, 2000.
36. ter Braake F: Direct endoscopic approach improves prognosis of septic-synovitis in the horse, *Tijdschr Diergeneeskd* 127:444, 2002.
37. Platt D: The role of oral disease-modifying agents glucosamine and chondroitin sulphate in the management of equine degenerative joint disease, *Equine Vet Ed* 262, 2001.
38. Brusie RW, Sullins KE, White NA et al: Evaluation of sodium hyaluronate therapy in induced septic arthritis in the horse, *Equine Vet J* 24:18, 1992.
39. Gayle JM, Cohen ND, Chaffin MK: Factors associated with survival in septicemic foals: 65 Cases (1988-1995), *J Vet Intern Med* 12:140, 1998.
40. Steel CM, Hunt AR, Adams LE et al: Factors associated with prognosis for survival and athletic use in foals with septic arthritis: 93 cases (1987-1994), *J Am Vet Med Assoc* 215:973, 1999.
41. Curtis PH: The pathophysiology of joint infection. *Clin Orthop Relat Res* 96:129, 1973.
42. Howard JB, Highgenboten CL, Nelson JD: Residual effects of septic arthritis in infancy and childhood, *JAMA* 236:932, 1976.
43. Smith LJ, Marr CM, Payne RJ et al: What is the likelihood that Thoroughbred foals treated for septic arthritis will race?, *Equine Vet J* 36:452, 2004.

7 Recognition and Resuscitation of the Critically Ill Foal

| Case 7-1 | Foal in Hemodynamic Shock | Jon Palmer |

'04 Revival was born on May 7 at 6 PM on day 338 of gestation to a multiparous mare after a normal gestation. The mare was expected to foal, but since she had not developed an udder, she was not watched closely. Signs of stage I parturition were not noticed. The mare was seen to break her water. Stage II parturition was 10 minutes or less, and stage III was approximately one hour. The placenta was edematous and meconium-stained. The foal was passing diarrhea as he was born which continued through the night. The foal was assisted to stand after one and a half hours and nursed from the mare. After watching the foal nurse, the farm manager left the barn for the evening, leaving further observations up to the "foal watcher," whose primary job was to observe the other pregnant mares for signs of impending parturition. During the night the foal was never vigorous. He got up once unassisted but only for short time and did not nurse. When the farm manager returned to the barn the next morning, she realized that the foal needed medical attention because he was weak, unable to stand, and had only nursed once. She immediately called her veterinarian, requesting referral to the Neonatal Intensive Care Service for evaluation and intensive care. As she waited for transport, she bottle fed '04 Revival 8 oz. of colostrum milked from the mare.

'04 Revival was admitted to the NICU when he was 15 hours old (Figure 7-1). The foal arrived recumbent and required transport to the NICU. As is the standard of practice, vital signs and essential organ function were rapidly evaluated while supportive therapy was initiated. This was done using a team approach. The following tasks were performed simultaneously: intranasal oxygen cannula placed, jugular vein prepared for catheterization, TPR data collected, rapid physical assessment of essential organ function made, arterial sample for blood gas and electrolytes obtained (before intranasal oxygen insufflation initiated as room air base-

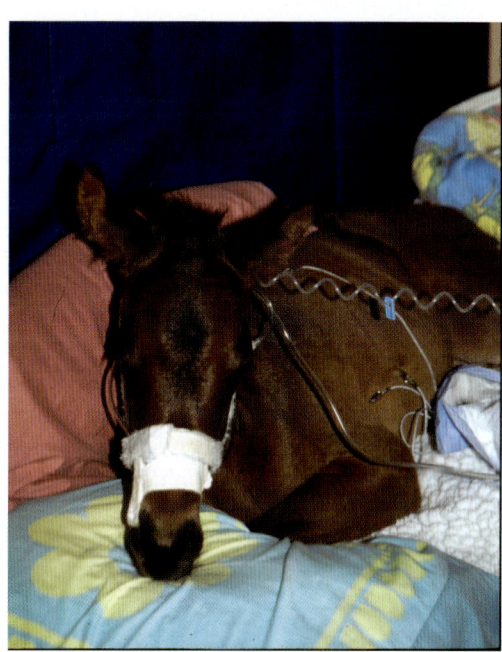

Fig. 7-1 '04 Revival receiving intensive fluid therapy soon after admission to the NICU.

line), and indirect blood pressures recorded. As the intravenous catheter was placed, blood for culture and laboratory analysis was obtained and intravenous fluid administration was initiated as the catheter was secured. This was accomplished within 10 minutes of arrival.

Vital parameters were: temperature (T) 100.4° F, heart rate (HR) 96 bpm, respiratory rate (RR) 24 bpm, blood pressure (BP) 88/50 (61)—systolic/diastolic (mean), packed cell volume (PCV) 44%, total protein (TP) 6.1 g/dl, venous dextrose (VD) 44 mg/dl (2.44 mmol/l), body weight (BW) 54 kg (119 lb).

Initial examination of essential organ function: Oral, nasal, and scleral membranes had mild to moderate large-vessel and small-vessel injection and all had

121

marked icterus. Multiple oral petechiae were present as well as marked lingual erythema. Normal respiratory pattern was present with little respiratory effort and no abnormal lung sounds. Normal cardiac rhythm with a relative bradycardia (90 to 96) was present considering that shock was evident. There was an apparent temperature gradient from periphery to core with ice-cold hooves, cold lower legs, and cool nose, ears, and upper legs. The foal had very weak pulses, poor arterial fill, and poor arterial tone. There was evidence of recent urination. Abdominal auscultation revealed few, quiet borborygmi, but the abdomen was primarily silent. On abdominal palpation, meconium was found in the right dorsal colon but little elsewhere. The foal had a history of fetal diarrhea which appeared to be subsiding at the time of admission. The foal was somnolent with occasional struggling, but the struggling appeared meaningful. The foal was able to be aroused and responsive to stimuli, but was subdued.

Supportive therapy was initiated concurrent with the examination by beginning intranasal oxygen insufflation at 10 liters/minute within three minutes of arrival and establishment of a jugular catheter placed aseptically within 10 minutes of arrival. Administration of dextrose 5% in water was administered at a rate to deliver 4 mg/kg/minute of dextrose, which was increased to 8 mg/kg/minute after two hours. One-liter boluses of a strong ion-balanced replacement crystalloid (Normosol-R, Abbott Laboratories, Abbott Park, IL) were given over 10 to 20 minutes with re-evaluation of cardiovascular status after each bolus. A plasma transfusion was given for both its colloid value and for the biologically active proteins including immunoglobulins. The foal was also placed on intravenous ticarcillin 100 mg/kg and clavulanic acid at 3 mg/kg repeated q6h.

Neonates that have inconsistent or lack of nursing behavior, are weak or develop progressive weakness, and become recumbent are critically ill and require immediate intervention with supportive therapy. In our practice, 70% to 80% of our neonates present within the first 48 hours of birth. Of the neonates that don't survive, 70% die within this initial 48 hours. Recumbent neonates presenting during this critical period require immediate attention. Rapid referral, immediate assessment of essential organ function, and immediate directed supportive therapy are essential. The most powerful therapeutic modality in the NICU is the well-coordinated care delivery team. These cases demand a team approach to insure rapid delivery of lifesaving supportive therapy.

Essential organ function during critical states is focused on delivery of oxygen and other nutrients to vital tissues and removal of waste products. The initial physical assessment of the neonate should focus on the respiratory and cardiovascular systems. Secondary organ function should also be assessed during the initial rapid examination both to detect major organ failure so that early directed therapy can be initiated and also to establish a baseline to help assess response to initial resuscitation with repeat examination. Rapid assessment of neurologic status, renal function, gastrointestinal function, and metabolic status should be performed. The initial assessment should be thorough but rapidly performed beginning during the transport to the hospital stall and completed within the first 10 minutes after admission, concurrent with placing the neonate on intranasal oxygen, placing an intravenous catheter, and obtaining initial blood samples for analysis and culture.

The object of the cardiovascular examination is to assess effective perfusion. In the critical case, both macro and microperfusion is of vital importance, but the assessment and intervention largely targets macroperfusion. Physical examination signs of hypoperfusion include cold extremities as blood is shunted centrally. In early compensated shock, the more distal areas are colder than the proximal areas with ice cold hooves, cold lower legs, and cool proximal legs, nose, and ears. There is a significant core to periphery temperature gradient. As shock progresses, this gradient is not so distinct. The cold limbs should not be treated with active warming as this will defeat the circulatory compensation. Other important physical findings that help assess perfusion are pulse quality, arterial tone, and arterial fill. Careful assessment of pulse quality can help determine pulse pressure (the difference between systolic and diastolic pressures). Arterial tone is assessed by the amount of finger pressure required to feel the pulse and the amount required to eliminate the pulse. It can be helpful to feel the pulse along the same artery with both hands, with the proximal fingers slowly increasing pressure until the distal fingers no longer detect a pulse. In patients with very poor arterial tone (and usually BP), a pulse can only be felt with a very light touch. In patients with abnormally high arterial tone (and usually high BP), it may be impossible to eliminate the pulse with finger pressure. Arterial fill is assessed by feeling the size of the artery's lumen as finger pressure is applied. Arterial fill relates to the blood volume on the arterial side of the circulation.

BP is a vital sign that should be measured in all critical neonates (Figure 7-2). Except in cases with severe hypotension and vasoplegia, taking indirect measurements using the oscillometric technique is generally adequate. With this technique, as the pressure in the cuff falls below the systolic pressure, the artery begins to pulsate. These pulsations are transmitted to the cuff, and oscillations are sensed by a transducer. The pressure transmitting maximum oscillations closely correlates to the mean BP. The pressure at which the cuff oscillations begin is recorded as the systolic pressure,

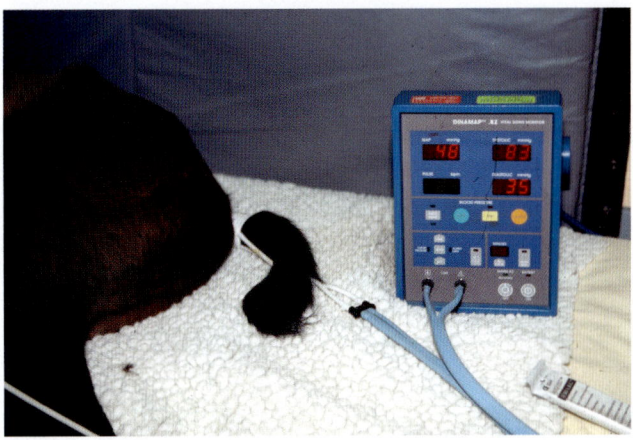

Fig. 7-2 Indirect blood pressure measurement using the tail artery.

and the pressure at which the oscillations stop decreasing is recorded as the diastolic pressure. The instrument eliminates internal artifacts by maintaining the level of cuff pressure deflation until two consecutive oscillations of equal amplitude are detected. Although the technology differs somewhat between monitors from different manufacturers, once the mean pressure is identified, algorithms are used to fine-tune systolic and diastolic values and eliminate artifacts.[1] However, it cannot differentiate external stimuli, so it is best to use when the patient is in a resting state.[2,3] When used correctly, BP measurements obtained by this method correlate well with direct, intra-arterial recordings unless the neonate is suffering from severe hypotension and vasoplegia, in which case it may be impossible to obtain a reading.[4-6]

To minimize errors of noninvasive BP measurements, careful attention to technique is important. First, the cuff should encircle at least 80% of the part's circumference (100% or more is best), and the width should be at least 40% (up to 70%) of the part's circumference. The same size cuff should be consistently used to minimize variation from artifacts. The cuff should be placed on the same body part each time and should have the same vertical relationship to the heart. In the foal, the tail is the most convenient site. The BP should be measured during a quiet or sleep state. BP values obtained during activity, full arousal, and especially when standing or heavily restrained have little relationship to the physiologic state of perfusion. It may take some perseverance to obtain readings while minimally disturbing the patient. Because of the likelihood of artifacts, at least three measurements should be taken to ensure consistent results. If the results are not consistent, more should be obtained until consistent results are found. The mean value is less likely to be erroneous compared to systolic and diastolic pressures.[3] BP values will tend to decrease with repeated measurements, but the differences will be small in magnitude.[4]

BP is related to perfusion (flow ≈ pressure/resistance), and since objective numbers are obtained with a BP measurement, it is frequently used as a surrogate for perfusion. However, this is a dangerous assumption when peripheral resistance is changing as it does in the neonate. The neonate is in a transition state from a low pressure fetal circulation to a normal pressure pediatric circulation, making normal BP values a moving target. The fetus depends on low systemic BP to maintain fetal physiology. Because of low vascular resistance, the low BPs are vital to maintain balanced fluid fluxes in and out of the interstitium and to maintain fetal blood flow patterns. This low BP is primarily due to low precapillary tone and a low baroreceptor set point, attenuating the baroreceptor response. Near birth, there is a decrease in circulating and local vasodilators and a simultaneous increase in vascular sensitivity to circulating and neurogenic vasopressors. This results in an increase in precapillary tone and thus an increase in peripheral resistance as the transition from fetal to pediatric cardiovascular function begins. During this period, an increase in BP is vital to maintain tissue perfusion. This is accomplished by a shift in baroreceptor sensitivity resulting in a progressive increase in BP matching the increase in peripheral resistance.[7] This process begins before birth and slowly progresses during the neonatal period, being most evident during the first week of life. It is also import to note that the transition does not proceed simultaneously in all tissues. This means that tissue perfusion and thus susceptibility to hypoperfusion is not uniform in all tissues. Because of this transition and the variability between individuals, there is no one critical BP. Rather, the critical BP is a moving target.[8] A normal neonatal foal with good perfusion may have a BP of 59/35(45), as is our frequent clinical experience, and another may have hypoperfusion (shock) with a BP of 73/55(61). Low BP should not be treated alone unless there are coexisting signs of hypoperfusion such as cold extremities; poor arterial pulses, fill, and tone; oliguria; metabolic acidosis; or other signs of organ hypoperfusion. BP numbers should not be given more weight in directing therapeutic interventions than any other physical examination finding.

The final assessment of the cardiovascular system is auscultation to detect cardiac rhythm, rate and the presence of murmurs. It should be noted that prominent flow murmurs without clinical significance are often present during the first 30 days of life (see Chapter 13). Flow murmurs can usually be identified by their soft quality and variation in loudness with heart rate and body position. The presence of a persistently loud, coarse murmur should raise the suspicion of a significant congenital defect that will require further investigation. Transient cardiac arrhythmias are not unusual during the first hours after birth. Persistent atrial or ventricular arrhythmias are occasionally present and suggest significant myocardial damage secondary to hypoxic ischemic damage, sepsis, or trauma (e.g., contusions or lacerations secondary to fractured ribs). The most common arrhythmia is an inappropriate bradycardia in the face of hypoperfusion. That is, although the heart rate may be within the expected normal range, when significant hypoperfusion is present, it would be more appropriate to respond with tachycardia. This inappropriate response is likely a failure of the baroreceptor response secondary to autonomic failure. Failure of the autonomic nervous system is a frequent and significant problem in the neonate and requires careful attention.[9-12]

A rapid evaluation of the respiratory system should include assessment of respiratory rate, rhythm, depth, air movement throughout the lungs, presence of abnormal lung sounds, and presence of fractured ribs. Admission blood gas on room air and a repeat blood gas on intranasal oxygen insufflation within an hour of admission, after initial resuscitation has begun, is the best method for pulmonary evaluation. Neurologic examination should include level of awareness, responsiveness, body tone, respiratory pattern, and the presence of seizurelike behavior. Rapid abdominal evaluation should include evidence of meconium passage, presence of borborygmi, abdominal fill, and abdominal palpation, including assessment for quantity and location of retained meconium, thickened bowel, pneumatosis intestinalis, intussusception, internal umbilical hematoma, bladder size, kidney size and texture, and the presence of hepatomegaly. Renal assessment includes noting the timing of the first urination, which should occur at about 6-12 hours of age. Early urination suggests serious renal impairment, prostaglandin dominance, or vasopressin exhaustion; delayed urination suggests failure of fetal-neonatal renal transition, vasopressin predominance, or very rarely anuric renal failure. Evaluation of fractional excretion of sodium may be helpful but will be confounded by fluid boluses. Obtaining a baseline plasma creatinine value is very important as the neonate will be creatinine-loaded and the slope of the decrease in plasma creatinine will be an accurate predictor of glomerular filtration rate (GFR). Following drug clearances, such as measuring aminoglycoside trough levels, is also very useful. Finally, it is vital to evaluate the metabolic status of the neonate by measuring blood glucose levels and following the response to therapy.

INITIAL THERAPEUTIC INTERVENTIONS

Immediate supportive therapy should begin as soon as the neonate has been transported to the hospital stall.

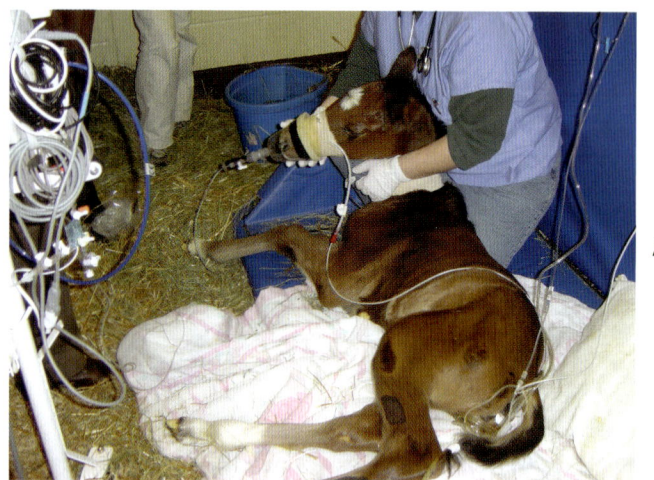

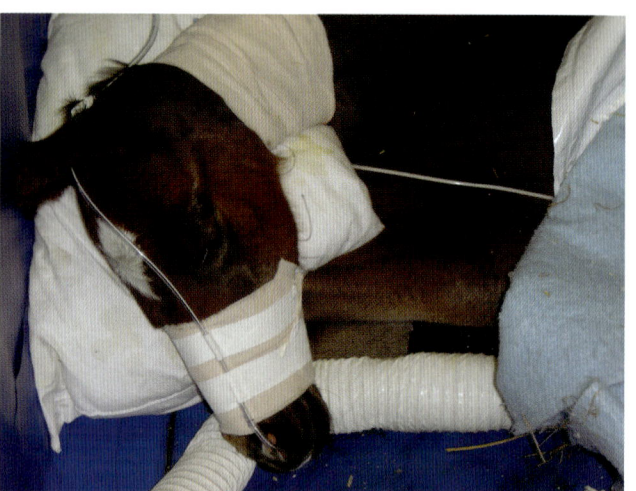

Fig. 7-3 Administration of oxygen through a mask, *A*, or intranasal tube, *B*, is an important initial step in increasing tissue oxygen delivery.

The most important goal of early therapy is assuring tissue oxygen delivery by maximizing pulmonary loading of hemoglobin, guaranteeing sufficient blood oxygen content and returning lung and tissue perfusion to normal. The neonate should be placed on intranasal or mask oxygen insufflation immediately (Figure 7-3, *A* and *B)*. As the intranasal oxygen line is being placed, but before oxygen is delivered, it is my routine to draw an arterial sample for blood gas analysis while the neonate is still breathing room air. This will be compared to a second sample taken after initial resuscitation. The intranasal oxygen flow is generally begun between 5 and 10 liters/minute to compensate for mismatching if present and also for hypoventilation allowing maximal blood oxygen loading. If the neonate is anemic (PCV <25%), a blood transfusion should be seriously considered. Currently available hemoglobin-based blood substitutes have significant adverse effects in cases such as this and are contraindicated.

Hypoperfusion in the critical neonate is usually secondary to hypovolemia due to poor vascular tone. Sick neonates are almost never dehydrated during the first 48 hours of life unless there is significant diarrhea, reflux, or GI tract pooling of fluids, in rare cases of polyuria, or when there are high insensible losses as in extremely hot weather when tachypnea is present. In fact, when neonates have been subjected to intra-uterine stress, because of fluid shifts, they are usually born overhydrated. Critical neonates presenting during the first 48 hours of life are often hyperhydrated but hypovolemic. So when approaching fluid therapy, it is essential to optimize by not only administering high enough volumes to correct the hypovolemia but also to use care not to give excessive fluid volumes that will further exacerbate the hyperhydration.[13]

There is no compelling evidence that shows an advantage in using crystalloids or colloids when treating hypovolemia.[14] I generally use both with crystalloids playing the dominant role. When choosing a crystalloid, particular attention should be paid to the tonicity and the strong ion difference of the fluid. Since large volumes will be used, there will be a tendency for the plasma osmolarity and strong ion balance to move toward that of the fluids. I prefer isosmotic fluids with a strong ion balance approximating normal plasma. '04 Revival was given Normosol-R (Abbott Laboratories). Delivering 20 ml/kg boluses of fluids over 10 to 20 minutes allows delivery of fluids in a timely manner but also imposes a set time for reassessment (after completion of each bolus) so as to achieve rapid return of perfusion while avoiding excessive fluid delivery (Figure 7-4). Thus, in a typical 50 kg foal, a 1-liter bolus is given rapidly (usually over 10 minutes with the aid of a pressurized cuff) and once delivered, a rapid assessment of return of perfusion (peripheral body temperature, pulse quality, return of signs of organ function) is used to decide if the bolus should be repeated. One or more liters of plasma are also given for its colloid properties and for the bioactive proteins it contains.

An intravenous line was established within 10 minutes of arrival, and '04 Revival was given a 1 liter bolus of Normosol-R (Abbott Laboratories) over 10 minutes with the use of a pressurized cuff to treat the hypovolemia in an attempt to reverse the cardiovascular collapse. Reassessment of signs of perfusion showed increase in leg temperature but no change in pulse parameters and a BP of 65/45(50). The fluid bolus was repeated with reassessment after each bolus until a total of 5 liters (90 ml/kg) was given. By that time, one hour after admission, the foal had also received 1 liter of plasma for a total fluid load of 110 ml/kg. At that point, the temperature gradient from periphery to core had decreased remarkably. '04 Revival's nose, ears, and upper legs were warm, his lower legs were

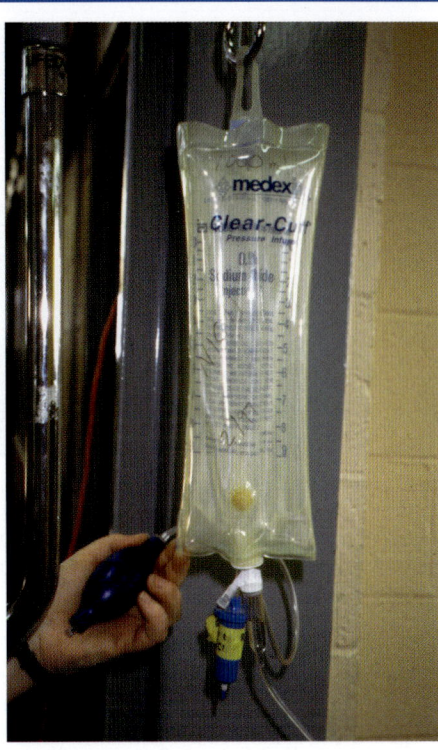

Fig. 7-4 Using a pressure cuff around a 1-liter fluid bag facilitates fluid delivery so that the entire 20 ml/kg bolus can be given within 10 to 20 minutes.

still cool, and hooves were cold. He had not yet made urine and had become minimally responsive to tactile and auditory stimuli. His peripheral pulses were moderately strong; he had good arterial fill but poor arterial tone. His BP was 58/35(45). Dobutamine was initiated as a continuous rate infusion (CRI) of 10 mg/kg/minute. After 10 minutes, the foal's leg temperature had improved, but his legs were still cool. The other signs of perfusion had not changed. His BP was 69/35(48). CRI vasopressin was initiated at 0.5 mU/kg/minute. Within 15 minutes, '04 Revival's hooves and legs were warm, his peripheral pulses were strong, and he had excellent arterial fill and very good arterial tone. His BP was 75/40(55). He actively changed from lateral to sternal recumbency, he held his head up, looked around, and vocalized. He also urinated 200 to 300 ml and did so several more times in the first hour after initiating therapy.

Inopressor Therapy

If there is inadequate return of perfusion after four to six fluid boluses or if the patient is deteriorating despite the fluid loading, inopressor therapy should be initiated[15] (Figure 7-5). The drugs used most commonly in support of perfusion are adrenergic agonists (usually dopamine, dobutamine, norepinephrine, or epinephrine) and vasopressin, although physiologic doses of corticosteroids, naloxone, and NOS blockers

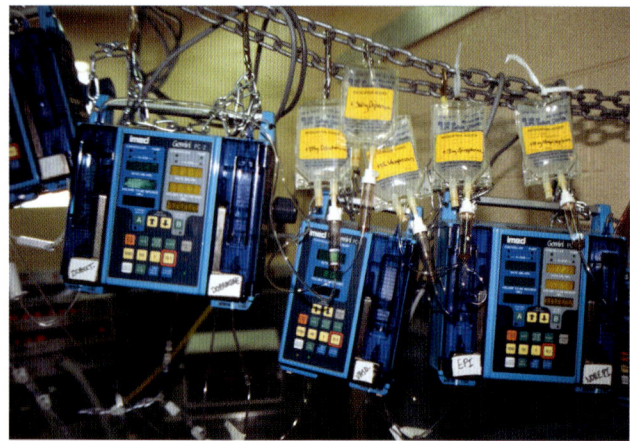

Fig. 7-5 Dobutamine, dopamine, epinephrine, norepinephrine, and vasopressin being infused together. Inotrope and pressor therapy requires carefully controlled infusions, best accomplished by using intravenous infusion pumps. Sometimes combination therapy is useful achieving profusion goals.

(methylene blue) have also been used. Some of these drugs have more inotropic (increases contractility) effects, while others are more inopressors (increase vascular resistance). When choosing drugs to support the cardiovascular system, it is important to ensure cardiac output. If pressors are used without inotropic support, there is danger that cardiac output and perfusion will decrease (despite an increase in BP numbers). For this reason, inotropes are almost always indicated when pressors are used. Mixed inotropic and pressor support or inopressor support can best be achieved by selecting an inotrope, such as dobutamine or medium-dose dopamine, as part of the initial therapy.[16]

When adrenergic agonists are used, each patient is a pharmacokinetic experiment. This is due to the variation in plasma half-life, receptor density, receptor affinity, receptor reactivity, and the effect of plasma pH on all of these factors. The dose must be tailored to the individual by monitoring for signs of improved perfusion during continuous rate infusion (CRI) and adjusting the dose accordingly. Because of the short half-life, the effect of new doses is readily evident within 10 to 15 minutes. The individual may change with time depending upon many confounding factors, so the delivered dose may also need to be adjusted. The goal is to withdraw therapy as soon as possible.

Whenever the cardiovascular system is supported by pharmacologic doses of adrenergic agonists, there may be both an increase in perfusion and, simultaneously, an increase in the maldistribution of that perfusion. There is a balance between improved perfusion and exaggerated malperfusion.[17] When beginning aggressive support, keep in mind that the goal is to return perfusion to minimally acceptable levels and not to try to achieve normal or supranormal perfusion. Doing so can result in disastrous effects.

No matter what drug is used, diluting the drug using the "rule of 6" can be very useful. The rule of 6 is a method of calculating how much drug should be placed in infusion fluids so that it is easy to determine the infusion dose based on the infusion rate. Thus 6 × body weight (kg) will equal the number of milligrams of drug that should be added to 100 ml of infusion fluids. Then for each 1 ml/hour of infusion, the patient will receive 1 µg/kg/minute of the drug. For drugs with infusion rates in the 0.1 to 1 µg/kg/minute range, 0.6 should replace 6; for each 1 ml/hour of infusion, the patient will receive 0.1 µg/kg/minute of the drug. With the rule of 6, accurately changing the infusion rate becomes simple. As long as patient weight, initial calculation, and drug addition to the infusion are accurate, errors in dosing are avoided. Efforts of human hospital quality-control organizations to standardize drug infusion concentrations have been met by vocal resistance from neonatologists who feel that moving away from the rule of 6 will more likely introduce errors in fluid overload and pump programming. But such moves in human medicine may make it more difficult to find stock drug solutions useful in making infusion fluids using the rule of 6.[16,18]

Dobutamine has primarily β_1 activity at low to moderate doses and thus is a good inotrope. In humans, some α_2 activity may result in mild vasodilation, but in general α_1 and α_2 stimulus is well balanced so is clinically not important. In horses, α_1 activity appears as the dose increases, causing significant vasoconstriction. Thus dobutamine could be classified as an inopressor at high doses. When patients need support but are not in shock, a good starting dose is 5 µg/kg/minute, followed by titration to the effective dose. When the neonate is suffering from shock, a good starting dose is 10 µg/kg/minute, followed by titration to the effective dose. The dose range is 2 to 20 µg/kg/minute, with occasional cases needing as high a dose as 50 µg/kg/min. Adverse reactions include tachycardia and occasional arrhythmias[16,19] (Table 7-1).

Dopamine has dopaminergic activity at low doses, β_1 and β_2 activity at moderate doses, and α_1 activity at high doses. It causes norepinephrine release from nerve terminals, which has lead to the suggestion that this is its major mode of action at high doses and the suggested limitation in critical patients who become depleted. Dopamine can be classified as an inopressor. When patients need support but are not shocky, a good starting dose is 5 µg/kg/minute, followed by titration to the effective dose. When the neonate is suffering from shock, a good starting dose is 10 µg/kg/minute, followed by titration to the effective dose. The dose range is 2 to 20 µg/kg/minute. At doses over 20 µg/kg/min, intrapulmonary shunting may occur, which limits the high end of the dose range. Adverse reactions include occasional arrhythmias. Dopamine

Table 7.1

Drug	Starting Dose	Range of Dose	Adverse Effects
Dobutamine	5 μg/kg/minute	2–20 μg/kg/minute	Tachycardia, occ. arrhythmias
Dopamine	5 μg/kg/minute	2–20 μg/kg/minute	occ. arrhythmias
Norepinephrine	0.3–0.5 μg/kg/minute	0.1–3.0 μg/kg/minute	occ. arrhythmias
Epinephrine	0.3–0.5 μg/kg/minute	0.1–2.0 μg/kg/minute	occ. arrhythmias, hyperglycemia, lactatemia
Vasopressin	0.25–1.0 mU/kg/minute	0.25–1.0 mU/kg/minute	Possible hyponatremia

has complex effects on the gastrointestinal tract and many other organ systems[16,20] (Table 7-1).

Norepinephrine has α_1 and β_1 activity, but variable β_2 activity resulting in potent vasopressor activity; it has both inotropic and chronotropic activities, but its chronotropic affect is usually blunted by vagal reflex slowing the heart rate induced by the rise in BP. There is an increase in myocardial oxygen consumption due to cardiostimulation and increased afterload. It has been thought of primarily as a pressor, and its use has been advocated in septic shock. It is frequently used in combination with either dopamine or dobutamine to enhance the inotropic effect because of the strong pressor effect. Although frequently used, it appears to suffer more from maldistribution of blood flow than the other adrenergic agonists. A good starting dose is 0.3 to 0.5 μg/kg/minute with further titration to an effective dose. The dose range is from 0.1 to 3.0 μg/kg/minute with a few difficult cases requiring 4 to 5 μg/kg/minute. The major adverse reactions are occasional arrhythmias. These are rare unless there is pre-existing myocardial damage such as in hypoxic ischemic asphyxial disease or secondary to sepsis[16,21] (Table 7-1).

Epinephrine has α_1, α_2, β_1, and β_2 activity. Beta activity is predominant resulting in increased cardiac output and decreased peripheral resistance at low doses, making it an attractive inotrope at low doses with inopressor activity as the dose increases. It has been associated with hyperglycemia and increased lactate production. The increase in lactate is rapid and may be dramatic but is easily reversible. When given for its inotropic effect, a good starting point is 0.3 to 0.5 μg/kg/minute with further titration to an effective dose. The dose range is from 0.1 to 2.0 μg/kg/minute with a few difficult cases requiring 3 to 4 μg/kg/minute. The major adverse reaction (in addition to the metabolic derangements) is occasional arrhythmias. These generally occur when there is pre-existing myocardial damage such as in hypoxic ischemic asphyxial disease or secondary to sepsis[16] (Table 7-1).

Vasopressin at physiologic levels has been used in the treatment of hypotension associated with septic shock.[16,22] Recent studies have suggested a deficiency in vasopressin levels in patients who succumb to septic

shock.[23] The current approach to therapy has been suggested to be in essence replacement therapy and not pharmacologic therapy. Vasopressin receptors are currently classified into V1 vascular receptors, V2 renal receptors, V3 pituitary receptors, oxytocin (OTR) receptors, and P2 purinergic receptors. V1 receptors are found in high density on vascular smooth muscle, causing vasoconstriction through calcium fluxes, nitric oxide synthase (NOS) inhibition, and by resetting ATP gated potassium channels. It is also found on cardiac myocytes, in the kidney, CNS, and many other tissues. V2 receptors are responsible for the antidiuretic effect and have only definitely been identified on renal collecting tubules. V3 receptors are found in the pituitary gland and cause secretion of ACTH. OTR has equal affinity for vasopressin and oxytocin. It is found in high density on vascular endothelium, triggering activation of NOS leading to vasodilation and is found in the heart where activation stimulates the release of atrial natriuretic peptide and may have a positive inotropic effect. Vasopressin stimulates the P2 class of purinoreceptors resulting in increased synthesis and release of prostacyclin and nitric oxide. This causes vasodilation, and an increase in cardiac contractility resulting in inotropy not accompanied by a positive chronotropic effect and thus without the expense of a rate-related increase in myocardial oxygen demand.[23]

The actions of vasopressin on the heart are complex. Depending upon the species, dose, and circumstances, vasopressin can cause coronary vasoconstriction or vasodilation and exert positive or negative inotropic effects as well as metabolic effects on the heart. There appears to be a difference between the "normal" and stressed heart in response to vasopressin. Vasoconstriction is seen in the normoxic state, and vasodilation is seen during hypoxia. In hypoxemic states, low doses appear to result in a directed pressor response and simultaneously increase coronary perfusion, act as an inotrope, and increase cardiac output. But with high doses, there is a significant decrease in coronary flow, myocardial oxygen consumption, and left ventricular peak systolic pressure.[22]

Vasopressin is a unique vasoactive hormone that is important in control of vascular tone and has myocardial effects. Vasopressin, in low, physiologic doses, can restore vascular tone in refractory vasodilatory shock states due to closure of ATP gated potassium channels, inhibitory action on NOS, and potentiation of endogenous and exogenous vasoconstrictors. In addition, it will cause selective vasodilation and increased cardiac output resulting in a more physiologic return of perfusion.[22] Infusion of exogenous vasopressin at a rate of 0.25 to 1.0 mU/kg/minute causes an increase in arterial pressure in many of our hypotensive patients (Table 7-1). There may even be a modest increase in our normotensive neonates. In some patients, BP may be maintained with vasopressin alone without the administration of exogenous adrenergic agonists. The clinically apparent positive effect of vasopressin on perfusion has become consistent enough that I have begun to use vasopressin has a first-line therapy, rather than just a rescue intervention. The feeling is that at the very low doses being used, this is primarily a replacement therapy and we are treating a vasopressin deficiency. Returning vasopressin to its physiologic levels allows endogenous BP regulation mechanisms to cope with the challenges facing the neonate. Urine flow rates increase significantly during administration of vasopressin in patients in septic shock.

Although our experience has been positive for the most part, caution should be exercised in treating neonates with vasopressin, since all metabolic ramifications of this intervention are not clearly understood. In several cases of severe refractory hypotension that have responded to vasopressin treatment, we have seen development of hyponatremia. These cases are at high risk of hyponatremia for many reasons, including difficulty handling water loads, predilection for sodium losing nephropathies, and development of depletional or redistribution hyponatremia. In these cases, it is unlikely that hyponatremia is secondary to inappropriate antidiuresis since the urine is not concentrated. It is unclear whether vasopressin has played a role in the development of hyponatremia or whether hyponatremia is secondary to other therapeutic interventions and confounding pathologic influences. In similar cases, hyponatremia has occurred when vasopressin has not been part of the therapeutic regime.

Neonates with marginal perfusion who are hypothermic should not be treated with active external warming as part of thermal management until the BP is stable. Active external warming will cause cutaneous vasodilation, which can lead to further hypoperfusion. Heat conservation techniques such as blankets to capture body heat can be useful, but active warming such as hot-water circulating pads, hot-water bottles, or forced warm air should be avoided until the patient is stable.

'04 Revival's admission venous glucose level was 44 mg/dl. As soon as vascular access was available, he was started on 5% dextrose in water at a rate of 259 ml/hour, which delivered 4 mg/kg/minute of glucose. Within one hour, the blood glucose had increased to 74 mg/dl. After two hours, it was 89 mg/dl. The concentration of the dextrose solution was increased to 10% so that the foal was receiving 8 mg/kg/minute of glucose.

Dextrose Therapy

All compromised neonates will benefit from exogenous glucose support. The main challenge is convincing the neonate's physiology to accept exogenous glucose without becoming hyperglycemic. Many clinicians confuse blood glucose levels with a gauge of adequate glucose stores. Blood glucose levels are a summation of glucose mobilization and glucose utilization. Before birth, the normal fetus is receiving all of their glucose needs through the placenta. Transfer rate of glucose from the placenta to fetus vary somewhat between species but generally is between 4 and 8 mg/kg/minute (fetal foal 6.8 mg/kg/minute, fetal calf 5 mg/kg/minute).[24] With fetal distress because of placentitis or because of lack of nutrient transfer from the dam, the fetus born with active glucogenesis may develop a high resting glucose. The normal fetus is born before glucogenesis begins, usually with low blood glucose (neonatal foal 25 to 45 mg/dl, 50% to 60% of the maternal value at birth). The glucose continues to drop for the first few hours of life until either glucogenesis is initiated or enteral nutrition provides a source of glucose. The low point of blood glucose levels is usually two to four hours after birth. The normal foal will begin glucogenesis without a problem, but the neonate suffering from perinatal disease may not make the transition to glucogenesis and may become dangerously hypoglycemic, compounding the neonate's problems. In either case, whether the neonate has precocious glucogenesis or no glucogenesis, supplementing the neonate with exogenous glucose decreases the catabolic state and supports recovery. In '04 Revival's case, the admission venous dextrose was 44 mg/dl. At 15 hours, this is clearly below the expected value at that age and reflects abnormal glucose kinetics with either poor glucogenesis, lack of nutrient ingestion, increased metabolic demands, or a combination of all three. Lack of production could represent hypoxic ischemic stress, intrauterine distress, or sepsis/SIRS. Increased utilization could reflect sepsis/SIRS.

When delivering glucose therapy, a rate of 4 to 8 mg/kg/minute should be the goal.[25] Neonates tolerate exogenous glucose best if the infusion is begun at the low rate and gradually increased over the first hours of therapy. Even when the blood glucose is too low to register, I still feel beginning at 4 mg/kg/minute is a good starting dose. Blood glucose levels can be followed, and the infusion rate of dextrose increased rapidly if necessary. In foals with severe sepsis or septic shock, the infusion rate often must be increased above 8 mg/kg/minute and may even need to be as high as 20 mg/kg/minute. When giving high exogenous glucose loads, addition of thiamine to the fluids may help ensure proper metabolism.

'04 Revival became hyperglycemic on the glucose infusion of 8 mg/kg/minute. By six hours of hospitalization the foal's glucose had increased to 176 mg/dl. By 12 hours of hospitalization the glucose level was 225 mg/dl, and by 18 hours it was 326 mg/dl. '04 Revival began spilling glucose in his urine (glucosuria 500 to 1000 mg/dl). He was started on a CRI of regular insulin.

Glucose intolerance may occur because of failure to adapt to the exogenous glucose load.[25] The normal fetus does not need to regulate its glucose level but rather relies on maternal regulation. So another transition that occurs at birth is regulation of glucose levels. The insulin response to high blood glucose levels may be somewhat sluggish in the neonate, especially the neonate who has had significant perinatal stress. The hope of administering exogenous glucose is to spare endogenous calorie stores. Occasionally the neonate will continue glucogenesis despite the delivery of exogenous glucose resulting in hyperglycemia. Hyperglycemia may also occur if glucose administration is in excess of utilization in the absence of an adequate insulin response. A third reason for hyperglycemia is iatrogenic glucose overload because of errors in calculations or administration of glucose containing fluids as boluses.[25] If the neonate becomes hyperglycemic, the clinician should double-check the infusion rate, ascertain whether the intolerance might be secondary to sepsis, and also be patient, allowing time for the neonate to develop an insulin response. Hyperglycemia without an insulin response may result in a degree of cellular dehydration, but the major adverse effect is a glucose diuresis with subsequent fluid and electrolyte wasting. If the neonate is only mildly hyperglycemic (<250 mg/dl) and there is no significant glucose diuresis, I prefer to give the neonate some time (hours) to develop its own innate insulin response. If there is a glucose diuresis or the blood dextrose is persistently high without apparent adaptation, I prefer to initiate insulin therapy rather than decreasing glucose infusion, since decreasing glucose infusion will not address the energy needs of the neonate. Recently Van den Berghe's group presented evidence that tight glucose control with intensive insulin therapy decreases mortality in human cardiac surgery cases.[26] No similar studies have been done in pediatric or neonatal populations. Certainly glucose and insulin kinetics is much different in growing neonates than in adults. The implications of supplementation in the face of a neonate's attempt to develop control of stable metabolism are certainly different than in adults who have lost control of their metabolism. Insulin's effect on growth hormones such as insulinlike growth hormone 1 and its modulating effects on inflammation are complex and not well understood.[27] Until strict glucose control is shown to be beneficial (outweighing the advantage of glucose fluctuations in the development of normal insulin responsiveness) and the benefits outweigh the danger of hypoglycemia (which frequently occurs in pursuit of strict control), any managed change directed by such studies should be done with caution.[28]

If exogenous insulin is required, continuous infusion of regular insulin is well tolerated by most neonates and allows more control of glucose kinetics than other forms. In most cases, rather than being insulin-insensitive, neonates will respond to surprisingly low doses. This suggests an insulin deficit as opposed to insulin resistance. This is true even in most cases of sepsis. The amount of regular insulin required usually ranges between 0.00125 and 0.2 U/kg/hour with most cases responding with <0.05 U/kg/hour. I usually began at 0.0025 U/kg/hour and double the rate every 4 to 6 hours until the glucose is controlled or the infusion rate is > 0.04 U/kg/hour, at which time I more slowly increase the rate. Care should be taken not to increase the rate too quickly. The response to the infusion is not seen immediately, and it is easy to increase the infusion rate too soon and place the neonate on a glucose roller coaster. When preparing the insulin infusion, special care should be taken. First, it should be no more than three months since the insulin bottle was first used. Insulin is a suspension and should be gently rocked or rolled to resuspend the insulin but *never* shaken. Insulin adheres to both glass and plastic. Adherence can be decreased with albumin-containing solutions or other special diluents, or careful pretreatment of IV lines. Insulin should be diluted in saline in a glass bottle, by infusing the insulin into the saline and not allowing the undiluted insulin to run down the glass where it will adhere. I generally make up a 0.1 U/ml solution in 100 to 150 ml of saline. The insulin-containing solution in the final dilution should be used to treat all plasticware from the insulin line to the neonate by running 40 to 60 ml of the solution through the line and then flushing the line with solutions not containing insulin. Some studies suggest that having the insulin retained in the line for 24 to 72 hours may be more efficacious but this is certainly not practical. If the insulin is given after a plasma transfusion, albumin in the plasma may have already bound some of the sites on the plastic where insulin would normally adhere. If the lines are not pretreated or if there's a line change and the new lines are not pre-treated, the insulin kinetics may be erratic due to lack of delivery (as insulin binds to the lines) and then a sudden increase in delivery (once the sites are occupied).

Maintenance Fluids

Once the cardiovascular system is stable, the fluid therapy should be governed by the glucose needs, electrolyte needs, and fluid requirements. The most common iatrogenic problem with maintenance fluid therapy is fluid overload and sodium imbalance. The fluid volume required for maintenance of fluid balance depends upon a number of variables that are clinically difficult to quantitate. These include metabolic rate, the degree the metabolism is supported by catabolism, and insensible water loss. Metabolic rate varies with surface area to mass ratio, which heavily influences nonrespiratory insensible water loss secondary to heat loss. The volume of insensible water loss will also depend upon the ambient temperature, ambient humidity, respiratory rate, and body temperature. Tachypnea can significantly affect respiratory water loss as will other pathologic conditions such as hyperthermia or hypothermia. Urine osmotic load is also important. It can be increased by many medications, with hyperglycemia, and with catabolism. Along with the osmotic load, the kidneys' ability to concentrate this osmotic load (the amount of water required to excrete the osmotic load) is important. Finally, the gastrointestinal water loss can be quite variable ranging from none in foals with meconium retention to large volumes in foals with loose feces. Because all of these variables differ from one individual to another, there is no "correct" maintenance fluid rate. Thus the clinician must guard against being locked into a fluid rate based on tradition, but rather should seek a starting rate that suits most cases with the willingness to be flexible guided by the presence of confounding influences.

One way to calculate an initial maintenance fluid rate is with the Holliday-Segar formula.[29,30] This formula can meet the maintenance needs of most neonates over a broad weight range from 1 kg to 80 kg, making it ideal for neonates of all species. Using this formula, 100 ml/kg/day (approximately 4 ml/kg/hour) is given for each of the first 10 kg body weight; 50 ml/kg/day (approximately 2 ml/kg/hour) is given for each kilogram of body weight between 11 and 20 kg; and 25 ml/kg/day (approximately 1 ml/kg/hour) is given for each kilogram of body weight above 20 kg. This formula calculates a "dry" fluid rate for most foals. This is preferred since with most neonates fluid overload is more of a problem than mild fluid restriction once volemia has been ensured, especially when renal compromise is present. Partially restricting fluids will spare compromised kidneys the extra work of excretion of unnecessary fluids. The Holliday-Segar formula acknowledges that maintenance fluid needs are related to basal metabolism. Metabolism produces heat that must be dissipated by insensible evaporation and produces solute by-products that must be excreted in the urine.[30] Insensible losses and urinary losses are the two major sources of basal fluid requirements in a neonate without high gastrointestinal losses.

The glucose infusion rate for a 50 kg neonate is more than 2.5 times the calculated fluid maintenance rate using the Holliday-Segar formula (the larger the foal the greater the difference). It is my routine to have foals on the glucose infusion rate for 24 hours or less. By 24 hours, critical foals who cannot receive enteral nutrition are placed on parenteral nutrition and the non-nutritional fluid rate is slowed to maintenance levels.[31] Those on enteral nutrition will receive adequate fluids in their milk ration. Thus, during the initial 24 hours the neonate may be fluid loaded, often receiving plasma, bolus fluids, and glucose at a high infusion rate. But in the most critical foals who are likely to have significant renal compromise, the fluid rate is slowed to a dry maintenance rate (plus parenteral nutrition infusion and medication infusions) within the first 24 hours, sparing the neonate further fluid challenge.

It is important to guard against sodium overload of the neonate when formulating maintenance fluids. By combining 5% dextrose in water with sodium-containing fluids, fluid volume and sodium requirements can be delivered independently. Rehydration and maintenance of all fluid compartments are more readily achieved by using sodium dilute fluids than sodium isotonic fluids.[32] Also, many critically ill neonates tend to have a significant osmolar gap. Adding free water may be important in clearing the unidentified osmolytes.

It is easy to sodium overload or deplete a neonate because of their innate sodium conserving physiology and because perinatal disease impairs renal sodium handling.[33] Sodium overload is a common sequela to indiscriminate fluid therapy with sodium-containing fluids. Neonatal physiology is preprogrammed to optimize sodium conservation, probably because the neonate's diet of sodium-poor fresh milk.[33] The normal nursing foal receives 2 mEq Na/kg/day from mare's milk. The neonate requires about 1 mEq Na/kg/day for growth. The normal neonate's kidneys avidly conserve sodium so that the low dietary sodium intake will meet the neonate's needs. Initially this sodium conservation will occur irrespective of sodium intake. Thus sodium overload is a common unintentional sequela of therapy with sodium-containing fluids. The goal of sodium replacement is to limit daily sodium intake to <3 mEq/kg/day to mimic the normal sodium intake from milk while preventing overload that can cause excessive fluid retention and edema formation. In the typical 50 kg foal, 1 liter of balanced ionic fluids or 1 liter of plasma will deliver its daily sodium requirement. Foals that have been treated with plasma and fluid boluses for hypovolemia during the first 24 hours may not require additional sodium for several days because of the unavoidable sodium loading. Foals receiving 2 g/kg/day of amino acids in parenteral nutrition formulas may be receiving up to 1 mEq Na/kg/day. Foals will receive additional sodium with continuous rate infusion of a variety of drugs, including inopressors, insulin, and antimicrobials as well as bolus infusion of drugs such as antimicrobials and associated saline flushes. Careful attention to sodium intake will help with sodium balance and avoid the fluid overload and accompanying edema secondary to sodium overload.

Although neonates are born conserving sodium, probably in anticipation of a sodium-poor diet of fresh milk, if exposed to a high-sodium diet, sodium conservation will subside and sodium regulation will become more effective.[33] This transition may occur within days of birth, but in the compromised foal this transition may not occur this quickly. So a normal foal placed on milk replacer (which is much higher in sodium than mares' milk and may provide 10 mEq/kg/day of sodium when fed in a standard manner) can adapt to the high sodium load quickly and not develop edema, whereas a sick foal with a high sodium load in intravenous fluids (who does not make the transition and who has marginal fluid excretion because of renal and vascular compromise) may develop massive edema interfering with perfusion.

Some foals have a high sodium requirement rather than a tendency for sodium overload. Neonatal nephropathy is a common perinatal problem usually secondary to hypoxic ischemic insults or SIRS. In these cases, renal sodium wasting with high sodium clearance and high fractional excretion of sodium is common. Pathologic renal losses will result in high sodium requirements. Clinically, without gastric reflux and without diarrhea, urine is the only source of sodium loss. In cases with neonatal nephropathy, sodium can be balanced by matching sodium delivery to urinary losses plus sodium growth requirement (1 mEq/kg/day). Urinary sodium loss can be measured with total urine collection and calculation of daily sodium excretion. Total urine collection usually requires maintaining a urinary catheter, which can result in a serious nosocomial infection. When total urine collection is not available, sodium requirements can be estimated from spot urine sodium concentrations and fractional excretion results. Although the critical foal with normal renal function requires sodium restriction to prevent sodium overload, foals with renal sodium wasting can have such high losses that they may rapidly become dangerously hyponatremic. It is critical to follow the sodium balance carefully in these cases. Another source of excessive sodium loss is diarrhea. Foals with diarrhea require sodium-containing replacement fluids to match their excessive gastrointestinal losses. They should not be sodium restricted. Hyponatremia in the critical neonate is often a combination of excessive sodium loss and increased water retention secondary to antidiuresis and increased transfer of fluids to the interstitium, which occurs commonly in neonates.[13]

Maintenance potassium requirements are difficult to estimate. They will depend on renal losses, anabolic requirements (new cells require large quantities), catabolic potassium release, and intracellular shifts associated with the effect of insulin and epinephrine on sodium/potassium pump activity secondary to sepsis. Any neonate not consuming milk, with its high potassium content, will require supplemental potassium. When delivering a high fluid rate, such as with glucose therapy, empirical supplementation with 10 to 40 mEq/liter fluids is usually sufficient. When delivering fluids at the dry maintenance rate, higher concentrations in the range of 20 to 60 mEq/liter will be required. If the patient is allowed to become hypokalemic because of lack of potassium supplementation, very aggressive replacement therapy in the range of 80 to 100 mEq/liter may be necessary to "catch up." Most critical neonatal foals require 4 to 6 mEq K/kg/hour, but a select few may require up to 10 to 12 mEq K/kg/hour. Since it may be difficult to maintain potassium infusion at the necessary rate when it is placed the maintenance fluids, a separate potassium infusion containing 1 mEq K/mL can be useful. However, extreme caution must be used to ensure well-regulated infusion via fluid pump and at all costs avoid free flow of this infusate.

OTHER THERAPEUTIC INTERVENTIONS

Other therapeutic interventions important in a case like '04 Revival's include treatment for a possible septic cause of shock. As bacterial infections often play an important role, antimicrobials targeted at possible pathogens should be initiated as soon after admission as possible (before initial blood analysis is available). Although most bacterial isolates from blood cultures in neonatal foals are Gram negative, over 30% are gram positive and 15% of neonates may have multiple isolates.[34] Empiric choice for initial antimicrobial therapy should be broad-spectrum with a range that includes *E. coli, Enterobacter, Pantoea, Actinobacillus, Streptococcus, Enterococcus,* and *Staphylococcus.*[34] In '04 Revival's case, an antimicrobial (ticarcillin with clavulanate), which I do not usually consider as a first line choice, was used based on the severity of the infection and the antimicrobial use patterns on the farm leading to an educated guess about possible resistance patterns. In addition to antimicrobials, the biologically active ingredients in plasma can also aid in treating sepsis, and plasma is already administered as part of cardiovascular support.

The initial laboratory data for '04 Revival had some significant abnormalities. The foal had a significant leukopenia (800 cells/µl) with neutropenia (496 cells/µl) and lymphopenia (302 cells/µl) without left shift. This suggests acute, severe ongoing sepsis. This was later confirmed with an admission blood sample culture positive for Pantoea agglomerans. *He had a hyperfibrinogenemia of 461 mg/dl (normal range at birth 150 ± 50 mg/dl) at 15 hours old which was suggestive of intrauterine infection. An elevated creatinine of 3.46 was found on the serum chemistry. At admission '04 Revival had hyperlactatemia with a blood lactate level of 6.3 mmol/liter. Other important admission laboratory findings included an increased blood urea nitrogen (BUN) (36 mg/d)l, increased bilirubin (7.5 mg/dl), and abnormal blood gas values (pH (7.339), PaO$_2$—43.2 tor, PaCO$_2$—59.8).*

Laboratory Analysis

The initial laboratory results can be very helpful in understanding the magnitude of the underlying disease process, identifying organ systems involved, and understanding how many of the problems have prenatal origins. '04 Revival had evidence of both established sepsis and active sepsis. Since the rise in fibrinogen stimulated by a cytokine storm (primarily Il-6) usually requires one to two days, this finding indicates intrauterine sepsis. Thus '04 Revival's inflammatory stimulus began well before his birth. This is supported by the presence of chorionitis of the fetal membranes. Foals with established intrauterine sepsis usually have leukocytosis at or soon after birth, but '04 Revival had a neutropenia indicating an active ongoing SIRS.

'04 Revival's plasma creatinine was 3.46 mg/dl at 15 hours. Normal foals usually have a birth creatinine between 2 and 4 mg/dl, which quickly decreases. Foals born after fetal distress or who have suffered from placentitis can have a birth creatinine as high as 40 mg/dl but usually have levels, when increased, in the range of 6 to 20 mg/dl. This increase in creatinine level does not reflect renal function, but rather a redistribution of fluid and creatinine from the allantoic cavity, which normally has a creatinine level between 160 and 200 mg/dl.[31] The rapidity of the decrease in creatinine

after birth does reflect renal function and more specifically GFR. It is important to measure an early baseline value so that the decline can be observed. The initial height may indicate the severity of the intrauterine insult. However, it is not prognostic as it seems to be part of a compensatory response, which if effective may protect the fetus from the insult. '04 Revival's creatinine at 24 hours was within normal limits, but because of the rapidity of the decrease, his creatinine at birth may have been well above normal. It is interesting to note that the creatinine can drop significantly before the first urination.

'04 Revival had hyperlactatemia at admission with a blood lactate level of 6.3 mmol/liter. In many critical neonates, production of the strong ion lactate is an important cause of acidosis. The origin of lactic acid often has been misinterpreted in the past. Traditionally the amount of lactate produced has been linked to total oxygen debt, magnitude of hypoperfusion, and severity of shock. However, there are a number of other underlying causes of increased lactate production. When these are ignored and attempts are made to treat increased lactate production, to the exclusion of the other possible causes, poor outcomes can result.[35] Besides tissue hypoxia, hypodynamic shock, and organ ischemia, high lactate levels will result from hypermetabolism, as with increased aerobic glycolysis (from epinephrine), increased protein catabolism and increased muscle activity, decreased lactate clearance as with liver failure or shock, inhibition of pyruvate dehydrogenase as with thiamine deficiency or SIRS (secondary to cytokine enzyme inhibition), and activation of inflammatory cells as with ARDS.[36-38] It is also well to remember that lactate is an important carbon shuttle from the placenta to fetus, so at birth normal lactate levels are about 3 mmol/liter.[24] Also, the shivering neonate may have a sudden increase in blood lactate levels associated with muscle activity. In most cases it appears that elevated aerobic metabolism is more important than metabolic defects (pyruvate dehydrogenase inhibition) or anaerobic metabolism in increasing lactate.[39] Epinephrine, whether given exogenously or if stimulation results in endogenous increases, stimulates an increase in lactate levels by stimulating cellular metabolism (e.g. increased hepatic glycolysis). This effect does not occur with dobutamine or norepinephrine and is not related to tissue perfusion. Increased lactate, no matter what the underlying pathogenesis, should be taken as a sign of the critical state of the neonate. It is important to remember that although high lactate cannot be equated to poor perfusion and anaerobic metabolism (as this is only one possible cause), correcting hypoperfusion if present in the face of lactatemia is vital. However, once correct, efforts at super resuscitation in pursuit of normalizing lactate levels will cause more harm than good. It is also well to consider that since there are multiple reasons for an elevated lactate, during different stages of the disease process, these causes have different importance in producing the observed plasma lactate level. Lactate clearance is more important in predicting survival of the neonate than the absolute lactate value.[36]

In '04 Revival's case, he had a positive clearance with a 25% decrease in lactate during the first hour of hospitalization, over a 60% decrease during the first 10 hours of hospitalization, and a 75% clearance during the first 24 hours to a normal level of 1.6 mmol/liter.

The foals's admission BUN was 36 mg/dl. Because there is little catabolism occurring in the fetus, BUN at birth is generally quite low in normal foals (8 to 12 mg/dl)[24] However, with fetal distress, placentitis, or sepsis, the fetus will become catabolic and BUN will rise. '04 Revival's BUN of 36 mg/dl reflects established intrauterine catabolism, supporting a prenatal origin to at least some of his problems. The increased bilirubin (7.5 mg/dl) is also an indication of intrauterine distress. Although there are a number of possible explanations of birth hyperbilirubinemia, such as an intrauterine coagulopathy with intravascular hemolysins, intrauterine bleeding, or intrauterine sepsis with the release of bacterial hemolysins or toxins that cause cholestasis, a very likely explanation is stress-induced precocious maturation of enterocytes. Throughout gestation, conjugated bilirubin is deposited in the intestinal lumen, giving meconium its characteristic dark color. It cannot be absorbed, so it is effectively stored there until birth when it is passed with meconium.[40] Intrauterine stress will stimulate accelerated maturation of many body systems. It can induce the production of mucosal cell deconjugase that will liberate the bilirubin so it can be adsorbed, resulting in hyperbilirubinemia.

The major problem indicated by the admission arterial blood gas is a moderate hypoxemia (PaO_2 43.2 torr, SAT 77.1%, O_2 content 13.3 ml/dl) with the foal breathing room air. A significant part of this was mismatch, as indicated by the response to intranasal insufflation with 10 liters/minute of oxygen (PaO_2 144.2 torr, SAT 100%, O_2 content 14.9 ml/dl). Foals of this age frequently have $PaCO_2$ up to 60 probably due to a lack of sensitivity of the central respiratory center, either induced by perinatal damage or as part of natural maturation. In '04 Revival's case, his $PaCO_2$ of 59.8 is well balanced by a mild metabolic alkalosis, so the pH (7.339) is not significantly abnormal. This is often the case in neonates. The metabolic alkalosis is not renal compensation for the respiratory acidosis as it is often present at birth. It appears to be associated with catabolism and strong and weak ion shifts. I feel the metabolic alkalosis and the respiratory acidosis in these foals are independent but concurrent abnormalities

that are usually well balanced. Clinical experience shows that if these foals are ventilated so that the $PaCO_2$ is in the 40s, metabolic alkalosis will continue to progress; likewise, if the metabolic alkalosis is corrected, they continue to have high $PaCO_2$ levels.

In summary, the history, rapid admission examination, response to initial stabilization, and admission blood analysis showed that '04 Revival suffered from a significant intrauterine challenge, and presented in septic shock with a high lactate and an active infection. Although there was no direct evidence at admission, the foal was at high risk for neonatal encephalopathy and neonatal nephropathy. The history of intrauterine meconium passage followed by fetal diarrhea suggested neonatal enteropathy. How extensive this problem would become was not yet evident.

By four hours of hospitalization '04 Revival's cardiovascular status was stable. The foal had warm legs, consistent urine production, good arterial fill, excellent arterial tone, strong pulses, and consistent BP. He was responsive to his environment, and he was able to assume sternal recumbency without assistance, hold his head up, and look around.

'04 Revival's initial stabilization was successful, but over the course of his 18-day hospital stay, multiple problems had to be addressed. They included bacteremia, neonatal encephalopathy, enteropathy, nephropathy, urachitis, hepatomegaly, linear dermal necrosis, patent urachus, and angular limb deformity.

Critically ill foals often manifest with a new problem daily. Owners should be counseled about this probability at presentation because these foals will put them on an emotional "roller coaster." '04 Revival survived all of his problems, and after a slow start became a useful athlete (Figure 7-6).

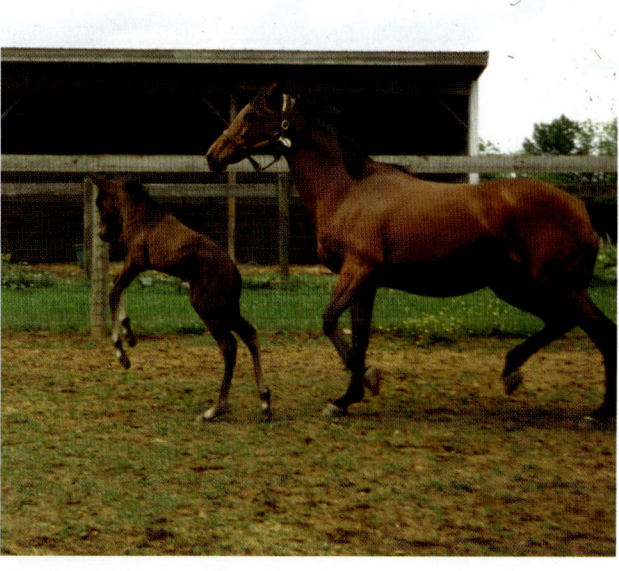

Fig. 7-6 '04 Revival after recovery.

REFERENCES

1. Lin CT, Liu SH, Wang JJ et al: Reduction of interference in oscillometric arterial blood pressure measurement using fuzzy logic, *IEEE Transactions on Biomedical Engineering* 50:432, 2003.
2. Nwankwo UM, Lorenz JM, Gardiner JC: A standard protocol for blood pressure measurement in the newborn, *Pediatrics* 99:e10, 1997.
3. Nuntnarumit P, Yang W, Bada-Ellzey HS: Blood pressure measurements in the newborn, *Clin Perinatol* 26:981, 1999.
4. Colan S, Fujji A, Borrow K et al: Non-invasive determination of systolic, diastolic and end systolic blood pressure in neonates, infants and young children. Comparison with central aortic pressure measurements, *Am J Cardiol* 52:867, 1983.
5. Park MK, Menard SM: Accuracy of blood pressure measurement by the Dianamap monitor in infants and children, *Pediatrics* 79:907, 1987.
6. Kimble KJ, Darnall RA, Yelderman M et al: An automated oscillometric technique for estimating mean arterial pressure in critically ill newborns, *Anesthesiology* 54:923, 1981.
7. Segar JL: Neural regulation of blood pressure during fetal and newborn life, in Polin RA, Fox WW, Abman SH, eds: *Fetal and neonatal physiology,* ed 3, Philadelphia, 2004, WB Saunders.
8. Engle WD: Blood pressure in the very low birth weight neonate, *Early Hum Dev* 62:97, 2001.
9. Sawaguchi T, Franco P, Groswasser J et al: Relationship between arousal reaction and autonomic nervous system in the sudden infant death syndrome, *Am J Forensic Med Pathol* 22:213, 2001.
10. Kravtsov IuI, Aminov FKh: Autonomic alternations in mature newborns with hypoxic damage of brain, *Zhurnal Nevrologii i Psikhiatrii Imeni S.S. Korsakova* 97:74, 1997.
11. Zeskind PS. Marshall TR, Goff DM: Cry threshold predicts regulatory disorder in newborn infants, *J Pediatr Psychol* 21:803, 1996.
12. Baska RE: Hypothalamic-midbrain dysregulation syndrome, *J Child Neurol* 7:116, 1992.
13. Palmer JE: Fluid therapy in the neonate: Not your mother's fluid space, *Vet Clin North Am Equine Pract* 20:63, 2004.
14. Rizoli SB: Crystalloids and colloids in trauma resuscitation: A brief overview of the current debate, *J Trauma* 54:S82, 2003.
15. Delinger RP: Cardiovascular management of septic shock, *Crit Care Med* 31:946, 2003.
16. Palmer JE: When fluids are not enough: Inopressor therapy, Proceedings of the Eighth International Veterinary Emergency and Critical Care Symposium, San Antonio, 2002.
17. Stopfkuchen H: What is a sufficient blood pressure in the preterm newborn? *Klinische Padiatrie* 215:16, 2003.
18. McLeroy PA: The rule of six: Calculating intravenous infusions in a pediatric crisis situation, *Hosp Pharm* 29:939, 1994.
19. Majerus TC, Dasta JF, Bauman JL et al: Dobutamine: Ten years later, *Pharmacotherapy* 9:245, 1989.
20. Subhedar NV, Shaw NJ: Dopamine versus dobutamine for hypotensive preterm infants, *Cochrane Database Syst Rev* 3:CD001242, 2003.
21. Theilmeier G, Booke M: Norepinephrine in septic patients—friend or foe? *J Clin Anesth* 15:154, 2003.
22. Holmes CL, Landry DW, Granton JT: Science Review: Vasopressin and the cardiovascular system part 2—clinical physiology, *Crit Care* 8:15, 2003.
23. Holmes CL, Landry DW, Granton JT: Science Review: Vasopressin and the cardiovascular system part 1—receptor physiology, *Crit Care* 7:427, 2003.
24. Fowden AL, Silver M: Glucose and oxygen metabolism in the fetal foal during late gestation, *Am J Physiol Regul Integr Comp Physiol* 269: 1455, 1995.
25. Kliegman RM: Problems in metabolic adaptation: Glucose, calcium, and magnesium. In Klaus MH, Fanaroff AA, eds: *Care of the high-risk neonate,* ed 5, Philadelphia, 2001, WB Saunders.
26. Van den Berghe G, Wouters P, Weekers F et al: Intensive insulin therapy in the critically ill patient, *N Engl J Med* 345:1359, 2001.
27. Groeneveld ABJ, Beishuizen A, Visser FC: Insulin: a wonder drug in the critically ill? *Crit Care* 6:102, 2002.
28. Vincent JL: Evidence-based medicine in the ICU, important advances and limitations, *Chest* 126:592, 2004.
29. Holliday MA, Segar WE: The maintenance need for water in parenteral fluid therapy, *Pediatrics* 19:823, 1957.
30. Chesney RW: The maintenance need for water in parenteral fluid therapy, *Pediatrics* 102:399, 1998.
31. Palmer JE: Practical approach to fluid therapy in neonates, Proceedings of the Eighth International Veterinary and Critical Care Symposium, San Antonio, 665, 2002.
32. Magder LS: Physiologic principles of fluid therapy, *Pediatr Crit Care Med* 2: S4, 2001.
33. Feld LG, Corey HE: Renal transport of sodium during early development. In Polin RA, Fox WW, Abman SH, eds: *Fetal and neonatal physiology,* ed 3, Philadelphia, 2004, WB Saunders.
34. Marsh PS, Palmer JE: Bacterial isolates from blood and their susceptibility patterns in critically ill foals: 543 cases (1991–1998), *J Am Vet Med Assoc* 218:1608, 2001.
35. James JH, Luchette FA, McCarter FD et al: Lactate is an unreliable indicator of tissue hypoxia in injury or sepsis, *Lancet* 354:505, 1999.
36. Nguyen HB, Rivers EP, Knoblich BP et al: Early lactate clearance is associated with improved outcome in severe sepsis and septic shock, *Crit Care Med* 32:1637, 2004.
37. De Backer D: Lactic acidosis, *Minerva Anestesiol* 69:281, 2003.
38. Levraut J, Ichai C, Petit I et al: Low exogenous lactate clearance as an early predictor of mortality in normolactatemic critically ill septic patients, *Crit Care Med* 31:705, 2003.
39. Levy B, Gibot S, Franck P et al: Relation between muscle Na+K+ ATPase activity and raised lactate concentrations in septic shock: A prospective study, *Lancet* 365:871, 2005.
40. Chen JY, Ling UP, Chen JH: Early meconium evacuation: Effect on neonatal hyperbilirubinemia, *Am J Perinatol* 12:232, 1995.

8 Noninfectious Respiratory Problems

Case 8-1	Immature Lungs in a Foal with Maternal Stress	Melissa R. Mazan

| Case 8-2 | Premature Lungs in a Foal from an Emergency C-Section | Melissa R. Mazan |

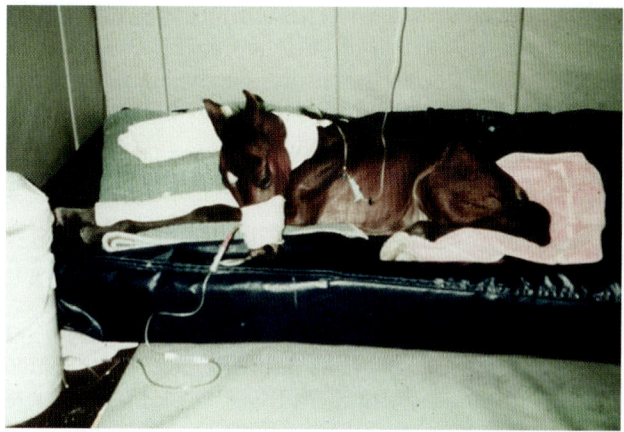

Fig. 8-1 '03 Surf's Up, a 305-day gestational age foal, presented with signs of moderate respiratory compromise.

'03 Surf's Up arrived into the world at 305 days of gestation, 35 days before her due date (Figure 8-1). A Thoroughbred with gilded bloodlines, she had been destined for great things, and there was no doubt about her breeding date. The night watchman found her in the stall early that morning. It was a good thing, because she would not have survived for very long in the chill of upstate New York in February. The farm veterinarian had been worried that the foal might arrive early, as the mare had developed signs of placentitis at eight months of gestation. The mare had been treated with trimethoprim-sulfa and altrenogest since that time, but no one thought the foal would arrive this early. The farm veterinarian didn't hesitate in deciding to send the foal to a referral hospital. She quickly administered colostrum via nasogastric tube, as well as 5% dextrose, penicillin, and amikacin intravenously, and sent the foal on her way.

On arrival at Tufts at six hours of age, the foal was weak, but surprisingly bright and alert. She had obvious signs of prematurity: a thin, silky haircoat, floppy ears, and lax tendons. The perionychium was still attached to the bottoms of her feet, showing that she had not been able to rise and walk. Her temperature was low—96.5° F, heart rate was 120 beats/minute, and respiratory rate was 60 breaths per minute. Her nostrils flared with each breath, but she showed no other signs of abnormal respiratory effort.

On another farm, '03 Last Gasp was being delivered by emergency C-section at 330 days of gestation. '03 Last Gasp's birth had also been lovingly anticipated. His dam's progress had been monitored every step of the way—no ultrasounds, vaccinations, or physical examinations had been spared. Her health had appeared perfect. Even as close to parturition as she was, Last Gasp usually came in eagerly from the pasture, ready for her evening meal. But today, she was nowhere to be found. Finally, they found her down, her left radius obviously shattered. The vet arrived in haste only to confirm what the owner's suspected—the mare could not be saved. The only thing to be done was to try to save the foal. The mare was anesthetized in the field for an emergency C-section.

The foal was small, and somewhat weak, but his ears were erect and his fetlocks appeared only mildly hyperextended. They dried him off, brought him to the barn, and prepared to rear an orphan foal. He seemed to have a strong suckle, and eagerly drank first the banked colostrum and then the milk replacer that was offered. He stood with difficulty in six hours, and when he did, his fetlocks sank almost to the ground. He tired quickly. The owners were happy to sleep in the barn in order to feed the foal every two hours, and the veterinarian agreed to

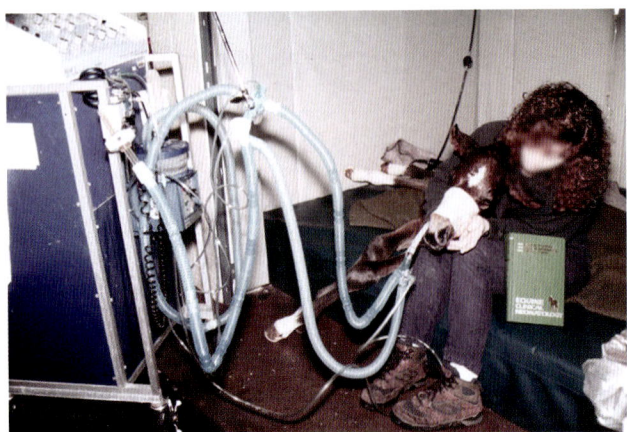

Fig. 8-2 '03 Last Gasp, a 330-day gestational age foal, was delivered by emergency C-section.

see them first thing in the morning. When the veterinarian arrived, she found a very different foal. He was recumbent, weak, and trembling. His nostrils flared with every breath, and his body rocked with the effort of his breathing. He grunted audibly at the end of each expiration. The owners reported that he had been eager to nurse until about two in the morning, when he appeared tired. He had not gotten up again.

Upon arrival at Tufts at 16 hours of age, his temperature was 97.0° F, heart rate was 160 beats/minute, and respiratory rate was 65 beats/minute. The foal's mucus membranes were muddy, and capillary refill time was >3 seconds. His respiratory effort had not improved (Figure 8-2).

HISTORY AND PHYSICAL EXAMINATION

'03 Surf's Up and '03 Last Gasp were chosen for this chapter to introduce the concepts of prematurity, readiness for birth, maternal stress, and the effects of these states on the maturation of the pulmonary system of the equine fetus/foal. Traditionally, a premature foal has been defined as being born before 320 days of gestation. However, the gestation period of the equid is markedly variable (320 to 360 days).[1] Some foals may be surprisingly mature at 320 days of gestation, while others meant to be born at 360 days of gestation but taken earlier, may be premature at 330 days of gestation. A syndrome of *dysmaturity*, wherein the foal is recognized to have the attributes of prematurity despite having achieved a gestational age of >320 days, is also recognized.[2]

These definitions are somewhat artificial and not always useful in considering the foal born before its respiratory system is ready for life outside the uterus. This chapter will focus on the neonatal lung, rather than the myriad of other systemic problems that can affect the premature foal, and will consider the lung of the foal that is completely unready to exist outside the uterus *premature*. In foals with a gestation length of <320 days that have non-life threatening, non-infectious pulmonary dysfunction, we would call the lungs *immature*. Length of gestation must take into account the normal gestational length for a *specific mare* and, while important, must share equal billing with the prenatal intrauterine environment in determining whether a foal is born with what we consider truly premature and therefore dysfunctional lungs, or with immature lungs.

Foals that experience "maternal stress," *in utero*, such as placentitis or twinning, appear to have accelerated maturation of their pulmonary system. This is also true in human pregnancies. These foals are "ready for birth" at an early gestational age and actually signal the parturition process. "Readiness for birth" is a term coined by Rossdale that denotes signaling from the foal to produce parturition.[2] These foals may have some respiratory clinical signs of immature lungs or mild pulmonary hypertension from persistent fetal circulation.

In contrast to the early foal with long-term "maternal stress," the foal that is delivered by C-section or is induced without the proper signs of impending parturition (gestational age >345 days, colostrum in udder, relaxation of pelvic ligaments, increased milk Ca^{2+} levels) may experience all the problems of pulmonary prematurity.

Another way to look at this is that failure of the lungs to mature by the time of birth in foals can be considered of endogenous or exogenous origin. The *endogenously* premature foal is one that has experienced considerable physiological intrauterine stress, resulting in a uterine environment that is no longer capable of supporting the foal. These foals are generally born before day 320 of gestation. There is often a history of placentitis (as was the case with '03 Surf's Up), twinning, or other systemic disease.[3] The *exogenously* premature foal, on the other hand, is one that has had a completely normal gestation up to the time of parturition: an external event, such as a C-section mandated by acute trauma to the mare or early induction, determines the early parturition. The exogenously premature foal may be born after 320 days, and must be considered premature regardless of earlier definitions of prematurity (i.e., earlier than 320 days).

The obvious outward attributes of prematurity are those that indicate that even if the foal has reached the requisite 320 days, it is functionally premature; these foals are generally small, their ears are floppy, their carpi and tarsi are often lax due to insufficient cartilage development, and their hair coats are short and silky.[4] The most important and alarming finding on physical examination of the premature foal, however, is difficult breathing. Both endogenously and exogenously premature foals may show early signs of respiratory system impairment, ranging from nostril flare to paradoxical breathing at birth; in others, subtle nostril flare is merely a precursor for subsequent respiratory failure. The exogenously premature foal is far more likely to lapse early into overt respiratory failure, while the endogenously premature foal more frequently avoids this scenario.[2]

As seen in Chapter 6, physical examination of the respiratory system in foals can be fraught with inconsistencies. Auscultation of the lungs can be normal despite widespread consolidation. Abnormal crackles and wheezes may be normal in the foal immediately after birth as the foal takes its first breaths and dissipates the residual fluid in the lung. If a recumbent foal is in lateral recumbency, then abnormal fluid sounds are often heard in the down lung due to atelectasis. Respiratory rate can be elevated for several nonpulmonary reasons as well. Excitement and acidosis can be causes of hypernea. The most reliable sign of respiratory problems in the equine neonate is increased respiratory effort. The foal with pronounced nasal flare, marked abdominal effort, expiratory grunting, or the appearance of paradoxical breathing is in respiratory distress.

In the case of the foal in respiratory distress, the need for immediate treatment must outweigh the desire for a meticulous physical examination and pursuit of clinical laboratory data. Cyanosis is often absent in the presence of severe hypoxemia,[5] so the appearance of pink mucous membranes alone should not lead the clinician to the conclusion that the respiratory system is functioning properly. Even in the case of apparent eupnea, it is important nonetheless to obtain an arterial blood gas. Koterba found that although only 4 out of 38 septic foals in one study appeared to be in respiratory distress, 83% were hypoxemic.[6] If there is more than one able hand present, one person may obtain a sample for arterial blood gas analysis while the other begins nasal insufflation of oxygen. As long as the foal is breathing, nasal insufflation of oxygen is usually sufficient for preliminary resuscitation. At this point, the careful physical examination may commence.

PATHOGENESIS

The foal that is born with premature lungs has multiple reasons for developing respiratory distress and failure: surfactant deficiencies, inadequate development of the lung parenchyma, excessive compliance of the chest wall, pulmonary hypertension in the presence of fetal circulation, and general weakness. In order to understand the devastating effect of the combination of these factors on the proper functioning of

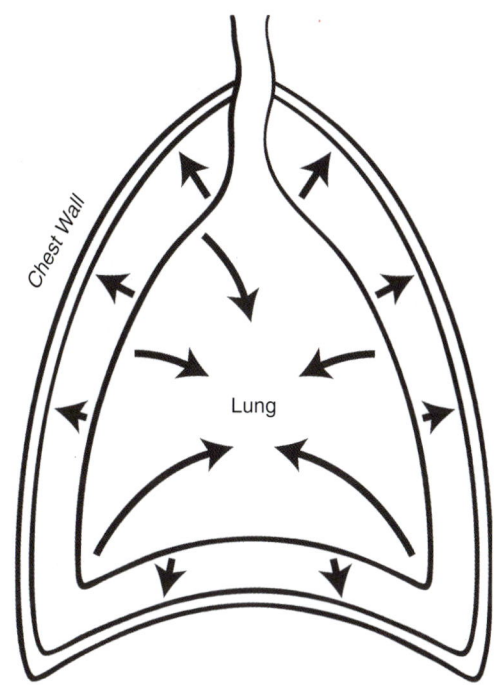

Fig. 8-3 Chest wall counteracts the tendency of the lungs to collapse.

the respiratory system, it is necessary to understand the basic physiology of the respiratory system of the neonate, particularly the mechanics of the respiratory system.

In both the normal and abnormal foal, the tendency of the lung to collapse is counteracted by the tendency of the chest wall to spring outward (Figure 8-3). The meeting place of the two determines the functional residual capacity (FRC), which is the natural resting place of the lung.[7] The FRC acts as an important reservoir of air, helps to prevent collapse of the lung with each breath, and is critical in preventing the very high work of breathing that accompanies cyclic lung collapse. We can see this on a quasi-static pressure volume (PV) curve (Figure 8-4). Picture the lung at residual volume—the very smallest volume that the lung can achieve. If we then inflate the lung by increments, we see that at the earliest portion of the inflation curve, increasingly high pressures are needed to elicit a change in volume. At the end of this portion of the curve, the PV curve becomes relatively linear. The beginning of this linear phase is known as the lower inflection point (LIP), and represents the point at which collapsed alveoli begin to open.[7] Breathing below the LIP requires a high level of work of breathing—neonates should not have to repeat this work after the first postpartum breaths. The premature neonate, lacking a relatively stiff chest wall to counteract the inward elastic recoil of the lung, must employ other strategies to preserve its FRC.[8] One such strategy is to breathe against a closed glottis,

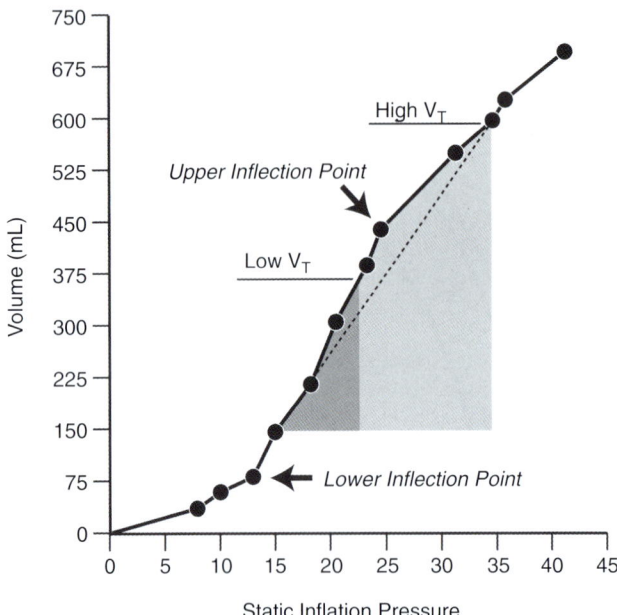

Fig. 8-4 PV curve. High pressures are needed to change the lung volume in the beginning of the curve. The point where the curve becomes more linear is the lower inflection point.

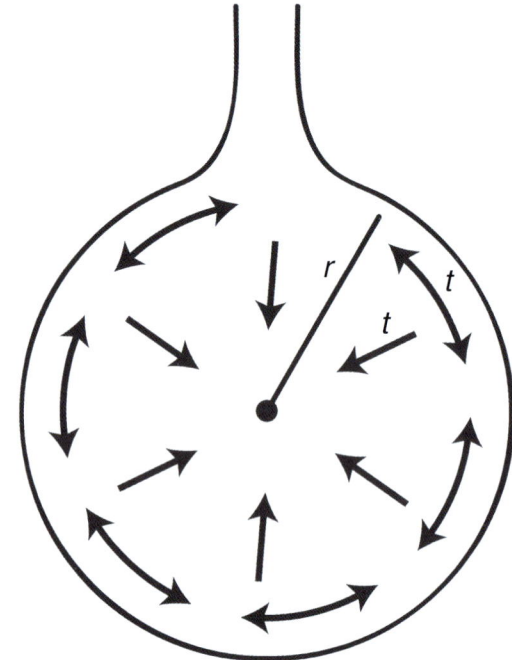

Fig. 8-5 According to Pierre-Simon Laplace, if surface tension does not vary, then a decrease in the radius of an alveoli will increase the pressure within that alveoli.

which allows the foal to trap air at end-expiration, or "auto-PEEP," (positive end expiratory pressure) and also elicits the characteristic grunt often heard from foals in respiratory distress. Although the neonate of all species has higher chest wall compliance than the adult, this difference is far less in the normal neonatal foal, which has an impressively stiff chest wall in comparison to other neonates. This helps the neonatal foal to preserve its FRC.[9]

The physics of the chest wall really pale in comparison to the physics of the alveoli and surfactant. Indeed, surfactant is the *sine qua non* of the respiratory system. A sufficient understanding of the Laplace relationship: $P = 2T/R$ (where P = pressure within the alveolus, T = surface tension of the alveolus, and R = the radius) helps to clarify the situation. This equation implies that if surface tension is not allowed to vary, then as radius decreases (as with a small alveolus), pressure within the alveolus becomes linearly greater. Imagine that an alveolus is attached to a second alveolus of twice the radius; the pressure in the larger alveolus will be one half that of the smaller alveolus. Thus, to equalize the pressure, the air from the smaller alveolus will flow into the larger alveolus (Figure 8-5). Thus, the natural tendency of the lung is to allow the smaller alveoli to collapse in favor of emptying into larger alveoli, with an overall decrease in surface area and volume of the lung.[10]

Now picture the neonate with insufficiently developed lungs. The chest wall alone would predispose the premature foal to respiratory failure; the less developed, more compliant chest wall of the premature foal,

combined with muscle weakness, will inevitably result in a decreased FRC as inward recoil of the lung overcomes the outward spring of the chest wall, resulting in difficult breathing.[8] It would seem that the Laplace relationship, in conjunction with the high compliance of the neonatal chest wall, would result in a lung that continually returns to residual volume even in the term foal, thus entailing enormous work of breathing with every breath.[10] It is important to know that surfactant turns the Laplace relationship topsy-turvy. It not only reduces surface tension at the air-liquid interface in the alveolus, but it allows this surface tension to vary with the diameter of the alveolus.

WHAT IS SURFACTANT, AND WHY IS IT SO IMPORTANT IN PRETERM FOALS?

Pattle first described the stability of pulmonary foam,[11] and Avery and Mead soon discovered that surfactant deficiency was the cause of hyaline membrane disease in premature infants.[12] The majority of surfactant is a combination of phospholipids, the most abundant of which is phosphatidylcholine (PC), or lecithin. Approximately 50% of PC is saturated, or dipalmitoylphosphatidylcholine, known as DPPC. DPPC is most critical for decreased surface tension in the airways.[13] While DPPC can form a surface layer devoid

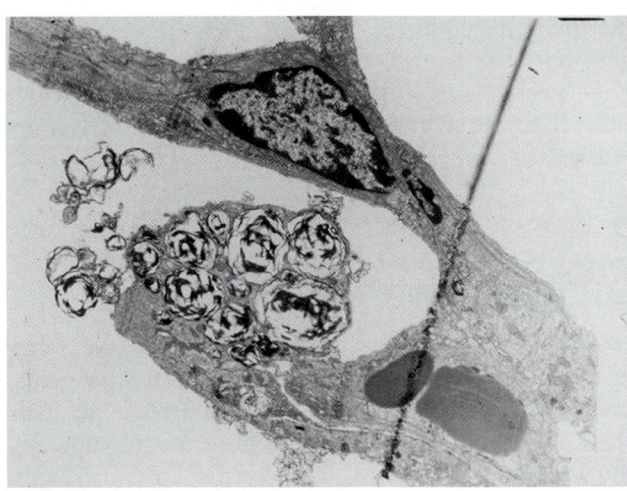

Fig. 8-6 Lamellar bodies in type II pneumocytes make and store surfactant.

of surface tension, it is not effective *in vivo* on its own; rather, it requires other lipids and especially surfactant-associated proteins to adhere to the lining of the lung. These proteins are also important in modulating inflammation and immune responses in the lung.[14] The proteins discovered to date have been named surfactant protein (SP)-A, SP-B, SP-C, and SP-D; without SP-B, in particular, the individual cannot survive.[15]

The lamellar bodies of type II pneumocytes make and store surfactant (Figure 8-6). The surfactant is subsequently released into the airways by the process of exocytosis, at which point, DPPC forms a lattice structure called tubular myelin in the presence of SP-A, SP-B, and Ca^{2+}. DPPC is an amphipathic molecule, and its polar head associates with the aqueous phase lining the airways and acts as a tether for the molecule.[16] The lipid portion faces the alveolar air; it is this portion of DPPC that resists film collapse at end expiration, and thus resists lung collapse. The low surface tension also ensures that the net flow of fluid is from the alveoli to the interstitium, thus counteracting pulmonary edema. As alveoli enlarge and stretch, each DPPC molecule is further from the next, thus resisting film collapse less. In this way, surfactant confers greater ability to resist collapse on smaller alveoli, which are in need of this neat trick.[15]

Surfactant also contains four other phospholipids: phosphatidylglycerol assists the surface activity of PC, but the function of the others is not known. However, in the majority of mammals, phosphatidylinnositol is the primary acidic phospholipid during the early stages of lung maturation; this changes to phosphatidylglycerol when the lung is fully mature.[15] Unfortunately, the horse does not seem to adhere to these general principles. Paradis and coworkers investigated the amniotic fluid of premature and term foals,

and found that neither DPC/sphingomyelin ratios nor the presence of phosphatidylglycerol were dependable in differentiating between preterm foals with respiratory distress syndrome (RDS), preterm foals without RDS, and term foals, unlike in the human.[16,17]

HOW DOES SURFACTANT DIFFER BETWEEN PREMATURE INDIVIDUALS AND TERM INDIVIDUALS?

First, the absolute amount of surfactant in term infants is almost 10 times that of premature infants, and the time from synthesis to secretion is slower in prematurity.[15] The surfactant is less biophysically functional in the premature individual, and is more sensitive to inactivation by inhibitors, probably because the protein level is decreased. Lung injury itself further decreases the alveolar pool of surfactant, and the surfactant's biophysical function becomes yet more diminished. This cascade of events is further compounded by dilution of surfactant with edema fluid.[18]

The clinical sequela of surfactant deficiency is neonatal respiratory distress syndrome (NRDS), formerly known as hyaline membrane disease. The acute problem with surfactant deficiency is loss of lung volume, with continuous lung collapse and re-expansion. Lung expansion is increasingly less successful, and results in marked atelectasis. The resulting ventilation perfusion inequalities lead to a high degree of pathologic development of dead space and a high level of intrapulmonary shunt.

The most important thing to note is the effect of surfactant deficiency on respiratory mechanics in the preterm lung. When the clinician conducts pressure-volume curves on preterm lungs, they do not begin to open before 25 cm H_2O. One of the biggest problems with surfactant-deficiency–associated lung injury is that there is massive heterogeneity in the lung. More collapsed units with smaller alveoli may require 40 to 50 cm H_2O of pressure to open; this may generate sufficient volume to rupture other, more compliant units. The higher critical opening pressures and higher volumes in the few alveoli that remain inflated result in considerable damage, which is known as NRDS. Hyaline membrane disease refers to the sequela of NRDS found on pathology; these membranes form consequent to the exudation of protein and fluid into the alveoli, and grossly, the lungs appear liverlike (Figures 8-7 and 8-8).[12] Surfactant allows us to avoid this sequela by decreasing surface tension, maintaining lung volumes, improving ventilation/perfusion matching, and thus oxygenation, all while decreasing the work of breathing.[5]

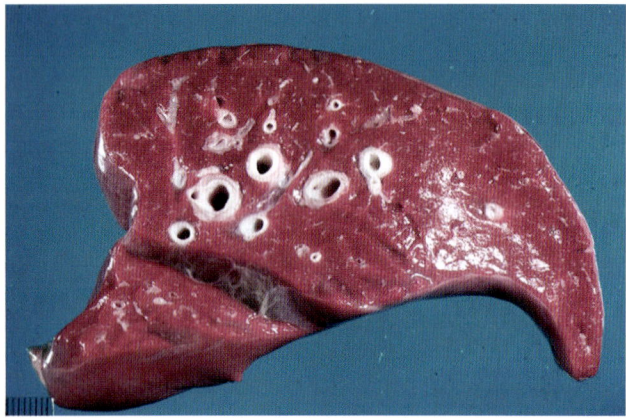

Fig. 8-7 Lungs from a foal with NRDS. Note the edema present.

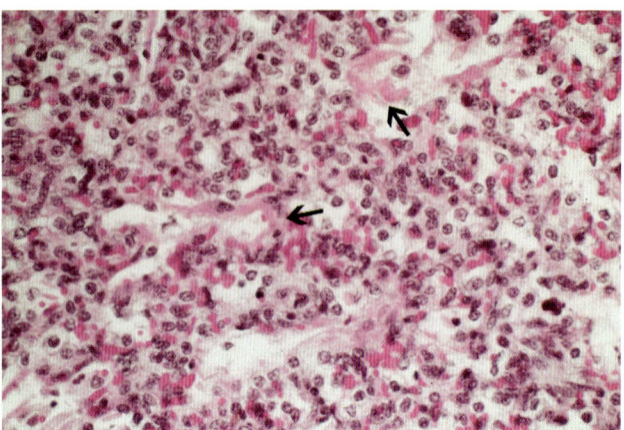

Fig. 8-8 Hyaline membranes refer to the eosinophilic membranes that line the alveoli in NRDS.

WHAT DO WE KNOW ABOUT SURFACTANT IN FOALS?

Soon after Pattle discovered the stabilizing properties of surfactant, he published an account of surfactant deficiency in a foal.[19] Barnard and colleagues were successful in showing that the lungs of the foal show considerable maturation relatively early in gestation, and that alveolar development began by 260 days, or 80% of gestation, similar to humans, wherein alveolarization begins at approximately 84% of gestation.[20,21] Type II pneumocytes, which produce surfactant, were clearly differentiated and contained osmophilic lamellar inclusions by 260 days, but nonsecretory forms were still seen at 320 days in some foals. By 320 days, alveoli were more numerous than the larger respiratory bronchiole spaces. When Barnard and colleagues looked at the elastin and collagen content of dysmature foals, they found that content of both was lower than in controls. Arvidson and coworkers demonstrated that an increase in total phospholipids occurs between days 100 and 150, and, finally, Pattle and coworkers demonstrated that surfactant begins to mature in the equine lung when approximately 88% of gestation has been completed; however, maturation is generally not complete until full term, and before full term, the activity of existing surfactant may be reduced.[22,23]

WHAT IS THE EVIDENCE FOR SURFACTANT DEFICIENCY IN PREMATURE FOALS?

In one study of naturally occurring premature foals, Rossdale found that the lungs of four of the foals showed evidence of severe atelectasis, macroscopically the lungs appeared red and liverlike in consistency, and that cut pieces sank in fixative.[24] The bubble method, which has now been superseded by more sensitive and specific methods, demonstrated reduced surfactant activity in one foal.[15] Macroscopic examination revealed widespread atelectasis, congestion in the capillaries, and desquamation of bronchiolar epithelium.[24] Dubielzig observed pulmonary lesions of neonatal foals that died at less than five days of age, and found patchy atelectasis in 35% (some of which may have been due to NRDS) and hyaline membranes in 5.4%. In another study, hyaline membranes were observed on microscopic examination.[25] Indirect evidence for surfactant deficiency in premature foals is also found in clinical studies of induced premature foals. When Rose and coworkers looked at foals induced between 270 and 320 days, the most striking clinical finding was respiratory distress and hypoxemia from the moment of birth.[26]

A second study by Rose and Hodgson examined the response of premature foals to oxygen, and found that they had a very poor response to nasal insufflation of oxygen, implying a high degree of shunt, likely intrapulmonary.[27,28] After this promising start, an extensive review of the literature reveals that the study of surfactant in the term and premature foal has been largely neglected and, although we can infer from our knowledge in other species that respiratory distress and failure in a premature foal is most likely associated with surfactant deficiency, more extensive pathologic and physiologic studies must be conducted in order to fully to understand this problem in the foal.

The initial workup on '03 Surf's Up included arterial blood gas, chemistry profile, immunoglobulin assessment, and blood cultures. The CBC revealed neutrophilic leukocytosis (15,000 WBC/μl, 13,000 segmented neutrophils/μl) and elevated fibrinogen of 600 mg/dl. The chemistry profile revealed mild azotemia (creatinine 3.2 mg/dl). Her immunoglobulins were between 400 and 800 mg/dl, reflective of the colostrum administered by the referring veterinarian. The foal was normoglycemic.

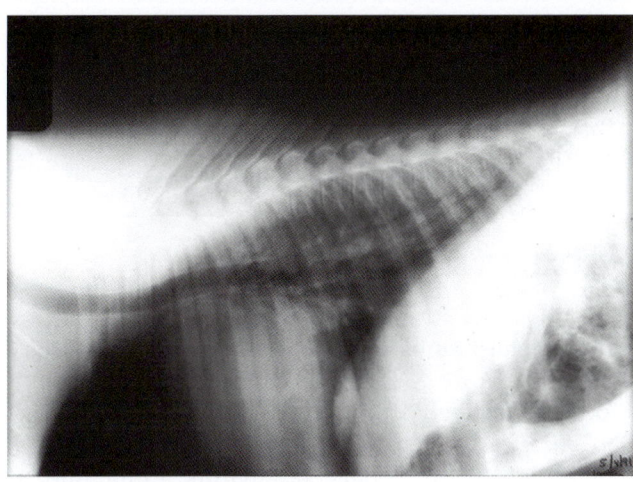

Fig. 8-9 A mild, diffuse interstitial lung pattern is seen on '03 Surf's Up's chest radiographs.

Her blood gases revealed marked hypoxemia (48 mm Hg) with mild hypocapnia (32 mg/dl) and a normal pH (7.34). Her calculated sepsis score was 14.

A calculated A-a (alveolar-arterial) gradient when breathing room air was 63.3. Immediate nasal insufflation of oxygen resulted in an arterial oxygen tension of 160 mm Hg and $PaCO_2$ of 45 mm Hg. Although it was not possible to have an exact calculation for administered fraction of O_2 with nasal insufflation, if we estimate that the FiO_2 was 35%, then the calculated A-a gradient with oxygen supplementation was 36 mm Hg.

Radiographs of the chest revealed a mild diffuse interstitial pattern (Figure 8-9). Radiographs of the carpi and tarsi revealed poorly ossified cuboidal bones. There was no growth on blood cultures.

On the second day, FRC measured under light sedation with midazolam by the helium rebreathing method was 1200 ml (lower than expected).

DIAGNOSTIC TESTS

The high neutrophil count and fibrinogen level indicate that '03 Surf's Up had been subjected to considerable inflammatory insult *in utero.* The high sepsis score supported a suspicion that the inflammation was accompanied by a possible active infection. The radiographs were suggestive of pneumonia and possible surfactant deficiency or functionally immature surfactant.[29] Both before and after oxygen, the A-a gradient was consistent with considerable V/Q mismatch, as well as mild shunt, either intra-pulmonary secondary to partial atelectasis or a focus of pneumonia, or potentially due to pulmonary hypertension with reversion to fetal circulation. The FRC was mildly reduced, consistent with moderate restrictive lung disease, such as pneumonia or patchy atelectasis. The mildly elevated

creatinine may have reflected placental pathology, prerenal disease, or intrinsic renal disease. The extent of prematurity was attested to by the poor cuboidal bone ossification. Nonetheless, '03 Surf's Up was not showing severe signs of respiratory distress. How can this be explained?

LUNG MATURITY AND INFLAMMATION

Chorioamnionitis, which correlates with pro-inflammatory cytokines IL-6, IL-1B, and TNF-alpha in amniotic fluid, is common in human preterm births, and is highly associated with decreased risk of RDS.[21] Recent studies in rabbits show that pro-inflammatory cytokines can influence lung maturation.[30] These investigators also found that IL-1 alpha increased surfactant lipids, and improved pressure-volume curves in a dose-dependent fashion. Moreover, in the lamb, the fetal lung responds to injection of endotoxin *in utero* into amniotic fluid, by increased mRNAs for SP-A, SP-B, SP-C, and SP-D within one day. In this study, SP mRNAs increased 100-fold over control values by seven days; DPPC increased in concert, linearly.[31] Similarly, LeBlanc and colleagues found elevated levels of pro-inflammatory cytokines in the amniotic fluid of mares with ascending placentitis.[32] The ability of the fetal lung to mature in response to inflammatory cytokines may explain the clinical impression of many internists that the endogenously premature foal has a better overall chance of survival than does the exogenously premature foal.

The initial workup on '03 Last Gasp was similar, but the results were quite dissimilar. The CBC revealed neutropenic leukopenia with mild lymphocytosis, with 1500 neutrophils/ml and 3,000 lymphocytes/ml. Fibrinogen was 200 mg/dl. IgG was 400 mg/dl, indicating partial failure of passive transfer. Chemistry profile revealed marked hypercreatininemia (5.2 mg/dl) and hypoglycemia (40 mg/dl). An arterial blood gas revealed PaO_2 of 37 mm Hg, $PaCO_2$ of 50 mm Hg, and pH of 7.20. The calculated A-a gradient was 53 mm Hg. Immediate nasal insufflation of oxygen resulted in an O_2 tension of 95 mm Hg and $PaCO_2$ of 75 mm Hg, resulting in a calculated A-a gradient of 65. FRC-helium measurements were stunningly low at 700 ml. Radiographs showed a marked alveolar pattern with air bronchograms throughout (Figure 8-10). A sepsis score was elevated at 18. Radiographs of the carpi and tarsi showed moderate cuboidal bone ossification.

'03 Last Gasp had marked clinical evidence of respiratory distress and severe hypoxemia to match. Although his CO_2 was only mildly elevated at presen-

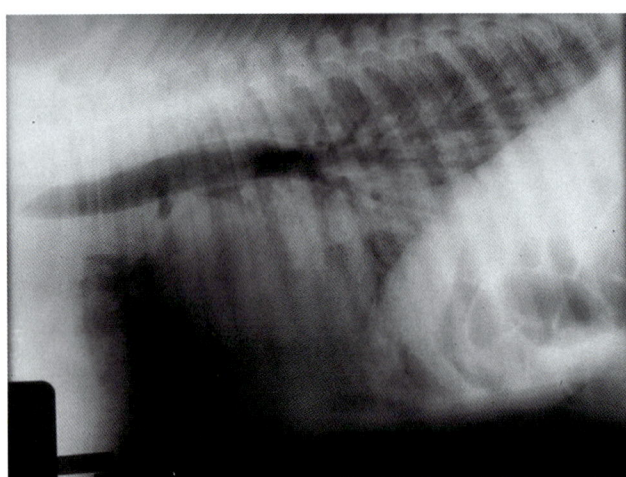

Fig. 8-10 A severe, diffuse, alveolar pattern in seen on '03 Last Gasp's chest radiographs. Note the air bronchograms.

tation, in the face of tachypnea, it ought to have been somewhat low. The elevated $PaCO_2$ after nasal insufflation of oxygen indicated that '03 Last Gasp had lost his sensitivity to elevations in CO_2 and was relying on hypoxic drive for the stimulus to breathe. When he received supplemental O_2, he decompensated this hypoxic drive. The A-a gradient was markedly elevated, compatible with considerable V-Q mismatch. The venous admixture was compatible with shunt of intrapulmonary or cardiac origin, and in this case, we suspected that there might be secondary pulmonary hypertension present. The very low FRC measurements were concerning, as it reflected serious loss of end-expiratory lung volume. Although the ossification of the cuboidal bones was compatible with a foal that was not technically premature, the severe, diffuse, alveolar pattern was strongly suggestive of primary surfactant deficiency.[29] The CBC was also compatible with prematurity; unlike '03 Surf's Up, this foal had neither neutrophilia nor elevated fibrinogen. Instead, the leukogram was suggestive of lack of adrenocortical influence in producing the more usual elevated neutrophil-to-lymphocyte ratio in the normal term foal. The neutropenia may also have been reflective of sepsis. The hypercreatininemia was compatible with intrinsic renal disease, placental pathology, or transplacental passage of elevated maternal creatinine.

Veterinarians are considerably hampered in their ability to monitor and predict prematurity in foals. Moreover, even if we have a strong clinical suspicion that the foal may be born premature, as with '03 Surf's Up, we lack good tests for determining whether the foal's respiratory system will be mature. The most commonly used method for determining respiratory maturity in humans is the lecithin (DPPC) to sphingomyelin ratio, however, it has relatively poor specificity and sensitivity.[16] Unfortunately, one of the better tests in humans, the lecithin to PG ratio, has shown conflicting results in horses.[17] Until we have more extensive research into the composition and function of surfactant in the equine neonate, it is unlikely that we will be able to progress in the prediction of lung maturity in the premature foal.

HYPOXEMIA BEYOND SURFACTANT

During fetal life, blood flow through the pulmonary circulation is low—less than 10% of cardiac output. Blood is effectively shunted away from the pulmonary bed because the fetus's hypoxic state results in constriction of the pulmonary vasculature. In the normal foal, pulmonary vascular resistance drops dramatically, and essentially all of the cardiac output flows with ease through the pulmonary bed. This situation can be altered by both primary pulmonary hypertension, (known as "black lung" PPHN, and relatively rare in human neonates) or by secondary pulmonary hypertension (known as "white lung" PPHN, and commonly seen as a complication of pulmonary vasoconstriction secondary to hypoxia in neonates).[33] The monikers black lung PPHN and white lung PPHN refer to the presence of infiltrates seen on chest radiographs in secondary PPHN, versus the typically clear radiograph seen in primary PPHN. It is important to image the lung either with radiographs or computed tomography; however, without this critical information it is impossible to determine if the PPHN is of primary origin or, as is much more common in human neonates, secondary to parenchymal disease.[34] Cardiac ultrasonography can be useful in further documenting whether there is right-to-left shunting of blood across the ductus arteriosus or foramen ovale, and to estimate right-sided vascular pressures.

Treatment for PPHN comprises primarily oxygen supplementation and frequently mechanical ventilation, in addition to treating acidosis, which may reinforce the abnormal circulatory pattern. Nitric oxide (NO), a vasodilator, has also been used successfully in infants with pulmonary hypertension, as well as in cases of suspected PPHN in foals.[34,35] Sildenafil, a common drug used for erectile dysfunction in men, is a phosphodiesterase-5 inhibitor that has also been used in foals to treat with PPHN (personal communication Dr. Pamela Wilkins).

Pulmonary hypertension probably contributed to '03 Last Gasp's hypoxia and subsequent decrease in response to oxygen therapy. Severe consolidation of the lung parenchyma on radiographs would be compatible with "white lung" or secondary pulmonary hypertension. A milder form of PPHN may also have been present in '03 Surf's Up causing initial hypoxemia, but responded to oxygen administration.

WHAT DO WE KNOW ABOUT THE PHYSIOLOGY OF PREMATURE FOALS?

The majority of our knowledge about premature foals is derived from the work by Rossdale and coworkers, who developed a model of prematurity in the horse. Surfactant development is dependent upon appropriate adrenocortical activity.[15] Rossdale's group found that in normal term foals, there was a marked increase in plasma cortisol in the two hours after delivery, whereas the levels were low and unchanging in the premature animals, suggesting that significant maturation may take place in even the postnatal period.[36] This inadequate corticosteroid response also compounds the prematurity of the hematological system; induced premature foals had much lower neutrophil counts, with neutrophil/lymphocyte ratios of 1:3, vs the normal ratio of >2.5.

Premature induced foals have significantly lower plasma glucose concentrations at birth than full-term foals, and there is delayed insulin response to glucose infusion in premature foals.[37] This likely compounds the weakness and hypoventilation that is seen in respiratory distress in premature foals. Finally, premature foals may be septic, complicating the difficulties of the physiology of prematurity.[6]

Both of the above foals were at high risk for sepsis and had high sepsis scores. FPT and the possibility of infection *in utero* for '03 Surf's Up make this a real probability. However, it should be remembered that the use of the sepsis score in the premature foal may not be a reliable indicator of sepsis. Many of the parameters such as neutropenia, hypoxemia, hypothermia, hypoglycemia, and gestational age that receive high values in a septic foal also receive high scores in the premature foal, but for different reasons.

'03 Surf's Up appeared to respond well to nasal insufflation of oxygen. As our goal was only to keep her PaO_2 in the 70 to 100 mm Hg range, we reduced the insufflated oxygen to 5 liters/minute. She was treated with 1 liter hyperimmune equine plasma to redress her immunoglobulin deficiency. We also began treatment with polyionic intravenous fluids at a rate of 66 ml/kg/day. As the foal was quite active, she kept herself in sternal position the majority of the time. As her sepsis score was high, she was further treated with broad-spectrum antibiotics (potassium penicillin and amikacin) until her CBC and fibrinogen were within normal limits. As her suckle was still somewhat weak, she was fed via an indwelling nasoesophageal tube. Because her cuboidal bones were strikingly immature, casts were placed on all four limbs to stabilize the bones as soon as she was able to walk.

By day three, '03 Surf's Up's chest radiographs no longer showed a diffuse interstitial pattern. On day four, helium FRC measurements revealed a marked increase, at 1600 ml (40 ml/kg). On day six, '03 Surf's Up's CBC had markedly improved (WBC = 10,000/μl, PMNs = 6500/μl, fibrinogen = 400 mg/dl), and her breathing effort appeared much less labored. We challenged '03 Surf's Up by removing nasal oxygen insufflation, and after two hours, found that PaO_2 remained at 70 mm Hg, with $PaCO_2$ at 40 mm Hg, a very favorable response. '03 Surf's Up still had a long road to travel until her legs became fully competent and she would be ready to live as a "real horse," but her respiratory system appeared well on the way to maturity.

After initial treatment with nasal insufflation, '03 Last Gasp was given 2 liters of hyperimmune plasma over a 24-hour period, and polyionic intravenous fluids with 5% dextrose, again at a rate of 66 ml/kg/day, were initiated. Central venous pressures remained within normal limits, and urine output was adequate. '03 Last Gasp also had a suspicious sepsis score, and treatment with broad-spectrum antibiotics was initiated, avoiding amikacin as we did not yet know the cause of the high creatinine.

Unfortunately, as treatment progressed, '03 Last Gasp's work of breathing was subjectively very high, and his response to nasal insufflation of oxygen was poor, so we decided to place him on mechanical ventilation. Mechanical ventilation was started with a tidal volume of 6 ml/kg (300 ml), and a rate of 20 breaths per minute using synchronized intermittent mandatory ventilation (SIMV), for a minimum minute ventilation of 6 liters/minute, and 5-cm H_2O positive end expiratory pressure (PEEP). Plateau pressures remained below 25 cm H_2O. Oxygen levels were set at 60%. The foal appeared to resist ventilation, and arterial blood gas analysis after one hour showed a worsening of hypoxemia and hypercapnia. Simultaneous measurement of end-tidal CO_2 (EtCO) and $PaCO_2$ showed a marked discrepancy, with $EtCO_2$ at 28 mm Hg, and $PaCO_2$ at 75 mm Hg. As the foal fought ventilation even in SIMV mode, we began a constant rate infusion of low-dose midazolam.

This resulted in mild sedation, and we were able to measure FRC-helium and construct a pressure volume curve using the ventilator to change tidal volume and measure plateau pressures. This revealed a strikingly low FRC (700 ml for a large foal), and an elevated lower inflection point of the PV curve. Based on these findings, we decided to titrate our PEEP levels in an effort to keep more of the lung open. We gradually increased PEEP until the compliance of the lung (tidal volume/plateau pressure) was optimal: this resulted in a PEEP of 12 cm H_2O. These changes resulted in an improvement in blood gases: $PaO_2 = 350$, $PaCO_2 = 50$, pH = 7.24, but with a calculated A-a gradient of 300 mm Hg!

TREATMENT

Foals such as '03 Surf's Up, with a history of maternal stress and premature birth, often will require pulmonary care in the form of intranasal oxygen. Other supportive care includes that which is necessary for any weak, possibly septic foal, such as intravenous plasma and crystalloid fluids, antibiotics, and nutrition. If PaO_2 levels do not respond to intranasal oxygen, then a diagnosis of pulmonary hypertension should be entertained. The administration of inhaled nitric oxygen has been used successfully in cases of unresponsive hypoxemia in foals.

In the case of '03 Last Gasp, not only was the response to intranasal oxygen poor, the foal's $PaCO_2$ increased significantly. Mechanical ventilation was needed to decrease $PaCO_2$ levels. An FRC of 700 ml indicates considerable loss of end-expiratory lung volume, consistent with atelectasis and pulmonary edema. The shunt fraction was high enough to be pathologic, and was compatible with intrapulmonary shunting, due to both atelectasis and pulmonary edema, as well as potential pulmonary hypertension. When the foal's respiratory parameters worsened despite mechanical ventilation, we theorized that either the foal's respiratory system was increasingly impaired or our ventilation strategy was inappropriate. In this case, it is important to assess the foal visually and to assess the ventilator data critically. Subjectively, the foal was fighting the ventilator, so mild sedation was appropriate.

We used a lower fluid rate than we might in a term foal (80 to 100 ml/kg/day) despite our desire to diurese the foal in an effort to address hypercreatininemia (as we had a tentative diagnosis of NRDS) and concern not to flood the lungs by overzealous fluid administration. The approach to fluid management in RDS has changed significantly in the past several years. The goal is to avoid worsening of pulmonary edema, and thus to have a reasonable reduction in right ventricular preload without decreasing cardiac output.[5] However, it is critical to realize that this does not mean that pulmonary edema is avoided at the cost of decreased perfusion. Thus, it is important to continuously monitor urine output, skin turgor, PCV/total solids, mean arterial pressures, and central venous pressures, as well as mental status.

WHAT WAS THE SIGNIFICANCE OF THE DECREASED ETCO₂?

CO_2 is produced and stored in the body, and must be transported by the cardiovascular system to the lungs where it is exhaled. It thus reflects metabolism, circulation, and ventilation. If there is little VQ mismatch, then $EtCO_2$ should be only slightly less than the $PaCO_2$. As VQ mismatch worsens, for instance, due to atelectasis, pneumonia, or pulmonary embolism, $EtCO_2$ will be markedly less than $PaCO_2$. Hypoventilation (either iatrogenically from inadequate alveolar ventilation during mechanical ventilation, or secondary to atelectasis) will also increase the $PaCO_2$-$EtCO_2$ gap.[38] With this evidence in hand, as well as hypoxemia, we knew that we needed to change the ventilator settings. The most likely cause of the VQ mismatch and hypoventilation was excessively low end-expiratory lung volumes due to loss of FRC, which is why we chose to increase PEEP. By increasing the PEEP, we were able to help restore the FRC, thus keeping a larger portion of the lung open for ventilation and avoiding further atelectrauma.

HOW DO MECHANICAL VENTILATION, SURFACTANT, AND THE DAMAGED LUNG INTERACT?

The pathology of acute lung injury is alveolar edema, decreased FRC and total lung capacity (TLC), and decreased compliance.[18] The goal of treatment, therefore, is to reverse alveolar edema, increase FRC and TLC, and increase compliance. To a large extent, physicians can hope to do all of the above with surfactant. Without surfactant, we are hugely handicapped in the case of primary surfactant deficiency. However, surfactant cannot necessarily cure a damaged lung; this is where mechanical ventilation must play a role. Mechanical ventilation must prevent collapse in a lung that is already damaged and may not be able to show an optimal response to surfactant. The irreversible damage that can be induced by suboptimal ventilator strategies was shown by a study that observed the response of the preterm lung to ventilation with 14 ml/kg tidal volume to yield $PaCO_2$ values of 25 to 30 mm Hg for one hour; thereafter, the lung was unable to respond to surfactant despite optimal mechanical ventilation.[39] Numerous animal studies have shown that it is volume, not pressure *per se* that causes lung injury. If the chest wall is constrained such that high pressures cannot produce a high tidal volume, then lung injury does not ensue.[40] Each breath is a critical moment for the premature neonate. Both atelectasis due to lung collapse, and stretch injury from volutrauma, can begin the preterm neonate on the road to NRDS.

High tidal volumes can produce damaged pulmonary capillaries even in normal animals being mechanically ventilated, resulting in fluid and blood leaking into the alveolar space. This, in turn, disrupts surfactant, creating the beginning of a vicious circle. The high transcapillary pressures that ensue lead to ever-increasing pulmonary edema and exudates.[40] If we add to this the inflammatory cytokines called forth by volutrauma, and the possible distal organ effects as the lung blood volume travels throughout the body, it seems impossible that any surfactant-deficient neonate could survive.

Optimal use of PEEP certainly has been shown to minimize lung collapse and improve oxygenation. When choosing tidal volumes for ventilation, it is important to remember the *effective* lung volume in an RDS lung. If we consider that one third of the lung with RDS may be completely atelectatic, one third may be recruitable, and one third may be functioning with some semblance of normalcy, it is clear that the lung is effectively only one third its normal size for initial ventilation. It is easy to see that if we try to push a calculated volume of 10 ml/kg into that lung, we will create volutrauma in the one third of the lung that is capable of accepting any volume. Thus, if mechanical ventilation appears necessary, it is best to go forward in the spirit of the ARDSNet trial, using a small tidal volume of 6 ml/kg, and accepting the consequence that hypercapnia and what we ordinarily might consider hypoxemia may occur.[41]

Currently, in human medicine, there has been an upsurge of interest in continuous positive airway pressure (CPAP) in the delivery room, as well as for more chronic therapy, in order to avoid intubation and ventilation. Of great interest to the veterinary world, wherein surfactant is often unavailable due to exorbitant cost, is the finding that use of CPAP greatly reduces the need for surfactant in infants that would otherwise have been so treated. In infants with birth weight <1200 g, only 10% of those treated with CPAP at birth needed surfactant, whereas 45% needed surfactant when they were intubated and ventilated.[42]

Other studies have shown that ventilator strategies associated with the loss of FRC and increased lung injury decreased the efficacy of surfactant therapy. When CPAP is combined with surfactant, studies have shown that surfactant as a rescue treatment needs to be administered only once in the majority of patients, as opposed to the multiple treatments that are often needed with mechanical ventilation.[43]

Interestingly, noninvasive mechanical ventilation has been studied in foals, using a mask and assist-control mode; this could easily be adapted to CPAP.[44] The authors found that $PaCO_2$ was significantly higher using this mode of ventilation vs endotracheal intubation; however, the increased level (62.0 + 6.5 vs 46.0 + 6.1) is certainly within the bounds of what is currently considered acceptable in human medicine.[45] Koterba and colleagues reported on a single case of a premature foal with respiratory distress treated with CPAP using a double-pronged nasopharyngeal tube. Although the procedure resulted in rapid improvement in blood gases and respiratory effort, it also resulted in accumulation of abdominal gas and resultant colic; the authors suggested that an indwelling nasogastric tube might be necessary to effectively apply CPAP.[46]

WHY DIDN'T WE TREAT '03 LAST GASP WITH SURFACTANT?

Unfortunately, we neither stocked surfactant nor were the owners able to afford it if we obtained it from a local human hospital. Would it have helped to use surfactant? With the current state of knowledge regarding prematurity and the respiratory system in the foal, it is impossible to state with certainty. If we use results from humans and all other animals that have been studied, it is most reasonable to assume that foals born prematurely are deficient in surfactant.[15] Does surfactant work in premature foals? There are no data available to make a scientific conclusion. An informal poll of board-certified veterinary internal medicine diplomats working in neonatal intensive care units suggests that surfactant is used infrequently, and when used, it is often used late, in inadequate doses, and at insufficient frequency due to high cost. There is considerable evidence in humans and other animals to show that when surfactant is used as an immediate prophylaxis rather than as a "rescue therapy," there is significantly improved lung volumes, improved oxygenation, and less lung injury.[47,48] Moreover, surfactant must often be used every 12 to 24 hours for one to three days, again, becoming prohibitively expensive in the neonatal foal.[43]

WHAT ARE THE OPTIONS FOR SURFACTANT TREATMENT?

There are multiple types of exogenous surfactants; however, natural surfactants, which contain most of the phospholipids and surfactant proteins, have been shown to be the best in treatment of surfactant deficiency.[49] Multiple studies have shown that surfactant is most effective when it is given prophylactically, within 30 minutes of birth, rather than as a rescue treatment. Even so, it may be necessary for the neonate to receive multiple doses (up to four to six) in a 48-hour period.[49] Information concerning the efficacy of surfactant therapy in neonatal foals is entirely anecdotal. It has been suggested that clear long-term benefits have not been seen when surfactant replacement therapy was used in high-risk large animal neonates such as calves.[3] This is clearly an area that requires much work.

The outcome for '03 Last Gasp was not as happy as for '03 Surf's Up. Despite initial improvement on the ventilator, on day two, the foal's blood gases deteriorated further. Radiographs of the lungs were retaken, and the severe, alveolar pattern had worsened. Measurements of FRC indicated further decreases, likely due to worsening of atelectasis and pulmonary flooding. The owner did not wish to pursue further treatment. On autopsy, the lungs were red, rubbery, and did not float in fixative. Histopathology of the lung showed classic hyaline membrane formation.

INDUCTION OF PARTURITION

In general, one would prefer not to induce parturition in the horse. Gayle and coworkers found that foals with a history of induced parturition were significantly less likely to live.[50] Rossdale and coworkers convincingly showed that induced parturition was associated with significantly reduced survival, and that fetuses induced at less than 320 days did not survive.[26] However, in certain situations, such as with '03 Last Gasp, it is necessary on an emergent basis. If there is a situation in which continuing the pregnancy puts the mare at risk, yet there is still a desire to save the foal, it is very important to know when the foal has the best chance of surviving in the extrauterine environment.

The timing of the "readiness for birth" of the equine fetus is very hard to gauge. In most other species, there is an increase in fetal adrenocortical activity for several weeks before birth, whereas in the equine, there is minimal adrenocortical activity until 24 to 48 hours before birth.[51] Also, it appears that very important final maturation occurs during these few days. Purvis indicated that a minimum gestational length of 330 days was necessary, but this is heavily dependent upon the individual mare and the day length.[52] In addition, there should be mammary development and secretions, with calcium levels rising before birth (>10 mmol/liter), along with an inversion of the sodium/potassium ratio.[53] This may be less reliable in maiden mares.[54] Calcium increases prematurely, as well, in mares with placental pathology; 16 out of 17 foals in one study with prematurely elevated mammary secretion calcium had placental pathology, and 63% of these foals either died shortly after birth or were delivered stillborn.[55] Thus, in the very animals one is monitoring, the results may need to be viewed with caution. What method is optimal? Pashen gave low-dose oxytocin (2.5 to 10 IU IV) and concluded that it was ineffective unless the foal was in its final maturation stage.[56] Although there is clear evidence that corticosteroid treatment in the 48 hours before parturition in humans helps to mature the lung, there is no evidence to support this in horses.[57] Recent work by Ousey and colleagues showing that repeated treatment with exogenous ACTH causes sustained plasma cortisol levels in the mare, as well as elevating plasma progestagen and premature delivery of viable foals, suggests that this may be optimal prior to induction of parturition.[36]

OUTCOME

There are few case reports and no case studies concerning the clinical course and outcome in premature foals. The most complete evidence as to the outcome of premature foals comes from the almost 60 foals, gestational age 292 to 319 days, induced by Rossdale and colleagues in 1970.[24] Rossdale suggested that there were two different groups of premature foals, regardless of gestational age—one that is vigorous and goes on to mature normally, and another that makes no progress or makes progress for a short time, then deteriorates in terms of the respiratory, metabolic, and neurologic systems.[24] This further supports the idea that gestational age is not linearly associated with lung maturity. Nonetheless, Rossdale also observed that no foals survived that were induced before 320 days of gestation. Individual case reports are few, but suggest that surviving premature foals require expensive, intensive care.[46,58,59,60] Evidence of prematurity certainly features in accounts of pulmonary lesions in foals, survival in neonates in intensive care, and prognostic variables for survival of foals with radiographic evidence of pulmonary disease; however, no information beyond that provided by Rossdale's group is available.[28,29,61] It must be kept in mind, of course, that Rossdale and coworkers did not afford any sort of intensive care to the premature foals in their studies, and the improved critical care and ventilatory strategies available in the intervening years likely improve the outlook for these foals.[62] Certainly, the evidence discussed above from human infants suggests that a gentler mode of mechanical ventilation may well allow us to effectively help foals that died even a few years ago. What would happen if we had adequate quality and amount of surfactant with which to treat these foals, especially if we used surfactant as a prophylactic rather than as a rescue treatment? Surfactant made a stunning difference in the treatment of premature infants—the mortality rate was reduced by at least 50%.[63] There is also a different mandate in treating human infants, wherein every life has worth. Of some real concern, however, to an equine practitioner interested in promoting the survival of athletically functional animals, is the finding that preterm baboons ventilated for seven days with 100% oxygen have fewer and larger alveoli when evaluated as young adults, and that surfactant-treated preterm lambs that are chronically ventilated with just sufficient pressure to maintain normal gas exchange (using supplemental O_2 less than 50%) have an arrest in vascular and alve-olar development.[64,65] Thus, it is possible that short-term success in these foals might be obviated by long-term problems. It will require much study before we are able to make any definitive statement of long-term success in premature foals.

REFERENCES

1. Hintz HF, Hintz RL, Lein DH et al: Length of gestation periods in Thoroughbred mares, *J Equine Med Surg* 3:289, 1979.
2. Rossdale PD, Ousey JC, Silver M et al: Studies on equine prematurity 6: Guidelines for assessment of foal maturity, *Equine Vet J* 16:300, 1984.
3. Costa L, Eades S, Goad M et al: Pulmonary surfactant dysfunction and lung maturation in neonatal foals: Therapy, prevention, and prognosis, *Compend Cont Ed* 467, 2004.
4. Hardy J, Latimer F: Orthopedic disorders in the neonatal foal, *Clin Tech Equine Pract* 2:96, 2003.
5. Murray N: *Textbook of respiratory medicine,* Philadelphia, 2000, WB Saunders.
6. Koterba AM, Brewer BD, Tarplee FA: Clinical and clinicopathological characteristics of the septicaemic neonatal foal: Review of 38 cases, *Equine Vet J* 16:376, 1984.
7. Lumb AB: *Nunn's applied respiratory physiology,* Oxford, Butterworth Heinemann, 2000.
8. Koterba AM, Kosch PC: Respiratory mechanics and breathing pattern in the neonatal foal, *J Reprod Fertil* (Suppl)35:575, 1987.
9. Koterba AM, Wozniak JA, Kosch PC: Respiratory mechanics of the horse during the first year of life, *Respir Physiol* 95:21, 1994.
10. Ganong W: Medical Physiology, ed 17, Norwalk, Conn., 1995, Appleton and Lange.
11. Pattle RE: Properties, function and origin of the alveolar lining layer, *Nature* 175:1125, 1955.
12. Avery ME, Mead J: Surface properties in relation to atelectasis and hyaline membrane disease, *Am J Dis Child* 97:517, 1959.
13. Poynter S, LeVine A: Surfactant biology and clinical application, *Crit Care Clin* 19:3, 2003.
14. Krauss AN: New methods advance treatment for respiratory distress syndrome, *Pediatr Ann* 32:585, 2003.
15. Jobe AH, Ikegami M: Biology of surfactant, *Clin Perinatol* 28:655, 2001.
16. Torday J, Rehan V: Testing for fetal lung maturation: A biochemical "window" to the developing fetus, *Clin Lab Med* 23:361, 2003.
17. Paradis M: Lecithin sphingomyelin ratios and phosphatidyl glycerol in term and premature equine amniotic fluid, 5th Ann Vet Internal Med Forum, Washington, 789, 1987.
18. Jobe AH, Ikegami M: Update on mechanical ventilation and exogenous surfactant, *Clin Perinatol* 28:3, 2001.
19. Rossdale PD, Pattle RE, Mahaffey LW: Respiratory distress in a newborn foal with failure to form lung lining film, *Nature* 215:1498, 1967.
20. Barnard K, Leadon DP, Silver M: Some aspects of tissue maturation in fetal and perinatal foals, *J Reprod Fert* (Suppl)32:589, 1982.
21. Jobe AH, Ikegami M: Antenatal infection/inflammation and postnatal lung maturation and injury, *Respir Res* 2:27, 2001.
22. Arvidson G, Astedt B, Ekelund L et al: Surfactant studies in the fetal and neonatal foal, *J Reprod Fert* (Suppl)23:663, 1975.
23. Pattle RE, Rossdale PD, Schock C et al: The development of the lung and its surfactant in the foal and in other species, *J Reprod Fert* (Suppl)2:651, 1975.
24. Rossdale PD: Some parameters of respiratory function in normal and abnormal newborn foals with special reference to levels of PaO_2 during air and oxygen inhalation, *Res Vet Sci* 2:270, 1970.
25. Mahaffey L, Rossdale P: *Vet Rec* 69:1277, 1957.
26. Rose J, Rossdale PD, Leadon DP: Blood gas and acid-base status in spontaneously delivered, term-induced, and induced premature foals, *J Reprod Fert* (Suppl)32:521, 1982.
27. Rose J, Hodgson D: Effect of intranasal oxygen administration on arterial blood gas and acid base parameters in spontaneously delivered, term induced, and induced premature foals, *Res Vet Sci* 34:159, 1983.
28. Dubielzig: Pulmonary lesions of neonatal foals, *J Equine Med Surg* 1:419, 1977.
29. Bedenice D, Heuwieser W, Solano M et al: Risk factors and prognostic variables for survival of foals with radiographic evidence of pulmonary disease, *J Vet Intern Med* 17:868, 2003.
30. Bry K, Lappalainen U, Hallman M: Intraamniotic interleukin-1 accelerates surfactant protein synthesis in fetal rabbits and improves lung stability after premature birth, *J Clin Invest* 99:2992, 1997.
31. Jobe AH, Newnham J, Willet K et al: Intra-amniotic IL-1 alpha treatment alters postnatal adaptation in premature lambs, *Biol Neonate* 72:370, 1997.
32. LeBlanc M, Giguere S, Brauer K: Premature delivery in ascending placentitis is associated with increased expression of placental cytokines and allantoic fluid prostaglandins E2 and F2alpha, *Theriogenology* 58:841, 2002.
33. Newman B: Imaging of medical disease of the newborn lung, *Radiol Clin North Am* 37:1049, 1999.
34. Abman SH: New developments in the pathogenesis and treatment of neonatal pulmonary hypertension, *Pediatr Pulmonol* (Suppl)18:201, 1999.
35. Wilkins P: Persistent pulmonary hypertension of the neonate, Proc 22nd ACVIM, Minneapolis, MN 178, 2004.
36. Ousey JC, Rossdale PD, Palmer L et al: Effects of maternally administered depot ACTH(1-24) on fetal maturation and the timing of parturition in the mare, *Equine Vet J* 32:489, 2000.
37. Fowden AL, Silver M, Ellis L et al: Studies on equine prematurity 3: Insulin secretion in the foal during the perinatal period, *Equine Vet J* 16:286, 1984.
38. Bhende M: End-tidal carbon dioxide monitoring in pediatrics: Concepts and technology, *J Postgrad Med* 47:153, 2001.
39. Ikegami M, Kallapur S, Michna J et al: Lung injury and surfactant metabolism after hyperventilation of premature lambs, *Pediatr Res* 47:398, 2000.
40. Auten RL, Vozzelli M, Clark RH: What is it, and how do we avoid it? *Clin Perinatol* 28:505, 2001.
41. Slutsky AS, Ranieri VM: Mechanical ventilation: Lessons from the ARDSNet trial, *Respir Res* 1:73, 2000.
42. Van Marter L, Allred E, Pagano M: Do clinical markers of barotrauma and oxygen toxicity explain interhosptial variation in rates of chronic lung disease? *Pediatrics* 105:1194, 2000.
43. Verder H, Albertsen P, Ebbesen F et al: Nasal continuous positive airway pressure and early surfactant therapy for respiratory distress syndrome in newborns of less than 30 weeks' gestation, *Pediatrics* 103:E24, 1999.
44. Hoffman AM, Kupcinskas RL, Paradis MR: Comparison of alveolar ventilation, oxygenation, pressure support, and respiratory system resistance in response to noninvasive versus conventional mechanical ventilation in foals, *Am J Vet Res* 58:1463, 1997.

45. Upadhyay A, Deorari A: Continuous positive airway pressure—a gentler approach to ventilation, *Indian Pediatrics* 41:459, 2004.

46. Koterba AM, Haibel G, Grimmet J: Respiratory distress in a premature foal secondary to hydrops allantois and placentitis, *Compend Cont Ed* 5:S121, 1983.

47. Kendig W, Otter R, Cox C: A comparison of surfactant as immediate prophylaxis and as rescue therapy in newborns of less than 30 weeks' gestation, *NEJM* 324:865, 1991.

48. Morley C: Systematic review of prophylactic v. rescue surfactant, *Arch Dis Child* 77:70, 1997.

49. Suresh GK, Soll RF: Exogenous surfactant therapy in newborn infants, *Ann Acad Med Singapore* 32:335, 2003.

50. Gayle JM, Cohen ND, Chaffin MK: Factors associated with survival in septicemic foals: 65 cases (1988-1995), *J Vet Intern Med* 12:140, 1998.

51. Silver M, Fowden A: Prepartum adrenocortical maturation in the fetal foal: 48 hours before birth, *J Endocrinol* 142:417, 1994.

52. Purvis A: Elective induction of labor and parturition in the mare, Proc 18th Annual Conv Am Assoc Eq Pract 113, 1972.

53. Ousey JC, Dudan F, Rossdale PD: Preliminary studies of mammary secretions in the mare to assess foetal readiness for birth, *Equine Vet J* 16:259, 1984.

54. Macpherson ML, Chaffin MK, Carroll GL et al: Three methods of oxytocin-induced parturition and their effects of foals, *J Am Vet Med Assoc* 210:799, 1997.

55. Rossdale PD, Ousey J, Cottrill C: Effects of placental pathology on maternal plasma progestagen and mammary secretion calcium concentration, and on neonatal adrenocortical function in the horse, *J Reprod Fert* (Suppl) 44:579, 1991.

56. Pashen R: Low doses of oxytocin can induce foaling at term, *Equine Vet J* 12:85, 1980.

57. Bolt RJ, van Weissenbruch MM, Lafeber HN et al: Glucocorticoids and lung development in the fetus and preterm infant, *Pediatr Pulmonol* 3276, 2001.

58. Mazan M, Paradis MR: Bypassing the oral cavity: The use of tube esophagostomy for long-term enteral nutrition in a foal, *Vet Emerg Crit Care* 10:7, 2000.

59. Lloyd K, Kelly A, Dunlop C: Treatment of respiratory distress in a prematurely born foal, *J Am Vet Med Assoc* 193:560, 1988.

60. Bain FT, Brock KA, Koterba AM: High-frequency jet ventilation in a neonatal foal, *J Am Vet Med Assoc* 192:920, 1988.

61. Hoffman AM, Staempfli H, Willan A: Prognostic variables for survival of neonatal foals under intensive care, *J Vet Intern Med* 6:89, 1992.

62. Rose R, Rossdale PD, Leadon DP: Blood gas and acid-base status in spontaneously delivered, term-induced and induced premature foals, *J Reprod Fert* (Suppl)32:521, 1982.

63. Halliday HL: Surfactant replacement therapy, *Pediatr Pulmonol* (Suppl)11:96, 1995.

64. Coalson JJ, Winter V, deLemos RA: Decreased alveolarization in baboon survivors with bronchopulmonary dysplasia, *Am J Respir Crit Care Med* 152:640, 1995.

65. Albertine KH, Jones GP, Starcher BC et al: Chronic lung injury in preterm lambs. Disordered respiratory tract development, *Am J Respir Crit Care Med* 159:945, 1999.

Case 8-3	**Aspiration Pneumonia Secondary to Dysphagia**	**Mary Rose Paradis**

'05 HardToSwallow, Thoroughbred filly, was normal at birth with the exception of somewhat upright front pasterns. She stood and nursed within three hours of birth and was seen to urinate and pass meconium within the first 12 hours of life. The mare had lost her previous foal to **Rhodococcus equi** *at one month of age. In an attempt to prevent this from happening again, the referring veterinarian transfused the foal with hyper-immune R. equi plasma at two days of age. Because of her upright pasterns, the foal was also treated with high levels of oxytetracycline to see if they would come down into a normal conformation. At three days of age, the owner reported that the foal appeared to have milk coming from her nose after nursing. The foal appeared somewhat depressed and her breathing was somewhat labored. Because of the history of respiratory problems in the previous foal, the owner was very worried about this foal and decided to ship the foal to a referral hospital.*

On presentation, the foal was bright and alert (Figure 8-11). Her temperature was 101° F, and her heart rate was 90 beats/minute. Her respiratory rate was rapid at 60 breaths per minute, and her respiratory effort was

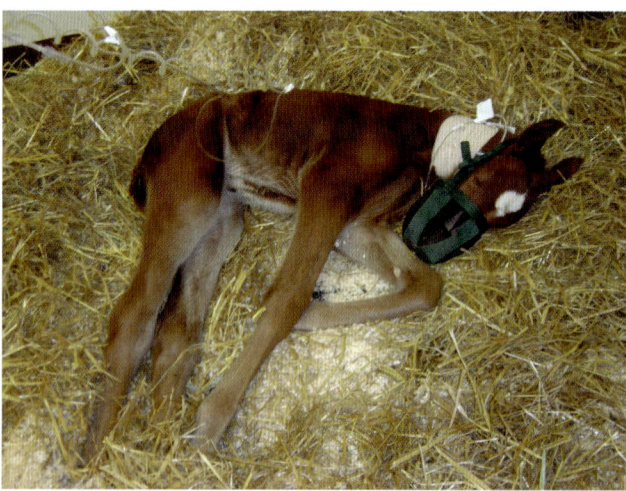

Fig. 8-11 '05 HardToSwallow, a three-day-old Thoroughbred filly, presenting with aspiration pneumonia. The foal was muzzled to prevent nursing.

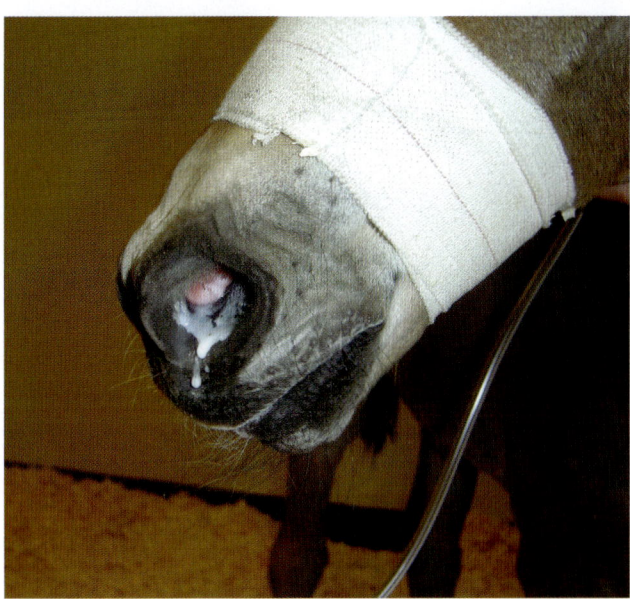

Fig. 8-12 Dysphagia in the foal is clinically manifest as milk regurgitation from the nares soon after nursing.

increased with noticeable rib excursion and slight nostril flare. Wheezes were heard on auscultation of her right lung field. Following nursing, milk was observed coming from both her mouth and nostrils (Figure 8-12).

Aspiration of foreign material is another cause of noninfectious pneumonia in the neonatal foal. Meconium is the most common material aspirated by the foal *prenatally*. Meconium is the first feces produced by the foal. It may be released prepartum into the amniotic fluid in times of fetal distress such as in dystocia. The normal foal's lungs are bathed in amniotic fluid before birth. If meconium is released into the fetal fluid, then the foal, as it gasps, will inhale the particles of meconium into the lung. Meconium is a sterile substance, but the large particles will cause airway obstruction, regional lung atelectasis, and chemical pneumonitis in the foal.[1,2] Signs of respiratory impairment occur soon after birth.

Milk is the most common material aspirated *postnatally* in the newborn foal. The most common causes of milk aspiration in the foal are related to dysphagia, which manifests itself externally as milk regurgitation from the foal's nares after nursing. **Milk regurgitation should not be ignored.** Milk in the nostril must be differentiated from external splashing of milk on the foal's nose as a result of the streaming of milk from the mare and true regurgitation. Regurgitation represents a disruption in the foal's ability to transport milk from the oral cavity to the esophagus and ultimately to the stomach. When milk regurgitation from the nares occurs right after nursing, it is usually secondary to dysphagia. In some cases, milk reflux from the nares can

occur due to esophageal dysfunction. In these foals, the appearance of the milk at the nares is usually not right after nursing but occurs when the foal lowers its head.

In the normal foal, nursing begins by the foal wrapping its tongue around the mare's teat, compressing it against the hard palate and creating a negative pressure to draw milk into the oral cavity. The milk bolus is then transported through the oropharynx to the nasopharynx, and from the nasopharynx to the esophagus by a series of highly coordinated events.[3] Any disruption of these events can result in dysphagia. Milk regurgitation usually results from a failure of the soft palate to form a seal with the dorsal pharyngeal wall.

Dysphagia in the foal is clinically noted as reflux of milk from the nose and results in aspiration of milk into the lungs. The degree of milk regurgitation and aspiration determine the affect on the foal. Foals with mild dysphagia can be normal in appearance. If large amounts of milk are aspirated, then the pneumonia becomes severe. As aspiration pneumonia develops, wheezes and crackles may be heard on auscultation of the lungs. As the pneumonia progresses, these abnormal sounds may fade as the lung become fully consolidated. A rattle in the trachea from the aspirated milk can often be felt after the foal suckles. If obstruction of the upper airways occurs as part of the dysphagia, stridor, increased upper respiratory noise, and increased inspiratory effort may be prominent clinical signs (Table 8-1). Though non-infectious in origin,

Table 8.1	Causes of Upper Airway Dysfunction in Foals Categorized by Presenting Sign of Stridor
Stridor	**No Stridor**
Subepiglottic cyst	Dorsal displacement of the soft palate (simple)
Dorsal pharyngeal cyst	Pharyngeal weakness secondary to perinatal asphyxia, sepsis, prematurity, nutritional myodegeneration (white muscle disease)
Bilateral laryngeal paralysis	Cleft palate
Arytenoiditis	Esophageal dysfunction—megaesophagus, congenital anomalies
Pharyngeal collapse complicated with dorsal displacement of the soft palate and rostral displacement of the palatopharyngeal arch	

aspirated milk is not sterile and will develop into a bacterial pneumonia.

DIFFERENTIAL DIAGNOSIS FOR DYSPHAGIA

The differential diagnoses for dysphagia in the foal are many and can include the following: cleft palate, subepiglottal and pharyngeal cysts, bilateral laryngeal paralysis, arytenoid chondritis, dorsal displacement of the soft palate, rostral displacement of the palatopharyngeal arch, and megaesophagus (see Table 8-1).

Gross anatomic impairments to nursing or swallowing may include a cleft palate (either hard or soft) and the presence of subepiglottic or dorsal pharyngeal cysts. Unlike humans, where orofacial clefts, congenital fissures in the median line of the palate, are a common birth defect, cleft palate in the foal is very rare.[4-6] The heritability of the cleft palate in the horse is unknown.[7] Defects in the palate prevent the development of negative pressure in the oral cavity during nursing and allows milk to immediately flow from the mouth to the nasal passage or the pharynx. The milk regurgitation is noted during the first nursing bout.[3]

Subepiglottic and dorsal pharyngeal cysts may also interfere with the swallowing mechanism in the foal and cause upper airway obstruction. Though these cysts are thought to originate from the thyroglossal and craniopharyngeal ducts, respectively, reports of subepiglottic cysts have been in older foals and were histologically found to be inflammatory.[8,9] Large cysts may lead to obstruction of the larynx, resulting in severe respiratory stridor and respiratory distress.

Bilateral laryngeal paralysis and arytenoid chondritis have also been recognized in the newborn foal.[3] Clinically, these foals presented with stridor, respiratory distress, and aspiration pneumonia. Laryngeal paralysis has been associated with cerebral diseases such as congenital hydrocephalus (Figure 8-13).[10] Arytenoid chondritis appears as an enlargement of the arytenoid cartilages. The inflammation of the arytenoids may decrease their ability to move and it can mimic laryngeal paralysis. The etiology of the inflammation is thought to be septic and/or traumatic. Both conditions can prevent a tight seal of the larynx during swallowing and result in aspiration of milk.

In a study of 38 foals with milk regurgitation/upper airway problems, 13 presented with dorsal displacement of the soft palate (DDSP).[11] In DDSP, the soft palate is located above the epiglottis instead of under it. DDSP can be seen alone or in conjunction with other abnormalities such rostral displacement of the palatopharyngeal arch, redundancy of the soft palate, pharyngeal cysts, or a persistent epiglottal frenulum.[3,12,13] Prematurity, perinatal asphyxia, and white muscle disease may

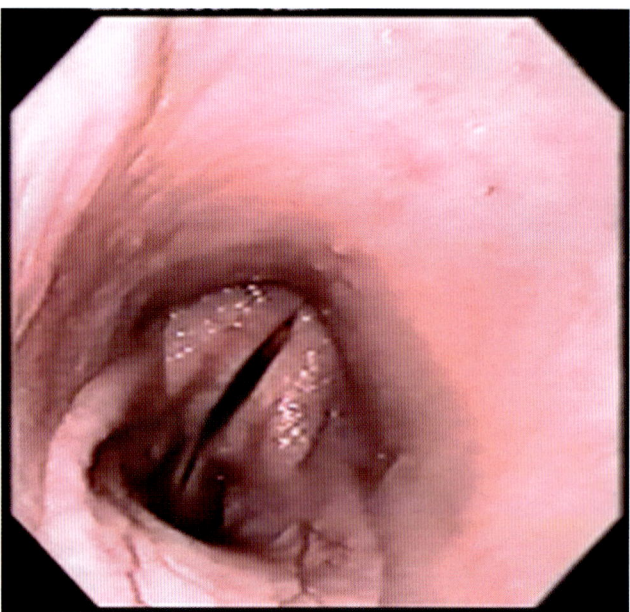

Fig. 8-13 Bilateral laryngeal paralysis prevents the effective sealing of the larynx during swallowing.

be risk factors for the development of DDSP. Cerebral or brain stem disease, such as in neonatal encephalopathy and head trauma, may also play a part in the foal's ability to swallow. Muscular weakness and depression may cause poor pharyngeal tone and disrupt the palatolaryngeal seal. The negative pressure created when nursing can exacerbate pharyngeal collapse, further increasing the dysphagia.[3] Generalized pharyngeal weakness resulting in the collapse of the pharyngeal walls may lead to upper airway obstruction, stridor, and respiratory distress.

Diagnostic tests that were performed on '05 Hard-ToSwallow at presentation included a CBC, chemistry profile, IgG analysis, arterial blood gas analysis, upper and lower airway endoscopy, and radiographs of the chest and throat latch region. Rostral displacement of the palatopharyngeal arch and a dorsally displaced soft palate were seen on endoscopy (Figure 8-14). When the scope was placed in the trachea, milk could be seen flowing down into the major bronchi (Figure 8-15). The DDSP was also confirmed on the lateral radiograph of the larynx. A severe consolidating pneumonia was found in the caudal ventral lung field on the lateral radiographs of the chest (Figure 8-16).

Leukopenia (WBC = 3,400 cells/ml) with slight neutropenia (2,176 cells/ml) was found on the CBC. The prominent abnormalities in the serum chemistry included an elevated AST (7121 U/L), CK (35,427 U/L), phosphorus (8 mg/dl), hypochloremia (94 mEq/dl), and mildly elevated lactate (3.3 mmol/liter). IgG levels were >800 mg/dl. Hypoxemia (53 mm Hg) was noted on the arterial blood gas analysis.

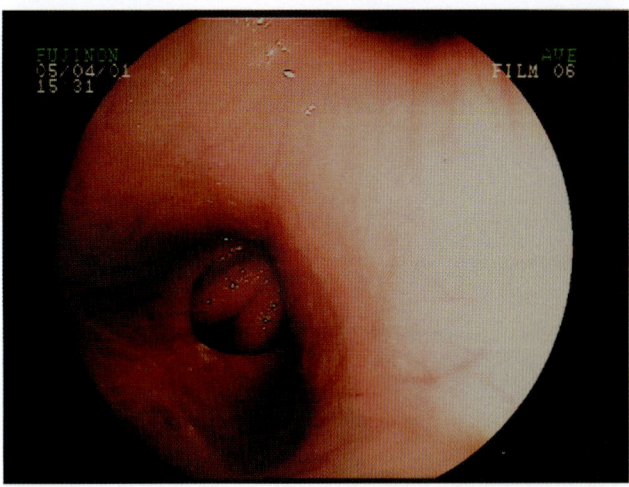

Fig. 8-14 Endoscopic view of '05 HardToSwallow's pharynx. Note the displacement of the soft palate and the mild rostral displacement of the palatopharyngeal arch.

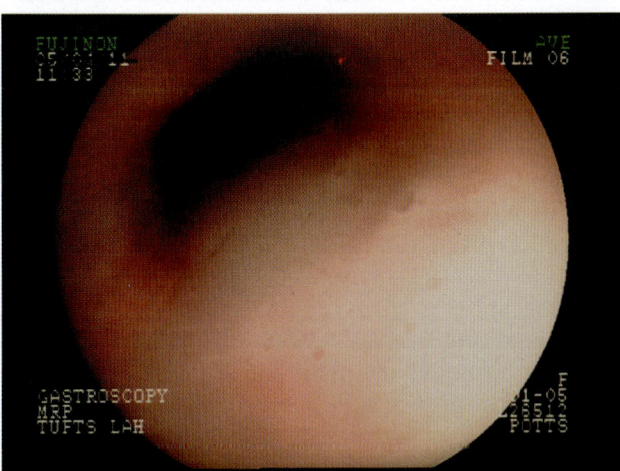

Fig. 8-15 Endoscopic view of '05 HardToSwallow's trachea following nursing. Note the presence of milk in the ventral trachea.

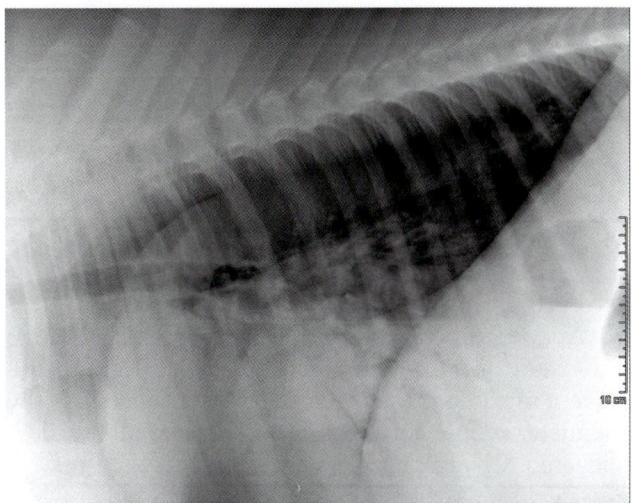

Fig. 8-16 A severe consolidating pneumonia was found in the caudal ventral lung field on the lateral radiographs of '05 HardToSwallow's chest.

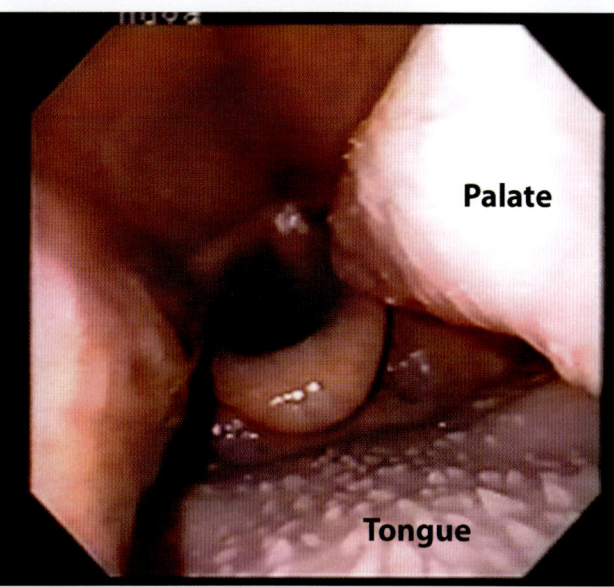

Fig. 8-17 Endoscopic visualization of a cleft hard and soft palate of a neonate from the perspective of the nose. Note the base of the tongue.

DIAGNOSTIC TESTS

Upper airway endoscopy is the most rewarding diagnostic test for finding the origin of the milk regurgitation. It is best performed with manual restraint of the foal because sedation may affect the findings. A 1 meter, a 1 to 1.5 cm diameter, endoscope can easily be passed in a >40 kg foal. It is sufficient to visualize the nasal cavity and pharyngeal region, and pass down the esophagus and trachea. Milk in the trachea is evidence that aspiration is occurring.

In a complete cleft palate, involving the hard and soft palate, one may observe it on a simple oral examination. If the cleft involves the caudal hard palate and soft palate, then use of endoscopy or a long-bladed laryngoscope is necessary for the diagnosis. Visualization of the oral cavity (such as the tongue) with the endoscope in the nares is evidence of a hard and soft cleft palate (Figure 8-17). Clefts of just the caudal portion of the soft palate may be less readily seen, especially if the epiglottis is in the correct position.

Dorsal pharyngeal cysts seen with the endoscope appear as a fluid-filled mass originating from the dorsal pharyngeal wall. It may fill your field of view obstructing the visualization of landmarks (Figure 8-18). Subepiglottic cysts will appear as a mass originating from the ventral pharynx and may also obscure the epiglottis from view. Upper respiratory distress may prevent a safe endoscopic examination of these foals until a tracheotomy is performed. Radiographic examination of the pharyngeal region may be helpful in determining the location and size of the cyst.

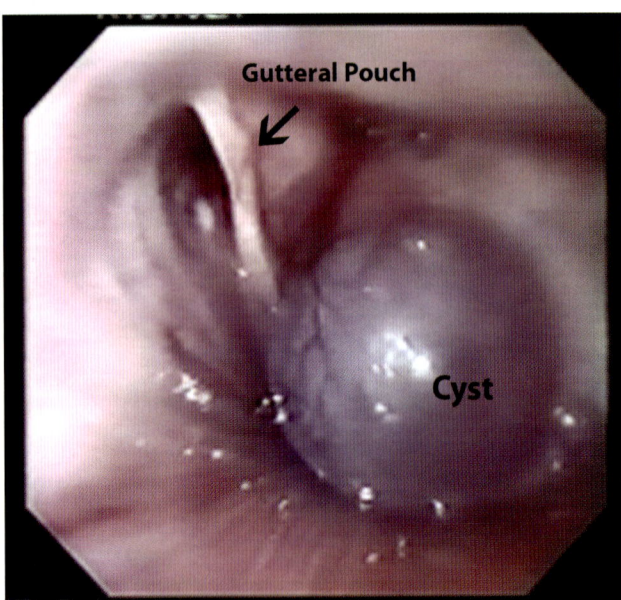

Fig. 8-18 Endoscopic view of a dorsal pharyngeal cyst. Note the lack of visualization of the larynx.

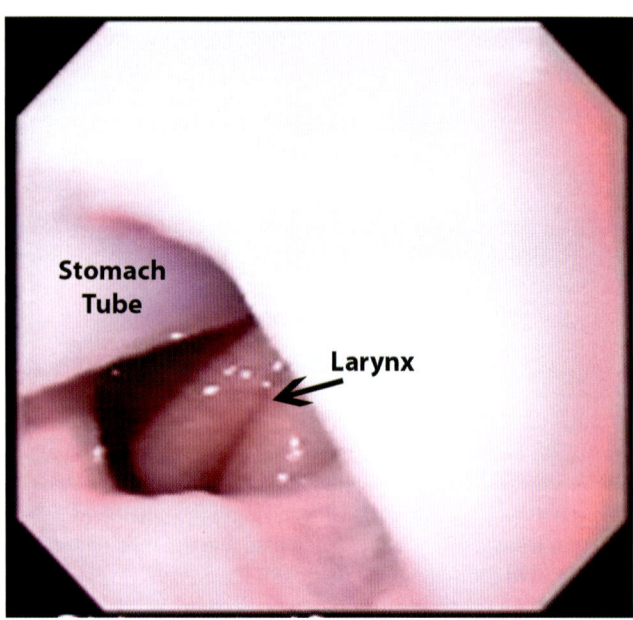

Fig. 8-19 Collapse of the pharyngeal walls prevents visualization of the larynx.

Paralysis of the larynx and arytenoid chondritis can be seen endoscopically as lack of movement of the arytenoids. In arytenoid chondritis, the arytenoids appear swollen and inflamed. Lack of movement of the arytenoids is best emphasized by holding off the foal's breath for a few seconds. The normal foal should abduct his arytenoids in response to lack of air, while foals with paralysis of the larynx and arytenoid chondritis will not respond. The slap test performed in adults to assess arytenoids movement is not consistently present in the newborn foal, therefore, it is not helpful in these diseases.[10]

DDSP is readily apparent on endoscopic examination if there are no other abnormalities. The normal triangular-shaped epiglottis is hidden under the soft palate. When DDSP is accompanied by other abnormalities such as rostral displacement of the palatopharyngeal arch and collapse of the walls of the pharynx, it may be difficult to orient oneself to the larynx (Figure 8-19). In small foals, such as mini foals, the presence of an endoscope in the nares may actually create enough rostral obstruction to increase negative pressure and artificially displace the soft palate during scoping. Lateral radiographs of the throatlatch of the head will often be diagnostic of DDSP. In DDSP, the free edge of the soft palate can be seen on radiographs (Figure 8-20, A and B)

Radiography is the best diagnostic for determining the extent of the aspiration pneumonia. If the foal has aspirated meconium, a caudoventral and caudal dorsal granular infiltrate is usually found in radiographs. Brown-tinged fluid in the trachea of the foal may be seen with the endoscope.[14] A heavy interstitial to alveolar pattern in the caudal ventral lung field is often found in milk aspiration. This location correlates with the accessory lobe of the lung, which is the first bifurcation from the right major bronchi and most subject to disease because of gravity.

Radiography is also helpful in the diagnosis of esophageal problems. A dilated esophagus can sometimes be apparent on plain films, especially if it is dilated with air. Caution should be used if contrast material is placed in the esophagus because of the possibility of aspiration into the lungs. Esophageal anomalies have been recognized and may be visualized with an endoscope.

Sampling of lung fluids by transtracheal aspiration or bronchoalveolar lavage for culture and sensitivity are not generally warranted in milk aspiration in foals. The results of the procedure do not warrant the risk of performing these tests on a critically ill foal. It can be assumed that a variety of bacteria that normally inhabit the oral cavity are present in the lung.

A minimum database consisting of IgG levels, a CBC, a chemistry profile, and an arterial blood gas analysis is important in these foals. If the dysphagia is severe, then the foal may have failure of passive transfer. Abnormalities in the CBC may help to determine the extent of the pneumonia or may indicate a concurrent sepsis as a cause of generalized weakness. The chemistry profile abnormalities in '05 HardToSwallow (elevated CK and AST) were highly suggestive of muscle disease. Nutritional myodegeneration or white muscle disease is a well-recognized cause of muscle weakness in foals.[15] Other abnormalities in routine bloodwork that may result in disruption of the foal's

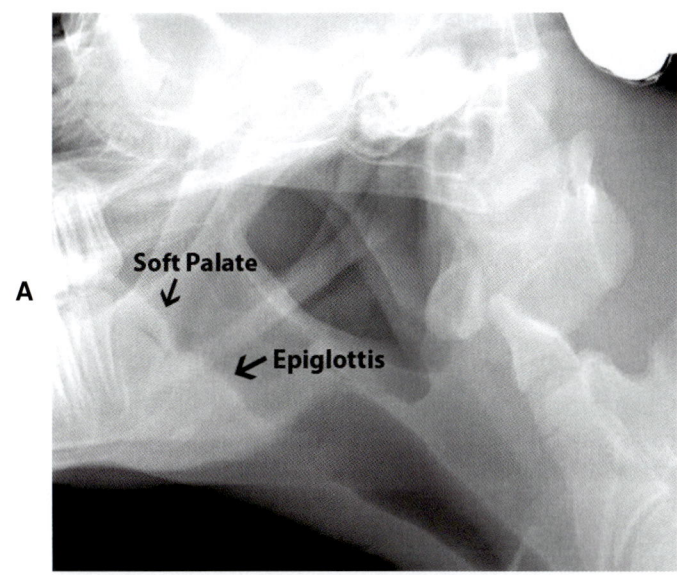

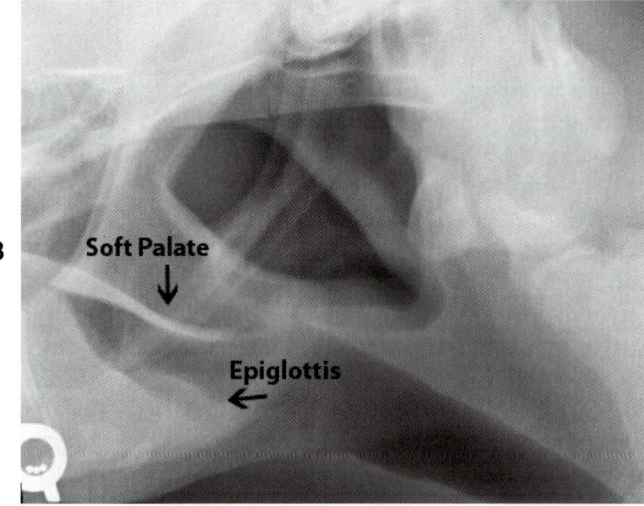

Fig. 8-20 A, Lateral radiograph of the pharyngeal region of a normal foal's head. Note the soft palate is under the epiglottis. **B,** Lateral radiograph of the pharyngeal region of a normal foal's head. Note the free edge of the soft palate is visible over the tip of the epiglottis.

swallowing ability include electrolyte deviations and hypoglycemia. An arterial blood gas analysis is helpful in directing specific respiratory therapy.

NUTRITIONAL MYODEGENERATION (WHITE MUSCLE DISEASE) AND DYSPHAGIA

In a review of 29 cases of nutritional myodegeneration (NMD) in foals, 52% (15) of the foals presented with dysphagia as one of the clinical signs.[16] Dysphagia may be the only clinical sign that is evident. NMD has been reported in foals from birth to one year of age. Clinical signs besides dysphagia vary in severity. They may include profound muscular weakness with recumbency, a stiff stilted gait, painful muscles, tachy-

cardia, arrhythmias, and aspiration pneumonia. Affected foals have elevated creatinine kinase (CK), aspartate transferase (AST), and lactate dehydrogenase (LDH) levels. CK levels are elevated proportionately to the degree of muscle damage and decrease rapidly after muscle damage ceases.[15-18] Because of this, it is a useful test to determine whether treatment is effective. Hyperkalemia, hyponatremia, hypocalcemia, and hyperphosphatemia are common electrolyte abnormalities found in affected foals.[17] Hyperkalemia is thought to be secondary to release of intracellular potassium from damaged muscles. This elevation in potassium can be life-threatening. Myoglobinuria may also be seen in affected foals.[15]

The pathogenesis of NMD is inadequate nutritional intake of selenium and/or vitamin E during the gestation period by the mare. Vitamin E and selenium work synergistically to prevent peroxide formation by tissues. Foals at highest risk for NMD are from areas of the country that have selenium-deficient soils.[15,16] These include the New England states, the Pacific Northwest, the Great Lakes region, and the southeastern United States.

A presumptive diagnosis of NMD can be made on the clinical signs plus an elevated CK and low vitamin E and selenium levels. Blood glutathione peroxidase (a selenium-containing enzyme) levels may also be helpful in determining the diagnosis. Selenium levels <0.06 ppm and glutathione peroxidase levels <15 units suggest selenium deficiency.[15] Reference levels may vary by laboratory. Prognosis for affected foals is guarded. Pale discoloration of the muscle and white streaks parallel to the muscle fibers are gross lesions seen postmortem on foals that fail to survive. Tongue lesions of myodegeneration have been reported in foals that had dysphagia as a clinical sign.[15]

'05 HardToSwallow was muzzled to prevent suckling and further aspiration of milk. An indwelling nasogastric tube was placed for feeding the foal initially at 10% body weight (combination of mare's milk and milk replacer). Broad-spectrum antibiotics (ceftiofur and amikacin) were administered to treat the concurrent aspiration pneumonia, and maintenance intravenous crystalloid fluids were delivered to support the foal and decrease lactate levels. Vitamin E/selenium supplementation was administered for treatment of possible nutritional myodegeneration. Nasal oxygen was instituted to improve the foal's oxygenation.

TREATMENT

Treatment of meconium aspiration can be very unrewarding. If the birth is attended by a knowledgeable team and it is recognized that fetal distress has occurred, then immediate action may prevent aspiration of meconium into the distal airways. Amniotic fluid from at-risk foals is yellow-brown in color, and the foals are stained with this material. In human infants with meconium staining, the hospital team clears the airways with deep suctioning before the infant takes the first breath. Unfortunately, in veterinary medicine, births are generally attended by laypersons with no equipment to accomplish this. Holding the foal by its hindlimbs and applying rapid coupage (striking the chest with a cupped hand) may help in loosening aspirated material from the airways. General respiratory support with oxygen is useful. Mechanical ventilation should be avoided if possible because it may drive meconium deeper into the lungs. Tension pneumothorax has been a complication in infants with meconium aspiration, especially with ventilation.[14]

Treatment of milk aspiration pneumonia is both general and specific. General treatment is focused on the immediate cessation of aspiration, the provision of nutrition to the foal, antibiotic therapy to eliminate any bacterial infection, and respiratory therapy to support the foal's oxygenation. Specific treatment is directed at the cause of the aspiration.

Because the aspiration of milk is secondary to dysphagia, cessation of the aspiration is accomplished by stopping the foal from nursing. This is most easily done by placing a muzzle on the foal. The use of specifically designed "bras" for the mare also prevents access to the udder by the foal. The foal will continue to attempt to nurse with either of these methods, bumping the udder and stimulating milk let-down. Foals can be very clever in trying to dislodge muzzles and mare "bras," so they should be checked frequently. The mare should be examined daily for signs of mastitis. Constant stimulation without nursing provides an excellent media for bacterial growth. An alternative to muzzling would be to separate the foal from the mare. Because regurgitation of milk can be a temporary problem in most cases, orphaning the foal should be a last resort.

Provision of nutrition for the foal with dysphagia is best accomplished through an indwelling nasogastric tube (see Chapter 4). The normal volume of milk for the foal is approximately 25% to 30% of its body weight in liters, divided into every two- to four-hour feedings over a 24-hour period. One may wish to start at a lower percentage body weight of milk such as 10% until the foal becomes adjusted to the abnormal feeding schedule.

Occasionally a foal will not tolerate the presence of a nasogastric tube and will hypersalivate—continuing to aspirate saliva into the lungs. Total parenteral nutrition may be an option (see Chapter 4). Placement of an esophagotomy tube bypassing the oropharynx may be a less expensive alternative of providing nutrition. Placement of an esophagotomy tube can be done under sedation and a local block.[19] A nasogastric tube is placed in the esophagus to define where to place the incision. It is usually placed in the upper third of the neck. Once the area is clipped and aseptically prepared, a one-inch incision is made over the indwelling tube. A second tube is then passed through the incision, down the esophagus, and into the stomach as the indwelling tube is withdrawn. This second tube is secured to the side of the neck with stay sutures, and the wound is wrapped with a bandage. The wound should be cleaned daily. Over a period of one week, a granulation bed will form around the incision. Healing of the incision is rapid once tube feeding is no longer needed. The tube is simply pulled and the incision cleaned daily. Some milk will leak through the site until it is completely sealed.[19]

Antibiotic therapy should provide broad-spectrum coverage. Generally an aminoglycoside for Gram-negative coverage plus a beta lactam or a celphalosporin for Gram-positive coverage is adequate (see Chapter 5). One can expect a mixed bacterial component due to the nature of the aspirated milk. The degree of respiratory support needed in these foals is related to the degree of aspiration that has occurred. If caught early, foals may need little in the way of oxygen. A foal that has aspirated large amounts of milk may have significant consolidation of the ventral lungs fields. Arterial blood gas analysis is helpful in deciding the necessary treatment. Usually intranasal oxygen is the extent of respiratory support needed, but occasionally hypercarbia will dictate the use of mechanical ventilation (see Cases 8-1 and 8-2).

Specific therapy for milk regurgitation depends upon the cause of the dysphagia. In cases in which there is severe stridor and upper airway obstruction, an emergency tracheotomy may be necessary. This may be done before you have made your diagnosis. This is most often seen in foals with pharyngeal cysts, arytenoiditis, bilateral paralysis of the arytenoids, and severe pharyngeal collapse. A tracheotomy is performed in the middle third of the neck. If possible, the area is clipped and aseptically prepared. A vertical, one-inch incision is made through the skin over the palpable trachea. This is followed by blunt dissection through the subcutaneous tissues. Once the trachea is exposed, a horizontal incision, approximately one third of the tracheal diameter, is made between the tracheal rings. An appropriate-size human tracheotomy tube is inserted through the incision into the trachea (Figure 8-21). The foal's stridor should immediately abate if the diagnosis of upper airway obstruction is correct. This allows time to further investigate and treat the cause of the obstruction. Care of the

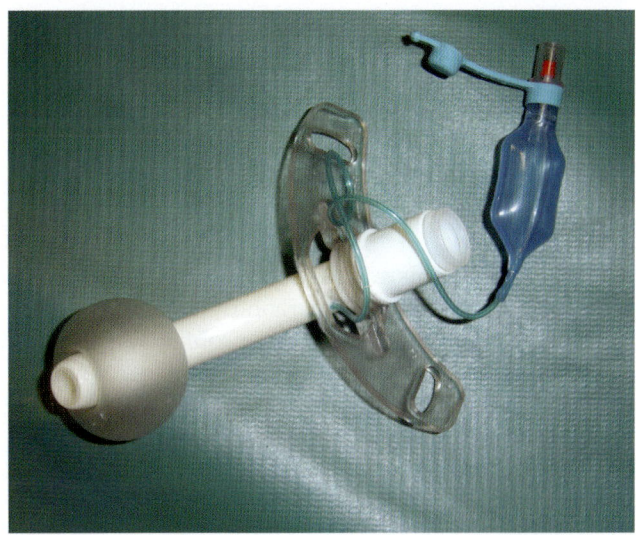

Fig. 8-21 Commercial tracheotomy tube used in human medicine. Different sizes are compatible with most foals.

tracheotomy tube involves daily cleaning. This can be accomplished by removing and replacing the tube daily. This can be problematic in an active foal. Some human tracheotomy kits have a removable sheath that allows cleaning without complete removal of the device.

In the case of pharyngeal cysts, surgical removal has been performed through a laryngotomy or pharyngotomy approach.[9] Transendoscopic laser surgery has also been successful and perhaps less traumatic than traditional surgical approaches. For immediate relief of the airway obstruction involved in the dorsal pharyngeal cyst, one can use an endoscopic biopsy instrument to puncture and drain the cyst. The remnants of the cyst wall may still impair swallowing, so follow-up removal of this tissue with a laser is needed.

Foals presenting with bilateral paralysis of the larynx or bilateral arytenoiditis are uncommon. The placement of a laryngeal prosthesis that fixes the arytenoid cartilage in abduction may be helpful in increasing the airway of a foal with laryngeal paralysis. If the paralysis is related to cerebral disease, then surgically increasing the airway will do nothing to improve the dysphagia. There is a risk of further complicating the dysphagia and aspiration pneumonia because of an inability to guard its larynx. Arytenoiditis is treated with antibiotics and anti-inflammatory drugs. Some people advocate the use of a nasopharyngeal spray consisting of DMSO, nitrofurazone, prednisolone, and glycerin.[20] Surgical excision of the body and corniculate process of the affected arytenoid has been performed in affected adults, but again a complication may be a worsening of the aspiration pneumonia. Prognosis for both of these conditions is not favorable.

Surgical repair can be attempted for the correction of cleft palates in the foal but the prognosis is poor. It is

difficult to obtain adequate visualization without a mandibular symphysiotomy. Complications include dehiscence of the repair, chronic nasal discharge, stunted growth, and osteomyelitis of the mandibular symphysis.[7]

If DDSP is accompanied by rostral displacement of the palatopharyngeal arch and collapse of the pharyngeal walls resulting in severe dyspnea, then a tracheotomy may be needed to ease the respiratory distress. As discussed earlier, etiology of DDSP in the neonatal foal has been attributed to redundant soft palate tissue, persistent epiglottic frenulum, prematurity, perinatal asphyxia, and NMD (white muscle disease). Many times no etiology can be found. Surgical approaches have been recommended in cases of redundant soft palate and persistent epiglottic frenulum, but with rest and supportive care many foals with simple DDSP will resolve on their own in two to four days.[21] Because of this, it is probably prudent to treat medically first. If the pharyngeal muscular weakness is secondary to prematurity or perinatal asphyxia, then treatment of the primary problems are important.

Specific treatment for NMD is the administration of a vitamin E/selenium supplement (E-Se®) by intramuscular injection (1 ml/45 kg). This can be repeated in three and eight days. Because the amount of vitamin E in the above preparation is minimal, additional vitamin E supplementation can be given. The role of vitamin E in NMD is controversial, but it does act synergistically with selenium to stabilize muscle cell membranes.[15] Foals should be confined to the stall, and all physical exertion minimized. Dill reports that foals who survive regain strength and the ability to swallow gradually in two to six days. The diagnosis of NMD in a foal may be reflective of a low selenium status in the herd. Feed supplementation can be given to pregnant mares, and prophylactic administration of vitamin E/selenium to newborn foals may prevent further problems.[15]

Over the next two days, '05 HardToSwallow's CK decreased to 1163 U/liter and was in the normal range by day eight of hospitalization. The AST decreased (1647 U/liter) but continued to be above normal at this time. The foal responded to the nasal oxygen (flow rate 7 liters/minute) by increasing the PaO2 to 221 mm Hg. Her lactate levels decreased to 1.8 mmol/liter. Clinically the foal was bright and alert and becoming more rambunctious.

On day four of hospitalization, endoscopic re-evaluation was performed on '05 HardToSwallow. DDSP was still present, but there appeared to be less collapse of the dorsal pharyngeal wall. Radiographs showed improvement in the caudal ventral alveolar pattern. The foal's weight was maintained at 51 kg.

By day six of hospitalization, '05 HardToSwallow's owner was becoming frustrated with the foal's progress.

Treatment options and prognosis were discussed. It was decided to remove the nasogastric tube and train the foal to bucket feed. It was felt that this may decrease the negative pressure in the pharynx and allow the foal to replace the soft palate. The foal was carefully monitored for tracheal rattling, coughing, milk regurgitation from the nose, and increased auscultation abnormalities after drinking. No milk was noted in the trachea after bucket feeding.

By day 11 of hospitalization, the foal continued to thrive. She had adapted to the bucket feeding regime and was gaining weight. Improvement of the aspiration pneumonia was evident on thoracic radiographs. Radiographs of the larynx showed a properly placed soft palate. Endoscopy of the upper airway confirmed a normal placement of soft palate. The foal was allowed to nurse for two minutes and rescoped. The DDSP and milk in the trachea were again evident.

Because nursing still induced the DDSP, the owner decided to separate the mare and foal, raise the foal as an orphan, and continue to bucket feed her. One month following discharge, the foal was growing well. There was no evidence of respiratory compromise.

OUTCOME

As opposed to foals with meconium aspiration, foals with milk aspiration do surprisingly well. In a survey of 38 foals with upper airway problems/aspiration pneumonia, only seven did not go home recovered or improved with medical care and support.[10] Those that were euthanized had the following diagnoses: bilateral laryngeal paralysis, bilateral arytenoiditis, septic pneumonia, and congenital heart defect. A study on the long-term outcome of surviving foals has not been done. Anecdotal reports have been favorable, but athletic performance has not been evaluated.

REFERENCES

1. Tyler DC, Murphy J, Cheney FW: Mechanical and chemical damage to lung tissue caused by meconium aspiration, *Pediatrics* 62:454, 1978.
2. Lopez A, Bildfell R: Pulmonary inflammation associated with aspirated meconium and epithelial cells in calves, *Vet Pathol* 29:104, 1992.
3. Barton MH: Nasal regurgitation of milk in foals, *Compend* 15:81, 1993.
4. Batstone JHF: Cleft palate in the horse, *Br J Past Surg* 19:327, 1966.
5. Mason TA, Speirs VC, Maclean AA et al: Surgical repair of cleft soft palate in the horse, *Vet Rec* 100:6, 1977.
6. Orka SW: Epidemiology and genetics of clefting: With implications for etiology. In Cooper HK, Harding RL, Krogman WM et al, eds: *Cleft palate and cleft lip: A team approach to clinical management and rehabilitation of the patient,* Philadelphia, 1979, WB Saunders.
7. Bowman KF, Tate LP, Evans LH et al: Complications of cleft palate repair in large animals, *JAVMA* 180:652, 1982.
8. Stick JA, Boles C: Subepiglottic cyst in three foals, *JAVMA* 177:62, 1980.
9. Hardy J: Upper airway obstruction in foals, weanlings, and yearlings, *Vet Clin North Am* (Equine Pract) 7:105, 1991.
10. Green S, Mayhew I: Neurologic disorders, in Koterba AM, Drummond WH, Kosch PC, eds: *Equine clinical neonatology,* Philadelphia, 1991, Lea & Febiger.
11. Paradis MR: unpublished data.
12. Shappell KK, Caron JP, Stick JA et al: Staphylectomy for treatment of dorsal displacement of the soft palate in two foals, *JAVMA* 195:1395, 1989.
13. Yarbtough TB, Voss E, Herrgesell EJ et al: Persistent frenulum of the epiglottis in four foals, *Vet Surg* 28:287, 1999.
14. Koterba AM, Paradis, MR: Specific respiratory conditions, in Koterba AM, Drummond WH, Kosch PC, eds: *Equine clinical neonatology,* Philadelphia, 1991, Lea & Febiger.
15. Dill, SG, Rehbun WC: White muscle disease in foals, *Compend Cont Educ Pract Vet* 7:s267, 1985.
16. Moore RM: Nutritional muscular dystrophy in foals, *Compend* 13:476, 1991.
17. Perkins G, Valberg SJ, Madigan JM et al: Electrolyte disturbances in foals with severe rhabdomyolysis, *J Vet Intern Med* 12:173, 1998.
18. Valberg SJ: A review of the diagnosis and treatment of rhabdomyolysis in foals, *AAEP Proceed* 48:117, 2002.
19. Mazan MR, Paradis MR: Bypassing the oral cavity, the use of tub esophagotomy for long term enteral nutritional support in a foal, *JEVCC* 10:7, 2000.
20. Ducharme NG, Hackett RP: Arytenoid chonditis. In Brown CM, Bertone JJ, eds: *The five minute veterinary consult equine,* Baltimore, 2002, Lippincott Williams & Wilkins.
21. Altmaier K, Morris EA: Dorsal displacement of the soft palate in neonatal foals, *Equine Vet J* 25:329, 1993.

9 Noninfectious Musculoskeletal Problems

Case 9-1	Foal with Flexural Deformity	Patricia Provost

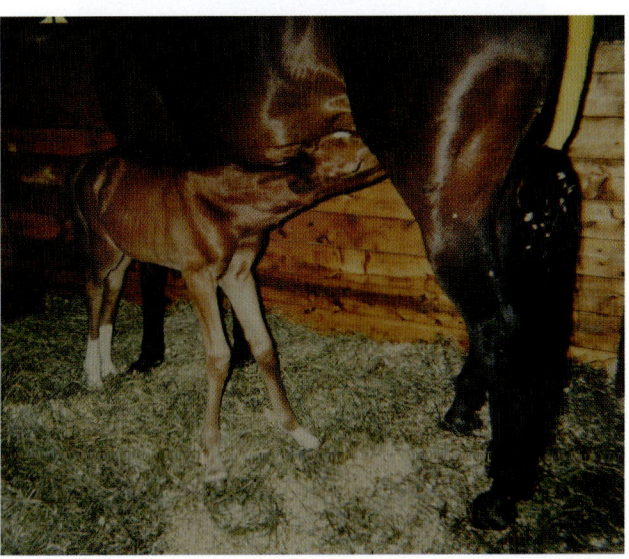

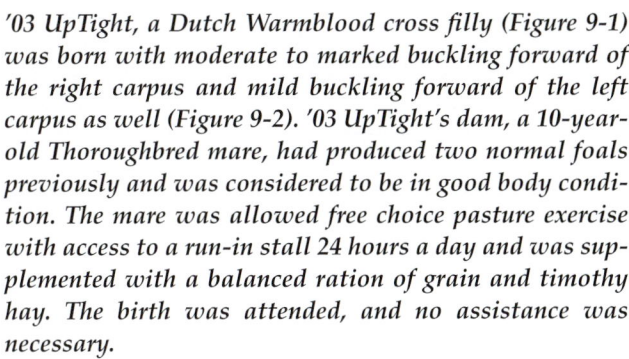

Fig. 9-1 '03 UpTight with flexural contracture of the right carpus.

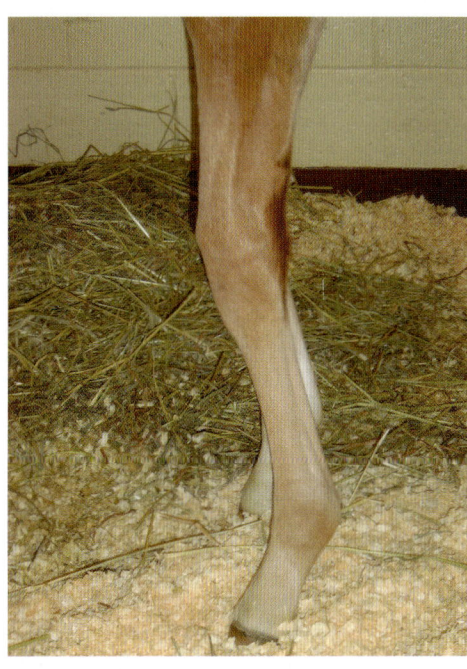

Fig. 9-2 '03 UpTight with mild buckling of the left carpus.

'03 UpTight, a Dutch Warmblood cross filly (Figure 9-1) was born with moderate to marked buckling forward of the right carpus and mild buckling forward of the left carpus as well (Figure 9-2). '03 UpTight's dam, a 10-year-old Thoroughbred mare, had produced two normal foals previously and was considered to be in good body condition. The mare was allowed free choice pasture exercise with access to a run-in stall 24 hours a day and was supplemented with a balanced ration of grain and timothy hay. The birth was attended, and no assistance was necessary.

The newborn foal was examined at the farm 36 hours after birth. She was bright and vigorous, and all vital parameters were within normal limits. A SNAP test (IDEXX Laboratories, Inc., Westbrook, ME) was performed, and IgG results were greater than 800 g/dl. The foal moved soundly around her stall with no difficulty in maneuvering. However, when she stopped and stood still, trembling of the forelimbs was noticeable when viewed from the side. Observation of her limbs revealed no conformation problems other than those associated with her carpi. Manual straightening of the overflexion to normal position was possible with the foal weight bearing in the left limb by pushing the carpus backward with a hand. The right carpus could not be straightened in this manner. No further diagnostics were done at this time, but conservative therapy was initiated with the application of a heavy bandage placed from her elbow to directly above the metacarpophalangeal joint of the right forelimb.

HISTORY AND PHYSICAL EXAMINATION

The term *flexural deformity* can be used to describe opposite types of flexor tendon disorders in the neonatal foal—hyperflexion and hyperextension. Traditionally, these disorders are discussed as tendon contracture and tendon laxity, respectively. This is a probably a misnomer as tendons don't technically contract or relax. For the purpose of this chapter, the terms will be used interchangeably.

Frequently there is nothing in the history that will predict flexural limb deformities. Answers to questions about the possible ingestion of toxic plants or exposure to known teratogens are usually negative. In cases of severe contractual deformity, dystocia may have occurred because the foal is unable to assume the correction position for delivery. A history of placentitis or twinning may result in a premature parturition and a foal with hyperextension. In any limb deformity, close questioning about the timing and amount of colostrum ingestion is important. Foals that have difficulty standing and nursing due to orthopedic reasons are at high risk for failure of passive transfer and sepsis (see Chapters 3 and 5).

The flexural deformity of the carpus in the above foal is hyperflexion, which is readily diagnosed at birth. The degree of overflexion may be very mild or it may be so severe as to result in dystocia and/or the inability of the foal to stand. The disorder may involve one limb or both. It may also be present in the metacarpophalangeal joint(s), and less commonly the distal interphalangeal (DIP) joint. Flexural deformity of the DIP joint may be present at birth but is much more common in foals older than four weeks of age.[1] Tarsal and metatarsophalangeal joint involvement have also been reported but are rare.[2]

Diagnosis is made through observation and physical examination. When this type of flexural deformity of the carpus is viewed from the side, there is a buckling forward of the carpus in the stance. At the trot or canter, the foal with mild to moderate hyperflexion may be able to completely extend the limb, but the hyperflexion returns when the foal slows to walk or stops. After exercise, trembling of the muscles may be apparent secondary to fatigue from trying to maintain limb extension. Lameness is uncommon; if present, joint sepsis should be ruled out first.

Similar to that described in the above case, manipulation of the limb is used to determine the severity. This can be done with the foal restrained and standing or with the foal in lateral recumbency. As above, the carpus is manually pushed backward as the cannon bone is held stationary (Figure 9-3). Mild deformities will often straighten easily with manipulation, but moderate to severe hyperflexures will rarely do so

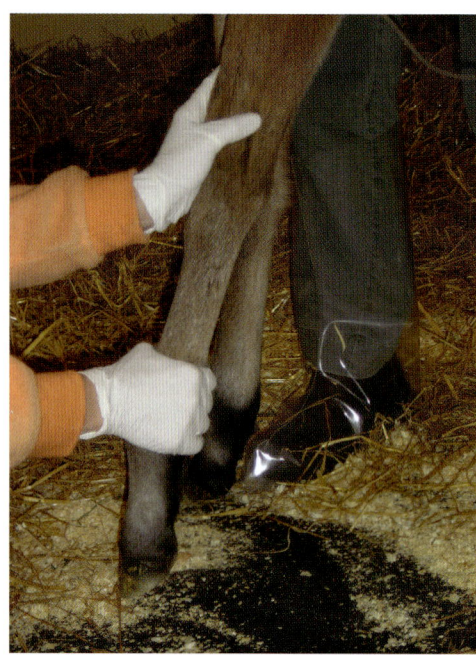

Fig. 9-3 Attempts to straighten the carpus helps to determine the severity of the flexural contracture.

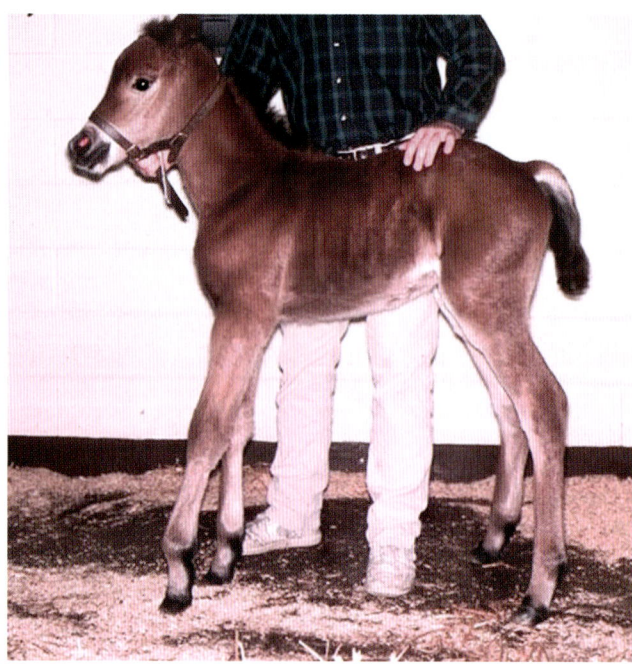

Fig. 9-4 A foal with metacarpophalangeal joint flexural deformity appears to knuckle over at the fetlock.

completely. The ability to fully flex the joint should also be determined. An uncomplicated flexural deformity will have normal flexion.

When observed from the side, foals with metacarpophalangeal joint flexural deformity appear to knuckle over at the fetlock (Figure 9-4). When severe, it is difficult for the foal to walk, and the foal may walk on the dorsum of the joint. When evaluating a foal with this type of deformity, it is important to check if the sole of the foot makes contact with the ground. Resolution is more difficult in those that don't.

Flexural deformity of the distal interphalangeal joint may also result in the foal walking on the toe. Differentiation between problems arising from the metacarpophalangeal joint and the distal interphalangeal should be made. With involvement of the third phalanx only, the foal will have normal angulation of the fetlock and first and second phalangeal alignment. The hoof wall angle, however, is more upright than the angle of the pastern. Over time, the heel length will grow and result in the classic clubfoot or boxy foot appearance (Figure 9-5, A and B). Treatment of a foal that is unable to place its foot flat on the ground has a greater chance of success if it is resulting from distal interphalangeal joint versus metacarpophalangeal flexural deformity.[3]

When performing the physical examination, it is also important to evaluate the common digital extensor tendon over the dorsolateral aspect of the carpus. A rupture should be suspected if there is swelling over the dorsolateral surface of the carpus and can be confirmed by digital palpation or ultrasound imaging of the separated tendon ends (Figure 9-6). Rupture of this tendon may occur in neonates leading to forelimb conformation that may be mistakenly diagnosed as a primary carpal or metacarpophalangeal flexural deformity. Tendon rupture may occur without any other orthopedic problem, or it can be secondary to either a moderate to severe primary carpal or metacarpophalangeal flexural deformity. When the tendon rupture is secondary to a flexural deformity, then manual extension of the limb is not easily achieved.

The second form of flexural deformity in the foal is caused by hyperextension or laxity in the foal's tendon/muscle unit. Hyperextension of the digit is quite common in neonates at birth and following prolonged recumbency associated with illness. The condition is characterized by dorsiflexion of the interphalangeal joints that results in the foal walking on the heel bulbs of the foot and in extreme cases, the palmar or plantar aspect of the phalanges and fetlock, with the toe elevated (Figure 9-7). Digital hyperextension is more common in the hindlimbs but can affect all limbs. Occasionally hyperextension of the carpus can be seen in foals. Fortunately most cases respond favorably over time with minimal intervention.

PATHOGENESIS

Flexural deformities of the limbs may either be congenital or acquired in origin. Acquired contractures in

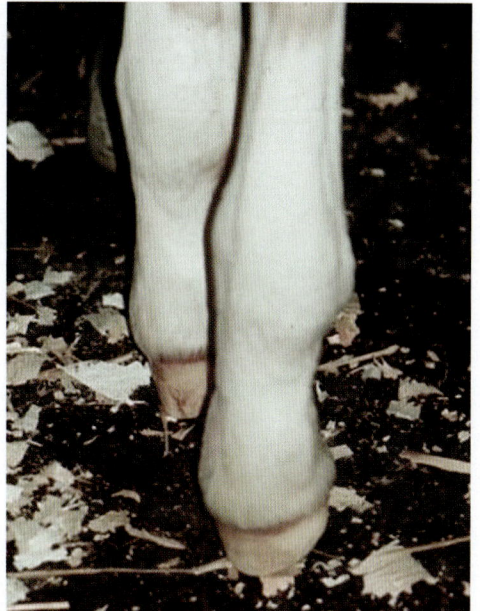

A

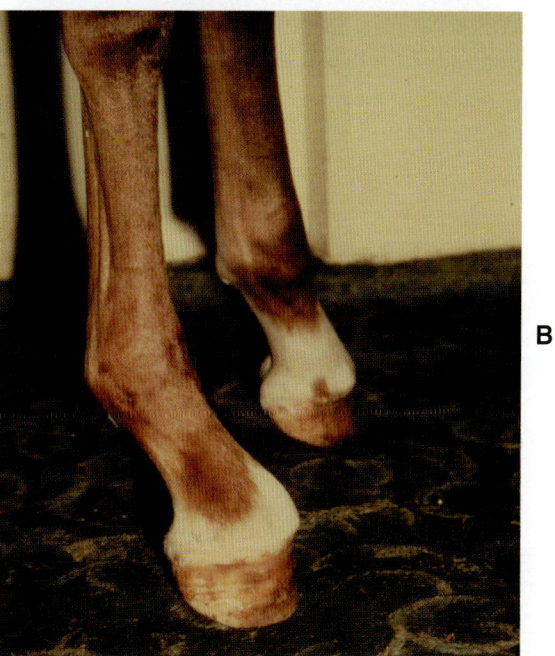

B

Fig. 9-5 A, This foal's conformation is a result of a flexural deformity at the fetlock level. **B,** This foal has a DIP flexural deformity that has resulted in a clubfooted appearance over time.

the neonate are rare unless the foal has been recumbent because of illness or is not fully weight bearing on a limb due to lameness. Much more common are deformities seen at birth, with the hyperflexed condition generally restricted to the carpus, the metacarpophalangeal joint, and less commonly the distal interphalangeal joint.[2,4] The most common hyperextension disorder occurs in the distal interphalangeal joint.

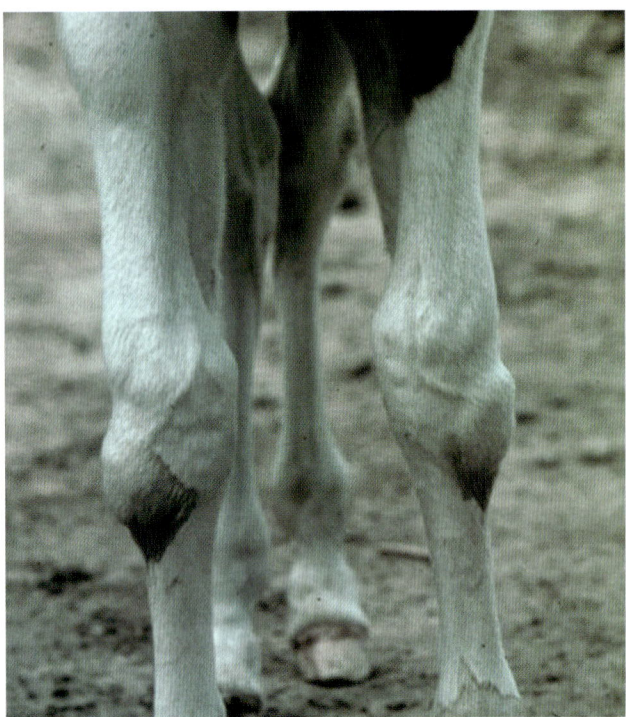

Fig. 9-6 Rupture of the common digital extensor tendon presents as a swelling over the lateral surface of the carpus.

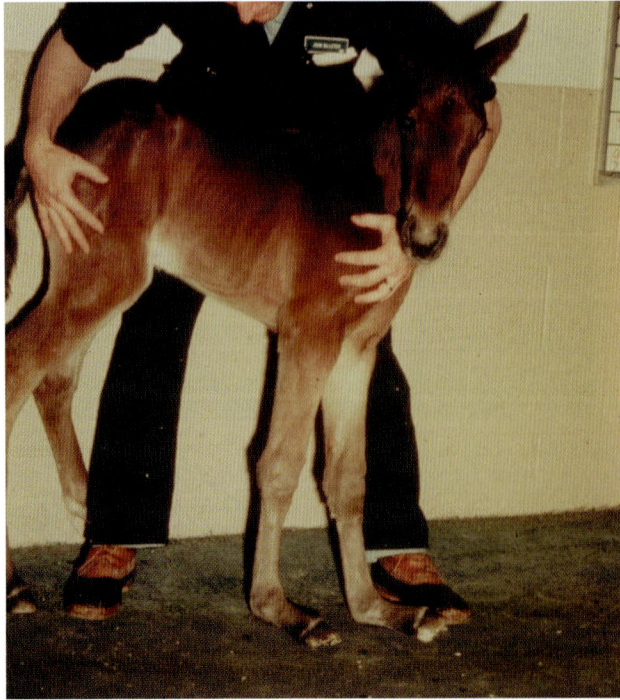

Fig. 9-7 Laxity in a foal's flexor tendon/muscle unit results in dorsiflexion of the interphalangeal joints. The toes of the foot are generally off the ground, and the foal may walk on the palmar or plantar aspect of the phalanges. This is a severe case.

The pathogenesis of congenital contractual flexural deformities is speculative. Several theories, including ingestion of teratogens, nitrates, sudan grass, or locoweed; neuromuscular disorders; lathyrism; and equine goiter or hypothyroidism have been proposed, but no one theory is supported.[5,6] Intrauterine positioning continues to be discussed and may be responsible in some but unlikely all cases as frequent repositioning of the fetus *in utero* occurs.[7,8] Body pregnancies are more likely to present with hyperflexion secondary to *in utero* positioning because the foal's movement is restricted in late gestation. Inheritance is less likely as many dams, similar to that in the above case, have had previously normal foals by the same stallion. As with many unknowns, a multifactorial etiology is likely.

Tendon hyperextension is commonly seen in the premature foal, twins, or the foal with intrauterine growth restriction (IUGR). Term foals with this condition have been described as dysmature, foals with normal gestation but have characteristics similar to the premature foal. The problem is assumed to be secondary to muscular weakness rather than an increased tendon length.

In both distal interphalangeal and fetlock hyperflexed deformities, pathology is typically restricted to an incongruity between the length of the flexor tendons and the skeleton.[9] In distal interphalangeal cases, the deep digital flexor tendon is involved; in fetlock contracture, both the superficial and the deep digital flexor muscle-tendon units are shortened. In some instances, shortening of the suspensory ligament may be primarily involved. This differs from that of carpal contracture in which rarely is a specific tendon-muscle unit involved. Instead, contracture of the carpal fascia and palmar ligament is more common, which makes treatment of severe cases much more difficult.[3]

DIAGNOSTIC TESTS

Few, if any, diagnostic tests are required for the management of neonatal flexural limb deformities of the carpus or metacarpophalangeal joint. Of primary importance is IgG determination to confirm adequate immunologic coverage. Foals that have difficulty rising and ambulating due to moderate to severe contracture are quite likely to have inadequate IgG concentrations, as well as dehydration and hypoglycemia due to inadequate nursing. Radiographic imaging of the affected joint(s) may be pursued but is not necessary in most foals. Exceptions include foals that are lame, have severe contracture, or are unable to flex the joint as well as extend it. Foals with flexural deformity of the DIP joint may also benefit from radiographic examination. Over time, pedal osteolysis develops in foals that have altered blood flow to the foot secondary to abnormal weight bearing.[10] Seedy toe and toe abscessation may occur if left untreated.[10]

Radiographs should also be obtained if the foal is premature with risk of incomplete ossification of the cuboidal bones or has a moderate to severe angular limb deformity (ALD) as well. Radiographs will generally be unremarkable in the majority of foals with mild to moderate congenital flexural limb deformities of these joints. However, radiographs would be warranted in a foal failing to improve with therapy.

Likewise, ultrasound imaging is generally not initially required but may be useful in the evaluation if it is suspected that a foal has common digital extensor tendon rupture, or the foal is lame, unable to flex the joint, or failing to respond to therapy.

Bandaging of the right forelimb was continued by the owner for three days. Temporary improvement of the flexural limb deformity was seen when the bandage was removed. However, on the following day, despite controlled exercise, the foal exhibited hyperflexion of the right forelimb, especially as she tired. Additionally, despite exercise, there was no overt improvement of the left forelimb. At one week of age, the foal was administered oxytetracycline intravenously, and both forelimbs were bandaged and then splinted caudally using PVC piping from the mid forearm to the distal metacarpus. The bandages and the splints were reset every other day for one week and then removed.

Although initially there was a marked improvement of the flexural limb carpal deformities for several days following bandage and splint removal, return of the contracture became increasingly more apparent at the end of the day as the foal tired and as time progressed. Extension of both forelimbs was completely normal when the foal walked, trotted, and galloped. Bandages and splints were reapplied by the owner eight days following removal of the first set and continued for an additional week. The foal was re-examined by the veterinarian at the end of this time. The foal's flexural limb deformity of the carpi had improved 50% since the time of birth. With the foal nearing five weeks of age, the decision was made to apply sleeve casts to both forelimbs in the hope of resolving the flexural deformities. The foal was sedated and anesthetized at the farm using injectable medication. Sleeve casts were applied that extended from just distal to the elbow to just proximal to the fetlock joint. The foal and dam were confined to stall rest.

The foal was re-anesthetized nine days later and the casts removed. Both limbs had visible carpal hyperextension. There were no cast sores. The foal and dam were allowed access to their paddock once again.

Over the next four weeks, the foal was bandaged and splinted three additional times by the owner for five- to seven-day intervals. When unbandaged during this month, the foal would initially remain normal for several days, then exhibit trembling of the limbs during the stance after exercise and intermittent mild hyperflexion (at the knee).

TREATMENT

Treatment of foals with flexural limb deformity should be initiated quickly, as early intervention is often more successful and implementable than that pursued as the foal ages.[11] Carpal and fetlock hyperflexures generally respond favorably to a combination of controlled exercise, bandaging with or without a splint, and use of intravenous oxytetracycline.[8,9,12] Mild contractures often improve within just a few days as the foal becomes stronger with exercise. Exercise should be restricted to firm footing to encourage tendon stretching and to a small paddock for frequent but short amounts of time. With extended periods of exercise, deformities may worsen due to fatigue of the muscles and tendons and the pain associated with their stretching. Ambulatory foals with mild deformities that are not rapidly improving or those with moderate or severe deformities require more aggressive treatment.

Application of a bandage and splint that extends from the elbow to directly above the fetlock is indicated. The compressed bandage thickness should be at least one inch prior to placement of the splint to prevent pressure sores. The splint can be fashioned from polyvinyl chloride piping (four-inch diameter, thick-walled PVC cut into thirds or halves) that has been cut to an appropriate width (that of the bandage posteriorly) and length (about three inches shorter than the bandage) for the specific patient. The PVC splint can be further customized using heat to bend it. Foam material or cotton is glued or taped to each end for extra padding protection.

The splint is centered over the caudal aspect of the bandage and secured in place with the limb in extension using a nonelastic tape such as duct tape or two-inch white tape. With this type of external coaptation, adequate padding is essential to avoid pressure necrosis of the skin. Skin areas at greatest risk are the medial and lateral malleoli of the distal radius, the accessory carpal bone, and that beneath the distal end of the splint. Ideally the bandages should be changed and the skin examined for sores daily but at minimum every two days. It should be changed more often if the splint slips or the bandage becomes wet. Patches can be fashioned using thick foam (two- to four-inch) to redistribute pressure away from pressure points. Improvement in the flexion of the carpus should be seen after several days. Discontinuation of the splints should be done once the carpus has a normal angle.

However, use of the bandages for several days beyond this is recommended as in some foals the flexural deformity will reappear otherwise.

Intravenous oxytetracycline (44 mg/kg per body weight) diluted in 1 liter of polyionic fluid given intravenously is a successful adjunct to bandaging and splinting and may also be effective when used alone to treat some cases.[12,13] The mechanism by which oxytetracycline works is not completely understood. Chelation of Ca^{++} within the skeletal muscle has been theorized, but measurement of Ca^{++} in clinical cases does not support this.[14] Neuromuscular blockade effected by oxytetracycline has also been suggested.[15] Neither theory explains why flexor tendon relaxation is targeted over that of extensor tendons.

Clinical and investigative studies have documented improvement in distal interphalangeal, metacarpophalangeal, and carpal joint angles in foals following oxytetracycline administration.[12] In 1992 Lokai reported its clinical use in 123 foals with congenital flexural deformities with a 94% success outcome.[12] Patients included foals that were less than 14 days of age that were able to place some part of the foot on the ground. A second dose of oxytetracycline was required in foals that did not significantly respond by 48 hours of the initial treatment. The effects of the oxytetracycline can be short-lived (~96 hours), so retreatment as well as continued support bandaging may be necessary to maintain the improvement. In a controlled study measuring metacarpophalangeal joint angles in normal foals following administration of oxytetracycline (44 mg/kg of body weight diluted in 10 ml of 0.9% normal saline), the initial significant change in metacarpophalangeal angle was not present by day four following administration.[14]

Oxytetracycline, at this high dose, can adversely affect renal function and thus it should be given only in the well-hydrated, nonseptic foal. Renal parameters should assessed prior to administration of additional doses. Oxytetracycline-induced acute nephrosis has been reported in a foal treated at one day of age with 70 mg/kg per body weight of the drug.[16] Although this foal's subclinical neonatal isoerythrolysis and hypovolemia may have been predisposing factors, the case points to the importance of patient selection and careful monitoring. This reaction appears to be idiosyncratic in nature. Studies looking at renal parameters of foals receiving this high dose of oxytetracycline showed no abnormalities. The diluting of the dose of oxytetracycline in a liter of balanced electrolyte fluid may help to avoid this reaction.

The use of sleeve casts (elbow to directly above the fetlock joint) can be substituted for bandaging and splinting if substantial and continued improvement is not made or in circumstances in which frequent rebandaging of the foal would be burdensome. General anesthesia is recommended for cast placement and allows the limb to be extended as far as possible without resistance from the foal. The use of Teflon® cast padding with a two-inch strip of orthopedic felt placed at each end has been successful in our hospital in eliminating rub sores caused by the cast.

Four layers of fiberglass cast tape (usually three inches in width) are used in light horse breed foals. Seven to ten days is usually adequate to observe marked improvement, and during this time the foal is stall rested with its dam. Anesthesia of the foal is recommended for cast removal. Again, continued bandaging may be necessary to maintain normal extension as was seen in the above case. Bandaging, splinting, and casts effect their action by improving the direction of the weight-bearing forces on the limb so that tension is applied to the flexors. Through an inverse myotactic reflex, relaxation of the muscle-tendon unit occurs.[3,17]

The use of controlled exercise, bandaging with splints, oxytetracycline, and casts have also been successful in the treatment of metacarpophalangeal flexural deformities.[8,12,13] Guidelines for their use are similar to those described for carpal contractures, however, placement of the bandage, splint, and cast are different. For foals with fetlock but no carpal involvement, only the limb below the level of the carpus is bandaged, splinted, or cast. In the latter, the foot is incorporated into the half limb cast. If both the carpus and the fetlock are involved, then a full limb bandage/splint or full limb cast is used.

For those foals with distal interphalangeal joint contracture, corrective farriery may be helpful. A toe extension is used for the treatment of DIP and fetlock flexural deformities.[4,9] This plus controlled exercise consisting of hand walking on a firm surface several times a day will generally correct mild deformities. Improvement following short-term use of a half-limb cast has also been reported.[4] In foals that fail to respond within one to two weeks or those with more severe flexion, surgical intervention is recommended.

Surgical intervention should be reserved for those foals with severe congenital contractures and those with acquired contractures that fail to respond favorably to conservative therapy. Surgical intervention in severe carpal flexural deformities requires an approach to the palmar aspect of the carpus through the medial aspect of the carpal canal by a surgeon familiar with the anatomy. The tendons are retracted caudally and then the radiocarpal and middle carpal joint capsules are transected in an attempt to straighten the limb. If the limb can be straightened, placement in a bandage with a splint or cast follows. If extension cannot be achieved, euthanasia is recommended as the prognosis for a normal limb is poor.[18]

Surgical treatment of deformities affecting the fetlock joint is approached in a stepwise fashion. Foals with congenital contractures often respond favorably to inferior check ligament desmotomy. Desmotomy of the superior check ligament may result in further improvement if necessary and can be completed during the same anesthetic. The degree of extension achieved with these desmotomies should be evaluated at the time of surgery, as it may be necessary in severe cases to proceed with severing the superficial digital flexor tendon or suspensory ligament or its branches.[9]

The tautest structure is severed first and then the foal recovered. Additional structures should be cut one at a time in subsequent surgeries, allowing sufficient time for observation of improvement. Arthrodesis of the metacarpophalangeal joint can be pursued in those foals with marked flexion and abnormal joint anatomy.[19] Pasture soundness can be obtained.

Most distal interphalangeal joint flexural deformities respond to desmotomy of the inferior check ligament.[8,9] Success is best achieved by combining this with use of orthopedic shoeing. In foals with a hoof ground angle greater than 90° that fail to improve following inferior check ligament desmotomy may require deep digital flexor tenotomy to achieve improvement.[8,9,20] The tendon can be transected either at the level of the midcannon or at midpastern within the tendon sheath. In foals, both may result in a cosmetic and athletic outcome.[9]

Foals with hyperextension of the digit will often correct themselves with controlled exercise. Bandaging and/or splinting the limb for support should be avoided, as this will result in further flexor laxity. Light dressings may be necessary to prevent or cover existing decubital sores.

In severe cases, corrective farriery can be an important component to the treatment of hyperextension of the digit.[21] Farriery treatment consists of trimming the heel to elongate the weight-bearing surface and to give a flat surface on which the foal can bear weight. In mild cases of flexor tendon laxity, this will reduce the foal's tendency to rock back onto its heel bulbs. For more severe cases, a caudal heel extension is necessary (Figure 9-8).

Selection of an appropriate extension will depend upon the materials that one has available. Ideally the extension should extend one to two inches behind the heel bulbs, and it should be made of material strong enough not to bend during weight bearing. The width should be similar to that of the foot. Curtis and Stoneham described the use of 5- to 7-mm-thick aluminum plating, but aluminum or steel hinges may be more readily obtainable.[3,22] The aluminum is bent to extend partway up the dorsum of the foot and then along the sole of the foot. Application of the rigid extension to the hoof is facilitated with the use of hoof

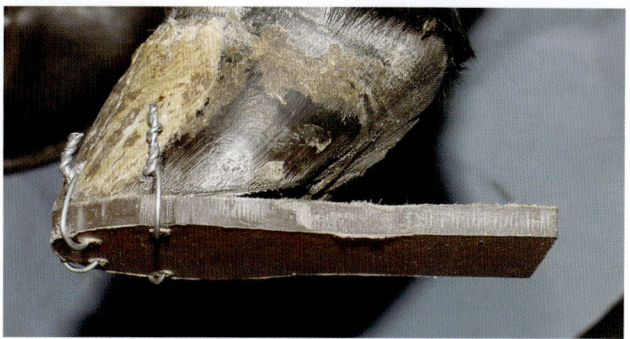

Fig. 9-8 Caudal heel extensions are helpful in reducing the foal's tendency to rock back onto its heels in cases of flexure tendon laxity.

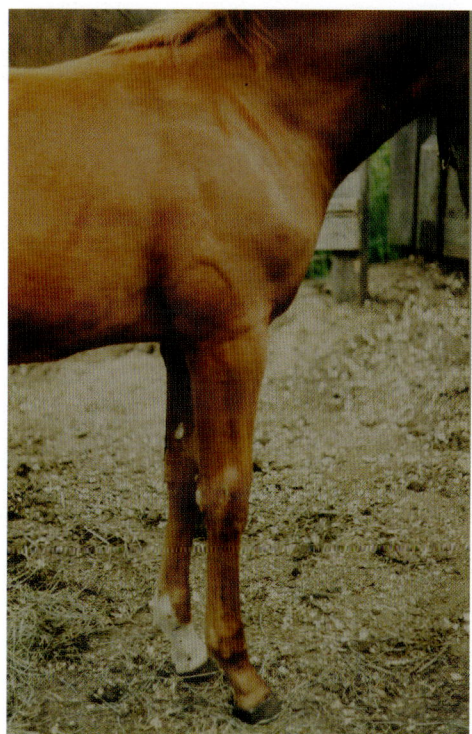

Fig. 9-9 '03 UpTight at three months of age.

repair composite with or without fiberglass strengthening cloth incorporated in it. Taping with elastic tape or duct tape may also be used, but generally results in the extension becoming loose and ineffective. Custom glue-on shoes (Baby Glu, Mustad, Inc.) may be devised. However, the need to use them has decreased with the available hoof wall composites. In the neonate, nailed-on or wired-on shoes can be problematic as there is little hoof wall to safely nail to.[22] Shoes attached in this manner often pulled off because of the softness of the hoof wall.

If caudal heel extensions are necessary on the forefeet, the length of the extension versus the risk of the foal overreaching with the hindlimb and removing the extension will need to be evaluated on an individual case basis. It may also be necessary to pad or bandage these forelimb caudal extensions so that they do not result in injury. Exercise will also hasten the correction.

Nonsteroidal anti-inflammatories should be used judiciously during the correction of congenital flexural deformities. Invasive as well as conservative treatments may result in pain, as shortened musculotendinous units, ligaments, and joint capsule is stretched.[1,8,9]

At 10 weeks of age, the foal's carpal flexural limb deformities had completely resolved. At three months of age, the foal's conformation was considered normal (Figure 9-9). White hair blemishes over her accessory carpal bones, secondary to bandaging pressure sores, are the only remaining remnants of her previous problem.

OUTCOME

Successful outcome is typical for mild to moderate carpal contractures although, as demonstrated by this case, perseverance may be necessary. Similar positive outcomes are seen in foals with mild to moderate deformities of the fetlock and distal interphalangeal joints treated conservatively and with those requiring inferior or superior check ligament desmotomy.[23-25] Outcome in foals with severe flexion of the carpus (carpal angle ≤90°) often will not improve regardless of treatment, including surgery.[9] Foals with hyperextension problems usually improve on a daily basis as the animal matures and strengthens. In some cases the foal continues to be hyperextended for weeks despite aggressive shoeing attempts. Again persistence is important. Special attention should be paid to maintaining hoof balance in these foals as they grow.

REFERENCES

1. Wagner PC, Reed SM, Hegreberg GA: Contracted tendons (flexural deformities) in the young horse, *Comp Cont Ed Pract Vet* 4:S101, 1982.
2. Embertson RM: Congenital abnormalities of tendons and ligaments, *Vet Clin North Am Equine Pract* 10:351, 1994.
3. McIllwraith CW: In Stashak TS, ed: *Adams' lameness in horses*, ed 5, Philadelphia, 2002, Lippincott Williams & Wilkins, 598.
4. Auer JA: Flexural deformities. In Auer JA, Stick JA, eds: *Equine surgery*, ed 2, Philadelphia, 1999, WB Saunders, 752.
5. Baker JR, Lindsay JR: Equine goiter due to excess iodine, *J Am Vet Med Assoc* 153:1618, 1968.
6. Pritchard JT, Voss JL: Fetal ankylosis in horses associated with hybrid sudan grass pasture, *J Am Vet Med Assoc* 150:871, 1967.
7. Rooney JR: Contracted foals, *Cornell Vet* 56:172, 1996.
8. Hay WP, Mueller POE: Flexural deformity. In Colahan PT, Mayhew IG, Merritt AM et al, eds: *Equine medicine and surgery*, ed 5, St Louis, 1999, Mosby.
9. Adams SB, Santschi EM: Management of flexural deformities in young horses, *Equine Pract* 21:9, 1999.
10. Arnbjerg J: Changes in the distal phalanx in foals with deep digital flexor tendon contraction, *Vet Radiol* 29:65, 1988.
11. Johnson JH: Contracted tendons, *Mod Vet Pract* 54:67, 1973.
12. Lokai MD: Case selection for medical management of congenital flexural deformities in foals, *Equine Pract* 14:23, 1992.
13. Lokai MD, Meyer RJ: Preliminary observations on oxytetracycline treatment of congenital flexural deformities in foals, *Mod Vet Pract* 66:237, 1985.
14. Madison JB, Garber JL, Rice BS et al: Effect of oxytetracycline on metacarpophalangeal and distal interphalangeal joint angles in newborn foals, *J Am Vet Med Assoc* 204:246, 1994.
15. Pittinger C, Adamson R: Antibiotic blockade of neuromuscular function, *Annu Rev Pharmacol* 12:169, 1972.
16. Vivrette S, Cowgill LD, Pascoe J et al: Hemodialysis for treatment of oxytetracycline-induced acute renal failure in a neonatal foal, *J Am Vet Med Assoc* 203:105, 1993.
17. Kelly NJ, Watrous BJ, Wagner PC: Comparison of splinting and casting on the degree of laxity induced in the thoracic limbs in young horses, *Equine Pract* 9:10, 1987.
18. Wagner PC: Flexural deformity of the carpus. In White NA, Moore JN, eds: *Current practice of equine surgery*, Philadelphia, 1990, JB Lippincott.
19. Whitehair KJ, Adams SB, Toombs JP et al: Arthrodesis for congenital flexural deformity of the metacarpophalangeal and metatarsophalangeal joints, *Vet Surg* 22:228, 1992.
20. Fackelman Ge, Auer JA, Orsini J et al: Surgical treatment of severe flexural deformity of the distal interphalangeal joint in young horses, *J Am Vet Med Assoc* 182:949, 1983.
21. Flecker RH, Wagner PC: Therapy and corrective shoeing for equine tendon disorders, *Comp Cont Ed Pract Vet* 8:970, 1986.
22. Curtis SJ, Stoneham S: Effective farriery treatment of hypoflexion tendons (severe digital hyperextension) in a foal, *Equine Vet Educ* 11:256, 1999.
23. Stick JA, Nickels FA, Williams MA: Long-term effects of desmotomy of the accessory ligament of the deep digital flexor muscle in standardbreds: 23 cases (1979-1989), *J Am Vet Med Assoc* 200:1131, 1992.
24. Wagner PC, Grant BD, Kaneps AJ et al: Long-term results of desmotomy of the accessory ligament of the deep digital flexor tendon (distal check ligament) in horses, *J Am Vet Med Assoc* 187:1351, 1985.
25. Sønnichsen HV: Subcarpal check ligament desmotomy for the treatment of contracted deep flexor tendon in foals, *Equine Vet J* 14:256, 1982.

| Case 9-2 | Foal with Forelimb Valgus Deformity | Patricia Provost |

| Case 9-3 | Foal with Incomplete Ossification of Cuboidal Bones | Patricia Provost |

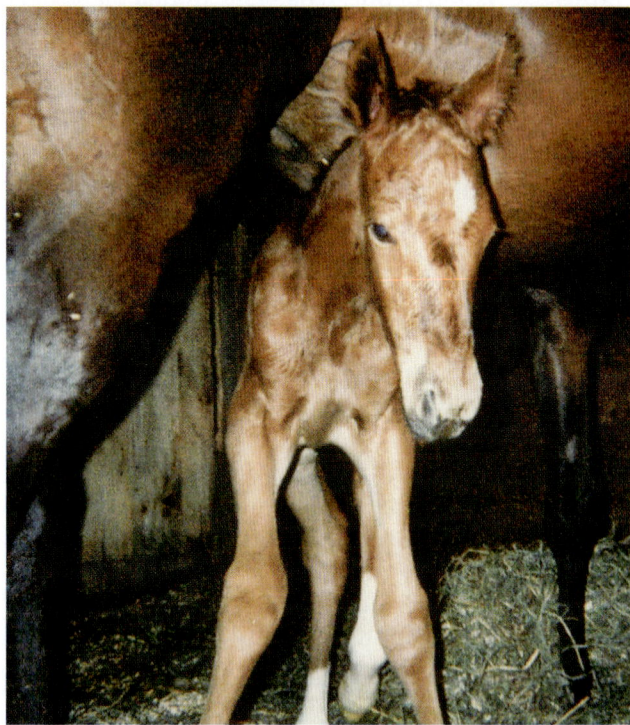

Fig. 9-10 '04 Crooked Mile born with bilateral valgus deformity of the carpi.

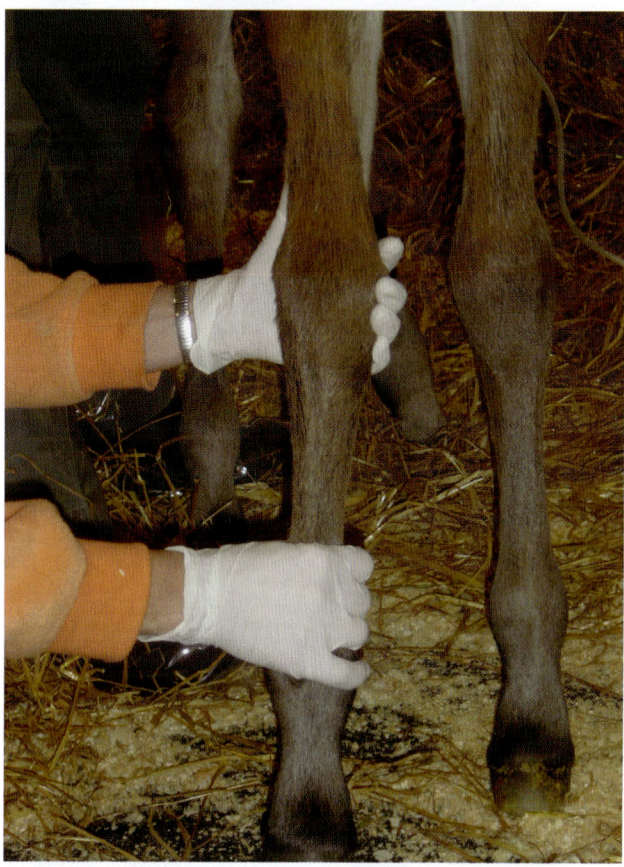

Fig. 9-11 To determine if the valgus deformity is secondary to ligament laxity, an attempt to manually straighten the leg should be made.

'04 Crooked Mile was an Arabian Warmblood cross filly who was born at term. Assistance during the foaling was necessary as the foal was presented with her head down. The foal however stood without assistance within an hour of foaling and nursed. At birth it was noted that the filly had a valgus angular limb deformity, involving both carpi (Figure 9-10). As the foal was able to rise on her own and nurse, a complete physical examination was not performed until the following day.

At 18 hours of age, the foal's vital parameters and IgG status were considered normal and adequate, respectively. The foal was active and sound, yet there was no improvement seen in the angular limb deviation since birth. An attempt was made to bring each limb into alignment, by placing one hand on the inside of the carpus and the other hand pushing the lower aspect of the cannon bone medially (Figure 9-11). Minimal improvement was gained, ruling out deviation secondary to ligament laxity. Radiographs were taken of the foal's forelimbs to determine the cause of the angular deviation.

On another farm across town, another foal had finally arrived after a long gestation. '04 Gumby, a Thoroughbred filly, was born at 367 days of gestation to an 18-year-old dam with chronic laminitis. The foaling was attended by the owner and proceeded without difficulty. Although the foal appeared vigorous, assistance was required to help her stand and nurse. She was noted to be "weak" on all four limbs, and her limbs appeared crooked (Figure 9-12, A and B).

At one day of age she was brought with her dam to the hospital for further evaluation. At presentation the foal was found to be in good health, although she was IgG deficient and small for her gestational age at 35 kg body weight. The foal's forelimbs and hindlimbs appeared to point outward while she stood or moved. The limbs, however, could be straightened manually. Laxity of the ligaments and tendons were suspected. The mare's illness, age, grain-restricted diet, and judicious use of phenylbutazone for pain control were speculated as a potential cause of the foal's problems. Based on the foal's size and

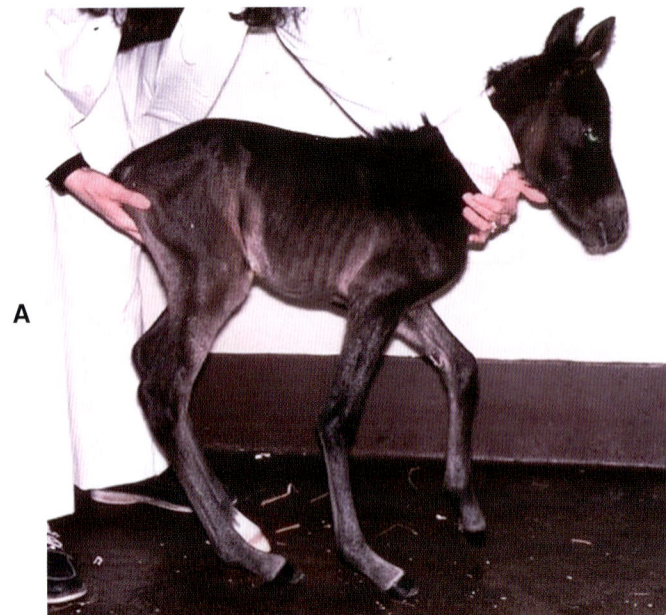

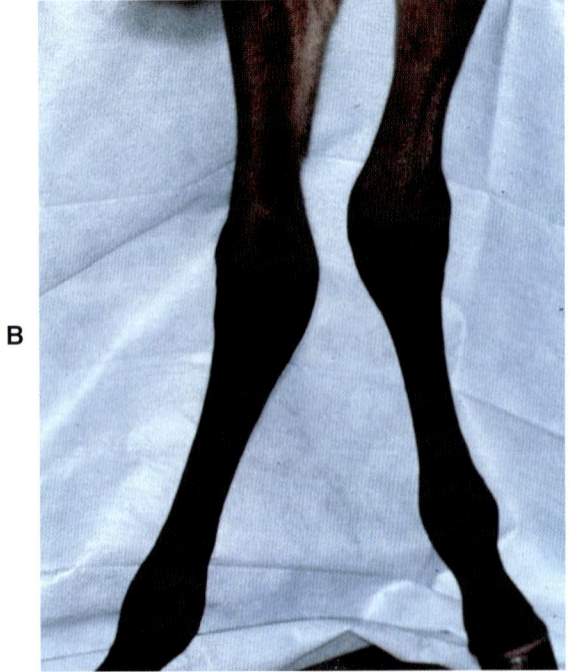

Fig. 9-12 **A,** '04 Gumby has the classic signs of intrauterine growth restriction. She is small for her gestational age of 367 days. Note the hyperextension in her forelimbs. **B,** '04 Gumby has valgus deformity of both front carpi.

the mare's history, the decision was made to obtain radiographs of her limbs. Exercise was restricted to the stall pending the imaging results.

HISTORY AND PHYSICAL EXAMINATION

All foals are born with some degree of angular limb deformity, ALD, a deviation in the long axis of the limb

recognized in the frontal plane. The job of the practitioner is to determine if the deviation is pathologic and ultimately if intervention is necessary. The above cases were selected to demonstrate two of the many different causes of ALD. Carpal valgus is the most common angular limb presentation. The distal limb deviates laterally (away from midline) from the level of the carpus. Deviation of limb axis in the frontal plane may also less commonly occur medially or toward midline (varus deformity), and either deviation may affect the carpus, tarsus and metacarpophalangeal/metatarsophalangeal joints.

In any foal with congenital malalignment of the limb axis in the frontal plane, as was seen in the above foals, two items need to be addressed at the time of presentation in order to avoid undo trauma to the neonate's joint. The first is assessment of periarticular ligament strength, and the second is assessment of the degree of ossification of the cuboidal bones that comprise the joint. Periarticular ligament laxity is easily diagnosed when present. Observe the foal standing on a level, firm, nonbedded surface by standing directly in front of the foal and then directly behind it, and observe as it moves about in the stall with its dam. A suspicion for periarticular laxity should arise if the foal's limbs sometimes look normal and at other times look crooked when the foal stops and stands. To confirm the suspicion, an attempt to manually straighten the limb should be made. This can be done with the foal standing or recumbent. Ligament laxity, with or without incomplete cuboidal bone ossification, is present if the limb can be manually straightened.

In premature (<320 days of gestation) and dysmature foals, incomplete ossification of the cuboidal bones should be suspected regardless of whether or not there is ligament laxity. Incomplete ossification of the cuboidal bones is a potential rule-out in the small '04 Gumby foal despite the gestational period of 367 days and its vigor. The dam of the foal suffered from chronic laminitis and spent many days recumbent, on medication, and on a restricted carbohydrate diet. It is possible that the health of the dam may have influenced the rate of foal maturity and prolonged gestation. The small size of the foal, despite prolonged gestation, is also suggestive of possible placental insufficiency and IUGR. Determination of cuboidal bone ossification is warranted and is rightly pursued prior to allowing the foal uncontrolled exercise to prevent cartilage damage. Determining cuboidal bone ossification should also be pursued in neonates born with moderate or severe ALD and in those that have normal conformation at birth but develop ALD shortly thereafter.

Additionally, during the physical examination the affected limb or limbs should be palpated for swelling and/or heat and the foal observed for lameness.

Trauma and/or infection should be suspected in limbs that are painful, and it should be investigated further rather than assuming that the foal has a simple ALD. At the completion of the examination, the veterinarian should have a feeling for the degree of deviation present (mild, moderate, or severe), the site of origin, and whether or not further diagnostics are warranted at the time.

PATHOGENESIS

The pathogenesis of congenital ALD has been classified as multifactorial in origin. Nutrition, placental blood flow, hypothyroidism, genetics, intra-uterine positioning, presence of twinning, and gestational age at birth have all been discussed as possible factors.[1-3] At birth, due to the narrow width of the foal's chest, carpal valgus deviation is anticipated. The point of the elbow adducts to rest against the chest wall, which results in the radius and distal limb rotating outward. The foal will stand with its front feet toed-out. In the presence of normal bone structure, as the foal's chest widens during growth, the elbow rests more laterally and the axis of the limb straightens. This process occurs in two phases. Partial correction of the limb occurs within four months of age followed by a hiatus until the foal is 8 to 10 months of age. At this time, there is a growth spurt in the lateral aspect of the distal radial physis.[4] This is normal bone growth in the average foal, and little intervention is necessary.

In a small subset of foals, aberrant bone development or bone growth exists or develops secondary to trauma that results in a more severe ALD or perpetuation of that present at birth. Long bone growth occurs primarily at the physis through the process known as endochondral ossification. Through this process, germinal cells develop and are later calcified through an elaborate process of ossification that is influenced by weight bearing.[5,6] All or just a few of the germinal cells within the physis can be affected and long bone growth interrupted. When germinal cells are injured on the lateral aspect of the physis, those located medially continue to produce bone at a normal rate and a valgus deformity develops. A varus deformity develops when the injury involves the medial aspect of the physis.

In the normal foal, the stress of weight bearing is distributed evenly along the physis, the epiphysis, and through the joint. In foals that are allowed unrestricted exercise and are born with ligamentous laxity, incomplete cuboidal bone ossification, or moderate to severe ALD secondary to pre-existing disproportionate physeal growth, the distribution of stress across the joint and physis is altered resulting in physeal and/or cuboidal bone injury. Excessive pressure within the physis affects the blood supply to both the epiphyseal and metaphyseal side of the physis.[5,6] Decreased growth occurs secondary to the retarded production of chondrocytes as well as retardation of the maturation and calcification process.

Ossification of the cuboidal bones that comprise the carpus and tarsus is a process that begins during the last two months of gestation and is completed when the foal is approximately one month of age. Ossification starts in the center of these bones at around 260 days and expands radially.[7,8] In general, by 300 days of gestation all bones of the carpus and tarsus are visible radiographically but they are still surrounded thickly with precursor cartilage and appear rounded radiographically. At term, bones have their normal adult shape morphologically, but have a wider appearing joint space radiographically as a result of the remaining precursor cartilage. Until ossification is complete, injury to these cartilaginous templates can occur secondary to compressive and shearing forces that occur normally during stance and exercise. Uneven load pressure can result in deformation of the bone, possible fracture (most common in the tarsus), and degeneration of joint cartilage with progression to arthritis.[9-11]

Acquired ALD may also occur in the newborn. Reported predisposing factors include poor conformation, improper nutrition, excessive exercise, increased weight bearing due to lameness in another limb, external trauma, and hematogenous osteomyelitis of the physis.[1] Any cause for abnormal weight distribution across the joint results in areas of increased stress concentration. Microfractures and compression or crushing of the physis may occur in these cases as well in foals subjected to excessive exercise. These injuries, classified as Salter Harris type V fractures, affect the hypertrophic and calcifying layers of the physis, causing an alteration of metaphyseal blood supply and subsequent failure of calcification and decrease in growth at the injured site.[12] The side of the physis that encounters these abnormal forces has a decreased rate in growth, while the other side continues at a normal rate, resulting in ALD.

Neither foal was found to be lame on the physical examination, therefore, trauma and sepsis were considered unlikely causes for their ALD. However, both presentations should raise concern that secondary injury to the joints or physes may occur. Visually, '04 Crooked Mile has moderate carpal valgus of the right forelimb and mild valgus of the left forelimb. Determination of the site of the deviation, especially in the right limb, can help to formulate a plan of action, which may possibly involve only conscientious observation, but the decision to do so becomes founded. '04 Gumby represents the opposite end of the spectrum. The foal is weak, small, and with liga-ment laxity is at the greatest risk of injuring her joints and physes. Further diagnostics are a requirement and not an option.

DIAGNOSTIC TESTS

So how does one decide if the degree of ALD present is within normal limits? Although the diagnosis of ALD is routinely based on clinical inspection, defini-tive diagnosis of the origin and extent of the deformity is based upon radiographic geometric and morpho-logic analysis.[13] Radiographs of the limb should be taken with the foal fully weight bearing. Allow the foal to stand normally without trying to improve the stance by manually placing the limb. At minimum, two views should be obtained, a dorsopalmar/plantar (DP) view and a lateral to medial view. Images should be obtained that include as much of the long bone above and below the joint as is possible. Seven-inch-wide by 17-inch-long cassettes are necessary for carpal and tarsal imaging. Shorter cassettes can be used for the fetlock region.

The DP images are used for geometric analysis, while morphologic analysis is facilitated using both views. In evaluating the carpus using the DP view, a clear acetate sheet is placed over the radiograph. Then one line is drawn to bisect the long axis of the radius, and a second line is drawn to bisect the long axis of the metacarpus. The point at which the two lines inter-sect is traditionally considered to be the "origin" of the deviation. The angle formed by these two lines (pivot point angle) is the degree of limb deviation (Figure 9-13). A 5° to 7° pivot point angle is generally consid-ered normal for the foal up to four months of age.[4] However, careful inspection of the carpus should be performed as significant changes in the shape of the bones can exist despite the foal having a "normal" pivot point angle.[14] Differential growth rates of indi-vidual cuboidal bones secondary to differences in bone compression during weight bearing can result in a variety of bony changes within the joint that may be thought insignificant if only the pivot point angle is determined.

Changes in limb angulation can be further defined through the measurement of deviation within each specific joint (e.g., carpometacarpal, middle carpal, and radiocarpal joint).[14] Lines are drawn on the acetate film through the distal radial physis and the radiocarpal, middle carpal, and carpometacarpal joints. An angle of deviation for each individual joint is then determined by measuring the angle formed from the intersection of a line bisecting the long axis of the metacarpal bone with those of each carpal joint and the physis (Figure

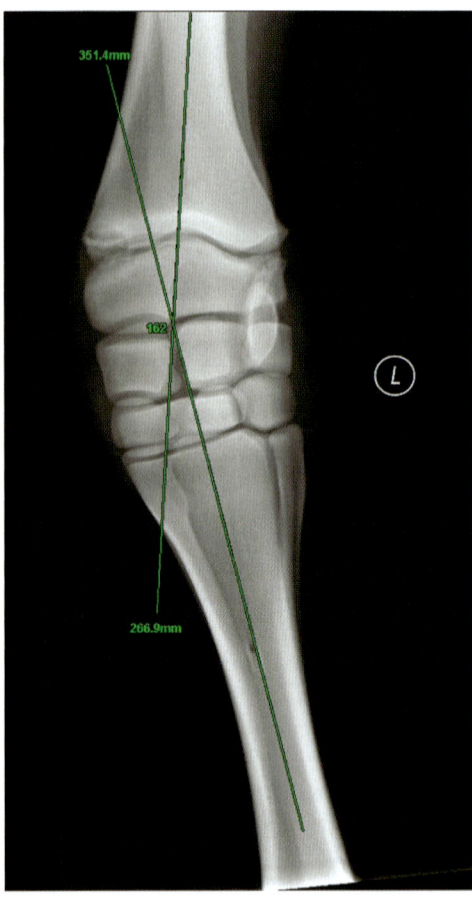

Fig. 9-13 Radiographs with the pivot point of the valgus defor-mity at the level of the radiocarpal joint by the traditional method of measurment.

9-14). Brauer and colleagues reported that 62% of their study cases had deviation occurring from within the carpal joints in addition to the physis.[14] Location of the origin of deviation is important as it may better eluci-date the reason for the deformity, which may affect prognosis as well as treatment.

Morphologically, several changes may be seen. These changes include asymmetric width of the distal radial physis, metaphyseal or epiphyseal flaring, asymmetric width of the epiphysis, diaphyseal remod-eling, incomplete cuboidal bone ossification, evidence of trauma, and remodeling of adjacent bones.[15] Addi-tional radiographic views are often required.

Determining deviation of the metacarpopha-langeal/metatarsophalangeal joints and the tarsus can be more challenging. In foals with carpal valgus, metacarpophalangeal valgus deformity can often be mistakenly diagnosed because of the foal's toed-out appearance. However, using similar methodology as above for the carpus, lines drawn to bisect the metacar-pus and the first phalanx will eliminate the confusion (Figure 9-15). Deviation originating at the level of the fetlock accounts only for approximately 12% of foal ALD, and most commonly this deviation will be

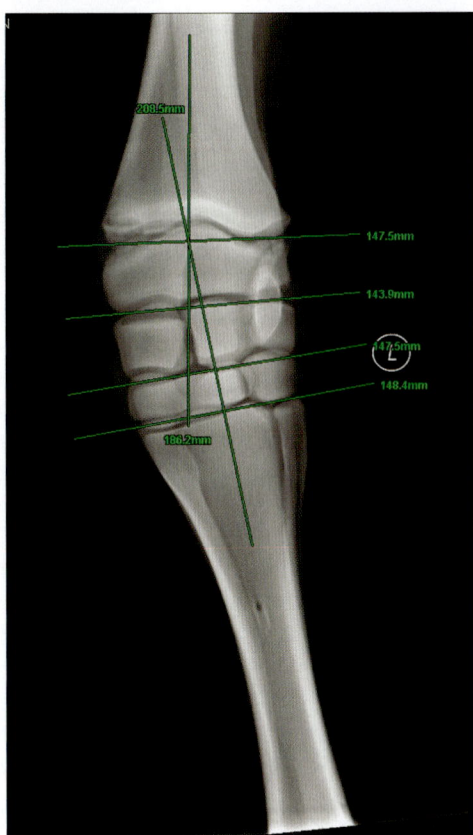

Fig. 9-14 Changes in limb angulation can be further defined through measurement of deviation within each specific joint in comparison to a line bisecting the metatarsus.

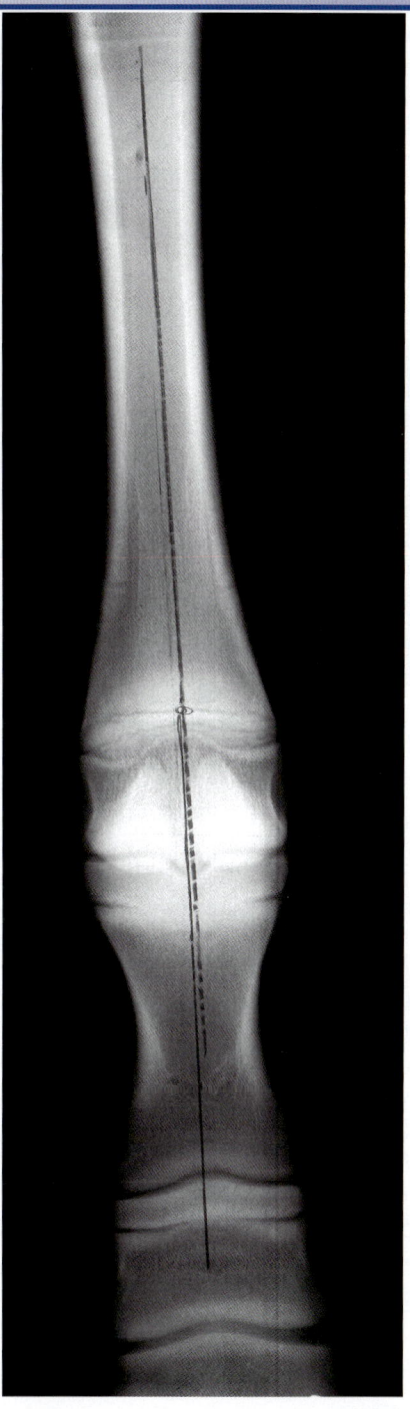

Fig. 9-15 The pivot point of deviation in the fetlock can be determined radiographically by the intersection of lines bisecting the metacarpus/metatarsus and the phalangeal bones.

varus.[13,16] A strong suspicion of fetlock varus should arise when observing any foal whose toes appear to point straight forward in the presence of carpal valgus.[1,4]

Radiographs of the fetlock region can be obtained with the foal weight bearing or with the foot elevated through support of the forearm. The latter view eliminates the influence of an unbalanced foot on fetlock angle in weight-bearing views. More than a few degrees of deviation at the fetlock is cause for concern because the window for nature or surgical intervention to correct the deviation is narrow.[17]

ALDs involving the tarsus are the least common. When present, the deviation is generally valgus.[13,16] Determination of the degree of angular deviation is difficult because the tibia, tarsus, and lower limb are not within the same frontal plane.[1] More important are the results of the lateral view. In the neonate, incomplete ossification of the tarsal bones can lead to wedging of the central and third tarsal bones and a curby appearance to the joint. Collapse or fracture of the central and/or third tarsal bone followed by osteoarthritis of the joint may develop if the condition goes undiagnosed[18] (Figure 9-16). Clinically the foal may appear to be sickle hocked and/or have tarsal valgus. Lameness in the form of a bunny hop gait may be present.[1] When examining for incomplete ossification, a lateral to medial radiograph should be obtained of both hocks as normal ossification in one does not preclude its absence in the other.[18] Oblique views are also important as collapse may only be seen on the anterior medial view.

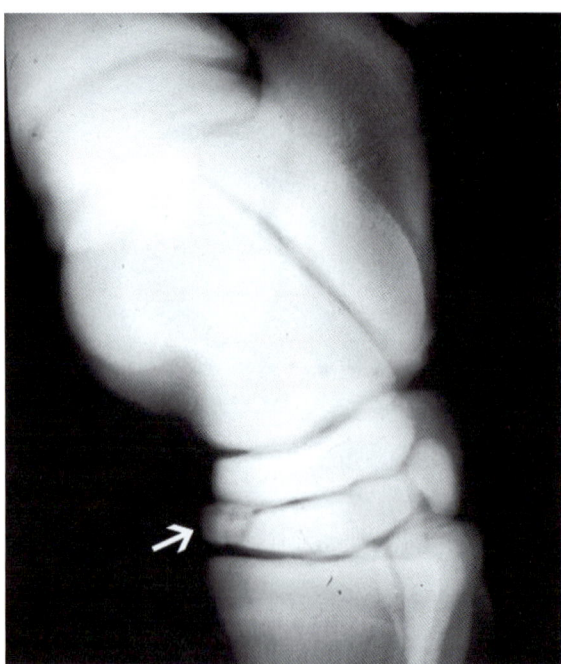

Fig. 9-16 Lateral radiographs of the tarsus with "crushing" of third tarsal bone.

Applying the above methodology to radiographs taken of '04 Crooked Mile's forelimbs, a 9° deviation was present at the level of the right front distal radial physis and a 6° deviation was present at the level of the left front distal radial physis. Radiographs were initially taken of '04 Gumby's carpi, but it became clear that views of her tarsi were also in order. Marked cuboidal bone hypoplasia is present. Due to the ligament laxity and the incomplete ossification, determination of pivot point intersection and angle is inappropriate (Figure 9-17, A).

TREATMENT

Determining the need for intervention can be simplified by following the outline below keeping in mind the age of the foal, the growth rates of the long bones involved, and the severity of the deformity. Hoof trimming or corrective shoeing is often an adjunct to either conservative or surgical therapy. The goal is to provide solar medial to lateral balance. With valgus deformities, the medial side of the hoof becomes worn down more quickly, and it is generally necessary to rasp or trim the lateral wall to balance the hoof. The opposite is true with varus deformities. Corrective shoeing using glue-on shoes or epoxy can be used but should not be used so that they create an imbalance to the hoof.[19,20]

1. Is the angular deformity a result of ligament laxity?
   - deformity present at birth
   - fluctuates between valgus, normal, and varus
   - no lameness
   - can manually straighten the limb axis
   - no radiographic abnormalities

   Treatment Goal: Prevent abnormal weight bearing on the physis and joint until ligamentous laxity resolves.

   Treatment: In mild cases of ligamentous laxity, exercise restriction is all that is necessary. The mare and foal should be allowed short periods (10 to 15 minutes) of small paddock (20 × 20 feet) exercise separate from others (or handwalked) several times a day, but should remain stalled the remainder of the time. A few days to one week usually suffices. With moderate to severe periarticular laxity, the affected joint(s) should be stabilized with splints or bandages until the laxity resolves (generally one to two weeks). Coaptation should extend from the elbow to directly above the fetlock, or stifle to directly above the fetlock if a hindlimb. The fetlock and foot are not incorporated to avoid flexor tendon laxity. Bandages and splints should be changed daily to avoid the development of pressure sores over bony prominences. If progressive improvement is not seen within 10 to 14 days, the case should be reassessed.

2. Is there incomplete ossification of the carpal or tarsal bones?
   - foal may be premature or dysmature
   - deformity may be present at birth or may develop shortly thereafter
   - ligamentous laxity may or may not be present
   - radiographically ossification is incomplete leading to the absence of calcified cuboidal bones or more rounded cuboidal bones and widened appearance of the joint spaces.

   Treatment Goal: Eliminate abnormal compressive and shearing forces on the immature bones until they ossify.

   Treatment: Foals with mild incomplete ossification and straight limbs can be managed successfully with stall rest alone. These foals should be observed daily for any change in their conformation that would necessitate a change in plans. They should be re-radiographed at two-week intervals. When ossification is sufficient, a normal exercise routine can begin. However, if there is a more pronounced lack of ossification, concomitant periarticular ligament laxity, or the foal does not have a straight limb, then more aggressive intervention is necessary. To prevent compression injury to the small cuboidal bones, it is necessary that the foal be placed in either bandages, bandages with

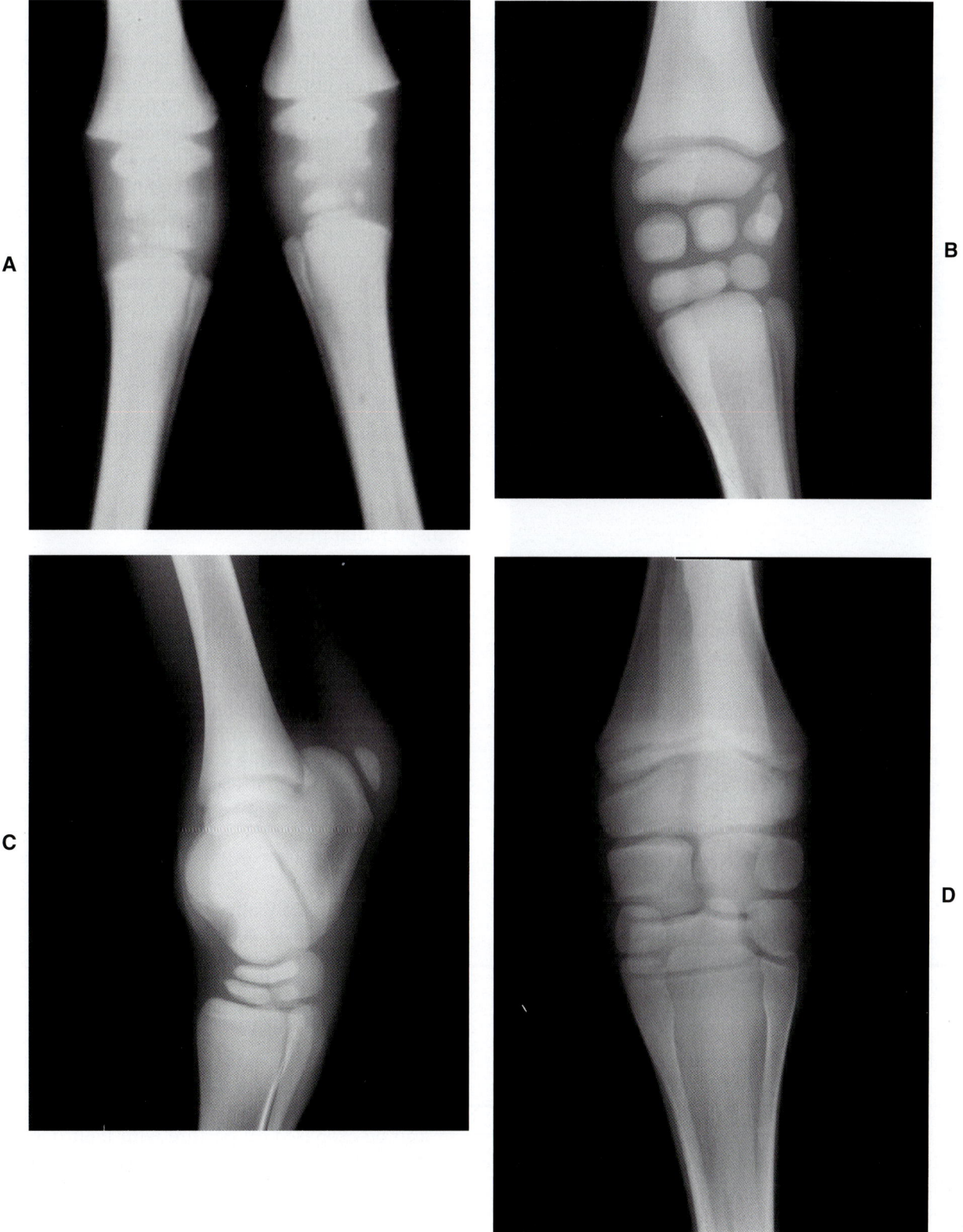

Fig. 9-17 Radiographs of '04 Gumby taken at birth, two weeks, and eight weeks of age. **A,** Incomplete ossification of carpal bones at birth. **B,** Incomplete ossification of carpal bones at two weeks. **C,** Incomplete ossification of tarsal bones at two weeks. **D,** Complete ossification of carpal bones at eight weeks.

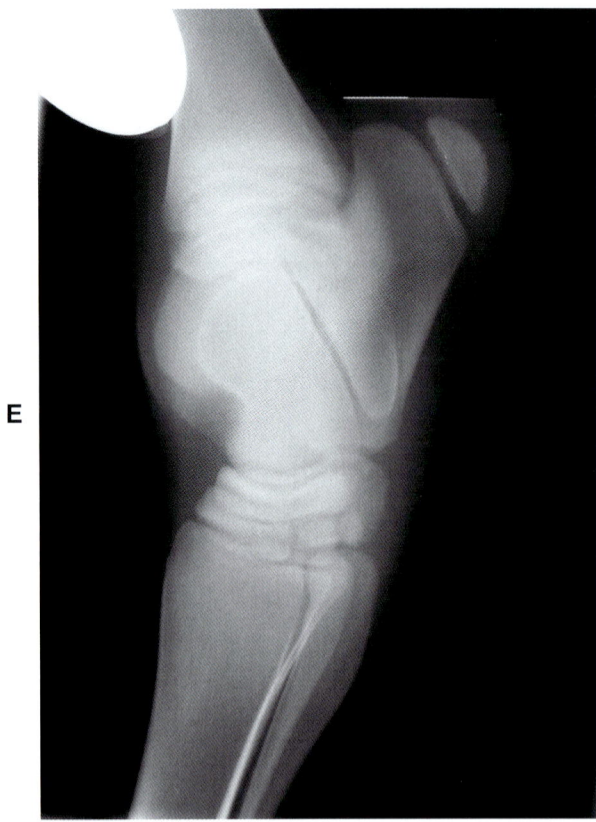

E

Fig. 9-17 E, Complete ossification of tarsal bones at eight weeks.

splints, or sleeve casts. Sleeve casts provide the most rigid support and the least amount of daily effort. However, cast sores can develop and remain undetected until removal of the cast. The use of Teflon® cast padding may decrease the risk of cast sores from developing. The foal that needs more than two limbs cast may also have a very difficult time getting up and down. Use of hindlimb casts in foals have also been associated with cox-ofemoral luxation.[21]

Bandaging the limb from the elbow to the fetlock or the stifle to the fetlock followed by placement of a rigid splint is another alternative. In the fore-limb, the splint should be placed on the palmar aspect of the limb and extend the length of the bandage. The bandage should be at least one inch thick to prevent pressure sores from developing at the top and bottom of the splint and over the palmar aspect of the accessory carpal bone. A hindlimb splint should be placed on the dorsal aspect of the limb and again is the length of the bandage. Splints may be constructed from PVC pipe cut in halves or thirds or made from fiberglass casting tape. PVC pipe can be bent with heat to match the contour of the hind limb. When con-structing a splint from fiberglass casting tape,

three- or four-inch cast material can be folded out lengthwise to the appropriate length and applied over the bandage in the appropriate position. Alternatively, a sleeve cast can be placed and then immediately cut in half and the appropriate half saved for use as a splint. Tape is then used to hold the splint in position. Bandages and splints should be changed at least every 48 hours.

With any method, close attention to the devel-opment of skin sores is imperative. Depending upon the degree of ossification, radiographs should be repeated at one- to two-week intervals. It is usually requires two to four weeks for suffi-cient ossification to occur. If using sleeve casts, the casts should be removed and replaced at two-week intervals. Additional conservative exercise for two to four weeks may be necessary following discontinuation of coaptation to allow soft tissues that will have become lax to strengthen.

3. Is the ALD a result of disproportionate growth at the distal radial physis?
   - Valgus (or less commonly varus) appearance to limb
   - Normal ligament strength
   - Radiographically normal cuboidal bones
   - Radiograph pivot point lines intersect within or adjacent to the physis

   Treatment Goal: Encourage return of synchronous physeal growth resulting in a straight limb before the time of growth plate closure.

   Treatment: The foal's age and severity of the defor-mity are important factors to consider when de-termining the management of this problem. Although closure of the distal radial physis does not occur until 22 to 36 months, the rate of growth declines substantially after six months of age.[17] During the first month of life, a foal with a physeal-based ALD should be managed conserva-tively using exercise restriction and close observa-tion. The degree of restriction will depend on the severity of the ALD. Based on the pivot point angle measurement, severity of deformity can be classi-fied as mild ($\leq 5°$), moderate ($5°$ to $10°$), or severe ($>10°$). Foals considered to have mild deformity can be exercised on pasture with their dams, but they should be observed at 30-day intervals to ensure that the limb is straightening and not becoming worse. As mentioned previously, foals with a $5°$ to $7°$ deformity at four months of age can be expected to have straight limbs as an adult.[4]

   Foals with moderate to severe carpal ALD at birth need to be confined to a stall or small paddock with their dam. This will prevent exces-sive stress/compression of the immature growth plate through uneven weight bearing during

exercise until physeal growth has a chance to respond to the forces of weight bearing.[6] In the rapid growth phase, the rate of correction (up to 0.5°/day) can be substantial just with rest alone.[5,17] Exercise restrictions can be altered as the limb straightens. If improvement is not seen within the first two to three months, surgical intervention may be necessary.

Until recently, hemicircumferential transection of the periosteum (HCTP or periosteal stripping) was the procedure of choice for foals that were less than four months of age and had moderate to severe ALD.[9] Reports surfaced in 2000 indicating that time and not the procedure's effectiveness are responsible for improvement in the limb.[22] In 2002, the outcome of a controlled study reported by Read and colleagues concluded that periosteal stripping did not alter the rate of improvement in ALD using a surgical model for physeal disproportionate growth compared to the untreated limb.[23] The 15° deformity that was created improved to 7° within eight weeks and 2.5° by 48 weeks for both the control and treated limbs. Based on practitioners' observations and results of Slone's and Read's studies, periosteal stripping is performed less commonly today.[19,22-24]

Transphyseal bridging has again become the procedure of choice for foals failing to respond as expected with conservative exercise over time and for foals that have a less than 15° ALD and are three months of age or older.[25] Intervention should also proceed if the foal is four months of age and has a more than 7° deviation. Rate of correction is considerably slower and has been estimated at 0.05° to 0.1° per day in foals 100 days of age.[5] Transphyseal bridging is most commonly achieved by placing a 4.5-mm wide, 30-mm–long cortical screw on either side on the convex side of the physis. The screws are placed through stab incisions. By tunneling beneath the skin between the two screws, two 1.2-mm (18 to 20 gauge) diameter wires are placed around the screws in a figure-eight manner. The wires are tightened to achieve tension across the physis, which in turns retards endochondral ossification. The implants are removed during a second surgical procedure (usually done in the sedated, standing foal) when the limb axis is close to being straight. Complications associated with the procedure include dehiscence of the overlying skin incision, infection at the implants, and overcorrection secondary to failing to remove the implants in a timely fashion.

Transphyseal bridging can also be accomplished using orthopedic staples placed across the physis or by using a small bone plate.[1,26] Although they are inexpensive, orthopedic staples have the disadvantage of being less cosmetic and more difficult to remove, and they have a tendency to back out of the bone.[13] Cosmetic results have been achieved with use of the orthopedic plates and the risk of implant failure is less than with screws and wires, but the cost is greater.[1]

4. Is ALD a result of disproportionate growth at the distal metacarpal/metatarsal physis or proximal phalangeal proximal physis?
   • Varus (or less commonly valgus) appearance to limb
   • Radiograph pivot point lines intersect within or adjacent to either the distal metacarpal/metatarsal physis or the proximal phalangeal physis
   Treatment Goal: Encourage synchronous physeal growth resulting in a straight limb before the time of growth plate closure.
   Treatment: The tenets of treatment are similar to those for disproportionate growth of the distal radial physis but are based on a different timeline. Effective longitudinal growth from the distal MC III/MT III physis and the proximal physis of P1 ceases by the time the foal has reached three months of age, and the period for rapid growth decreases by 10 weeks of age.[17] It is important to monitor the foal closely to have sufficient time to achieve correction of an ALD at this location. Surgery of the fetlock is best performed by one month of age in foals with a 5° deviation of and as early as one week of age in foals with a 10° or greater deviation.[25] Retrospective analysis of a two groups of foals treated by transphyseal bridging of the distal MC III physis indicated that after 60 to 80 days of age there was no improvement in the degree of deformity.[13,27]

   Using radiological assessment of long bone growth, Campbell and colleagues concluded that a maximum of 12° correction could be expected if transphyseal bridging was performed at two weeks of age.[28] Transphyseal bridging can be performed at the distal MC/T III physis and less commonly at the proximal P1 physis using the methods described above. Wedge osteotomy can be pursued in individuals with ALD unresponsive to transphyseal bridging either due to age or severity.[27,29,30]

5. Is there an ALD that arises from within the carpal joint?
   • Valgus or varus deformity
   • Possible history of ligamentous laxity
   • Possible history of incomplete ossification
   • Radiographic pivot point lines intersect within the carpus
   • Possible radiographic evidence of carpal bone wedging (C3, C4)

- Possible evidence of carpal and metacarpal bone displacement
- Possible evidence of osteoarthritis

  Treatment Goal: To minimize the effects of abnormal weight bearing through the carpal joints.

  Treatment: Identification that in part or in its entirety, the origin of deviation arises within the carpal joint is the initial step. Using methodology described by Fretz and Brauer, localization to one or all of the three joints can proceed.[13,14] However, a full radiographic series is often needed to determine which of the carpal bones are developing abnormally. Common morphologic alterations include incomplete cuboidal bone ossification, wedging of the third carpal bone, and carpal and metacarpal bone displacement.[10] Although Brauer and Bertone have published reports indicating that ALD originating totally or in part within the carpus may respond favorably to treatment directed at the physis, others still consider an intra-articular–based deviation to be associated with a poorer prognosis for athletic soundness.[4,5,15,19]

6. Is there an ALD that arises at the tarsus?
   - Most commonly valgus
   - Possible history of ligamentous laxity
   - Possible history of incomplete ossification
   - Possible radiographic evidence of central and third tarsal bone injury
   - Possible evidence of osteoarthritis

   Treatment Goal: Encourage synchronous physeal growth resulting in a straight limb before the time of growth plate closure. Eliminate abnormal compressive and shearing forces on the immature bones until they ossify.

   Treatment: ALD deformity of the tarsus is less common than deformities associated with the carpus and fetlock. The origin of the deformity may arise within region of the distal tibial growth plate or it may develop from within the joint itself. Growth discrepancies associated with the physis are treated initially with patience. Provided there is no associated pathology of the tarsal bones, disproportionate growth rates at the physis will self-correct over time to an acceptable degree of axial alignment in most instances. Similar to that of the distal radial physis, rapid growth from the distal tibial physis occurs during the initial six months, but growth plate closure does not occur until 17 to 24 months of age.[5]

   Transphyseal bridging should be considered for foals that fail to show improvement within four months of age and for those with ALD greater than 25°.[19] Incomplete ossification of the tarsal bones generally results in permanent damage to the central or third tarsal bone if undiagnosed and not treated early.[1,4,18] As mentioned above, treatment should be directed at controlling the foal's exercise and with splinting or application of sleeve casts until there is radiographically sufficient bone to withstand weight-bearing forces. If fracture or more than 30% collapse of the central and/or third tarsal bone is present, treatment is often unrewarding.[4,11,18]

7. Does the ALD arise within the diaphysis of the long bone?

   Diaphyseal deformities rarely occur but commonly involve the metacarpus or metatarsus. Recognizing that the origin of the ALD is within the diaphysis is important, as treatment with manipulation of physeal growth will not lead to improvement. In some neonates, four to six weeks of stall confinement will result in self-correction. A corrective osteotomy/wedge ostectomy may be warranted in some cases.[27,30]

'04 Crooked Mile was treated with just "close observation" once it was determined that the origin of severe ALD in her right limb arose from the physis and that her carpal bones in both knees were normal. Based upon the above guidelines for age and degree of deviation, it was likely that '04 Crooked Mile's limbs would improve over time just with the help of Mother Nature. The mare and foal were restricted to a small 1-acre field for the first month. Instructions were given to the owner to contact the veterinarian if the foal's conformation worsened; otherwise the foal would be re-examined when the mare was ready to rebreed. Visual inspection at the end of the month verified that the foal was improving as anticipated (Figure 9-18). At four months of age, the foal's forelimb conformation is improved significantly and can be expected to have normal adult conformation (Figure 9-19).

More intensive veterinary care was necessary for '04 Gumby. Due to the severity of cuboidal bone hypoplasia and presence of ligament laxity, it was necessary to protect the foal's joints immediately to prevent injury to the developing carpal and tarsal bones. Because all of the foal's limbs needed to be protected for at least several weeks, a decision was made to use splints and bandaging rather than placing the foal in four sleeve casts. Although ideal, the latter would have made it very difficult for her to get up and down without assistance. Using sheet cotton, four-inch gauze and Vetrap™, bandages were placed extending from the elbow/stifle to above the fetlock. PVC pipe was cut to make a palmar splint for each forelimb, and fiberglass casting tape was used to make a custom dorsal splint for each hindlimb. For the first two weeks, splinting was alternated between contralateral limb pairs on a daily basis with the opposite pair being more heavily bandaged. In this manner, the

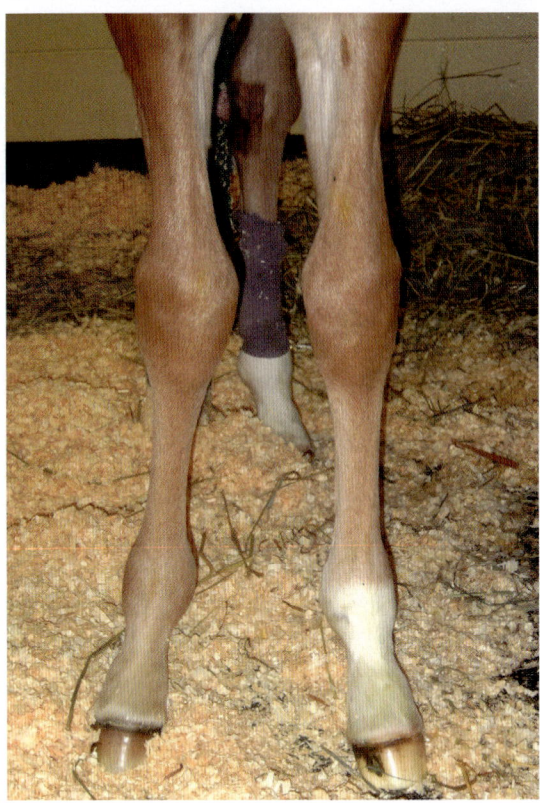

Fig. 9-18 '04 Crooked Mile at one month of age.

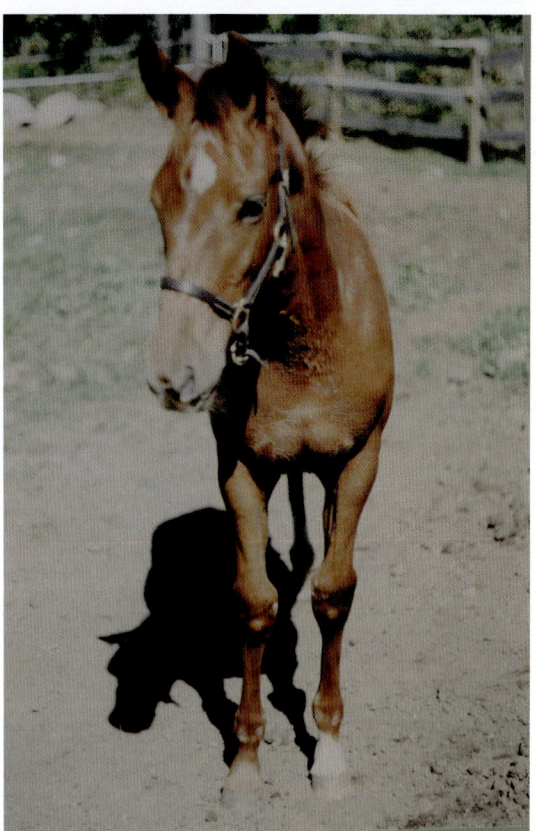

Fig. 9-19 '04 Crooked Mile at four months of age.

foal was able to rise with less assistance. Mare and foal were stall confined.

At two weeks, radiographs were taken (Figure 9-17, B and C). Improvement was greater in the carpi than in the tarsi. Ligament laxity in the forelimbs had also improved during the two weeks. For the following two weeks, bandages without splints were used on the foal's forelimbs, while both splints and bandages continued to be used on the hindlimbs. At four weeks of age, it was possible to discontinue splinting the hindlimbs. Light bandages were maintained for an additional week. Hand-walking with the dam started during this week, and the following week short periods of paddock turnout were begun. Radiographs were obtained at two months of age that revealed the presence of normal bone ossification and pivot point angles within normal limits (Figure 9-17, D and E). Although the foal is currently sound, arthritis secondary to cartilage injury from early weight bearing stress is still a potential possibility. Early intervention has hopefully minimized the risk.

OUTCOME

As is evident from the above cases and text, ALDs in the neonate vary in their origin and severity. Ultimately, whether or not a foal's limbs straighten and the

foal develops into an athletically sound adult is dependent upon many things the veterinarian and/or owner can influence, as well as things they cannot influence. Based upon our current level of knowledge, most foals born with an ALD have the ability for normal physeal growth and will require only conscientious observation and a restriction in exercise. Mother Nature does the rest. Studies that reported outcomes of ALD foals treated with periosteal stripping provide evidence of this. In a case series published by Bertone and colleagues, of 27 foals (41 limbs; 35-carpal region, 5-MT III, 1-distal tibia) the degree of ALD ranged from less than 5° to more than 20°.[31] When this case information is re-evaluated in light of today's current understanding of periosteal stripping, it can be inferred that improvement occurs, even in the absence of the more definitive surgery of transphyseal bridging: 12° carpal ALD present at two months of age, 20° carpal ALD present at two months of age, 29° carpal ALD present at three months of age, 10° carpal ALD at six months of age, 15° carpal ALD at seven months of age, and 25° carpal ALD at six months of age, etc. were classified as having straight limbs at follow-up.[31]

Although ALD involving the fetlock may improve with conservative exercise over time, a successful outcome is less likely because of the differences in the duration of effective long bone growth and growth plate closure. Transphyseal bridging of the distal MT/MC III physis is often necessary. To achieve success, Fretz recommended intervention with transphyseal bridging in foals before they reach four weeks of age and only when the ALD is less than 10°.[25] Bertone, however, reported improvement in foals older than four weeks of age that were treated with transphyseal bridging, and improvement even when pivot point angles exceeded 10°.[31] There is widespread agreement, however, that it is always better to proceed with surgery as early as possible when treating disproportionate growth of the distal MC/MT III physis.[4,19,32]

Axial realignment, however, does not always equal athletic success. Of 29 foals, Bertone reported 83% being sound for their intended use but only 59% were in performance training.[31] In a larger study of 199 Thoroughbreds treated by periosteal stripping, the results indicate that treated ALD foals did not have the same ability to start a race as did their siblings.[33] Additionally, the study indicated that starts percentile ranking between the treated and normal conformation foals was significantly less for foals treated with distal radius periosteal stripping and for foals requiring treatment of two anatomic sites when compared with their siblings. However, foals with ALD of the distal aspect of the MC/MT III were as successful as their siblings with presumed normal conformation.[33] It is unknown whether or not injury to immature carpal bones secondary to uneven weight-bearing forces in the neonate may have prematurely predisposed these racehorses to arthritis. Pharr and Fretz also reported more favorable results with fetlock ALD versus intercarpal ALD.[15]

In summary, the key to successful management of ALD in foals is understanding the potential complications associated with ligament laxity and cuboidal bone hypoplasia and providing prompt intervention when either or both are present. It is equally important to appreciate that some degree of ALD is normal in foals and these animals can mature into athletically sound adults.

REFERENCES

1. Auer JA: Angular limb deformities. In Auer JA, Stick JA, eds: Equine surgery, Philadelphia, 1999, WB Saunders, 736-752.
2. Shaver JR, Fretz PB, Doige CE et al: Skeletal manifestations of suspected hyperthyroidism in foals, Eq Vet Med 3:269, 1979.
3. Mason TA: A high incidence of congenital angular limb deformities in a group of foals, Vet Rec 109:93, 1981.
4. Bramlage LR, Embertson RM: Observations on the evaluation and selection of foal limb deformities for surgical treatment. In Proceedings, 36th Annu Meet Am Assoc Equine Pract 273, 1990.
5. Fretz PB: Angular limb deformities in foals. Vet Clin of North Am: Large Animal Practice 2:125, 1980.
6. Frost HM: Structural adaptations to mechanical usage. A proposed three way rule for bone remodeling, Vet Comp Ortho Trauma 2:80, 1988.
7. McLaughlin BG, Dioge CE: A study of ossification of carpal and tarsal bones in normal and hypothyroid foals, Can Vet J 23:164, 1982.
8. Soana S, Gnudi G, Bertoni G et al: Anatomo-radiographic study on the osteogenesis of carpal and tarsal bones in horse fetus, Anat Histol Embryol 27:301, 1998.
9. Auer JA, Mathers RJ: Hemicircumferential transection of the periosteum and periosteal stripping: Experimental and clinical evaluation of a new method for correction of angular limb deformities in foals, Proc Ann Mtg ACVS, San Diego, 1982.
10. McLaughlin BG, Doige CE, Fretz PB et al: Carpal bone lesions associated with angular limb deformities in foals, J Am Vet Med Assoc 178:224, 1981.
11. Dutton DM, Watkins JP, Honnas CM et al: Treatment response and athletic outcome of foals with tarsal valgus deformities: 39 cases (1988-1997), J Am Vet Med Assoc 215:1481, 1999.
12. Salter RB, Harris WR: Injuries involving the epiphyseal plate, J Bone Joint Surg 45A:587, 1963.
13. Fretz PB, Turner SA, Pharr J: Retrospective comparison of two surgical techniques for correction of angular limb deformities in foals, J Am Vet Med Assoc 172:281, 1978.
14. Brauer TS, Booth TS, Riedesel E: Physeal growth retardation leads to correction of intracarpal angular deviations as well as physeal valgus deformity, Equine Vet J 31:193, 1999.
15. Pharr JW, Fretz PB: Radiographic findings in foals with angular deformities, J Am Vet Med Assoc 179:812, 1981.
16. Gaughan EM: Angular limb deformities in the horse, Comp Cont Educ Pract Vet 20:944, 1998.
17. Fretz PB, Cymbaluk NF, Pharr JW: Quantitative analysis of long-bone growth in the horse, Am J Vet Res 45:1602, 1984.
18. Dutton DM, Watkins JP, Walker MA et al: Incomplete ossification of the tarsal bones in foals: 22 cases (1988-1996), J Am Vet Med Assoc 213:1590, 1998.
19. Greet TRC: Managing flexural and angular limb deformities: The Newmarket perspective, AAEP Proceedings 46:130, 2000.
20. Stashak TS, Hill C, Klimesh R et al: Trimming and shoeing for balance and soundness; Proper limb development in foals. In Stashak TS, ed: Adams' lameness in horses, ed 5, Philadelphia, 2002, Lippincott Williams & Wilkins, 1140.
21. Trotter GW: Coxofemoral luxation in two foals wearing hind limb casts, J Am Vet Med Assoc 189:560, 1986.
22. Slone DE, Roberts CT, Hughes FE: Restricted exercise and transphyseal bridging for correction of angular limb deformities, Proc Am Assoc Equine Pract 46:126, 2000.
23. Read EK, Read MR, Townsend HG et al: Effect of hemicircumferential periosteal transaction and elevation in foals with experimentally induced angular limb deformities, J Am Vet Med Assoc 221:536, 2002.
24. Wilson DG: Periosteal stripping: Does it work?, Proc 12th Ann Vet Symposium ACVS 142, 2002.
25. Fretz PB, Donecker JM: Surgical correction of angular limb deformities in foals: A retrospective study, J Am Vet Med Assoc 183:529, 1983.
26. Heinze CD: Epiphyseal stapling—a surgical technique for correction of angular limb deformities, Proc Am Assoc Equine Pract 15:59, 1969.

27. Bramlage LR: Step ostectomy: A surgical technique for correction of permanent angular limb deformities in horses, *Am Assoc Equine Pract* 111, 1994.

28. Campbell JR, Lee R: Radiological estimation of differential growth rates of the long bones of foals, *Equine Vet J* 13:247, 1981.

29. Fretz PB, McIlwraith CW: Wedge osteotomy as a treatment for angular deformity of the fetlock in horses, *J Am Vet Med Assoc* 182:245, 1983.

30. White KK: Diaphyseal angular limb deformities in foals, *J Am Vet Med Assoc* 182:272, 1983.

31. Bertone AL, Turner AS, Park RD: Periosteal transaction and stripping for treatment of angular limb deformities in foals: Clinical observations, *J Am Vet Med Assoc* 187:145, 1985.

32. Hunt RJ: Management of angular limb deformities, *AAEP Proceedings* 46:128, 2000.

33. Mitten LA, Bramlage LR, Embertson RM: Racing performance after hemicircumferential periosteal transaction for angular limb deformities in Thoroughbreds: 199 cases (1987-1989), *J Am Vet Med Assoc* 207:746, 1995.

10 Neurologic Dysfunctions

| Case 10-1 | Foal with Hypoxic Encephalopathy | Mary Rose Paradis |

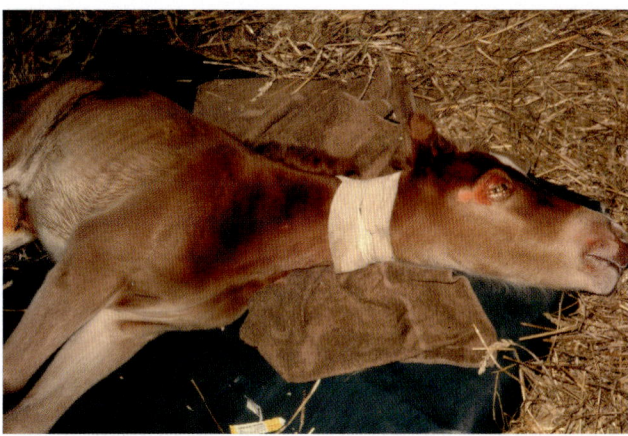

Fig. 10-1 '05 Carpe Diem seizing at presentation. Note the abrasions around his eyes.

'05 Carpe Diem was born without much fuss at 8 AM. In fact, the delivery was swift with the placenta being expelled within 10 minutes of parturition. The 50 kg colt was standing within 60 minutes and nursing by 90 minutes. The owner was relieved and left the mare and foal alone for a few hours to bond. When the owner returned, the foal was standing in the back of the stall looking a little dazed. When approached, the foal made no effort to escape and in fact did not appear aware of the owner's presence. Worried about what could have happened in her absence, she called her veterinarian to check out the foal.

It took the veterinarian approximately one hour to arrive at the farm. During that time, '05 Carpe Diem became recumbent and was seizing with his head thrown back in opisthotonus (Figure 10-1). The veterinarian administered 5 mg of diazepam and immediately referred the foal to a neonatal clinic for evaluation. Upon arrival to the clinic, the foal was somnolent and unresponsive. His heart rate was within normal limits, while his temperature was slightly elevated at 102.4° F. Though the foal's respiratory effort was normal, he appeared to have developed an apneustic (breath-holding) breathing pattern. Mucous membranes were pink with a capillary refill time of <2 seconds. The foal had multiple superficial abrasions around his eyes. A limited neurologic examination was performed because of the foal's mental status. During the examination, he began to show seizurelike activity manifested by extensor rigidity with opisthotonus and tonic/clonic marching activity.

NEUROLOGIC EXAMINATION IN THE NEONATAL FOAL

The goal of the neurologic examination in the neonatal foal is the same as that of the neurologic examination of the adult horse—lesion localization. Once the lesion is localized, possible etiologies can be explored. There are some unique differences in neurologic response in the neonate and the adult horse. Observation of any deviation from normal behavior patterns or timetable of behavioral events should be noted. As seen in Chapter 1, the newborn foal should assume sternal recumbency soon after birth, stand within two hours of birth and nurse within three hours of birth. The foal should be mentally alert during this time. Foals may exhibit submissive behavior when approached by a human or a horse besides its dam. Submissive behavior in the foal consists of raising its head and exhibiting a chomping motion with its mouth.[1] Deviations from a normal behavior pattern can be the result of many different origins, including perinatal asphyxia, intrauterine infection, prematurity, and congenital disease.[2,3,4]

179

Upon examination of the cranial nerves of the newborn foal, several differences should be noted. The newborn foal lacks a menace reflex. This is a learned reflex and generally develops over the first two weeks of life. The pupillary light reflex in foals may be affected by their level of excitement perhaps secondary to increased sympathetic tone, with the excited foal having a slightly slower constriction. This may be hard to evaluate in a struggling foal because they will not hold their heads still long enough for the examination. Foals normally have exaggerated head movements in response to external stimuli. The pupils of the foal appear to have a slight ventromedial deviation up until one month of age. Effective nursing generally indicates the normal functioning of cranial nerves 5, 7, 9, 10, 11, and 12.

In evaluating laryngeal function, it has been found that foals do not respond consistently to the "slap test" until about one month of age.[3] The test is performed by gently slapping the foal on the withers with a hand while either palpating the larynx or viewing it with an endoscope. A positive test would be the adduction of the arytenoid on the opposite side of the body from the slap. Foals may nicker or whinny right after birth, which is a sign of an alert foal.[1] It is not uncommon for foals to protrude their tongues to one side of their mouth or to suck on them. This is particularly seen in foals that have not been allowed to suckle or are orphaned. Tongue tone is normal in these foals and not a result of hypoglossal nerve damage. If the tongue lacks tone, then a neurologic deficit should be suspected in this nerve.

Gait analysis of the foal can be done as the foal moves freely about the stall or paddock. Restraint of the foal may actually get unexpected results. Many foals will collapse in the handler's arms as restraint is applied.[1-3] One's first reaction is to tighten the restraint and hold the foal up. Though it is counterintuitive, the actual lightening of restraint will cause the foal to bounce up and regain its normal standing posture. Foals will often assume a basewide stance. The newborn foal is obviously clumsy but develops a more coordinated gait within hours of birth. The gait tends to be choppy and dysmetric at first, but as the foal exercises more the gait assumes the more normal gait of the adult.[1-3] In foals that have been confined to a stall, the development of the more adult gait is delayed.

Spinal reflexes can be assessed in the recumbent foal. When manipulating the foal's limbs, one may encounter a strong extensor rigidity that should relax with continued passive motion. Limb reflexes are usually hyperreactive in the foal as compared to the adult. A crossed extensor reflex is commonly seen in the contralateral limb in response to the withdrawal reflex and may be present for the first three weeks of life.[1]

The most common neurologic presenting complaints in the newborn foal are changes in normal behavior, lack of suckle, depression, and seizures. Localization of the lesions causing these signs is centered in the brain, but other nonneurologic causes must be considered in evaluating the foal. These include septicemia, hypoglycemia, hypothermia, and hypovolemia. Behavioral changes that an owner may observe can be as subtle as the foal being somewhat quieter than normal. The foal may be slower to rise and to suckle. Foals generally form a close bond to their dams in the first 12 hours of life, staying within just a few feet of her for the first week. Foals with cerebral problems may be seen to wander away from their dams with no apparent affinity to her.

The suckle reflex is present in all normal foals and is never lost unless a disease process interferes.[6] Normal foals can be seen curling their tongue and making suckle movements within 10 minutes of birth. Suckling is instinctual and though the hypoglossal nerve is responsible for muscular coordination of tongue movement, seeking of the udder and actively suckling is probably under cerebral control as well. Loss of suckle is often the first neurologic sign that an owner may note, and it is usually the last sign to remain as the neurologic syndrome resolves.

Depression in the newborn foal is manifest by lack of response to external stimuli and increased periods of sleeping. The activity of normal foals falls into three categories—eating, sleeping, and running circles around their dams. A pattern of eating and sleeping is established early with the foal usually lying down after a meal. Normal foals are easily aroused from their sleep, while the depressed foal may not respond. When aroused, the depressed foal may stand and unenthusiastically udder-seek but lacks the playfulness or flight response from external stimuli. Depression can lead to complete loss of consciousness or coma.

Seizures are also a sign of cerebral dysfunction. They are caused by aberrant electrical activity in the brain. It is felt that foals may have a lower seizure threshold because of cortical immaturity.[3] Changes in the neuronal membrane, local tissue trauma, or systemic illness can also lower the seizure threshold further.[5] Seizures are often described as focal, subtle, or generalized clinical presentations that are dependent on the location and extent of the electrical activity. Subtle or focal signs in the foal may present as oral movements such as random chewing, suckling, or flemen. Rapid eye movements, muscle fasciculations, and apneustic breathing may be present.[3] More generalized clinical signs include thrashing, paddling, opisthotonus, extensor rigidity, and hyperthermia. Abrasions to the head and corneal ulcerations are common sequela to an uncontrolled generalized seizure.[3]

Spinal ataxia can also be seen in the newborn foal but is a less recognized problem than cerebral disease. If present at birth or soon after, then congenital malformations of the spine or spinal cord, vascular accidents during the birth process, and spinal trauma should be considered in the differential diagnosis.[2]

DIFFERENTIAL DIAGNOSIS FOR SEIZURE IN THE NEONATAL FOAL

Seizures in the first few days of life of the foal can be acquired or congenital in origin. Acquired etiologies are related to certain perinatal events such as perinatal asphyxia, infection, and trauma, while congenital causes may be due to malformation of neurologic or skeletal tissue or genetic defects.

Neonatal Encephalopathy

Neonatal encephalopathy (NE), also known as neonatal maladjustment syndrome, hypoxia ischemic encephalopathy, hypoxic encephalopathy, dummy foals, barker foals, and convulsives, is the most common cause of acquired seizures in the foal. In one retrospective study, 18% of foals presented to a neonatal referral center with neonatal maladjustment syndrome.[7] Affected foals may present with neurologic dysfunction immediately at the time of birth, or the clinical signs may have a delayed onset but usually within the first 24 hours of life. Hess-Dudan makes the distinction between these two groups of foals based on the onset of clinical signs. Foals that have a delayed onset of clinical signs are usually full-term, have a rapid, seemingly uncomplicated parturition, and have relatively normal postnatal behavior immediately after birth. They may stand and walk and may or may not have an effective suckle. Onset of neurologic signs is usually within six hours. Because the signs are not present immediately at birth, it is felt that the asphyxial trauma to the foal takes place during or immediately after the birth process. The progression of signs is variable, but in general foals lose their suckle reflex, wander away from their dam, become recumbent, and then begin seizing. Not all foals follow this entire process. Signs may only progress to the loss of suckle reflex. This variability in clinical sign progression may be related to the degree of perinatal insult in the foal.[8] In human neonatology, the degree of asphyxia (mild, moderate, and severe) is linked to metabolic acidosis with a base deficit >12 mmol/liter.[9]

Hess-Dudan's second category of foals with neonatal encephalopathy includes foals that exhibit abnormal behavior immediately after birth. The delivery and/or the placenta may have been abnormal. The neurologic signs may be similar to the first category of foals, but in addition these foals are weak and may show signs of prematurity. It is felt that these foals have experienced a more chronic insult in utero perhaps due to placental insufficiency.[8]

The etiology of NE is not simple. It is felt that an asphyxial event plays an important part in the process. This event could be secondary to chronic placental insufficiency or acute placental separation. Impaired oxygen delivery results in asphyxia, hypoxia, and sometimes ischemia. In times of low blood oxygen, the fetus tries to maintain blood flow to the brain and heart by redistributing it from the gut, kidneys, liver, and muscle. Brain injury occurs when this mechanism is insufficient. Though not directly studied in foals, studies in neonates of other species (rats, piglets, monkeys, and humans) show that neuronal cell death can be acute from high levels of neurotoxins such as glutamate (produced in response to the asphyxia) and influx of calcium into neuronal cells, or can be delayed as a result of reperfusion injury and release of oxygen radicals.[9-14] Reperfusion injury becomes evident hours after the original insult. This may explain why many foals with NE appear normal at birth but begin showing signs of neurologic compromise three to six hours after birth.

The neonate is adapted to handle short nonprogressive periods of hypoxia. Studies looking at a single continuous partial asphyxia in fetal monkeys near term demonstrated brain swelling with neuronal injury.[9] For neuronal injury to be sustained, the hypoxic insult must be progressive over a period of time. Injury has been produced by maintaining the hypoxic event for 60 minutes.[9] Possible parturition events that might result in progressive hypoxia that would meet this time criteria includes premature separation of the placenta during parturition, umbilical cord compression or torsion, and chest compression in the birth canal for prolonged periods of time.

Postmortem examination of affected foals may or may not be rewarding. Significant vascular accidents (SVA) comprising subarachnoid, parenchymal, and nerve root hemorrhages; cerebral edema; and ischemic necrosis have been described on postmortem examination of some foals that died subsequent to showing signs of neurologic disease.[15-18] High vascular pressures that peak at 400 mm Hg during delivery have been hypothesized as a possible cause of the SVA.[19]

There are many clinical manifestations of neonatal encephalopathy. The respiratory centers are a common target. Abnormal respiratory patterns seen include central tachypnea (midbrain lesion), apneusis (pontine lesion; breath-holding inspiratory pause with no expiratory pause), periodic apnea (midbrain lesion; defined as >20 seconds between breaths), cluster

(↑ production of oxidising species) Reactive O₂ species – disturbance in normal redox state
→ peroxides / free radicals
↓ antioxidant defenses

breathing (high medullary lesion; several rapid breaths followed by a respiratory pause or apnea), ataxic breathing (medulla; irregular timing of breaths) and Cheyne-Stokes breathing. These abnormal breathing patterns may or may not be accompanied by central hypercapnia. It is important to detect and treat hypoventilation as it occurs in the early hospital course. Hypercapnia must be detected by blood gas analysis, as often the abnormal respiratory patterns are not accompanied by changes in $PaCO_2$.[20] Though the central nervous system signs are the most prominent in cases of perinatal asphyxia, other systems are also affected. In human infants, mild asphyxia may affect systems such the cardiovascular, respiratory, and renal systems mildly or not at all. Moderate to severe asphyxia is more likely to have moderate to severe effects on these systems.[8] Renal compromise in the foal with NE may present as decreased urine production. Gastrointestinal effects of perinatal asphyxia may include colic, transient ileus, and necrotizing entero-colitis. Cardiac arrhythmias, edema, and hypotension may result from hypoxia of the myocardium.[16]

Bacterial Meningitis

Bacterial meningitis is an infrequent manifestation of septicemia in the neonatal foal.[21] Koterba found that approximately 10% of foals with confirmed septicemia presented with bacterial meningitis.[22] Foals usually have a history of failure of passive transfer and present with the signs of sepsis (see Chapter 5). Neurologic signs of depression, weakness, and anorexia must be distinguished from the generalized septic process in the foal and a more specific localization of meningitis. More specific neurologic signs that may suggest inflammation of the meninges would include cervical pain, proprioceptive deficits, intention tremors, opisthotonus, and coma. It is difficult to distinguish bacterial meningitis from NE because the signs are similar and sepsis often is present in the foal with NE.

The bacteria involved in bacterial meningitis are the same that are involved in sepsis—*E. coli, Klebsiella sp., Actinobacillus sp., Salmonella sp., Enterobacter sp., Strep-tococcus sp., Staphylococcus sp.,* and *Pseudomonas sp.* Bacteria gain entry to the meninges by the hematogenous route.[2] The central nervous system of the neonate has an incomplete blood-brain barrier. Open tubulocisternal endoplasmic reticulum components of the cerebral endothelial and choroids plexus epithelial cells are thought to be sites of bacterial seeding in the neonate.[23] Once bacterial entry has occurred, the cerebral spinal fluid acts as a good media for bacterial growth. Rapid multiplication of the bacteria is favored because of the inadequate humeral and phagocytic defenses of the CNS.[23]

Inflammation secondary to the activation of the cytokine cascade is a large component of the course of the disease. Brain edema and increased cerebral blood flow initially increase intracranial pressure. As the disease progresses, intracranial pressure increases resulting in a decrease of cerebral blood flow. Ischemia results in irreversible neuronal cell damage.[22,23]

Trauma

Head and neck trauma in the foal is fairly common in the history of foals with neurologic disease. Generally the history will present a foal that was clinically normal up until the incident of injury. Clinical signs are dependent on the severity and location of the trauma. Cerebral trauma will have signs of blindness, depression, seizure, head pressing and coma (Figure 10-2). Trauma to the brain stem may be accompanied with signs of nystagmus, facial paralysis, strabismus, and gait abnormalities.[2,3] Neck trauma results in signs of ataxia or paralysis.[25] Fractures of the frontal and parietal bones, the petrous temporal bone, and the basisphenoid bones are common. Intracranial hemorrhage can be parenchymal, subdural, or both. Subdural hematoma formation usually develops from bleeding by a damaged cortical artery or underlying parenchymal injury, or from tearing of a bridging vein form the cortex to a draining venous sinus. Small subdural hematomas often resolve spontaneously, but continued bleeding and expansion of the hematoma leads to increased intracranial pressure and deformation of the brain.[26]

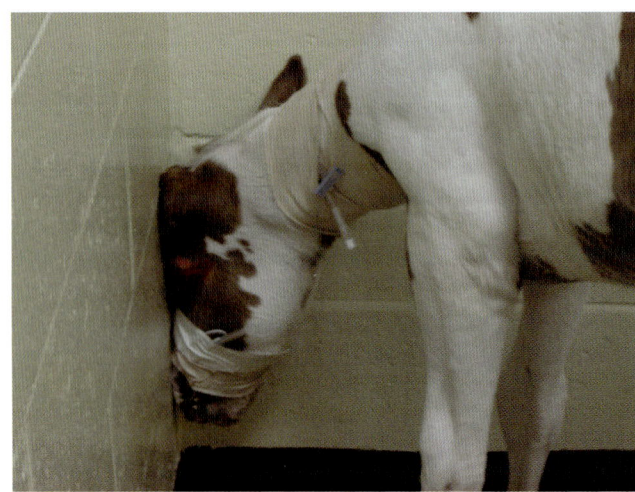

Fig. 10-2 Foal with head trauma exhibiting depression and head pressing.

Subarachnoid closed space.

Congenital Neurologic Problems

Several congenital neurologic problems have been noted in foals, particularly in Arabian foals. Benign pediatric epilepsy has been seen in Arabian and cross Arabian foals particularly from the Egyptian line. Foals are generally normal between seizures. Seizures are unpredictable and may be single or multiple in occurrences. Central blindness for an extended amount of time may be noted as a postical sign. Foals will often have evidence of trauma around the head. Foals appear to grow out of this problem.[3,27]

A recently emerging neurologic condition of the Egyptian Arabian foal is called Lavender Foal syndrome by breeders. The name is derived from the unusual dilute coat color present in these foals at birth. The foals are usually pale versions of grey, thus giving a lavender appearance. These foals experience continuous seizures or activity without the ability to rise. Extensor rigidity, paddling, and opisthotonus are prominent signs.[27,28] These foals do not appear to respond to anticonvulsant therapy. No extensive study has been conducted on this syndrome. Bowling reports that an anomalous choroids plexus has been found on postmortem examination and suggests that an autosomal recessive gene may be involved in the etiology.[28]

Cerebellar abiotrophy of Arabian foals is believed to be an inherited disorder in which there is degeneration of the Purkinje cells and thinning of the granular and molecular layers of the cerebellum. The cerebellum is grossly normal in size on postmortem. Clinical signs are not usually evident at birth but become progressively more evident as the foal ages. Clinically foals present with a hypermetric gait and intention tremors. A menace response is absent even in foals older one month of age.[3]

Occipitoatlantoaxial malformations have also been reported in Arabian foals and other foals.[29-31] The clinical syndromes associated with this malformation include foals that are stillborn, foals that are tetraparetic at birth, foals that have progressive ataxia, and foals that present with signs of cervical scoliosis or head deviation with no signs of spinal cord or brain disease.[29] Sometimes a palpable clicking sound/movement can be heard or felt when the foal moves it head and neck. Careful palpation of the base of the skull and cervical vertebrae 1 and 2 may reveal a deformity. If the brain stem is affected, then the foal may hypoventilate. Hypercarbia may be evident on arterial blood gases.

Narcolepsy is a sleep disorder that has been described in humans and other animals as excessive daytime sleepiness. Lunn reported the familial occurrence of narcolepsy in miniature horses. Signs were evident in affected animals at birth or within three days of birth. Foals would collapse particularly when stimulated by suckling or handling. Besides clinical signs of sudden onset of marked drowsiness, diagnosis can be confirmed through administration of intravenous physostigmine. Physostigmine administration causes an increase in clinical signs of affected animals. This can be reversed with the administration of atropine. Some affected foals have shown signs of resolution as they mature. A close familial relationship of two or three cases suggest a hereditary component to the disease.[32]

Internal hydrocephalus, the abnormal accumulation of cerebral spinal fluid (CSF) in the ventricles of the brain, has been reported in foals. Clinical signs depend upon the amount of hydrocephalus that is present. Foals may appear normal at birth but progressively become weaker. An enlarged dome-shaped forehead may be evident on presentation (Figure 10-3). The enlarged head may be cause for dystocia. Exopthalmos and ventrolateral strabismus are common in hydrocephalic animals. Most affected foals die soon after birth because of massive increased intracranial pressure.[3,33] Prognosis is poor with no recommended treatment. Though the cause of most cases is unknown, Ojala reported on the inheritance of hydrocephalus in a line of Standardbreds.[34]

Hydranencephaly, the complete or almost complete absence of cerebral hemispheres, has also been reported in the horse.[35] Holoprosencephaly, a defect characterized by the absence of the longitudinal cerebral fissure fusion of the the cerebral hemispheres and

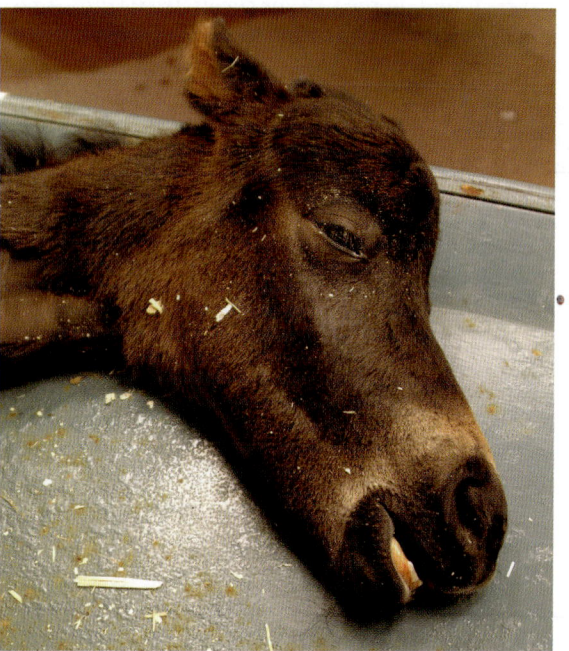

Fig. 10-3 Foal with a domed forehead secondary to hydrocephalus.

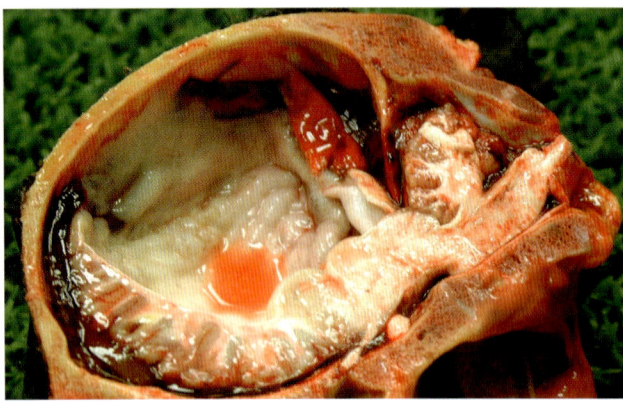

Fig. 10-4 Cranium of foal with possible holoprosencephaly (incomplete cleavage of forebrain during embryogenesis) or hydranencephaly (almost complete absence of cerebral) hemispheres.

one large ventricle, has also been seen a foal (Figure 10-4).

The seizure activity delayed the diagnostic workup of '05 Carpe Diem until treatment could be administered. Diazepam (5 mg) was administered intravenously as the foal was gently restrained from harming itself. The foal's body temperature at the time of seizure increased to 103.5° F, and metabolic/respiratory acidosis was noted on a blood gas analysis. The foal responded to the diazepam by cessation of the seizure and relaxation of its muscles. The foal's mental status remained unresponsive.

The initial diagnostic workup for the foal included a CBC, chemistry profile, IgG analysis, repeated arterial blood gas analysis, and a blood culture. No abnormalities were found on the CBC or chemistry profile. A resolving acidosis and a mild hypoxemia ($PaO_2 = 65$ mmHg) was present on the subsequent blood gas analysis, and the foal's IgG level was low at 400 to 800 mg/dl. Because of the neurologic signs, performance of a cerebral spinal tap was discussed but was delayed in order to further evaluate the foal's response to treatment.

DIAGNOSTIC TESTING

A minimum database of a CBC, IgG levels, blood gas analysis, and chemistry profile can be helpful in eliminating some causes of seizures immediately. In cases of sepsis and septic meningitis, an abnormal leucogram would be prominent. Depending upon the stage of the disease, either a neutropenia or a neutrophilia may be noted. IgG levels are usually insufficient, being below 800 mg/dl. Arterial blood gas analysis can identify severe hypoxemia or acidosis as contributing factors in the neurologic process. Finally, the chemistry profile would rule out hypoglycemia,

electrolyte abnormalities, and hepatic encephalopathy as likely causes of the seizures.

A cerebral spinal fluid (CSF) analysis is the diagnostic test of choice to confirm the diagnosis of septic meningitis. The procedure is not generally needed for the diagnosis of perinatal asphyxia, NE, or cerebral trauma. It may in fact be harmful if there is an elevated intracranial pressure. Sudden release of pressure may result in herniation of the brain stem at the tentorium. CSF can be obtained from the atlantooccipital (AO) space or the lumbosacral (LS) space in a foal. The landmarks are the same as those of the adult. While the AO tap is best done under anesthesia, the LS tap can be obtained under light sedation. The AO tap is preformed with the foal in lateral recumbency. A 10-by-10-cm area behind the poll of the foal's head is clipped and aseptically prepared. The puncture is made at the intersection of a line drawn from the anterior wings of the atlas and the midline of the dorsum of the neck. A three-inch spinal needle is inserted perpendicular to the midline, cautiously feeling for distinct "pops" as the needle penetrates the AO and dural ligaments. One should stop moving the needle forward at each pop, withdraw the stilet from the needle, and check for the presence of CSF. CSF should flow easily from this site but not stream.

The landmarks for the LS tap include the tuber sacrale and the midline of the back. The foal is best placed in a "frog leg" position on its sternum. The area is prepared in the same manner as above with clipping and aseptic scrub. The spinal needle is inserted perpendicularly in a small depression on the midline that is on the anterior edge of the tuber sacrale. Fluid does not flow as easily from this site and may need to be aspirated. Fluid flowing freely from this site may suggest elevated CSF pressure. The LS tap is the safer of the two sites to obtain fluid in the foal, both from the possibility of pressure changes in the cerebrospinal system but also from the possibility of causing harm by inadvertently damaging the spinal cord. Changes in the CSF reflective of septic meningitis will still be present in fluid from this site.

CSF should be analyzed within 30 minutes of obtaining a sample. Normal CSF has very few cells present, in the magnitude of 1 to 5 cells/μl.[3] The differential of these white blood cells are normally monocytes and lymphocytes. Neutrophils should never be seen in normal CSF. CSF protein levels in the neonatal foal have been reported to be higher than those in the adult. Protein levels of 138 ± 50 mg/dl have been reported in normal pony foals up to 40 hours of age.[36] It is felt that the immaturity of the blood-brain barrier in foals results in an increase in permeability that is more permissive of the crossing of proteins and bacteria into the brain. Another study reported a lower mean of approximately 82 ± 19 mg/dl in foals 10 days of age. This study found the albumin quotient of CSF (CSF albumin/serum albumin ×100) in the neonatal foal was approximately 1.85, and the immunoglobulin index (CSF IgG/serum IgG × serum albumin/CSF albumin) was approximately 0.50. Elevated CSF albumin quotients in the sick foal may indicate increased blood-brain barrier permeability, while an increased IgG index may be indicative of intrathecal IgG production that may occur in septic menigitis.[37] The level of glucose in normal CSF is generally 80% of the serum glucose. Glucose levels decrease in response to the presence of bacteria or to decreased serum levels.[3]

Grossly normal CSF is light yellow and clear. In septic meningitis, CSF can appear serosanginous and slightly cloudy. There is an increase in cells and protein, and differential of cells will include the presence of neutrophils. Gram stain of the fluid may reveal bacteria. In trauma, CSF may be xanthochromic or have a serosanginous appearance as well. The presence of hemorrhage will make it more difficult to know if the increase in cells and protein are secondary to the presence of blood or secondary to sepsis. Erythrophagocytosis indicates intrathecal hemorrhage as opposed to hemorrhage secondary to tap contamination. CSF from foals with NE is generally normal in appearance and analysis.

Diagnostic imaging may be helpful in the diagnosis of cerebral or spinal trauma or malformation. Radiographic examination of the head and neck for fractures can be somewhat problematic in the identification of nondisplaced fractures. The skull in particular has numerous suture lines that may be confused or misinterpreted as a fracture. Malformations of the spine, as seen in occipitoatlantoaxial abnormalities, are generally evident on palpation and standard radiography.[29] The use of myelography is not often needed.

The newer technologies of computed tomography (CT) and magnetic resonance imaging (MRI) are better methods of visualizing actual neuro-tissue and the boney structures surround the brain and spinal cord.[38-40] Accessibility and cost are limiting factors in the widespread use of these technologies (Figure 10-5). Normal brain anatomy has been reported in using MRI in the neonatal foal by Chaffin and colleagues.[40] The use of contrast material enables one to highlight damaged areas of the brain secondary to trauma, such a subdural hematomas and parenchymal hemorrhage (Figure 10-6). CT or MRI scanning has the potential for helping clinicians understand the neurologic disturbances in foals with NE that do not currently go to pathology. Because a high percentage of foals that present with signs of NE survive without noticeable permanent neurologic dysfunction, it is difficult to know if a clinician is dealing with the same pathology that is seen on postmortem of the foals with NE that

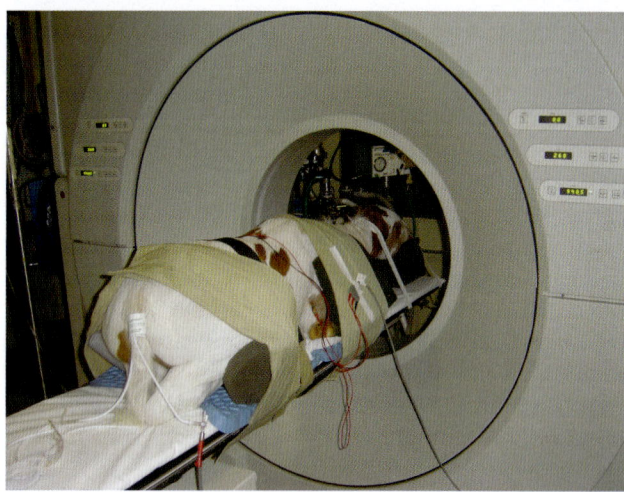

Fig. 10-5 A foal with evidence of head trauma having computed tomography performed.

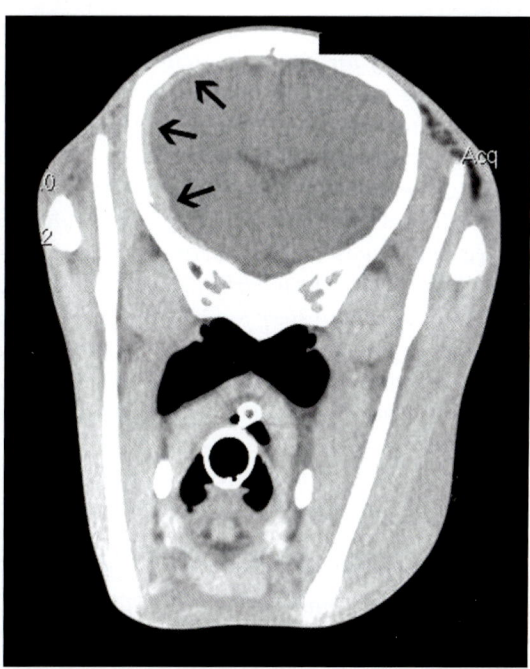

Fig. 10-6 Computed tomography image of a foal that suffered head trauma. Contrast material highlights an area of subdural hemorrhage (arrow).

don't survive. These advanced imaging techniques may give the clinician a "window" of insight into the pathophysiology of the disease.

Ultrasound is of little use in evaluating the CNS because the barrier of bone surrounding the tissue prevents visualization of the important structures. Foals do not normally have an open fontanel as is found in human infants. In one reported case of hydrocephalus in a foal with a boney defect in the skull, ultrasound was used to make the diagnosis.[33]

There is currently no specific test that will lead to the diagnosis of NE. Diagnosis is made through the history of CNS signs that develop within the first day of life with no observation of trauma, the absence of metabolic abnormalities such as hypoglycemia, elevated hepatic enzymes and electrolyte disturbances, and the lack of genetic clues such as diluted coat color in Arabian breed with Egyptian lines. The uncomplicated NE should have a normal CBC as well. Unfortunately, because of the early onset of seizures or decreased suckle reflex the NE foal often has evidence of failure of passive transfer and may currently develop CBC changes that are indicative of sepsis. Playing the odds, NE with concurrent septicemia is more common than septic meningitis. However, treatment of both possibilities simultaneously is prudent.

'05 Carpe Diem appeared systemically stable with the exception of continued breathing abnormalities, mental depression, and intermittent seizure activity. Repeated doses of diazepam were used to control the foal's seizures. Administration of 5 mg of diazepam would hold the seizures at bay for approximately 30 minutes before retreatment was needed. The foal was treated with intravenous phenobarbital (2 mg/kg dose) to see if a longer duration of seizure control could be obtained. Phenobarbital was given in an as-needed fashion until seizures were controlled. A total of 8 mg/kg of phenobarbital given over three hours was required before the seizures subsided. Following the phenobarbital administration, '05 Carpe Diem appeared to sleep for 24 to 36 hours. One liter of hyperimmune plasma was administered intravenously to provide adequate IgG. Cefotaxine, a third-generation cephalosporin, was given at a dosage of 40 mg/kg because of the possibility of septic meningitis.

Because the colt was unaware of his surroundings, all of his needs had to be provided by his caretakers. An indwelling nasogastric tube was placed to provide enteral nutrition. Because the mare had a large quantity of milk, she was used as the source of nutrition for the foal. She was milked every two hours and produced 500 to 800 ml at each milking. The colt was started on 10% of its body weight (40 kg × 0.10 = 4 liters), divided by 12 to give a volume of approximately 330 ml every two hours. An 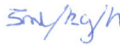 *initial intravenous fluid rate of 200 ml/hour was started with a crystalloid fluid to help maintain hydration.*

During the foal's earlier seizure activity, he had abraded the skin around his eyes. Fluorescein stain was taken up in the right cornea indicating the presence of a corneal ulceration. Initial therapy of the eye included triple antibiotic ointment and, because of bilateral miosis, two drops of atropine. The foal was carefully checked for signs of developing pressure sores, and none were found.

The owners reported that the foal had not been seen to pass meconium as of yet. There was urine wetness on the foal's abdomen and legs. A soapy water enema was administered and a large amount of meconium was

passed. The foal was finally cleaned and dried and placed on a foam mat covered with a faux sheepskin cloth. An attendant stayed with the foal continuously, gently restraining the foal if he began to struggle.

TREATMENT

Seizures not only cause increased demands for oxygen delivery, glucose utilization, and perfusion, all of which may be limited in the critical neonate, they are also associated with increased neurologic damage.[41,42] Thus, it is vital to control ongoing seizures and prevent recurrence. Diazepam or midazolam (0.11 to 0.44 mg/kg) are good choices for immediate seizure cessation. They are fairly safe and can be used even in systemically compromised foals. The disadvantage of these drugs is their short half-life. The effects will last five to 20 minutes depending upon the severity of the seizure.

Phenobarbital is the first line of long-term seizure-control therapy. The half-life of phenobarbital in some foals may be >200 hours (others may have faster clearance). Thus the sedation achieved may be prolonged. Low doses of phenobarbital (2 to 10 mg/kg) can be given repeatedly until seizures are controlled. It should be infused over 15 to 20 minutes with peak activity expected at 45 minutes. Once the seizures are controlled, usually no further doses are needed since there will be a prolonged effect that may span the seizure period. In rare cases, it may be necessary to repeat the dose in six to 12 hours because of the variability in clearance.[20]

High doses of phenobarbital will cause a drop in core body temperature, a decrease in respiratory drive possibly leading to hypercapnia, a decrease in pharyngeal tone possibly leading to upper airway obstruction, and may potentiate hypotension resulting in deterioration of perfusion.

Hypercapnia, whether produced by the apneustic breathing or the effect of phenobarbital, can be corrected through mechanical ventilation or through the use of caffeine as a respiratory stimulant. Caffeine helps to reset central respiratory centers so that they are more sensitive to $PaCO_2$ levels. Caffeine is effective only in cases in which the hypercapnia has produced a significant acidosis. Caffeine (loading dose of 10 mg/kg, maintenance dose of 2.5 to 3.0 mg/kg) is quite safe, having a high therapeutic index. It can be repeated as needed to help control hypercapnia without mechanical ventilation.[16,20]

Because NE foals have a higher risk of failure of passive transfer of maternal antibodies and subsequent development of septicemia, antibiotic coverage is prudent. Choice of antibiotics should be directed toward providing broad-spectrum coverage against Gram-positive and Gram-negative organisms normally seen in sepsis (see Chapter 5). If there is a suspicion that septic meningitis may be the cause of the neurologic signs, then the choice of an antibiotic that readily crosses the blood-brain barrier is important. Two factors may favor the entrance of antibiotics into the CNS of foals—meningeal inflammation secondary to the infection and an incomplete barrier due to immaturity. It has been suggested that 10 to 30 times the minimum bactericidal concentration in the CSF is needed for sterilization of bacterial meningitis.[43] Unfortunately, many first-line antimicrobials used in the treatment of septicemia in the equine neonate (aminoglycosides because of their high molecular weight, and beta-lactams because of their lipophobic and ionized nature) have poor penetration of the CNS, even in the inflamed state. Chloramphenicol, which crosses the blood-brain barrier, has been effective against some Gram-positive organisms. However, it is difficult to reach levels effective against most Gram-negative enteric bacteria found in neonatal septicemia.[43] Trimethoprim-sulfonamides (TMSs) also cross into the CNS readily. This is the drug of choice for sensitive bacteria. One problem with TMSs is the increasing developing resistance to the common bacteria of neonatal sepsis.

Third-generation beta-lactamase–stable cephalosporins have enhanced penetration into the CSF and are bactericidal against a broad spectrum of bacteria that are present in neonatal sepsis. In human Gram-negative meningitis, these drugs are helpful in sterilizing the CSF. Clinical reports of the use of cefotaxime sodium (40 mg/kg, IV, 4 times daily) in neonatal foal septicemia and meningitis show promise for the treatment of unresponsive bacteremia in the foal.[44] Cefotaxime and ceftazidime, a newer third-generation cephalosporin, should be held in reserve in the general treatment of septicemia, but in cases of suspect meningitis, they should become a first line of defense. Diarrhea occurs in about 1% to 2% of human patients treated with cefotaxime.[44]

The next step in the treatment of neurologic disease in foals, particularly NE, is to look at possible ways to reduce the edema formation in the brain/spinal cord and to protect the brain from the harmful effects of reperfusion injury. Agents that have been used to decrease cerebral edema include corticosteroids, osmotic diuretics, and dimethyl sulfoxide (DMSO). Dexamethasone has been used successfully in the treatment of human infants and children with bacterial meningitis.[45] Full-term foals have high endogenous steroids at birth. This plus the fear of further immunocompromising an already immunocompromised animal, tends to cause veterinarians to shy away from the use of steroids. Mannitol at a dose of 0.25 to 1.0 g/kg, as a 20% IV solution, is an osmotic diuretic that removes fluid from the extravascular space. Debate continues on whether it is safe to use in the face of cerebral hemorrhage. Without the routine use of CT or MRI, it is difficult to know whether the hemorrhage is a part of the pathology associated with all NE. DMSO (0.5 to 1 g/kg, as a 10% to 15% IV solution) has many attributes to its name. These include stabilization of membrane phospholipids, prevention of platelet aggregation, maintenance of vascular integrity of the spinal cord, increasing oxygen availability, and scavenging of free radicals.[46] Though the rational behind their use is sound, the actual beneficial effects of these drugs are debatable as there is no controlled research in foals regarding their use. Different equine neonatal centers use these drugs at different rates but have similar survival statistics, so it is difficult to know what their role is in the treatment of NE.

Various other drugs have been used to try to protect the CNS tissue from further damage. Thiamine has been used to help preserve aerobic brain metabolism at a dose of 1 to 20 mg/kg added to intravenous fluids.[16] Studies in infants with hypoxic ischemic encephalopathy (HIE) showed a correlation between low Mg^{2+} levels in cord blood and the severity of their neurologic signs.[47] The levels of N-methyl-D-aspartate (NMDA) increase with neuronal damage. It is felt that Mg^{2+} plays a role in blockading NMDA production and that Mg^{2+} supplementation can restore this blockade. There are conflicting studies in various species as to the actual benefits of Mg^{2+} administration as a neuroprotectant.[48] A recent study looking at the ability of administered Mg^{2+} to penetrate the blood-brain barrier of human patients with brain injury showed only marginal increases in CSF Mg^{2+}.[49] Naloxone, an opiate antagonist, has been advocated to diminish CNS depression. Ascorbic acid and alpha-tocopherol have been used in their roles as antioxidants in NE.[5] Again there are no controlled studies to verify the benefits from these treatments (Table 10-1).

After controlling the seizures and providing immunologic and antibiotic coverage, the most important therapy is the supportive care that the foal receives. Enteral feeding is best accomplished with an indwelling nasogastric tube. Nutritional support should begin at a reduced rate—perhaps 10% to 15% of body weight—in order to evaluate the gastrointestinal tract's ability to handle food. In perinatal asphyxia, ileus with gastric distension may become a problem. As the foal tolerates the enteral feeding, the amounts can be increased gradually to the normal 25% to 30% of body weight.

Adequate hydration and maintenance of normal blood pressure is important in the treatment of cerebral trauma. As the brain swells with edema, it will tend to compress the vascular structures in the

Table 10.1	Drugs Commonly Used in Foals with Neurologic Disorders*
Drugs	**Dosage**
Diazepam	0.11–0.44 mg/kg IV, as needed
Phenobarbital	2–10 mg/kg IV, as needed
Mannitol	0.25–1 g/kg IV as a 20% solution
DMSO	0.5–1.0 g/kg IV as a 10–15% solution
Caffeine	Loading dose: 10 mg/kg PO
	Maintenance dose: 2.5–3.0 PO q 24 hours
Naloxone	0.01–0.02 mg/kg IV
Magnesium sulfate	50 mg/kg/hour diluted to 1% slow IV, then decrease to 25 mg/kg/hour up to 24 hours
Thiamine	1–20 mg/kg q 12 hours IM
Ascorbic acid	50–100 mg/kg/day, PO
Alpha-tocopherol	500–1000 IU, PO daily

*Adapted from Vaala WE: Perinatal asphyxia syndrome in foals, Standards of care, Compendium 2:1, 2002.

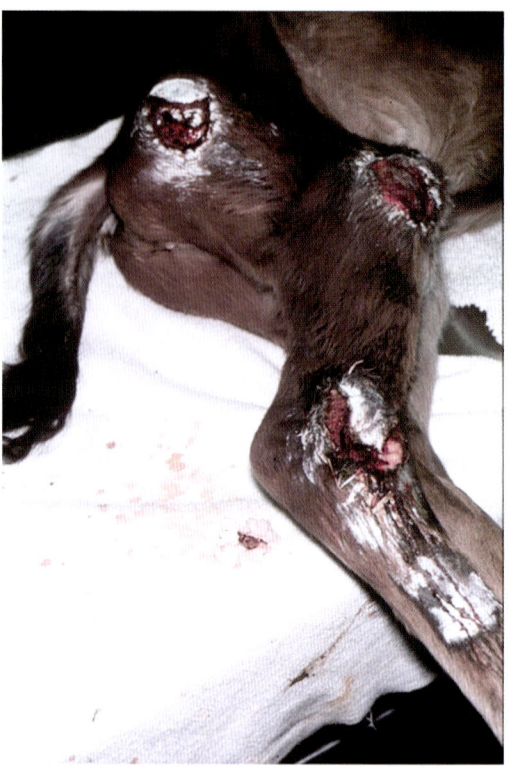

Fig. 10-7 Recumbent foals are susceptible to the development of decubital ulcers or pressure sores over bony prominences. These sores can develop rapidly—in a matter of 24 hours.

neuronal tissue, exacerbating the hypoxia to this vital tissue. Administration of crystalloid fluids and frequent monitoring of urinary output and indirect blood pressure all help in the assessment and maintenance of an adequate systemic blood pressure.

As seen earlier, the respiratory system can also be affected in a foal with perinatal asphyxia. Abnormal breathing patterns may be noted. If hypoxemia is present, then intranasal oxygen should be administered at a rate of 2 to 10 liters/minute. Caffeine may help to reset the respiratory centers. Because the foal has a compliant thoracic wall, it is important to keep the foal in sternal recumbency. This will decrease the amount of atelectasis that occurs in the down lung of a laterally recumbent animal and allow the foal to utilize both sides of its lungs.

A person willing to stay with the foal 24 hours a day is important for the reduction of self-trauma that the foal may undergo as it struggles. Foals will often develop pressure sores over the bony prominences of its body. Patches of skin over the hips, stifles, hocks, elbows, and carpi will thicken, die, and slough if one is not careful to provide adequate padding for the foal to lie on (Figure 10-7). Bandages can be applied to the lower limbs to prevent these decubital ulcerations from occurring. The placing of stay sutures around a decubital ulcer on the hip or elbow will allow padding and bandages to be laced onto these hard-to-bandage areas (Figure 10-8). Keeping the foal dry and warm may be a full-time job as the foal may urinate on itself in its unconsciousness.

Corneal ulceration is common sequelae to seizures and thrashing from affected foals. A padded helmet

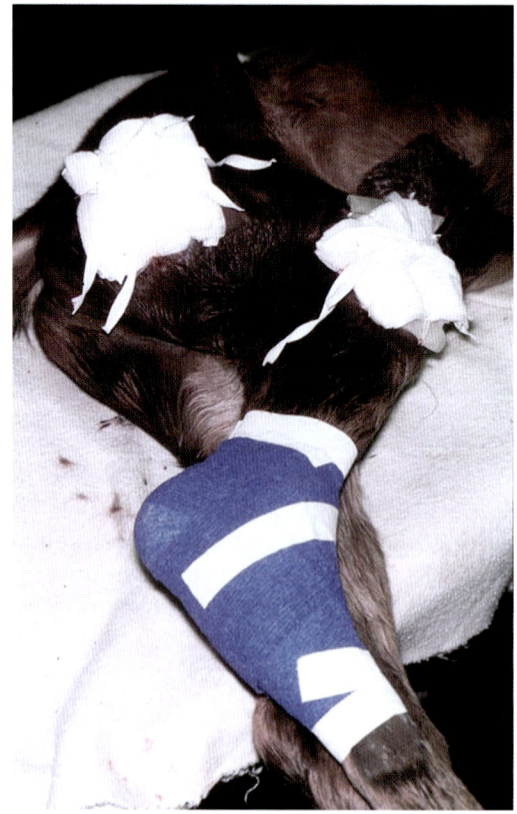

Fig. 10-8 Some areas can be difficult to bandage. The preplacement of stay sutures and the lacing of padding with umbilical tape can create an effective cover for the wound.

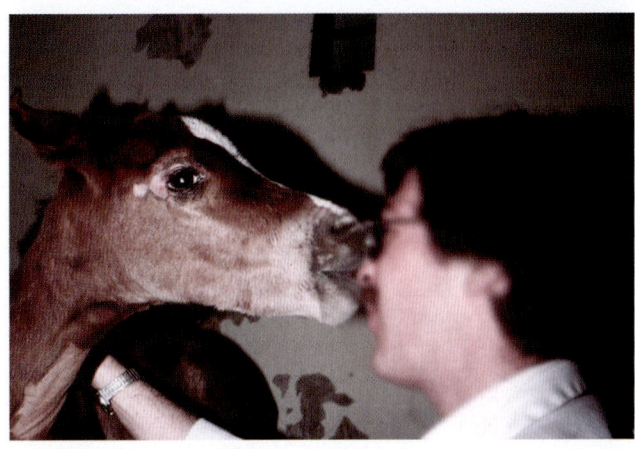

Fig. 10-9 On day six, '05 Carpe Diem developed a strong suckle reflex.

can be devised to prevent further head trauma. Foals have a decreased sensitivity to their corneas. Preventive application of a lubricant to the eyes will keep the corneas from drying out. Twice-daily staining of the eyes with fluorescein dye will help to identify any ulcerations that occur early. Ophthalmic antibiotic ointments should be applied in the presence of ulceration (see Chapter 14).

'05 Carpe Diem alternately slept and thrashed during the first 48 hours of his hospital stay. Gradually he became quieter and easier to handle. His nutrition was increased to 15% and then 20% of his body weight, and intravenous fluids were decreased accordingly. At the end of the second day, he actually lifted his head and appeared to be more aware of his surroundings. Despite bandaging of his legs, a decubital ulcer was noted on his left lateral hock. By day three, the foal was making attempts to stand. With help he could rise and support himself for five minutes. The foal continued to make progress. On day four he stood without assistance, On

day five he appeared to recognize his dam and developed a suckle reflex, and by day six his stomach tube was pulled and he was observed to suckle from his dam and from a bottle provided by his caretaker (Figure 10-9). Antibiotics were discontinued on day seven, and the foal was discharged on day eight. A follow-up report one month later found the foal to be normal in all ways that the owner could assess.

OUTCOME

The outcome of uncomplicated NE is generally good. The overall survival rate of these foals is between 70% and 80% depending upon the reporting center. Owners often ask the question about the mental capacity of the foals as they grow. Follow-up studies have not recognized any diminished training ability in the previously affected foals, and many have gone on to race successfully.[16] Foals that develop concurrent septicemia have a worse prognosis (see Chapter 5). Foals with septic meningitis have a poor to guarded outcome. The majority of foals with Gram-negative bacterial meningitis have not survived.[24] If a foal does survive, there is a chance that it will have a mental disability that may make it untrainable. With the more current use of third-generation cephalosporins, this picture may change.

Prognosis for foals that have received head and neck trauma depends upon the severity of the trauma and the lesion that it produces. Mild subdural hematomas may resolve with time and support, while compressing hematomas may lead to distortion of the brain and death.

Egyptian Arabian foals with epilepsy and American Miniature foals with narcolepsy seem to outgrow their neurologic problems with time. Lavender foals, on the other hand, have not survived.

REFERENCES

1. Adams R, Mayhew IG: Neurological examination of newborn foals, *Equine Vet J* 16(4):306, 1984.
2. Adams R, Mayhew IG: Neurologic diseases, *Vet Clin North Am Equine Pract* 1(1):209, 1985.
3. Green SL, Mayhew IG: Neurologic disorders. In Koterba AM, Drummond WH, Kosch PC, eds: *Equine clinical neonatology*, Philadelphia, 1990, Lea & Febiger.
4. Reed SM: Neurologic examination of neonatal foals and diagnostic testing useful to evaluate normal foals with neurological problems, *Proc. 8th ACVIM Forum* 601, 1990.
5. Vaala WE: Seizures, Coma in foals. In Brown CM, Bertone J, eds: *The 5-minute veterinary consult: Equine*, Baltimore, 2002, Lippincott Williams & Wilkins.
6. Rumbaugh GE, Cundy DR: Neonatal maladjustment syndrome in a foal with failure of passive transfer: A case report, *J Equine Med Surg* 1:344, 1977.
7. Ebben J: Neonatal intensive care: A retrospective study, *Minn Thoroughbred J,* 1989.
8. Hess-Dudan F, Rossdale PD: Neonatal maladjustment syndrome and other neurological signs in the newborn foal: Part I, *Equine Vet Educ* 8(1):24, 1996.
9. Low JA: Determining the contribution of asphyxia to brain damage in the neonate, *J Obstet Gynaecol Res* 30:276, 2004.
10. Myers RE, Beard R, Adamsons K: Brain swelling in the newborn rhesus monkey following prolonged partial asphyxia, *Neurology* 25:327, 1975.
11. Bickler PE, Fahlman CS, Taylor DM: Oxygen sensitivity of NMDA Receptors: Relationship to NR2 subunit composition and hypoxia tolerance of neonatal neurons, *Neuroscience* 118:25, 2003.
12. Acker T, Acker H; Cellular oxygen sensing need in CNS function: Physiological and pathological implications, *J Exp Biol* 207:3171, 2004.

13. Chiral M, Grongnet JF, Plumier JC et al: Effects of hypoxia on stress proteins in piglet brain at birth, *Pediatr Res* 56:775, 2004.

14. Mishra OP, Delivoria-Papadopoulos M: Effect of hypoxia on protein tyrosine kinase activity in cortical membranes of newborn piglets—the role of nitric oxide, *Neurosci Lett* 30:372, 2004.

15. Green SL: Current Perspectives on Equine Neonatal Maladjustment Syndrome, *Comp Contin Educ Equine Pract* 11:1550, 1993.

16. Vaala WE: Perinatal asphyxia syndrome in foals, standards of care, *Compendium* 2:1, 2002.

17. Palmer AC, Rossdale PD: Neuropathological changes associated with the neonatal maladjustment syndrome in the Thoroughbred foal, *Res Vet Sci* 20(3):267, 1976.

18. Mayhew IG: Observations on vascular accidents in the central nervous system of neonatal foals, *J Reprod Fertil Suppl* 32:569, 1982.

19. Rossdale PD, Jeffcott LB, Palmer AC: Raised foetal blood pressure and haemorrhage in the CNS of newly born foals, *Vet Rec* 99:111, 1976.

20. Palmer J: personal communication, January 2005.

21. Vaala WE: Peripartum Asphyxia, *Vet Clin North Am Equine Pract* 10:187, 1994.

22. Koterba AM, Brewer BD, Tarplee FA: Clinical and clinicopathological characteristics of the septicaemic neonatal foal: Review of 38 cases, *Equine Vet J* 16(4):376, 1984.

23. Foreman JH: Considerations in the Diagnosis and management of infectious neonatal neurological disease, *Proc 8th ACVIM Forum* 607, 1990.

24. White, SL: Retrospective on neonatal septic meningitis, Dorothy R. Havemeyer Foundation Septicemia Workshop II, Talliores, France, 16, 2001.

25. McCoy DJ, Shires PK, Beadle R: Ventral approach for stabilization of atlantoaxial subluxation secondary to odontoid fracture in a foal, *J Am Vet Med Assoc* 185(5):545, 1984.

26. Meagher RJ, Young WF: Subdural hematoma, *E Medicine*, 2002.

27. Knottenbelt DC, Holdstock N, Madigan JE: *Equine Neonatology medicine and surgery*, Philadelphia, 2004, Elsevier.

28. Bowling AT: *Horse genetics*, Wallingford, 1996, CAB International.

29. Mayhew IG, Watson AG, Heissan JA: Congenital occipitoatlantoaxial malformations in the horse, *Equine Vet J* 10(2):103, 1978.

30. Whitwell, KE: Craniovertebral malformations in an Arab foal, *Equine Vet J* 10(2):125, 1978.

31. Wilson WD, Hughes SJ, Ghoshal NG et al: Occipitoatlantoaxial malformation in two non-Arabian horses, *J Am Vet Med Assoc* 187(1):36, 1985.

32. Lunn DP, Cuddon PA, Shaftoe S et al: Familial occurrence of narcolepsy in Miniature horses, *Equine Vet J* 25(6):483, 1993.

33. Foreman JH, Reed SM, Rantanen NW et al: Congenital internal hydrocephalus in a Quarter Horse foal, *Equine Vet Sci* 3(5):154, 1983.

34. Ojala M, Ala-Huikku J: Inheritance of hydrocephalus in horses, *Equine Vet J* 24(2):140, 1992.

35. Leipold HW, Troyer DL: Congenital neurologic abnormalities, *Proc 8th ACVIM Forum* 607, 1990.

36. Rossdale PD, Cash RS, Leadon DP et al: Biochemical constituents of cerebrospinal fluid in premature and full term foals, *Equine Vet J* 14:134, 1982.

37. Andrews FM, Geiser DR, Sommardahl CS et al: Albumin quotient, IgG and IgG index determinants in CSF of neonatal foals, *Proc Third International Conference on Veterinary Perinatology*, Davis, Calif, 19, 1993.

38. Ragle CA, Koblik PD, Pascoe JR et al: Computed tomographic evaluation of head trauma in a foal, *Vet Radiol* 29:206, 1988.

39. Cudd TA, Mayhew IG, Cottrill CM: Agenesis of the corpus callosum with cerebellar vermin hypoplasia in a foal resembling the Dandy-Walker syndrome: Pre-mortem diagnosis by clinical evaluation and CT scanning, *Equine Vet J* 21:378, 1989.

40. Chaffin, MK, Walker MA, McArthur NH et al: Magnetic resonance imaging of the brain of normal neonatal foals, *Vet Radiol Ultrasound* 38:102, 1997.

41. Levene M: The clinical conundrum of neonatal seizures, *Arch Dis Child Fetal Neonatal Ed* 86:F75, 2002.

42. Miller SP, Weiss J, Barnwell A et al: Seizure-associated brain injury in term newborns with perinatal asphyxia, *Neurology* 58:542, 2002.

43. Jamison JM, Prescott JF: Bacterial meningitis in large animals—Part II, *Compend Contin Educ Pract Vet* 10:225, 1988.

44. Morris DD, Rutkowski J, Lloyd KCK: Therapy in two cases of neonatal foal septicaemia and meningitis with cefotaxime sodium, *Equine Vet J* 19(2):151, 1987.

45. Lebel MH, Freij BJ, Syrogiannopoulos GA et al: Dexamethasone Therapy for Bacterial Meningitis, *NEJM* 319:964, 1988.

46. Clabough DL, Martens RJ: Equine neonatal maladjustment syndrome, *Compend Contin Educ Equine Pract* 7:S497, 1985.

47. Ilves P, Kiisk M, Soopold T et al: Serum total magnesium and ionized calcium concentrations in asphyxiated term newborn infants with hypoxic-ischaemic encephalopathy, *Acta Paediatrica* 89:680, 2000.

48. Wilkins PA: Hypoxic ischemic encephalopathy. In Wilkins PA, ed: *Recent advances in equine neonatal care*, Ithaca, 2003, International Veterinary Information Service, available at www.ivis.org.

49. McKee JA, Brewer RP, Macy GE et al: Analysis of the brain bioavailability of peripherally administered magnesium sulfate: A study in humans with acute brain injury undergoing prolonged induced hypomagnesaemia, *Crit Care Med* 33:661, 2005.

11 Gastrointestinal Disease

| Case 11-1 | Colic in the Newborn Foal | Michelle Henry Barton |

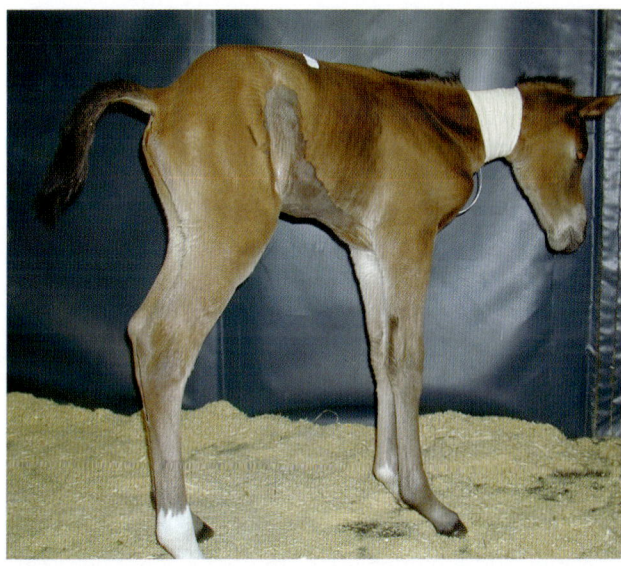

Fig. 11-1 Straining to defecate. '03 RockN'Roll at the time of presentation to the Veterinary Teaching Hospital at approximately 26 hours of age. The foal is exhibiting signs of straining to defecate: raised tail head, slightly arched back, hindlimbs slightly under the trunk. Note the meconium staining on the tail and perineum. The white tape on the foal's back was used as a landmark to serially measure the circumference of the foal's abdomen. Compare this foal's stance to the stance in Figure 11-4.

RockN'Roll, a 12-year-old Thoroughbred mare, foaled uneventfully at approximately 4 PM on April 14, 2004. '03 RockN'Roll stood within two hours of delivery and nursed. He passed meconium at approximately four hours of age, and he seemed bright and alert. On the morning of April 15, the owners found the foal straining to defecate. The local veterinarian was called for further evaluation and found a quiet but alert foal with a normal rectal temperature and heart rate. Meconium staining was noted on the tail. Gastrointestinal sounds were audible on both sides of the abdomen. A digital rectal examination was performed, and firm meconium was palpable in the rectal ampulla. A nasogastric tube was passed. No reflux was obtained, thus 30 ml of dioctyl sodium sulfosuccinate (DSS) was given. In addition, 50 mg of flunixin meglumine was given intravenously and a DSS and water enema was administered. The foal continued to strain and was intermittently recumbent, prompting referral to the University of Georgia's Veterinary Teaching Hospital.

At the time of presentation, '03 RockN'Roll was approximately 26 hours old. The foal was quiet, but tracked the mare well and was interested in nursing. The abdomen was slightly distended, and meconium staining was present on the tail and perineum. Shortly after admission, the foal was observed to raise his tailhead and strain (Figure 11-1). A small amount of urine was passed. The rectal temperature was 100° F, heart rate was 88 beats/minute, and respirations were 40 breaths/minute. Borborygmi were audible on both sides of the abdomen. A nasogastric tube was passed, and no reflux was obtained. A digital rectal examination confirmed the presence of firm meconium at the pelvic inlet. Palpation through the abdominal wall revealed at least a 12-cm segment of bowel in the left caudoventral abdomen that was approximately 3 cm in diameter and contained firm ingesta. Intermittent straining, as well as flank biting, continued. The foal then became recumbent and rolled up onto his back. There were no other significant physical findings. The major problems identified were straining to defecate, mild abdominal distension, acute abdominal pain (colic), and firm feces at the pelvic inlet.

DIAGNOSTIC APPROACH TO COLIC IN NEONATAL FOALS

According to the results of the National Animal Health Monitoring System report on colic in horses in the

United States in 1998 and 1999, the incidence of colic in foals less than six months of age was approximately 18 times less than the incidence in mature horses.[1] However, when considering aliments affecting foals, gastrointestinal tract problems and infection were most commonly reported.[2,3] Because some etiologies of colic are unique in the neonatal period, special consideration must be given to the evaluation of abdominal pain in this age group.

In some respects, the diagnostic approach to colic in neonatal foals is similar to that used in mature horses: rarely will any single fact be useful in determining the exact etiology. However, careful and simultaneous inspection of multiple historical, physical, and diagnostic findings may be formative in determining the anatomical location of the lesion (stomach, small intestine, large intestine, peritoneal cavity), the etiologic category (congenital, nonstrangulating obstruction, strangulating obstruction, inflammatory, or other), or even possibly the specific diagnosis (Table 11-1). In obtaining a history, particular attention should be given to the farm history, use of medications (especially analgesics), risk factors for septicemia or failure of passive transfer, and problems with other foals on the farm.

As some differentials are strictly age-dependent (see Table 11-1), knowing the age of onset of clinical signs is important. In the neonatal period, commonly reported causes of abdominal pain are meconium impaction, small-intestinal volvulus, enteritis or colitis, uroperitoneum, intussusception, gastric ulcers, and ileus secondary to prematurity, septicemia, or neonatal encephalopathy.[4-8] Clinical signs of lethal white syndrome, meconium impaction, and uroperitoneum most commonly manifest in the first 12 to 24 hours, 12 to 96 hours, and 48 to 96 hours of life, respectively. However, if uroperitoneum is the result of urachal or urinary bladder infection, clinical signs may be delayed until 7 to 14 days of age. Although the potential spaces created by congenital or traumatic umbilical, inguinal, and diaphragmatic hernias may be present since birth, incarceration of bowel into these spaces may occur at any age, if at all. Enteritis, colitis, intussusception of small intestine, small-intestinal volvulus, and clinically significant gastric ulcers may develop at any age.

The breed and sex of the foal may provide supportive evidence for certain differential diagnoses. Lethal white syndrome is most commonly reported in all-white to almost-all-white offspring of overo cross overo Paint Horses. In one study of 168 horses with congenital umbilical hernias, the incidence was two times greater in fillies compared to colts, and Thoroughbreds were twice as likely to have an umbilical hernia compared to Standardbreds.[9] In this later study, incarceration of bowel into the umbilical hernia

was not reported. Scrotal hernias most commonly occur in Standardbred and Tennessee Walking Horse colts,[8] and fecaliths are frequently reported in American Miniature foals.[6,10] In one study, meconium impactions occurred twice as often in colts compared to fillies.[11] Although the incidence of uroperitoneum is often quoted to occur more commonly in colts, in one recent study, the incidence was approximately equal among the sexes.[12] Additional historic information that should be carefully scrutinized is the general health of the dam, the foal's gestational age, the foaling history and general perinatal health, such as ingestion of colostrum, age at passage of meconium, nursing frequency (see Chapter 1 for review of normal perinatal health), and farm history of potentially infectious causes of enteritis or colitis (Salmonella, rotavirus, Clostridium). Most foals will have passed meconium within 9 to 12 hours of life; however, the gastrocolonic reflex stimulated by ingestion of colostrum frequently initiates earlier passage of meconium. Evacuation of meconium may be delayed (meconium retention) as the result of ileus secondary to another primary nongastrointestinal disease, such as septicemia or neonatal encephalopathy. In these cases, although passage of meconium may be slower than expected, the delay in passage may not be accompanied by clinical signs of abdominal pain. Passage of "milk feces" or yellow pasty feces does not necessarily indicate that all meconium has been removed from the colon.

CLINICAL SIGNS

Clinical signs of abdominal pain in foals can be highly variable, and the intensity of the signs is not necessarily indicative of the etiology. It is important to note that foals with inflammatory lesions of the intestinal tract or those suffering from general functional ileus secondary to systemic disease can act as violently painful as foals with obstructive or strangulating lesions of bowel. However, in general, foals suffering from uroperitoneum and gastric ulcers have less intense abdominal pain than do foals with inflammatory or obstructive lesions. Repeatedly thrashing or rolling from side to side is generally accepted as a highly representative clinical sign of abdominal pain. However, early signs of abdominal pain in neonatal foals may only manifest as reduced frequency of nursing and prolonged recumbency. Other subtle but significant signs of abdominal pain in foals include general restlessness, especially in recumbency, and/or frequent adjustment of recumbent positions (Figure 11-2). Often recumbent foals with abdominal pain will stretch their limbs, twist their head or neck, roll into dorsal recumbency (Figure 11-3), and make frequent attempts or

Table 11.1   Categorical Differentials for Colic in Foals

Category	Considerations	Common Causes	Less Common Causes
Congenital	Typically manifests signs in the first few days of life Pain without fever	None	**12- to 48-hour Foals** Atresia (ani, coli, recti) Ileocolonic hypogangliosis Chyloperitoneum[37] **Any Age Foal** Hernia (inguinal, scrotal, diaphragmatic) with incarceration Myenteric hypoganglionosis[38] Colon displacement or impaction Cecal impaction Small-colon obstruction by polyp or ovarian ligament[7]
Obstruction	More commonly present without fever	Meconium impaction (12 to 96 hours old)	**Older Foals** Ascarids (four to 24 months)[39] Fecalith in American Miniatures (typically >1 month old) Phytobezoar or Trichophytobezoar Duodenal stricture post ulcers (typically >1 month old) Sand enteropathy Ileal impaction
Strangulation	Intense pain without fever	**Any Age Foal:** Small-intestinal volvulus Intussusception	Large-colon volvulus Incarceration of bowel through mesodiverticular band Small-intestinal volvulus around Meckel's diverticulum or vitelloumbilical band Incarcerated hernia
Inflammatory	Variable pain, often with fever, diarrhea, or clinical evidence of sepsis	Necrotizing enterocolitis *Clostridium perfringens* *Rotavirus* *Salmonella*	*Cryptosporidia* (rare) *Giardia* (very rare) *Aeromonas* NSAIDS Antimicrobial-induced peritonitis Intra-abdominal abscess Adhesions **Older Foals** *Rhodococcus equi* intra-abdominal abscess or colitis *Lawsonia intracellularis* enteritis
Other	Mild to moderate pain without fever; diarrhea may be present with gastric ulcers	Gastric ulcers Uroperitoneum (typically two to seven days old) Functional ileus secondary to septicemia, prematurity, neonatal asphyxia, neonatal encephalopathy, overeating, milk replacer	Ovarian torsion—very rare[8,40] Hemoperitoneum[41]

strain to either defecate and/or urinate. In the standing foal, signs that are classically associated with straining to defecate include frequent tail swishing, a "water spout" tail, and a "camped under" leg stance with a dorsiflexed back (Figure 11-1). In contrast, a flat or ventroflexed back with the hindlimbs stretched backward and the tail held up is associated with urination (Figure 11-4). Other signs of abdominal pain include lip curling, flank biting or watching, pawing at the ground, and kicking at the abdomen. *It is important to recognize that often critically ill foals that are stuporus will not overtly demonstrate classic signs of*

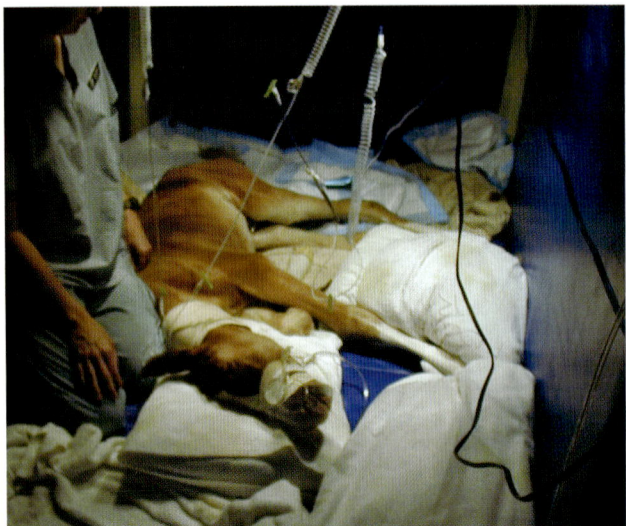

Fig. 11-2 Clinical sign of abdominal pain. There are various clinical signs of abdominal pain in the neonatal foal. This foal has neonatal encephalopathy with secondary intestinal ileus. His abdominal pain was low-grade and manifested by neck twisting, frequent stretching of the forelimbs, and general restlessness.

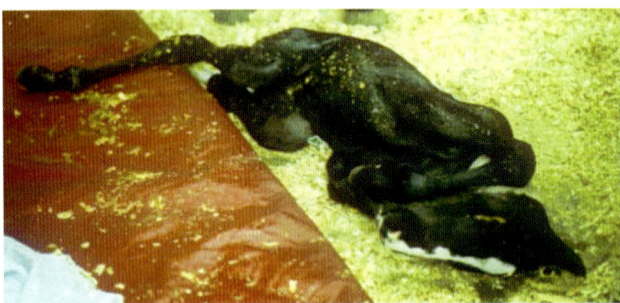

Fig. 11-3 Clinical signs of abdominal pain. This foal has acute enterocolitis and is demonstrating more classic and intense signs of abdominal pain: recumbency with rolling into a dorsal position and forelimbs retracted up over the neck and head.

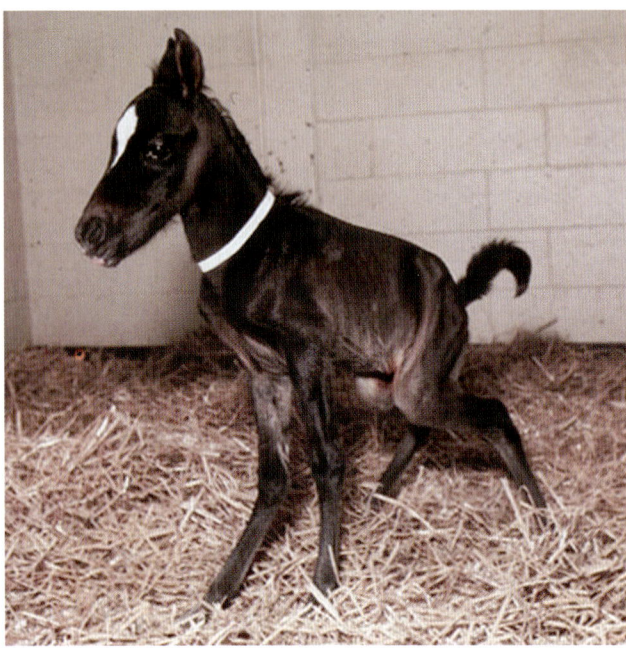

Fig. 11-4 Stance to urinate. This foal is demonstrating the typical stance seen with urination: tail straight up, back flat, hind limbs slightly stretched back. Compare this foal's stance to the stance in Figure 11-1.

abdominal pain, despite the presence of serious gastrointestinal disease.

The colicky neonatal foal should receive a thorough general physical examination with careful attention given to identification of clinical signs or physical evidence of sepsis (see Chapter 5). Sepsis may be directly associated with the primary etiology of the abdominal pain or it may develop secondary to bacterial translocation if the integrity of the gastrointestinal mucosa is compromised. The presence of fever, depression, petechiae, injection, synovitis, uveitis, or diarrhea may be cardinal clues that the abdominal pain has an inflammatory etiology. Although the presence of diarrhea may be an important sign of enterocolitis, intense abdominal pain frequently precedes the onset of diarrhea. Tachycardia and/or tachypnea are expected findings despite etiology. Persistent tachycardia (heart rate >120 beats per minute) has been suggested to be more commonly associated with surgical disorders of the abdomen, compared to medical etiologies.[13] Gross abdominal distension will develop with gas or fluid accumulation in the bowel or abdomen. Severe abdominal distension with intense pain that elicits high-pitched "pings" with percussion is consistent with gas-distended large intestine or cecum. Repeated measurement of the abdominal circumference may be helpful in more objectively determining the course of progression of abdominal distension. Typically, the absence of intestinal sounds is not helpful in determining etiology; however, increased borborygmi may be associated with enteritis or colitis. If diarrhea is present with signs of abdominal pain in a foal, additional fecal diagnostics may be indicated (see Case 11-3).

Unlike mature horses, transabdominal wall palpation can be performed in the neonate and may identify gastric distension, hepatomegaly, thickened or distended bowel, meconium, and the urinary bladder. The ventral abdomen and inguinal rings should be carefully examined for evidence of herniation. Ballottement or succussion of the abdomen may verify a fluid wave compatible with excess fluid in the peritoneal cavity. With adequate restraint or sedation, a careful digital rectal examination may identify meconium or ingesta in the pelvic inlet. A nasogastric tube should be passed in all foals with clinical signs of abdominal pain. Compared to mature horses, successful retrieval of gastrointestinal reflux can be frustrating in the neonate, even in the presence of proximal

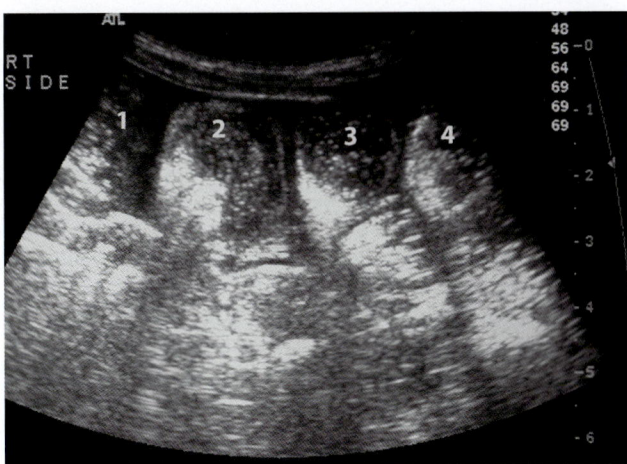

Fig. 11-5 Ultrasonographic image obtained on '03RockN'Roll at 26 hours of age with acute abdominal pain. This image was obtained using a 7-4 MHz curvilinear probe set to a depth of 6 cm. Note the four "balls" of meconium of mixed echogenicity in small colon (1, 2, 3, 4). This image was obtained from the left caudoventral abdomen.

intestinal disease. Frequently, nasogastric tubes that are designed for neonatal enteral feeding are of insufficient size for gastric decompression. With this in mind, the largest-bore tube that can be comfortably passed should be used, and persistent attempts should be made to obtain gastric reflux, either by suction or priming the tube with water.

A complete blood count and serum biochemical profile were obtained from '03 RockN'Roll. The PCV was normal at 32%. The total white blood cell count was 9,600/µl, characterized by a normal neutrophil count (6,582/µl) with a significant left shift (864/µl). The only significant abnormalities identified on the serum biochemical profile were hypoproteinemia (total serum protein 3.4 g/dl) with a normal albumin concentration of 2.2 g/dl and hyperglycemia 148 mg/dl. A SNAP test (IDEXX Laboratories, Inc., Westbrook, ME) was performed and confirmed hypogammaglobulinemia with an approximate IgG concentration of 400 to 800 mg/dl.

Blood was obtained for a blood culture, and a 16g polyurethane catheter was placed in the jugular vein. A transabdominal ultrasound examination was performed using a 7-4 MHz probe and revealed ingesta of variable echogenicity, surrounded by a gas pattern, in several sections of bowel in the left caudal dependent abdomen (Figure 11-5). The diameter of the bowel in this location was approximately 2 cm. There were no other significant findings on the transabdominal ultrasound examination. Based on the history, physical findings, and transabdominal ultrasound examination, meconium impaction was suspected. Based on the presence of a significant left shift and partial failure of passive transfer, the potential for secondary sepsis was increased.

CLINICAL PATHOLOGY

Changes in the leukogram or serum biochemical analysis may provide indirect etiologic evidence. Neutropenia, neutrophilia, a significant left shift, toxic changes within the neutrophils, and hyperfibrinogenemia are indicative of an inflammatory or infectious etiology and if present in the equine neonate, aseptic collection of additional blood for culture is recommended. Hypoglobulinemia is indicative of failure of passive transfer and should be verified by specific IgG testing (see case 3-1). Panhypoproteinemia is indicative of loss and may accompany severe inflammatory lesions of bowel. Azotemia, hyponatremia, hypochloremia, and hyperkalemia may occur with enteritis, colitis, or uroperitoneum. Marked acidosis most commonly occurs in foals with inflammatory lesions of the bowel.

Many clinicians are hesitant to perform an abdominocentesis on a neonatal foal as the risk for complications such as inadvertent enterocentesis or omental prolapse occur more commonly in foals undergoing an abdominocentesis, as compared to adult horses. *Many clinicians perform a transabdominal ultrasound examination first to assess potential risks of performing an abdominocentesis versus the likelihood of successfully obtaining peritoneal fluid.* If an ultrasound examination reveals widespread and/or grossly distended loops of intestine, and/or free peritoneal fluid is difficult to identify, the chances of an uncomplicated and successful abdominocentesis are reduced. An abdominocentesis may be completed on the standing foal or with the foal in lateral recumbency. In either position, proper restraint is imperative and is best facilitated by light sedation (Table 11-2).

The procedure for performing an abdominocentesis in a foal is similar to the adult horse, using either a 20- to 18-gauge 1.5-inch needle or a teat cannula to collect the peritoneal fluid. First, the hair from the ventral midline of the rostral abdomen should be clipped and the skin sterilely prepared. The subcutaneous tissue of the abdominocentesis site in the rostral midline of the abdomen should be infiltrated with 0.5 ml of 2% lidocaine. When a teat cannula is used, entry through the abdominal wall must be preceded by a stab incision made with a number 15 blade through the skin and external portion of the linea alba. Although use of an 18-gauge needle is expeditious, there may be a greater risk of inadvertent enterocentesis or bowel laceration; however, enterocentesis may also occur with a teat cannula if the intestine is grossly distended. Localized or generalized peritonitis may develop subsequent to an enterocentesis, and prophylactic use of parenteral antimicrobials is recommended.

Table 11.2 Analgesics and Sedatives for Abdominal Pain in Foals

Drug	Dosage	Route	Comments
Flunixin meglumine	0.25 mg/kg q 8–24 hours 1.1 mg/kg q 12–24 hours	IV	Avoid repeat dosing
Xylazine hydrochloride	0.1–0.5 mg/kg up to 1 mg/kg	IV IM	Causes GI stasis, bradycardia, hypotension; avoid repeat dosing
Detomidine	10 μg/kg	IV or IM	More potent than xylazine, thus its use is discouraged in neonatal foals
Diazepam	0.05–0.2 mg/kg	IV	For sedation
Butorphanol tartrate	0.01–0.04 mg/kg up to 1 mg/kg	IV IM	May cause excitation or incoordination; frequently combined with xylazine
Pentazocine lactate	0.3–0.4 mg/kg	IV or IM	Less effective than butorphanol
N-butylscopolammonium bromide (Buscopan™)	0.3 mg/kg	Slowly IV	Anticholinergic for spasmodic pain; not label- approved for nursing foals; may cause transient tachycardia; avoid repeat dosing

More commonly, use of a teat cannula results in inadvertent prolapse of omentum through the abdominocentesis site upon collection of peritoneal fluid or removal of the cannula. If this happens, the omentum should be sharply transected with a sterile blade at the abdominal wall and tucked back into the abdominal cavity with another sterile teat cannula.

Normal peritoneal fluid should be light yellow in color and clear. The normal mean nucleated cell count in the peritoneal fluid of healthy foals was reported to be 450 cells/μl (range 60 to 1,400 cells/μl) for 17 foals that were 13 to 134 days of age[14] and 1,400 cell/μl (±1077) for 32 Thoroughbred foals that were 14 to 75 days of age.[15] Both of these reference ranges for nucleated cell counts are lower than means reported for healthy adult horses. The mean protein concentration by biochemical biuret determination and refractive index in foals was reported to be 1.2 g/dl and 1.6 g/dl, respectively.[14] The interpretation of peritoneal fluid nucleated cell count and protein concentration is similar to adult horses with abdominal pain and does not necessarily definitively distinguish etiology or medical from surgical causes of colic. Sanguinous fluid can be present with either severe enterocolitis or strangulating lesions of bowel. Special attention should be given to the cytologic examination. The presence of degenerative neutrophils or bacteria is worrisome (Figure 11-6) and is indicative of loss of the mucosal integrity, bowel rupture, or primary sepsis in the peritoneal cavity. In one study, 78% of colicky foals with peritoneal fluid protein concentrations >2.5 g/dl that subsequently underwent an exploratory laparotomy were euthanized.[8] When uroperitoneum is suspected, the creatinine concentration of both peritoneal fluid and serum should be simultaneously assessed. A peritoneal fluid creatinine to serum creatinine ratio >2 is

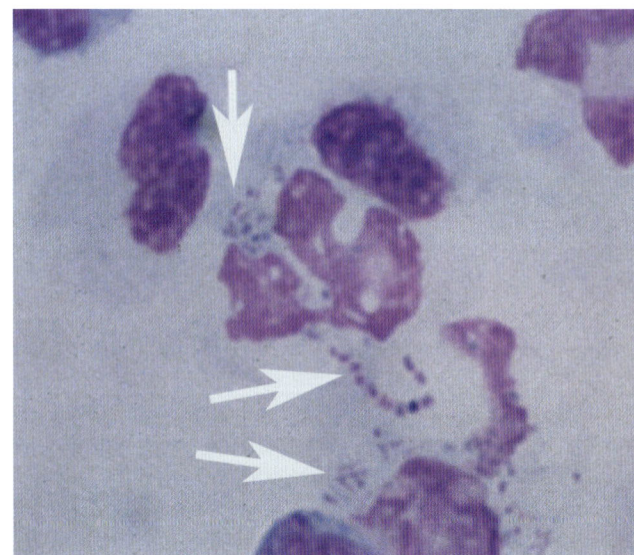

Fig. 11-6 Septic peritoneal fluid cytology. This peritoneal fluid was obtained by abdominocentesis from a 96-hour-old foal with acute abdominal pain and clinical signs of cardiovascular compromise. Note the degenerative neutrophils and the pleomorphic population of bacteria of various-sized rods and a chain of cocci *(arrows)*. The mixed population of bacteria is indicative of bacterial translocation across a severely compromised gastrointestinal wall, or gastrointestinal rupture. An exploratory celiotomy confirmed a perforated jejunal intussusception.

supportive evidence of uroperitoneum. When determining peritoneal fluid creatinine concentration on an automated chemistry analyzer, it is important to use plasma or serum methodology on the abdominal fluid. If urine methodology is used to determine the creatinine concentration on a peritoneal fluid sample, erroneously increased creatinine concentration may lead to an incorrect diagnosis of uroperitoneum.

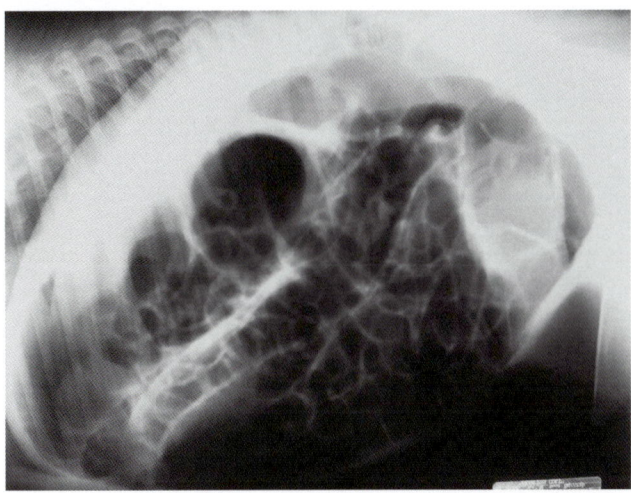

Fig. 11-7 Radiographic appearance of a strangulating obstruction. This abdominal radiograph was obtained from a four-day-old foal and reveals generalized gas distension in both the small and large intestine. A small-intestinal volvulus was identified at surgery.

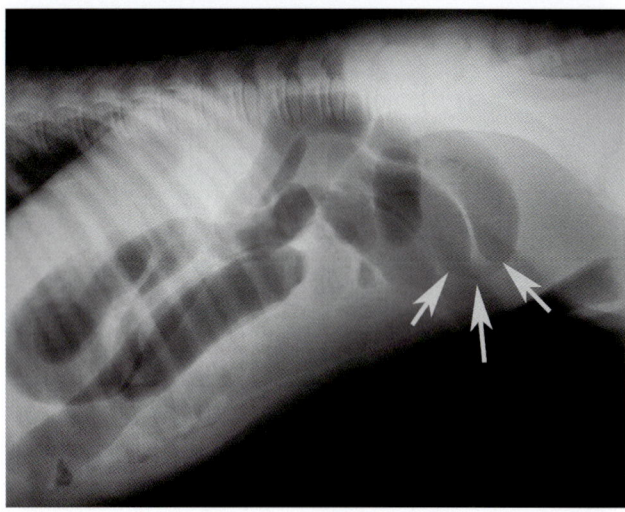

Fig. 11-8 Radiographic appearance of a small-intestinal obstruction. This neonatal foal had radiographic signs of small-intestinal obstruction, as evidenced by isolated loops of gas-distended small intestine that form a *U*-turn or "hairpin" turn *(arrows)*. An exploratory celiotomy confirmed a jejunal intussusception.

DIAGNOSTIC IMAGING

Unlike mature horses, abdominal radiography can provide useful information in a colicky neonatal foal. Grid, rare-earth screens and sufficient mAs (5 to 28) and kVp (80 to 120) should be used.[16] Radiographs may be taken with the foal either standing or in lateral recumbency; however, keep in mind that fluid-gas interfaces are easier to detect in the standing foal, when the radiographic beam is horizontal or perpendicular to the dorsoventral plane of the gas/fluid interface in the abdomen. Both right and left lateral views should be obtained as some structures will be more obvious, depending upon which side of the abdomen is closer to the film. Ventrodorsal views may only be possible in small foals or those that are stuporus, sedated, or anesthetized. This view will optimize identification of the pylorus, the descending duodenum, the base of the cecum, the left colon, and the transverse colon.[17] Some degree of gas is normally visible in the stomach, small intestine, cecum, and small colon.

In general, plain film abdominal radiology is more likely to provide information on the anatomic location of the problem than information directly leading to the exact etiology.[8,16,17] For example, gas distension of the small intestine is a nonspecific finding that may occur with enteritis, functional obstruction (ileus), or mechanical obstruction (Figure 11-7). However, if small-intestinal distension is accompanied by "hairpin" or "*U*-shaped" turns of the bowel (Figure 11-8) or multiple, uneven intraluminal gas-fluid interfaces (Figure 11-9), it is more likely associated with mechanical obstruction, though these findings can also

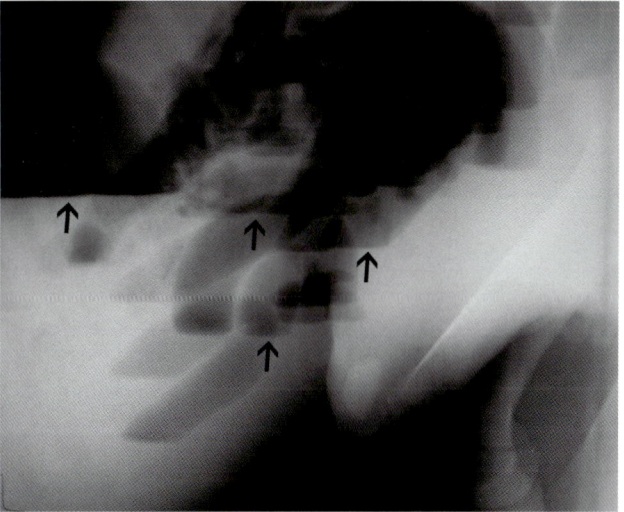

Fig. 11-9 Radiographic appearance of small-intestinal disease. The presence of multiple gas-fluid interfaces at different levels is often considered radiographic evidence of small-intestinal obstruction; however, it can also be seen in foals with intense ileus from enteritis, as was the situation for the foal depicted in this figure.

occur with enteritis or functional ileus. Thickened walls of small intestine may appear uneven or "corrugated" when caused by enteritis (Figure 11-10). Severe generalized gas distension of large intestine is more commonly associated with mechanical obstruction than with inflammatory lesions of large colon (Figure 11-11). Meconium frequently appears as granular contents in the ascending or descending colon (Figure 11-12). Pneumoperitoneum suggestive of bowel

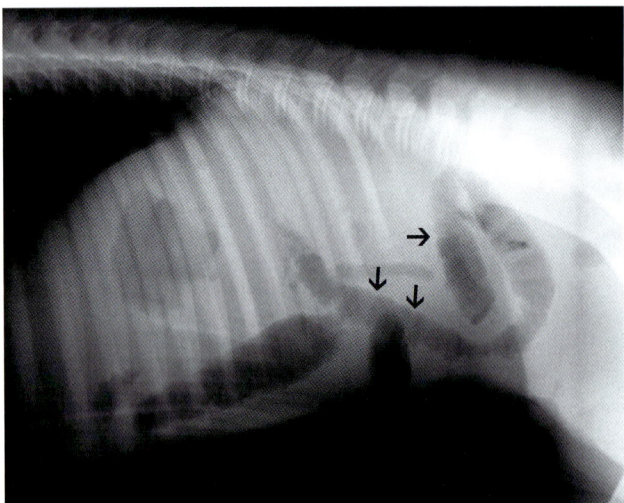

Fig. 11-10 Radiographic appearance of enteritis. Foals with enteritis may have numerous nonspecific radiographic findings, such as gas-distended small intestine and multiple gas-fluid interfaces. In the radiograph depicted here, the finding of individual loops of mildly to moderately gas-distended small intestine with irregular or "corrugated" walls is highly indicative of enteritis.

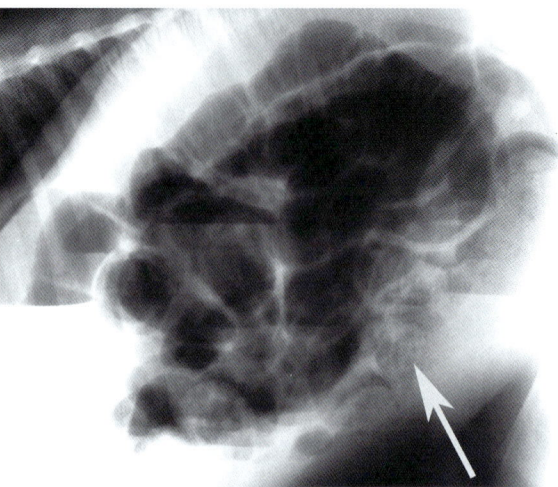

Fig. 11-12 Radiographic appearance of a meconium impaction. In addition to generalized gas distension of the large intestine, neonatal foals with meconium impactions may have radiographic evidence of excessive meconium, which often appears as granular contents within bowel in the ventrocaudal or caudodorsal abdomen *(arrow)*.

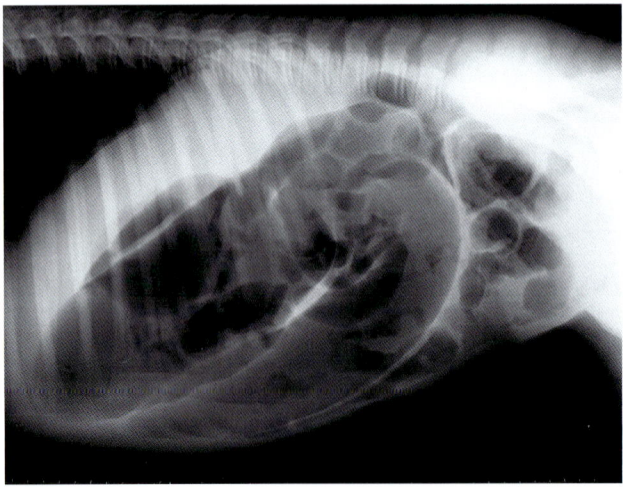

Fig. 11-11 Radiographic appearance of a large- or small-colon obstruction. Unlike small-intestinal gas distension, generalized gas distension of large colon is considered to be fairly specific for large- or small-colon obstruction. This foal had a distal meconium impaction.

rupture should be suspected if there is a gas cap in the dorsal aspect of the abdominal cavity, if the serosal surfaces of bowel are enhanced, or if visualization of the renal silhouettes is improved. Iatrogenic pneumoperitoneum should be considered if an abdominocentesis was performed prior to abdominal radiography.

Finally, abdominal radiography obtained on foals with necrotizing enterocolitis may demonstrate the pathognomonic sign of pneumatosis intestinalis, or intramural air. Radiographic signs of pneumatosis

intestinalis are spectacular and include localized cystic collections that appear as radiolucent "bubbles" in the bowel wall, or diffuse linear strips or flat oval-shaped areas of radiolucency in the bowel wall flanked by the radiopaque serosa and mucosa, when the bowel wall is viewed end-on.[18]

Contrast radiography also has some specific indications in neonatal foals. An upper gastrointestinal contrast study can be used to document delayed gastric emptying of older foals with suspected pyloric outflow obstruction.[16] Foals less than two weeks of age ideally should be fasted for four hours, and foals consuming solid feeds should be fasted for 12 hours prior to contrast radiography.[17] Barium is administered by gravity flow via a nasogastric tube (5 ml/kg as a 30% weight/volume solution), and abdominal radiographs are obtained every 30 minutes. If barium remains in the stomach for longer than two hours, delayed gastric emptying should be suspected but does not necessarily distinguish between mechanical or functional obstruction. Barium should normally reach the cecum and transverse colon by two hours and three hours, respectively, in 10- to 12-day-old foals.[16,17] Barium transit time to the transverse colon is five to eight hours in foals one to two months of age. In addition to documenting transit time, stenosis or abnormal bowel wall may be highlighted by the contrast (Figure 11-13). Lower-intestinal contrast studies (i.e., barium enema) have been reported to have 100% sensitivity and 100% specificity for identifying mechanical obstruction (meconium impaction, atresia coli) of the transverse colon or small colon in foals less than 30 days of age (Figure 11-14).[19] The foal should be restrained or lightly

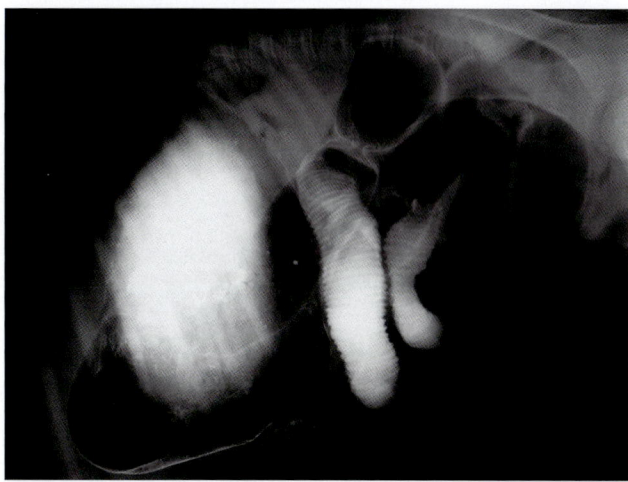

Fig. 11-13 Contrast radiographic evidence of enteritis. This abdominal radiograph was taken approximately 30 minutes after oral administration of barium to a foal with clinical signs of colic. Note the contrast highlighting the distended small intestine with distinctly abnormal loops of corrugated or thickened walls that appear as chains of rings in long axis.

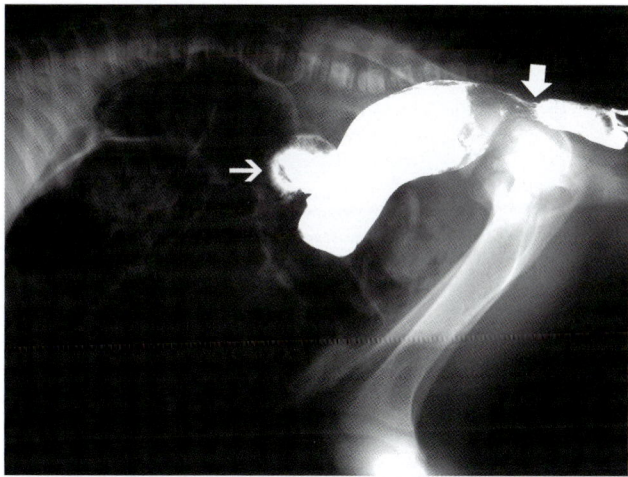

Fig. 11-14 Barium enema demonstrating distal obstruction. Administration of barium as an enema (see text) reportedly has 100% sensitivity and 100% specificity for identification of small or large-colon obstructions. The abrupt end of contrast in the small colon in this foal was highly indicative of atresa coli *(thin arrow)*, which was later confirmed at necropsy. Also note the stenosis of the rectum above the pelvis *(thick arrow).*

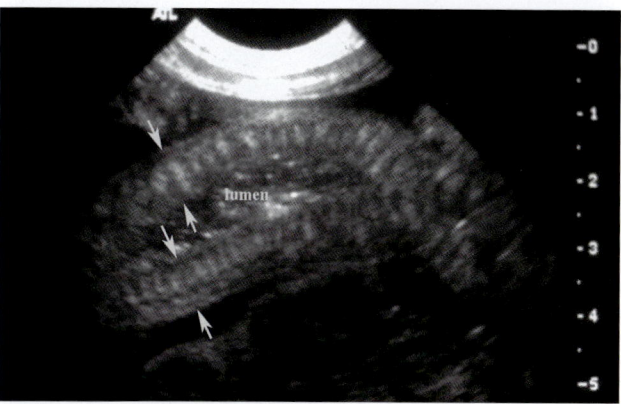

Fig. 11-15 Ultrasonographic appearance of enteritis. This image was obtained with a 7-4 MHz curvilinear probe set to a depth of 5 cm. Note the thickened and irregular wall of small intestine. Normal thickness of the jejunal wall is <4 mm. This foal's small-intestinal wall was almost 1 cm thick *(between arrows).*

sedated and placed in lateral recumbency. A 24-french Foley catheter is placed into the rectum and the bulb gradually inflated. By gravity flow, administer up to 20 ml/kg of 30% weight/volume barium.

Two-dimensional transabdominal ultrasonography is a valuable diagnostic tool in the colicky neonatal foal. Scanning techniques for the foal abdomen are extensively reviewed elsewhere,[20] though a brief review follows here. Standard linear array 4 to 7 MHz transducers are sufficient for visualization of most intra-abdominal structures in the neonatal foal; however a curvilinear transducer will optimize image quality. The foal may be scanned in either lateral recumbency or standing; however keep in mind that fluid-filled, thickened, or enlarged structures may descend to the dependent portion of the abdomen and could be overlooked if only the nondependent side of a recumbent foal is scanned. Furthermore, gas in non-dependent bowel, especially gas in large colon, may preclude examination of deeper structures in laterally recumbent foals. Visualization of intra-abdominal structures is facilitated by clipping the abdominal hair; however thorough wetting of the hair with water or alcohol, in addition to acoustic coupling gel, may be sufficient. In the colicky neonate, transabdominal ultrasonography can be used to identify fluid-distended structures (i.e. stomach, small intestine, large intestine, urinary bladder), gastric or intestinal wall thickness, abnormal intestinal contents (i.e. meconium, fecaliths, phytobezoars, or trichophytobezoars), peritoneal fluid, and to determine intestinal motility.

Normal gastric wall thickness in foals should be less than 7 mm, whereas intestinal wall thickness is 3 to 4 mm. Foals with gastritis or gastric ulcers may have a thickened or irregular gastric wall. Likewise, foals with enteritis or colitis will frequently have diffusely increased small and/or large intestine wall thickness (Figure 11-15). This feature alone does not definitively identify enteritis, as edematous bowel that develops as the result of strangulation (volvulus or intussusception) will also appear regionally thickened (Figure 11-16), with distended fluid-filled intestine proximally. The presence of gas echoes in the intestinal wall, a thickened hypoechoic wall that appears "wavy," or the presence of sloughed mucosa in the lumen are more consistent with a diagnosis of enteritis and should be

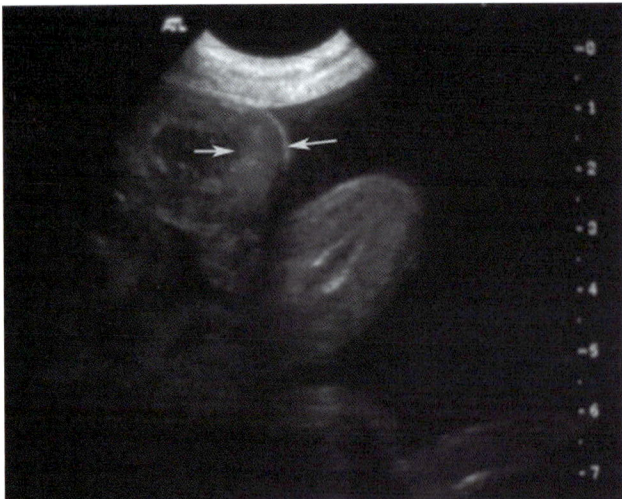

Fig. 11-16 Ultrasonographic appearance of edematous small intestine. This image was obtained with a 7-4 MHz curvilinear probe set to a depth of approximately 7 cm. Note the excessive anechoic peritoneal fluid that surrounds the small intestine with an approximate wall thickness of 1 cm *(between arrows)*. This foal had a small-intestinal volvulus.

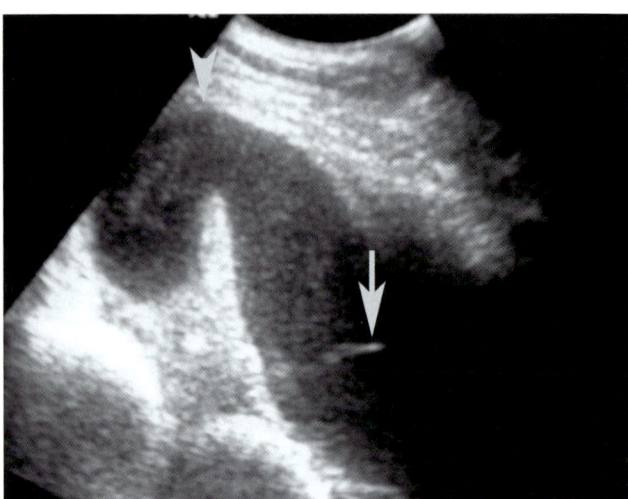

Fig. 11-18 Ultrasonographic appearance of small-intestinal obstruction. This image was obtained with a 7-4 MHz curvilinear probe set to a depth of 8 cm. Note the *U*-turn or hairpin turn in the fluid-distended small intestine *(arrowhead)*. This foal had an ascarid impaction that was confirmed with an exploratory celiotomy. Note the ascarids in the lumen of the distended small intestine *(arrow)*.

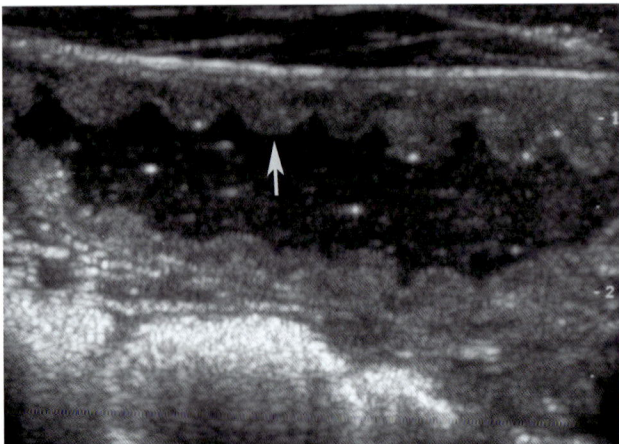

Fig. 11-17 Ultrasonographic appearance of enteritis. This image was obtained with a 7-4 MHz linear array probe set to a depth of approximately 3 cm. The wavy edge of the small-intestinal mucosa *(arrow)* in this long-axis view of fluid-distended small intestine is a finding that is most frequently detected in foals with enteritis.

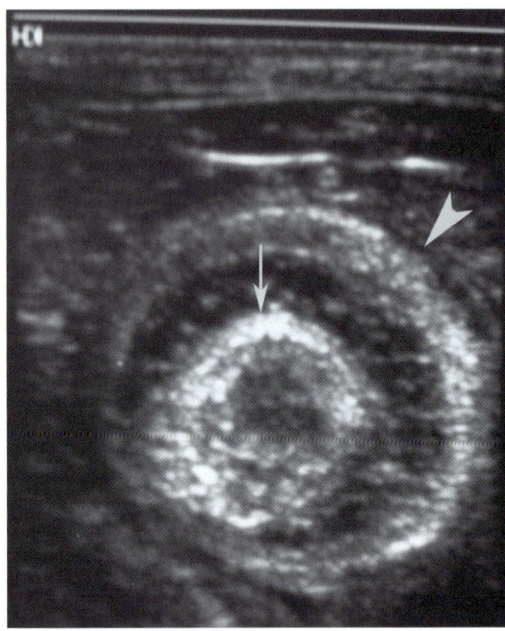

Fig. 11-19 Ultrasonographic appearance of an intussusception. This image was obtained with a 7-4 MHz linear array probe set to a depth of 4 cm. The "target" or "bull's-eye" appearance of concentric rings is created by the thickened and distended outer loop of small intestine *(arrowhead)* separated by fluid from the thickened entering loop of small intestine *(intussusception, arrow)*, as viewed in short axis.

considered as distinguishing features from strangulating lesions (Figure 11-17). Foals with enteritis or colitis may demonstrate either hypermotile or hypomotile bowel, whereas functional ileus and mechanically obstructed intestine more often will appear hypomotile. Neonatal foals with mechanical obstruction of small intestine may have hairpin or *U*-shaped turns of the small intestine when viewed in long axis (Figure 11-18). The unique regional presence of a double intestinal wall or what appears to look like a "bull's-eye" of multiple concentric rings in a short axis view of small intestine is consistent with an intussusception (Figure 11-19), which most commonly is seen in the dependent portion of the abdomen.

Meconium may appear hyperechoic, hypoechoic, or as a mixture of echogenicities in hypomotile intestine.

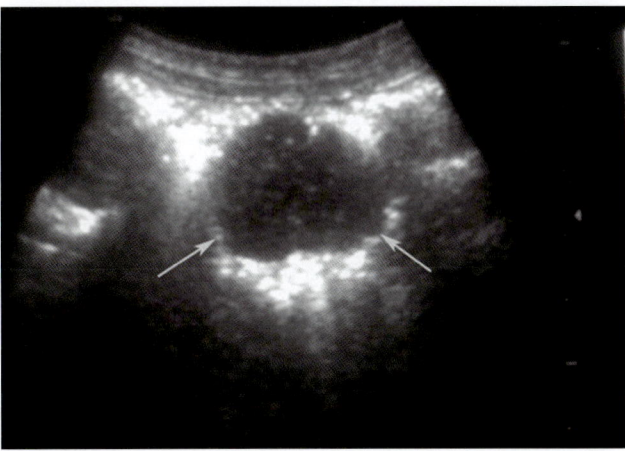

Fig. 11-20 Ultrasonographic appearance of meconium. This image was obtained with a 7-4 MHz curvilinear probe set to a depth of 6 cm and shows a single "ball" of fairly uniformly hypoechoic meconium *(arrow)*, surrounding by gas in the small colon.

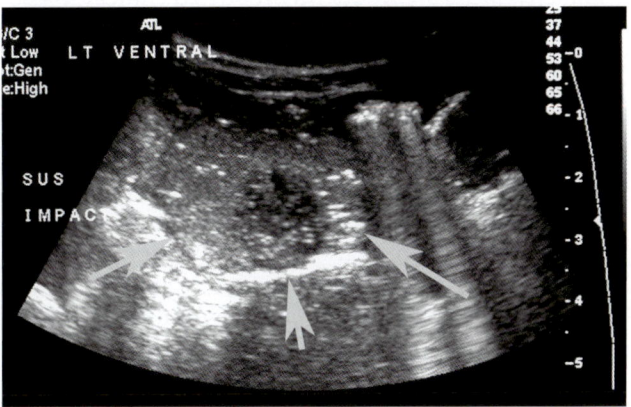

Fig. 11-21 Ultrasonographic appearance of meconium. This image was obtained with a 7-4 MHz curvilinear probe set to a depth of 5 cm and shows a single "ball" of meconium *(arrows)* with mixed echogenicity in the small colon.

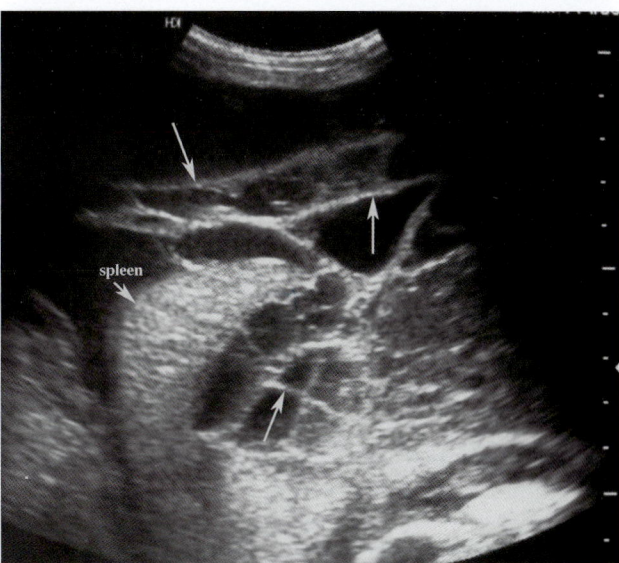

Fig. 11-22 Ultrasonographic appearance of intra-abdominal adhesions. This image was obtained with a 7-4 MHz curvilinear probe set to a depth of 11 cm. This foal developed septic peritonitis as a sequela to severe necrotizing enterocolitis. Note the excessive amount of peritoneal fluid containing numerous fibrin strands *(arrows)*, connecting loops of bowel, and the spleen. This foal was euthanized due to recurring bouts of abdominal pain, despite resolution of the enteritis.

Fluid- or gas-distended intestine may be present proximal to the obstruction (Figures 11-20 and 11-21). When present in the small colon, retained or impacted meconium often appears as a row of "balls" and is most easily identified in the dependent portion of the left caudal abdomen in the standing foal. It may be traceable dorsal to the urinary bladder and often is surrounded by a thin layer of hyperechoic gas in sacculated intestine (small colon). Meconium in large colon typically is more amorphous. Extensive gas in the large colon frequently hinders visualization of other intra-abdominal structures and can be associated with mechanical obstruction, though it may also occur with acute colitis. The sonographic appearance of abdominal abscesses is variable, but in the neonatal foal, intra-abdominal abscesses are often associated with umbilical remnants, previously devitalized bowel, or mesenteric lymph nodes. Finally, the presence of excessive anechoic fluid may be indicative of uroperitoneum (see Chapter 12), though anechoic transudate may also develop as a result of enteritis, colitis, or strangulation. Hyperechoic densities within peritoneal fluid may represent fibrin strands, leukocytes, or adhesions (Figure 11-22). The presence of gas echoes free within the peritoneal fluid is indicative of a ruptured viscus.

Gastroscopy may be accomplished with a 1-meter endoscope in a neonatal foal and is covered elsewhere in more detail later in this chapter (see Case 11-2). For most neonatal foals, suckling can be allowed prior to gastroscopy, but solid-feed consumption should be withheld for 6 to 10 hours.[21] Caution should be exercised in the interpretation of the clinical significance of gastric ulcers in foals, as up to 50% of young asymptomatic foals have gastric ulcers along the margo plicatus of the greater curvature of the stomach, and gastric ulcers may develop secondary to another primary gastrointestinal disorder.[22,23] However, multiple deeper ulcers, bleeding ulcers, ulcers along the lesser curvature or in the glandular mucosa, or those accompanied by clinical signs that are consistent with gastric ulceration should be considered clinically significant.

DIFFERENTIAL DIAGNOSIS

Most information on colic in the neonate is obtained from referral institutions or, more often, from foals undergoing exploratory celiotomy for acute abdominal pain; therefore the data may not precisely reflect the true incidence of each reported etiology. The only published study on 20 foals less than two weeks of age with acute abdominal pain reported that an exploratory celiotomy revealed functional ileus (45%), meconium impaction (25%), large-colon displacement (15%), small intestine displaced around the base of the cecum (10%), ruptured gastric ulcer, and small colon obstructed by the ovarian ligament.[7] Other retrospective studies of abdominal surgery in the foal include foals three to six months of age and thus it was difficult to ascertain the etiology of abdominal pain exclusive to the neonatal period. In 53 foals that underwent an exploratory celiotomy from birth to three months of age, meconium impaction, uroperitoneum, enteritis, small-intestinal strangulation (herniation with incarceration, small-intestinal volvulus, and intussusception), and enteritis accounted for 80% of the total cases.[4] In a study that reviewed 83 foals up to six months of age, the most commonly reported diseases identified at surgery were small-intestinal volvulus, meconium impaction, and intussusception.[8] These reports underscore the difficulty in definitively identifying the cause of abdominal pain prior to exploratory celiotomy in neonatal foals, as clearly some of these cases, such as enteritis and functional ileus, would not be considered to be predominantly surgical diseases. *Furthermore, it is noteworthy that if the etiology of the abdominal pain cannot be ascertained in the violently painful patient, an exploratory celiotomy may be indicated solely as a diagnostic tool.* The purpose of this section is to provide a brief review of the conditions most commonly reported in the neonatal foal. Table 11-1 provides a more comprehensive list of reported causes of acute abdominal pain in the young foal.

Meconium Impaction

Meconium is the sticky caramelized feces of the newborn foal that comprises intestinal secretions, swallowed amniotic fluid, and cellular debris. In one study of 30 newborn foals, it was reported that the total weight of meconium is equal to 1% of the foal's body weight.[24] Most foals will start to evacuate meconium shortly after the first ingestion of colostrum, which acts both as a laxative and stimulator of the gastrocolonic reflex. The majority of the meconium is evacuated within the first 12 hours of birth and is replaced by "milk" feces, which are pasty and yellow in appearance. However, concurrent disease such as neonatal asphyxia, prematurity, septicemia, and encephalopathy may delay passage. Meconium impaction implies failure to evacuate sufficient quantities of meconium with subsequent development of signs of colonic obstruction: pain, straining to defecate, and abdominal distension secondary to accumulation of gas in bowel proximal to the impacted meconium.

It has been suggested that meconium impaction is more likely to occur in colts[11] and in foals greater than 340 days of gestational age.[25] To the author's knowledge, prophylactic use of an enema at birth has not been shown to prevent meconium retention or impaction. Foals with meconium impaction are disinterested in nursing, strain to defecate, and typically stand with a slightly arched back and frequently "swish" their tail (Figure 11-1). Digital examination may detect meconium within the rectum. Colic, abdominal distension, tachypnea, general restlessness, and tachycardia are frequently reported clinical signs.[11] Intestinal borborygmi are usually present[11] and are not a reliable sign of obstruction. Meconium can usually be identified by either plain or contrast abdominal radiography or ultrasonography (see "Diagnostic Approach to Colic in Neonatal Foals" section above). In more severe obstructions, excessive amounts of gas may accumulate in the large colon, proximal to the obstruction. Rupture of the urinary bladder may occur in foals that strain excessively from meconium impaction.[11] Furthermore, extensive mural damage lends to bacterial translocation and secondary septicemia.

Lethal White Syndrome

Other causes of acute abdominal pain that closely mimic meconium impaction and primarily manifest during the first 24 to 48 hours of life are the rarely reported cases of ileocolonic aganglionosis, atresia coli, and atresia recti. Ileocolonic aganglionosis, or "lethal white" syndrome, is a fatal autosomal recessive disorder principally of overo cross overo Paint Horses that is caused by a point mutation in amino acid 118 in endothelin receptor B.[26] The endothelin receptor is critical for the proper development and migration of cells from the neural crest that ultimately form melanocytes in the skin as well as neurons in the intestinal tract. Thus, foals that are homozygous for the mutation are essentially all white (though some small areas of pigmentation can occur) and develop signs of functional ileus in the first few hours of life (Figure 11-23). Color patterns in the dam and sire that have the highest incidence of heterozygote carriers of the mutation are

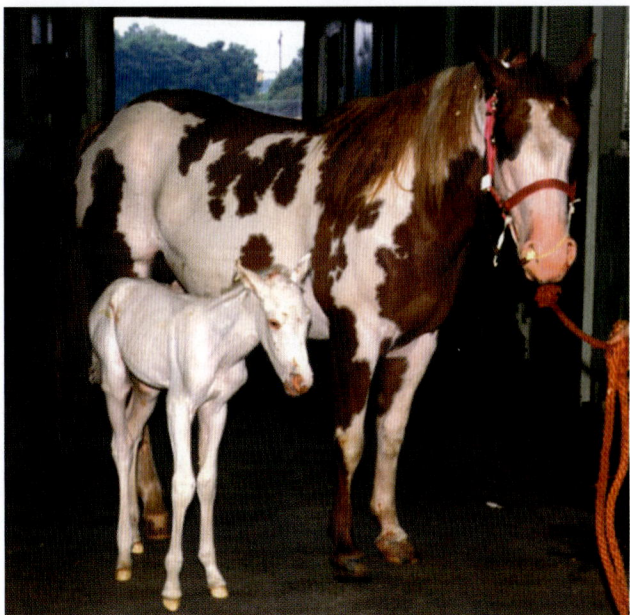

Fig. 11-23 Lethal white syndrome. This all-white foal born to an overo Paint mare that was bred to an overo Paint stallion was diagnosed with ileocolonic aganglionosis at necropsy. The defect is caused by an autosomal recessive point mutation in the endothelin B receptor.

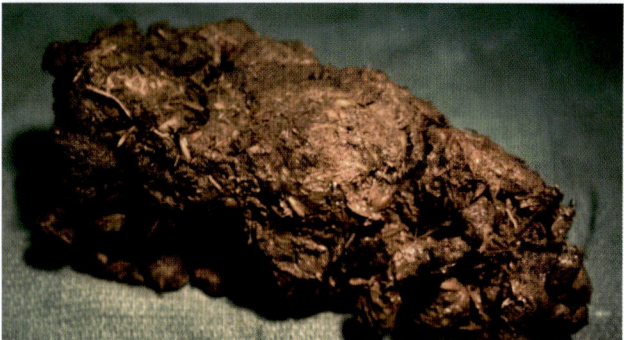

Fig. 11-24 Fecalith. This fecalith was removed by small colon enterotomy from a four-week-old American Miniature foal with acute abdominal pain and gross abdominal distension.

www.vgl.ucdavis.edu/service/horse/coatcolor.html. It should be noted that not all white foals of Paint lineage are lethal whites and when tested, these unaffected, rare, all-white Paint Horses are not homozygous for the mutation.

Other Differentials

Atresia coli, recti, or ani are rarely reported causes of colic in the newborn foal that may mimic meconium impaction, based on age of onset and signs of obstructive disease.[27] It may be possible to identify atresia recti on visual or digital examination of the rectum or by protoscopy. Retrograde contrast barium enema usually identifies an abrupt obstruction (see Figure 11-14), but definitive identification may require an exploratory celiotomy. Successful surgical repair has been described; however, other congenital abnormalities have been simultaneously reported and should be ruled out prior to consideration of surgery. The heritability of these defects is not fully known.[27]

Fecaliths are hard concretions of ingesta (Figure 11-24) that may also contain undigested material, such as hair. They most commonly occur in the American Miniature breed and have been reported in foals as young as 19 days of age.[6,10] Affected foals typically present with progressive unresponsive abdominal pain that is accompanied by gross abdominal distension. As fecaliths obstruct the small colon or rectal lumen, abdominal radiographs typically demonstrate gas distension of the large colon. Successful treatment almost inevitably involves a celiotomy with a small colon enterotomy.

Strangulating lesions of the small intestine that require surgery occur more frequently in neonatal foals, as compared to strangulating lesions of the large intestine. Volvulus of the small intestine is the most commonly reported strangulating lesion in foals less than three months of age.[8] Factors leading to development of

frame overo, highly white calico overo, and frame blend overo horses.[26] However, the heterozygote mutation has been occasionally rarely detected in other white-patterned Paints and "nonPaint" white-patterned bloodlines. It has not been detected in solid-colored breeding-stock Paint Horses without white, but heterozygote adult solid-colored Miniature Horses of Paint lineage and white-patterned horses of breeds other than the Paint Horse have been rarely identified.[26]

Lethal white foals typically are born "normal" in appearance and behavior, with the exception of the mostly white coat. Clinical signs of abdominal pain usually develop in the first few hours of life, after ingestion of colostrum, and progressively develop gross abdominal distension. Evidence of passage of meconium is often missing, though some meconium may be passed. The only way to definitively identify a lethal white foal is by DNA testing for the mutation or histopathologic demonstration of insufficient intestinal ganglia. Unfortunately, it can take weeks to obtain the results of DNA testing and hours to days to obtain the results of intestinal biopsies. Diagnosis is often initially presumptive, based on signalment, heterozygote parents, lack of response to symptomatic treatment, and rule out of other causes by additional diagnostics or surgical exploratory. Affected foals and heterozygote adults can be identified by submitting plucked hair with intact root bulbs from the mane (preferred sample) to the Veterinary Genetics Laboratory at the University of California, Davis, available at these lesions are undetermined, but alterations in motility may contribute. Intussusceptions are most commonly reported in three- to five-week-old foals[2] and may be acute or chronic and intermittent. Small-intestinal intussusceptions are most frequent, but ileocecal and cecocolic intussusceptions have been reported in young foals.[28] Most inguinal and umbilical hernias in foals resolve spontaneously without incarceration of intestine.[8,29-32] In a large retrospective study of 147 foals with umbilical hernias, only 13 required surgical repair.[29] Only 4 of the 13 foals that needed surgery had incarcerated bowel in the umbilical hernia. Although the hernias were present since birth, and strangulation may rarely occur shortly after birth, the majority of foals with strangulating umbilical hernias were not neonates, but most often, affected foals were presented in the first six months of life.[31] The most common presenting complaint in foals with an umbilical hernia with incarcerated bowel was an acute firm enlargement of the hernia that was sensitive upon palpation. Only 30% of foals with strangulated umbilical hernias presented with signs of abdominal pain.

In separate retrospective reports, inguinal hernias in neonatal foals that resulted in incarceration of small intestine that required surgical correction were exclusively found in newborn foals as a result of rents in the vaginal tunic (direct inguinal hernia).[30,32] Onset of clinical signs was typically within 48 hours of birth. Diagnosis should be suspected by the presence of an irreducible mass in the scrotal sac, edema in the scrotum and prepuce, and colic. Diagnosis of either an umbilical or scrotal hernia with incarceration can usually be confirmed by palpation and ultrasonography. It has been suggested that elective herniorrhagy should be considered if an umbilical hernia has been present in foals greater than six months of age or if the defect is larger than 10 cm.[31]

Diaphragmatic hernias are rare in foals and can result from failure of fusion of its embryonic components or from traumatic rupture of the diaphragm in utero, at birth, or after birth.[33] Affected foals can remain asymptomatic for prolonged periods of time, but the presenting complaint typically is acute abdominal pain. The intensity and onset of clinical signs is related to the amount of intestine that has herniated into the thoracic cavity and whether the herniated bowel is simply displaced or strangulated.[33] In addition to abdominal pain, tachypnea and/or dyspnea may be present. The diagnosis can be confirmed by either radiographic or ultrasonographic evidence of an incongruous diaphragmatic line, the presence of gas-fluid interfaces indicative of intestine in the thoracic cavity, and/or pleural effusion.

Enterocolitis, gastric ulceration, and uroperitoneum are commonly reported causes of abdominal pain in the neonate and are described separately later in this chapter and in Chapter 12. Functional ileus secondary to prematurity, sepsis, neonatal asphyxia, neonatal encephalopathy, electrolyte abnormalities, concurrent gastrointestinal disease, hypoxic or ischemia bowel, overfeeding, use of milk replacer, botulism, and many other concurrent diseases may induce significant abdominal pain in the neonatal foal. If these underlying conditions are present, careful consideration to additional diagnostics should be used to rule out more serious gastrointestinal disorders (see "Diagnostic Approach to Colic in Neonatal Foals" section above). Simple solutions, such as reducing or eliminating enteral feeding, changing the source of milk, or correction of electrolyte derangements and other underlying disorders should be tried first. However, it may be necessary to consider an exploratory celiotomy for definitive diagnosis and for therapeutic decompression of bowel before initiation of prokinetic therapy. Cecal impaction, large-colon volvulus, large-colon displacement, intestinal infarction, and ileal impaction are considered to be rare disorders of the neonatal foal.

For the suspected meconium impaction, 120 ml of mineral oil was given '03 RockN'Roll via a nasogastric tube. Lactated Ringer's solution was given at a rate of 100 ml/kg/day, as a continuous rate infusion. The foal was given 1 mg of butorphanol and 10 mg of diazepam intravenously. A 4% acetylcysteine retention enema was administered; 40 ml of 20% acetylcysteine was mixed with 160 ml of water. A 30-french Foley catheter was inserted into the anus, and the cuff was slowly inflated to prevent extraction. The acetylcysteine solution was given by gravity flow. After 45 minutes, the cuff was deflated and the Foley catheter was removed. Abdominal distension was monitored by periodically measuring the abdominal diameter using a tape measure. The foal was not allowed to nurse the mare and was continually observed by technical nursing staff.

To address the increased risk of sepsis, 1 liter of plasma was given intravenously and the foal was started on K penicillin (22,000 units/kg IV q 6 hours) and amikacin (21 mg/kg IV q 24 hours). Four hours after presentation, the blood glucose concentration decreased to 80 mg/dl and thus the LRS was supplemented with 2.5% glucose. The foal remained quiet and alert for the next several hours and was intermittently observed to strain. A small amount of meconium was passed six hours after admission. Approximately 10 hours after admission, the foal was observed to roll into dorsal recumbency. An abdominocentesis was performed using an 18-gauge needle. The peritoneal fluid was light yellow in color and had a nucleated cell count of 5,900/μl and a protein concentration of 2.6 g/dl. Cytologic examination revealed 95% nondegenerative neutrophils with occasional Dohle bodies, and 5% mononuclear cells. Microbes were not observed. The foal's TPR remained within normal limits

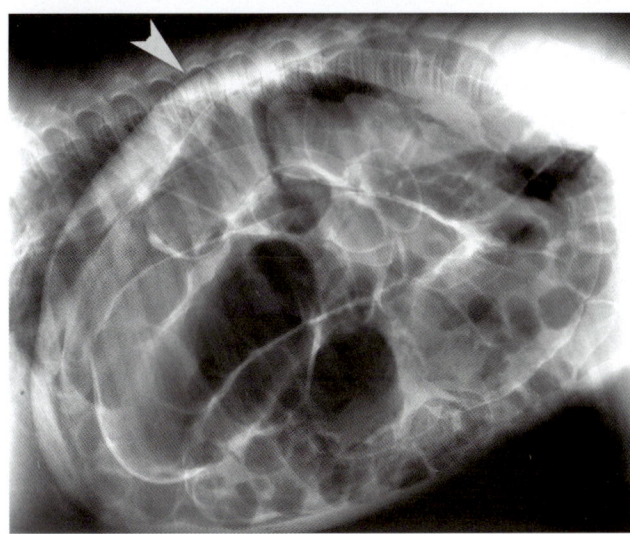

Fig. 11-25 Radiographs obtained from '03 RockN'Roll. These abdominal radiographs demonstrate diffuse gas-distended large intestine, with granular-appearing luminal contents in the caudoventral abdomen. The small amount of free gas visible ventral to the diaphragm *(arrowhead)* and the generalized increased radiopacity of the serosal surfaces are radiographic evidence of pneumoperitoneum.

until 12 hours after presentation, when the rectal temperature was 100.5°F, the heart rate was 176 beats/minute, and respiration was 24 breaths/minute.

A digital rectal examination revealed continued presence of ingesta at the pelvic inlet. Abdominal radiographs were obtained (Figure 11-25) and demonstrated generalized gas distension in the large colon with granular-appearing contents in the lumen. The serosal margin detail was increased, and free gas was noted in the peritoneal cavity. The radiographic findings were consistent with obstruction of the large colon with pneumoperitoneum. The tachycardia and radiographic findings prompted the decision to perform an exploratory celiotomy. An extensive and firm meconium impaction was confirmed in the small colon. Despite aggressive attempts to dislodge the impaction by injection of the impaction with carboxymethylcellulose, accompanied by external mural massage of the small colon, a small colon enterotomy was necessary to remove the impaction. Upon further exploration of the peritoneal cavity, a small full-thickness tear of the transverse colon wall was identified with focal adjacent fecal contamination. With this revelation, the foal was euthanized under anesthesia. A necropsy examination was not performed.

TREATMENT

Medical therapy for meconium impaction includes judicious use of analgesics, intravenous polyionic isotonic fluids, oral laxative therapy, and enemas. Foals with meconium impactions are expected to exhibit some degree of pain. Judicious use of analgesics (Table 11-2) is required to balance the necessity to provide relief from pain and the ability to appropriately assess the patient's progress. Mineral oil (4 to 8 ounces administered via a nasogastric tube) is used for its lubricating effect. Milk of magnesia (1 to 2 ounces) provides an osmotic laxative effect, but should be used sparingly as it may be dehydrating. The detergent dioctyl sodium sulfosuccinate can be quite irritating, and it should be avoided in both oral and rectal therapy.[8] Castor oil therapy has been described,[34] but can provoke violent abdominal pain in the foal.

Enemas are a mainstay of treatment for small-colon meconium impactions. Warm-water liquid detergent (i.e., Palmolive®) enemas (½ teaspoon liquid detergent to 500 ml water) are purportedly gentle to the rectal mucosa and effective. Commercial phosphate enemas (i.e., Fleet®) can also be used, but repeated administration may increase the risk of phosphate toxicity. Recently, acetylcysteine retention enemas have been reported to be a highly successful treatment for meconium impactions in foals.[11] It is hypothesized that the acetylcysteine cleaves disulphide bonds in the mucoprotein molecules in meconium, decreasing its overall tenacity.

A 4% acetylcysteine solution, pH 7.6, is made by adding 20 g of baking soda and 8 g of acetylcysteine to 200 ml of water. A 30-french Foley catheter with a 30 ml bulb is inserted approximately 2.5 to 5 cm into the rectum and, the bulb is slowly inflated to occlude the rectum. One hundred to 200 ml of the 4% acetyl cysteine solution is administered by gravity flow and retained for 30 to 45 minutes. The acetylcysteine retention enema was effective in eliminating 78% of meconium impactions within 12 hours.[11] If needed, the acetylcysteine therapy can be repeated in 12 hours, and was repeated up to three times in some cases before resolution of the impaction. Occasionally, repeated use of an enema generates significant rectal and small colon mucosal irritation that sustains signs of straining despite effective removal of the impaction. This continued straining may confound determination of successful treatment.

Surgical intervention should be considered if medical therapy is unsuccessful.[35,36]

When to Consider Surgery

Although there often is no single criterion that distinguishes the course of treatment in any particular case, an exploratory celiotomy should be considered in a foal with abdominal pain (of any etiology) if there is:

- Persistent pain that is unresponsive to analgesics

- Persistent tachycardia, especially a sustained heart rate greater than 120 beats/minute

- Progressive abdominal enlargement

- Increased peritoneal fluid protein concentration and/or nucleated cell count

- Sanguinous peritoneal fluid

- Evidence of sepsis in the peritoneal fluid, without known origin

- Radiographic or ultrasonographic evidence of obstruction

- Deterioration in the foal's condition with a definitive diagnosis not determined

- An owner that is well-informed of the cost and prognosis

OUTCOME

The prognosis for foals with a meconium impaction is generally considered good to excellent with short-term survival reported to be 100%[11] and long-term survival, following either medical or surgical treatment, reported to be 80% to 94%.[35,36] Most meconium impactions will resolve with medical intervention. At the University of California, Davis, from 1987 to 2002, 41 out of 44 foals (93%) with meconium impactions were successfully treated medically with acetylcysteine enemas.[11] About 40% of these former cases required more than one acetylcysteine enema, and in about 20% of cases it took more than 12 hours for the impaction to resolve. Once hospitalized, '03 RockN'Roll received one acetylcysteine enema and oral laxative and intravenous fluid therapy over 12 hours. Prior to surgery, the foal exhibited only mild to moderate signs of intermittent pain (straining to defecate with recumbency and rare dorsal recumbency) and his abdominal size did not significantly increase. The discovery of pneumoperitoneum before celiotomy was worrisome. However, because an abdominocentesis had been performed several hours prior to taking the abdominal radiograph, it was speculated that the pneumoperitoneum was iatrogenic from introduction of room air through the abdominocentesis needle into the peritoneal cavity. The subsequent detection of a ruptured transverse colon during surgery was an unexpected complication. Spontaneous rupture of the colon as a sequela to meconium impaction must indeed be rare, as there are no reports of its occurrence in the American literature. It remains unclear as to when the colon rupture occurred.

At presentation, the foal did not exhibit clinical signs of sepsis, though a small but significant left shift was present on the leukogram. This may have been a result of early sepsis from an unrelated cause or may have been the result of bacterial translocation across compromised mucosa along the colonic impaction. The foal did not exhibit intense signs of abdominal pain, in fact, he only showed signs of straining to defecate during the first 10 hours of hospitalization. Although he received an analgesic dose of flunixin meglumine prior to referral, he only received one other short-acting analgesic prior to surgery: 1 mg of butorphanol. The abdominocentesis was performed at approximately 10 hours of hospitalization, after the foal was observed to roll into dorsal recumbency. Although the nucleated cell count and protein concentration were both increased, there were no signs of sepsis cytologically. Either rupture had not yet occurred or it had already occurred and the peritoneal fluid sample obtained by abdominocentesis was not representative. In retrospect, the pneumoperitoneum seen radiographically at 12 hours of hospitalization most likely was indicative of a localized rupture. The decision to perform an exploratory celiotomy was based upon the lack of passage of a significant amount of meconium, the presence of extensive amounts of meconium in the colon (as seen ultrasonographically and radiographically), the presence of free air in the peritoneal cavity on abdominal radiographs, and the development of persistent tachycardia, with a sustained heart rate greater than 120 beats/minute.

Although the majority of foals with meconium impactions are treated medically, surgery is indicated in some cases. Postoperative intra-abdominal adhesion formation is the most common anticipated complication, thus surgery is often delayed for fear of poor long-term survival. Two short-term survival (i.e., survival until discharge) studies on foals undergoing exploratory celiotomy for meconium impactions had a combined survival rate of 90% (9 out of 10 foals).[4,6] Long-term survival to maturity was 67% (4 out of 6) for foals undergoing surgery with either enterotomy or manual reduction.[36] In a 2002 retrospective study in Germany on 42 foals undergoing an enterotomy for a meconium impaction, long-term survival to six months was 60%.[35] In general, for foals undergoing an exploratory celiotomy, the survival rate is better for foals with lesions of the large colon, compared to the small intestine.[8] Although studies before 1994 indicate that survival rate for foals undergoing surgery for colic is lowest for neonates, data from the early 1990s showed significantly higher survival rates, as compared to the 1980s.[4-6] With advancements in diagnostics and critical care, assuredly the long-term survival has continued to improve, though specific data is unavailable for recent years.

REFERENCES

1. Traub-Dargatz J, Kopral C, Seitzinger A et al: Estimate of the national incidence of and operational-level risk factors for colic among horses in the United States, spring 1998-1999, *J Am Vet Med Assoc* 219:67, 2001.

2. Platt H: Etiological aspects of perinatal mortality in the Thoroughbred, *Equine Vet J* 5:116, 1973.

3. Cohen N: Causes of and farm management factors associated with disease and death in foals, *J Am Vet Med Assoc* 204:1644, 1994.

4. Cable C, Fubini S, Erb H et al: Abdominal surgery in foals: A review of 119 cases (1977-1994), *Equine Vet J* 29:257, 1997.

5. Johnston G, Taylor P, Holmes M et al: Confidential enquiry of perioperative equine fatalities: Preliminary results, *Equine Vet J* 27:193, 1995.

6. Vatistas N, Snyder J, Wilson W et al: Surgical treatment for colic in the foal (67 cases): 1980-1992, *Equine Vet J* 28:139, 1996.

7. Adams R, Koterba A, Brown M: Exploratory celiotomy for gastrointestinal disease in neonatal foals: A review of 20 cases, *Equine Vet J* 20:9, 1988.

8. Bartmann C, Freeman D, Glitz F et al: Diagnosis and surgical management of colic in the foal: Literature review and retrospective study, *Clin Tech Equine Pract* 1:125, 2002.

9. Freeman D, Spencer P: Evaluation of age, breed, and gender as risk factors for umbilical hernia in horses of a hospital population, *Am J Vet Res* 52:637, 1991.

10. McClure J, Kobluk C, Voller K et al: Fecalith impaction in four miniature foals, *J Am Vet Med Assoc* 200:205, 1992.

11. Pusterla N, Magdesian K, Maleski K et al: Retrospective evaluation of the use of acetylcysteine enemas in the treatment of meconium retention in foals: 44 cases (1987-2002), *Equine Vet Educ* 16:133, 2004.

12. Kablack K, Hance S, Reimer J et al: Uroperitoneum in the hospitalised equine neonate: Retrospective study of 31 cases, 1988-1997, *Equine Vet J* 32:505, 2000.

13. Bernard W: Differentiating enteritis and conditions that require surgery in foals, *Comp Cont Ed for Pract Vet* 14:535, 1992.

14. Grindem C, Fairley N, Uhlinger C et al: Peritoneal fluid values from healthy foals, *Equine Vet J* 22:359, 1990.

15. Behrens E, Parraga M, Nassif A et al: Reference values of peritoneal fluid from healthy foals, *J Equine Vet Sci* 10:348, 1990.

16. Fischer A, Kerr L, Obrien T: Radiographic diagnosis of gastrointestinal disorders in the foal, *Vet Radiol* 28:42, 1987.

17. Campbell M, Ackerman N, Peyton L: Radiographic gastrointestinal anatomy of the foal, *Vet Radiol* 25:194, 1984.

18. Cudd T, Pauly T: Necrotizing enterocolitis in two equine neonates, *Comp Cont Ed for Pract Vet* 0(1):88, 1987.

19. Fischer A, Yarbrough T: Retrograde contrast radiography of the distal portions of the intestinal tract in foals, *J Am Vet Med Assoc* 207:734, 1995.

20. Reef V: Pediatric abdominal ultrasonography. In Reef V, ed: *Equine diagnostic ultrasound,* Philadelphia, 1998, WB Saunders, 364-403.

21. Chaffin M, Cohen N: Diagnostic assessment of foals with colic. In American Association of Equine Practitioners, 1999, Albuquerque, NM.

22. Murray M: Gastroendoscopic appearance of gastric lesions in foals: 94 cases (1987-1988), *J Am Vet Med Assoc* 195:1135, 1989.

23. Murray M, Murray C, Sweeney H et al: Prevalence of gastric lesions in foals without signs of gastric disease: An endoscopic survey, *Equine Vet J* 22:6, 1990.

24. Ganesan S, Bhuvanakumar C: Weighing meconium—an approach to prevent meconium retention in foals, *Centaur (Mylapore)* 10:23, 1993.

25. Lester G: The equine neonate: Special considerations. In Colahan P et al, eds: *Equine medicine and surgery,* St Louis, 1999, Mosby, 636-640.

26. Santschi E, Vrotsos P, Purdy A et al: Incidence of the endothelin receptor B mutation that causes lethal white foal syndrome in white-patterned horses, *Am J Vet Res* 62:97, 2001.

27. Young R, Linford R, Olander H: *Atresia coli* in the foal: A review of six cases, *Equine Vet J* 24:60, 1992.

28. Ford T, Freeman D, Ross M et al.: Ileocecal intussusception in horses: 26 cases (1981-1988), *J Am Vet Med Assoc* 196:121, 1990.

29. Freeman D, Orsini J, Harrison I: Complications of umbilical hernias in horses: 13 cases (1972-1986), *J Am Vet Med Assoc* 192:804, 1988.

30. Spurlock G, Robertson J: Congenital inguinal hernias associated with a rent in the common vaginal tunic in five foals, *J Am Vet Med Assoc* 193:1087, 1988.

31. Markel M, Pascoe J, Sams A: Strangulated umbilical hernias in horses: 13 cases (1974-1985), *J Am Vet Med Assoc* 190:692, 1987.

32. van der Velden M: Ruptured inguinal hernia in new-born colt foals: A review of 14 cases, *Equine Vet J* 20:178, 1988.

33. Bristol D: Diaphragmatic hernias in horses and cattle, *Comp Cont Ed for Pract Vet* 8:s407, 1986.

34. Bergman R: Retained meconium. In Robinson N, ed: *Current therapy in equine medicine,* Philadelphia, 1983, WB Saunders 260-262.

35. Sobiraj A, Herfen K, Bostedt H: Die mekoniumobstipation bei fohlen: Conservative und operative therapie unter besonderer berucksichitigung von komplikationen, *Tierarzti Prax* 28G:347, 2000.

36. Hughes F, Moll H, Slone D: Outcome of surgical correction of meconium impactions in 8 foals, *J Equine Vet Sci* 16:172, 1996.

37. Edwards G, Scholes S, Edwards S et al: Colic in 4 neonatal foals associated with chyloperitoneum and congenital segmental lymphatic aplasia. In The Fifth Equine Colic Research Symposium, Athens, GA, 1994.

38. Murray M: Megacolon with myenteric hypoganglionosis in a foal, *J Am Vet Med Assoc* 192:917, 1988.

39. Southwood L, Ragle C, Snyder J et al: Surgical treatment of ascarid impactions in horses and foals. In American Association of Equine Practitioners, Denver, CO, 1996.

40. Valk N Blackford J: Ovarian torsion as a cause of colic in a neonatal foal, *J Am Vet Med Assoc* 213:1454, 1998.

41. Green S, Specht T, Dowling S et al: Hemoperitoneum caused by rupture of a juvenile granulosa cell tumor in an equine neonate, *J Am Vet Med Assoc* 193:1417, 1988.

Case 11-2   **Gastric Ulcers and Esophageal Reflux (Endoscopy)**   Gary Magdesian

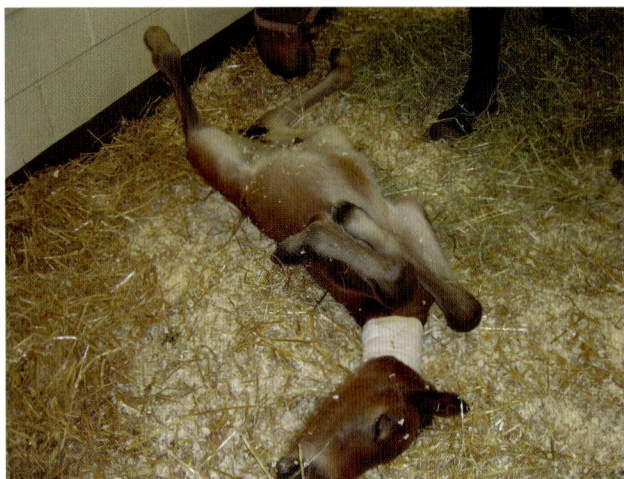

Fig. 11-26 '04 Belly Dancer, a three-day-old foal, in dorsal recumbency with signs of abdominal pain.

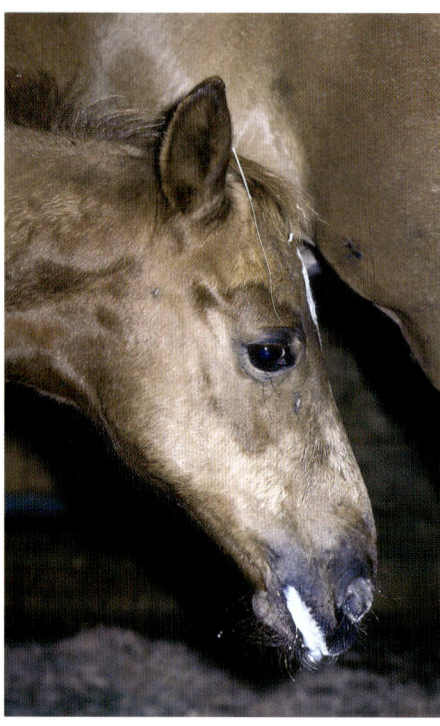

Fig. 11-27 Ptyalism in a foal with gastric ulceration.

'04 Belly Dancer, a three-day-old Quarter Horse filly, presented at the clinic for weakness, lethargy, and anorexia. Gestational history was unremarkable. The foal had congenital flexural deformity of the carpi, and had been treated with tetracycline (44 mg/kg, IV) for the contracture. She had been recumbent since birth, and had been assisted to stand to nurse or bottle feed in sternal recumbency. However, the foal had refused milk in the last 18 hours and she frequently assumed a dorsal recumbent position (Figure 11-26). On presentation the foal was in hypovolemic shock, as evidenced by tachycardia (166 beats/minute), cold extremities, weak peripheral pulse quality, and tacky mucous membranes. The foal was estimated to be 10% dehydrated. The carpi demonstrated mild contracture bilaterally.

After rehydration with lactated Ringer's and dextrose (2.5%), the foal's heart rate decreased and mentation improved. Upon increasing arousal, bruxism and ptyalism became apparent (Figure 11-27). Over the next several hours, the foal could rise with assistance and would attempt to nurse, but would stop nursing shortly after beginning. Dorsal recumbency became increasingly frequent.

HISTORY AND PHYSICAL EXAMINATION

Gastric ulceration has been diagnosed in foals as young as 24 hours of age and can been seen throughout the neonatal period and beyond.[1] The incidence of gastric ulceration in foals has been cited as high as 50%

in normal foals less than 50 days of age.[2,3] Because of this, it is difficult to know what role it plays in the health of the asymptomatic foal.[4] Stress has been implicated as a cause for gastric ulceration in the sick foal. In the neonate, ulcers are often present with concurrent diseases, such as enteritis or sepsis. The history should be utilized to determine if the foal had any prior illnesses, including diarrhea, colic, lethargy, or anorexia. Furr found that foals stressed by disease were more likely to have abnormal cortisol, T3, T4, and reverse T3 levels than age-matched normal controls foals. These stressed foals had a higher incidence of gastric ulceration than the normal foals.[4]

The clinical findings associated with ulcers can range from asymptomatic to death secondary to severe peritonitis from gastric rupture. A study in Japan of 40 foals with gastric ulceration found that the most prevalent clinical signs were depression and intermittent nursing (82.5% of affected foals) followed by diarrhea (65%), colic (37.5%), bruxism (10%), and ptyalism (7.5%).[5] Affected foals will often lay in dorsal recumbency trying to be more comfortable. Spontaneous gastric reflux from the nostrils can be seen on rare occasion. Foals with suspected or confirmed ulcers should be evaluated closely for sepsis or signs of peripartum asphyxia, as ulcers may develop secondary to these conditions. Some clinicians associate the stress of orthopedic disease in foals to be a risk factor for the development of gastric ulcerations.

Blood and urine from '04 Belly Dancer were submitted for analysis. A complete blood count showed a mild neutrophilia of 8,343/μl and a mild hyperfibrinogenemia of 500 mg/dl. A serum biochemistry profile and urinalysis were unremarkable. Because the foal's clinical signs were compatible with gastric ulceration, gastroscopy was performed. Hemorrhagic ulcers in both the squamous and glandular portions of the stomach were found. The duodenum and esophagus appeared unaffected. Abdominal ultrasonography was performed and the results were unremarkable. Abdominal radiography revealed mild to moderate gas distention of the intestines.

DIAGNOSTICS

Because of the role that other diseases may play in the development of gastric ulcers, the diagnostics surrounding the neonate with gastric and/or duodenal ulceration should include a thorough investigation of the systemic status of the foal, including complete blood count, serum biochemistries, and urinalysis. Blood cultures should be taken to evaluate for concurrent sepsis. Because of the potential role for hypoperfusion in the development of ulcer disease, perfusion should be monitored through serial blood pressure measurements (direct or indirect) and blood or plasma lactate concentrations.

Specific diagnostics for ulcer disease include gastroscopy or gastroduodenoscopy (including esophagoscopy for reflux esophagitis) as the most sensitive and specific means of diagnosing ulcer disease in the newborn. Usually this can be accomplished with a 1-meter endoscopy. The foal should be fasted for approximately two hours before scoping so that the gastric mucosa can be viewed better. The examination should be systematic being sure to view the distal esophagus and the squamous and glandular portions of the stomach. Lesions may vary from a mild hyperemia or gastritis to deep bleeding ulcerations (Figure 11-28, *A* and *B*). Another finding of gastroscopy in young foals is a desquamation of the squamous epithelia. This occurs in 80% of foals less than 35 days of age. Sheets of squamous epithelia shed during this time period. This can occur with or without ulceration (Figure 11-29).[6]

Radiographs of the abdomen may be useful in ruling out other causes of colic in the foal. The presence of free gas in the abdomen may be suggestive of a gastric perforation. Contrast radiography should be performed in foals with suspected gastric outflow obstruction (emptying disorders) such as those with

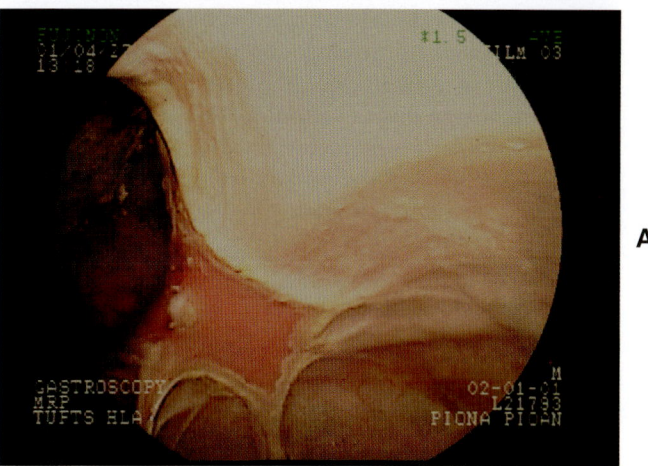
A

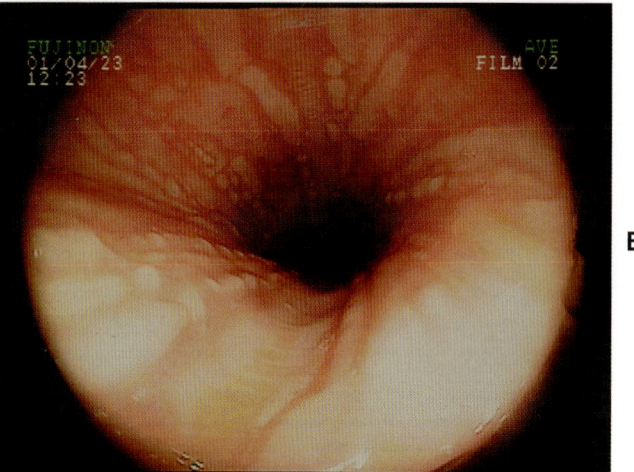
B

Fig. 11-28 A, Endoscopic view of ulceration of the squamous mucosa of a foal's stomach. **B,** Ulcerative esophagitis from gastric reflux. Note the "cobblestone" appearance of the mucosa.

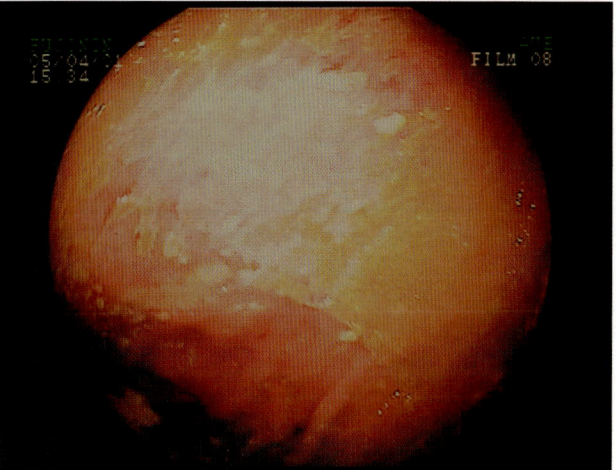

Fig. 11-29 Typical desquamation of squamous epithelia in a normal foal.

pyloric or duodenal ulceration (see Case 11-1). Delayed gastric emptying should be suspected if the barium is still in the stomach after two hours. Foals with ulcer disease should also have abdominal ultrasonography performed to evaluate for bowel wall thickness, ileus, and the possibility of peritoneal effusion. Ascites due to peritonitis in response to ulcers is a negative prognostic sign, and can mean perforation is imminent or has occurred.

Fecal or gastric occult blood may be suggestive of bleeding ulcers, but these tests are neither sensitive nor specific.

PATHOPHYSIOLOGY OF ULCER DISEASE

Neonatal ulcer disease occurs in a number of different syndromes, including silent ulcers, clinical or active ulcers, perforating ulcers, and duodenal ulcers. Silent ulcers are subclinical, but on occasion they have gone on to perforate. They may also be found incidentally on gastroscopy or postmortem examination. Clinical ulcers are consistent with the foal of this case; clinical signs included depression, partial anorexia, bruxism, ptyalism, dorsal recumbency, and colic. Ulcers can develop both in the glandular and nonglandular regions of the stomach. Duodenal ulcers, most common in the older (two- to five-month-old) foal, can result in pyloric strictures and gastric outflow obstruction and appear to represent a different syndrome than neonatal ulcers. These foals may develop reflux esophagitis as a result of the obstructive nature of this problem.

Healthy neonatal foals have an acidic baseline gastric pH, with an average pH of approximately 3.2 to 3.7.[7] They intermittently develop a gastric pH level below 1. Prolonged recumbency, greater than 20 minutes, results in a more acid gastric pH, often below 2.5 for prolonged periods.[7] Suckling milk raises the gastric pH to above 4.0, and sustains this high pH for several minutes.[7] This emphasizes the importance of frequent feedings in minimizing the potential for development of ulcers in the critically ill foal that is unable or not allowed to nurse.

The acid secretory profile of the critically ill foal is highly variable and differs widely from foal to foal. In one study, 43% of 23 hospitalized foals demonstrated alkaline profiles continuously, while another 43% had profiles typical of healthy foals.[8] The etiology of alkaline pH is unknown, but may represent parietal cell dysfunction as a consequence of hypoperfusion, or may alternatively reflect ileus with enterogastric reflux from the duodenum. Approximately 13% of foals have atypical profiles with periods of marked acidity.

The pathophysiology of gastric ulcer disease is multifactorial. In human infants, concurrent illness is strongly associated with gastric ulcers, with risk factors in some studies including mechanical ventilation (one of the most consistent risk factors), abnormal mode of delivery, delayed delivery, and hypotension.[9] Luminal factors that may predispose to ulcer formation include hydrochloric acid (HCl), pepsin, bile acids, and volatile fatty acids.[10] Additional pathophysiologic mechanisms for ulcer development include impairment of mucosal perfusion, reduction in mucus or bicarbonate secretion, neutrophil- and inflammation-mediated injury, and inhibition of nitric oxide.

Normal defenses of the mucosa vary anatomically. The squamous regions, including the esophagus, cardia, and fundus, are protected from acids by intercellular tight junctions. The glandular epithelium is protected by a mucous and bicarbonate barrier, prostaglandins, a rich mucosal blood supply, and rapid cellular restitution upon injury. Mucosal blood flow is highly dependent upon prostaglandins E1 and E2 as well as nitric oxide. Normal gastric and duodenal motility and duodenal sphincter tone are other protective mechanisms that minimize duodenal reflux of bile acids and other cytotoxins.

Ulceration in the squamous mucosa, particularly the region adjacent to the margo plicatus, must be interpreted with caution in terms of clinical significance because of the finding that up to 50% of clinically normal foals may have ulcers in this area.[2,3] Only 3% of these healthy foals had ulcers in the glandular mucosa. However, up to 40% of critically ill foals had glandular ulcers.[4] It appears that concurrent illness (sepsis, diarrhea, pneumonia) increases the incidence of glandular ulcers in the neonatal foal.

While luminal factors such as HCl may be the primary mechanisms of nonglandular mucosal injury, damage to the glandular mucosa may be multifactorial. Hypoperfusion and reduced oxygen delivery, as may occur with septic shock or hypovolemia, are believed to be important in the pathogenesis. Hyposecretion of sodium bicarbonate or mucus is also important, and these often occur secondary to hypoperfusion. Inflammatory mediators also play a role in mucosal injury. The use of nonsteroidal anti-inflammatory drugs, such as phenylbutazone, may lead to gastric ulceration as a consequence of prostaglandin E inhibition, leading to a reduction in mucosal blood flow, and bicarbonate or mucus secretion.[11,12] Candidiasis has been associated with gastric ulcers in neonatal foals, however in the author's opinion it is not clear whether they were primary or secondary invaders.[13]

'04 Belly Dancer was treated with a combination of supportive intensive care and gastric protectants. Supportive care consisted of crystalloid administration and parenteral dextrose administration, with a conservative approach to enteral feeding. Blood pressure was monitored

Table 11-3	Antiulcer Medication for Foals	
Drug	**Dosage**	**Action**
Sucralfate	10–20 mg/kg PO q 6–8 h	Mucosal adherent
Cimetidine	20 mg/kg PO q 6–8 h	Histamine-2 antagonist
	6.6 mg/kg IV q 6 h	
Ranitidine	6.6 mg/kg PO q 8 h	Histamine-2 antagonist
	1.5 mg/kg IV q 8 h	
Famotidine	2.8 mg/kg PO q 12 h	Histamine-2 antagonist
	0.3 mg/kg IV q 12 h	
Omeprazole	4 mg/kg PO q 24 h	Proton pump inhibitor
Metaclopramide	0.02–0.04 mg/kg/hour CRI	Prokinetic drug

and maintained with crystalloid therapy. Urine output was also monitored closely as a marker of renal perfusion. The foal was fed a combination of goat milk and mare's milk replacer through a small indwelling nasogastric tube. A total of 10% of body weight was fed per day, divided into small feedings every two hours. The foal was evaluated for gastric residuals via aspiration on the nasogastric tube with a syringe. Ceftiofur (6 mg/kg, IV) was administered because of the possibility of concurrent sepsis.

For ulcer treatment directly, omeprazole (4 mg/kg PO, q 24 h) was initiated. Oral sucralfate was also administered (20 mg/kg, PO, q 6 h). The sucralfate and omeprazole were staggered by several hours to prevent nonspecific binding of the omeprazole by sucralfate.

TREATMENT

Treatment of the neonatal foal with gastric ulcer syndrome consists of supportive care and the use of antiulcer medications. Supportive care consists of maintenance of fluid volume, pressure support, and supplementation of oxygenation through insufflation as necessary for hypoxemia. Acid-base and electrolyte disorders should be corrected. Antimicrobials should be administered to treat and/or prevent sepsis in the neonate. Nutritional support is also critical to the management of the neonate with gastric ulcers. Small, frequent meals of milk should be provided in order to buffer gastric acids and to maintain higher intraluminal pH.[7] Continuous rate infusions of milk can also be provided, but caution must be taken that the foal's stomach does not become overdistended.[14] The nasogastric tube should be intermittently checked for gastric residual accumulation.

Specific therapy of gastric ulcers includes mucosal adherents, histamine type 2 receptor antagonists, and proton pump inhibitors. Sucralfate, a hydroxy aluminum salt of sucrose called sucrose octasulphate, is a mucosal adherent. At acid pH (<2), sucralfate forms a viscous gel that binds ulcers. Sucralfate also inhibits pepsin, buffers acid, and stimulates the production of prostaglandin E. This latter action stimulates bicarbonate and mucus secretion.[10] Sucralfate also binds epidermal growth factor and thus may play a role in epithelial restitution. Suggested doses for sucralfate include 10 to 20 mg/kg PO q 6 to 8 h (Table 11-3).

Histamine-2 antagonists include cimetidine, ranitidine, and famotidine. These drugs decrease acid secretion by competitively binding to the histamine receptor, thereby reducing stimulation of gastric acid secretion by histamine (see Table 11-3). Suggested dosages include the following: cimetidine 20 mg/kg PO q 6 h or 6.6 mg/kg IV q 6 h; ranitidine 6.6 mg/kg PO q 8 h or 1.5 mg/kg IV q 8 h; famotidine 2.8 mg/kg PO q 12 h or 0.3 mg/kg IV q 12 h.[15] Because cimetidine is less potent, has variable absorption in horses, and is associated with inhibition of hepatic microsomal enzymes, it may be the least preferred drug compared to the other H-2 antagonists. Intravenous or oral administration of ranitidine significantly increased intragastric pH for four and eight hours, respectively, in healthy experimental neonatal foals.[7] However, in critically ill foals, ranitidine may have a blunted duration in terms of alkalinizing response.[8] In addition, these drugs will only be beneficial when gastric pH is acidic, which may not be the case in all foals.[8] Ranitidine and sucralfate have been shown to provide partial protection against clinical, clinicopathologic, and pathologic manifestations of phenylbutazone in foals.[16]

Proton pump inhibitors have been more recently added to the treatment options for gastric ulcers in horses. The most commonly used agent is omeprazole, which decreases acid production through irreversible binding to the hydrogen-potassium ATP pump of the parietal cell. Omeprazole has been studied in healthy neonatal foals.[17,18] An oral dose of 4 mg/kg resulted in an increase in gastric pH within two hours of administration (see Table 11-3).

For foals with delayed gastric emptying, prokinetic therapy may be in order. Metaclopramide is a dopaminergic receptor antagonist that can be given as a constant rate infusion (0.02–0.04 mg/kg/hour). Its actions are to tighten the esophageal sphincter, increase gastric motility, and relax the pyloric sphincter. Caution should be used, as overdosage can result in neurologic excitement (see Table 11-3).

While the therapy of ulcers certainly includes pharmaceuticals to raise gastric pH, prevention of ulcers through their use is controversial.[10,19] Some clinicians feel that alkalinizing the foal's stomach without evidence of ulceration may lead to increased survival of ingested bacteria and a risk of translocation of bacteria through the gastrointestinal mucosa. Also as stated above, the acid-secreting profile in the stomach of the critically ill foal may already be alkaline. Excellent supportive care along with intensive management of hemodynamics for the at-risk foal is at least as important to prevention of ulcers. Until research studies are available for defining the risks and benefits of the prophylactic use of antiulcer medications, definitive recommendations cannot be given.

'04 Belly Dancer was maintained in the hospital for approximately seven days, during which time the *bruxism, abdominal discomfort, and anorexia resolved. A recheck gastroscopy prior to discharge revealed the ulcers to be healing and no longer hemorrhaging. She was discharged with instructions to continue the omeprazole for 30 days. The sucralfate was discontinued.*

OUTCOME

The outcome of foals with gastric ulcers is highly variable. In a retrospective study by Taharaguchi, mortality from gastric ulceration ranged from 7.1% to 16.2% of deaths in foals between 1997 and 1999.[5] Foals with silent ulcers due to hemodynamic perturbations that go on to perforate have a grave prognosis. Foals with ulcers that do not progress to the point of perforation have a better prognosis, particularly those whose primary problem responds to therapy. Foals with duodenal ulcers have a guarded prognosis in general, because of the potential for duodenal strictures, fibrosis, and gastric outflow obstruction.[20]

REFERENCES

1. Lewis S: Gastric ulceration in an equine neonate, *Can Vet J* 44:420, 2003.
2. Murray MJ: Endoscopic appearance of gastric lesions in foals: 94 cases (1987-1988), *J Am Vet Med Assoc* 195:1135, 1989.
3. Murray MJ: Pathophysiology of peptic disorders in foals and horses: A review, *Equine Vet J Suppl*:S29:14, 1999.
4. Furr MO, Murray MJ, Ferguson DC: The effects of stress on gastric ulceration, T3, T4, reverse T3 and cortisol in neonatal foals, *Equine Vet J* 24:37, 1992.
5. Taharaguchi S, Okai K, Orita Y et al: Gastric ulceration in foals in the Hidaka District (1997-1999), *J Japan Vet Med Assoc* 54:435, 2001.
6. Murray MJ: Gastroduodenal Ulceration, In, Reed SM, Bayley WM, eds: *Equine internal medicine,* Philadelphia, 1998, WB Saunders.
7. Sanchez LC, Lester GD, Merritt AM: Effect of ranitidine on intragastric pH in clinically normal neonatal foals, *J Am Vet Med Assoc* 212:1407, 1998.
8. Sanchez LC, Lester GD, Merritt AM: Intragastric pH in critically ill neonatal foals and the effect of ranitidine, *J Am Vet Med Assoc* 218:907, 2001.
9. Kuusela AL, Maki M, Ruuska T et al: Stress-induced gastric findings in critically ill newborn infants: Frequency and risk factors, *Intensive Care Med* 26:1501, 2000.
10. Magdesian KG, Wilkins PA: Gastric and duodenal ulceration in the critical neonate. *Proc International Veterinary Emergency and Critical Care Society,* San Diego, CA 2004.
11. Carrick JB, Papich MG, Middleton DM et al: Clinical and pathological effects of flunixin meglumine administration to neonatal foals, *Can J Vet Res* 53:195, 1989.
12. Traub JL, Gallina AM, Grant BD et al: Phenylbutazone toxicosis in the foal, *Am J Vet Res* 44:1410, 1983.
13. Gross TL, Mayhew IG: Gastroesophageal ulceration and candidiasis in foals, *J Am Vet Med Assoc* 182:1370, 1983.
14. Paradis MR: Nutritional support: Enteral and parenteral, *Clin Tech Eq Pract* 1:87, 2003.
15. Buchanan BR, Andrews FM: Treatment and prevention of equine gastric ulcer syndrome, *Vet Clin North Am* 19:575, 2003.
16. Geor RJ, Petrie L, Papich MG et al: The protective effects of sucralfate and ranitidine in foals experimentally intoxicated with phenylbutazone, *Can J Vet Res* 53:231, 1989.
17. Sanchez LC, Murray MJ, Merritt AM: Effect of omeprazole paste on intragastric pH in clinically normal neonatal foals, *Am J Vet Res* 65:1039, 2004.
18. Murray MJ: Safety, acceptability, and endoscopic findings in foals and yearling horses treated with a paste formulation of omeprazole for twenty-eight days, *Equine Vet J Suppl* 29:67, 1999.
19. Barr BS, Wilkins PA, Del Piero F et al: Is prophylaxis for gastric ulcers necessary in critically ill equine neonates: A retrospective study of necropsy cases 1995-1999. Proc 18th American College Veterinary Internal Medicine Scientific Forum, *J Vet Intern Med* 14:328, 2000.
20. Acland HM, Gunson DE, Gillette DM: Ulcerative duodenitis in foals, *Vet Pathol* 20:653, 1983.

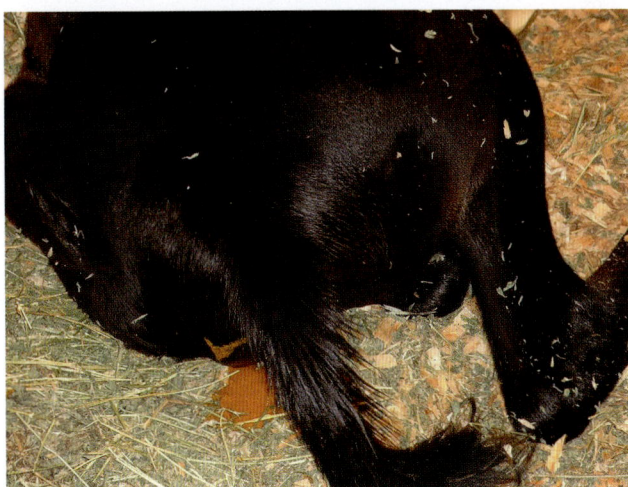

Fig. 11-30 '03 Liquid Assets, an eight-day-old Warmblood foal that presented with diarrhea.

'03 Liquid Assets, an eight-day-old Warmblood foal, was presented for lethargy, pyrexia, and signs of mild abdominal discomfort. The foal and its dam were pastured with other horses and one additional foal that were reportedly healthy. The foal had been clinically normal since birth. Gestation and parturition were unremarkable. The foal had been nursing well until that afternoon, when he preferentially sought out water. The owner monitored the foal's temperature that afternoon, and noted fevers as high as 103° F.

On presentation to the Veterinary Medial Teaching Hospital, the foal was found to be lethargic, alert, and ambulatory. A systemic inflammatory response syndrome was evident, as it was tachycardic (p = 115 beats/minute), tachypneic (80 beats/minute), and febrile (T = 102.2° F). The foal's body condition score was estimated to be 4/9, and mild abdominal distention was present. It was estimated that the foal was 5% dehydrated. Yellow mucoid feces were passed during the examination (Figure 11-30).

HISTORY AND PHYSICAL EXAMINATION

The peripartum history and history of the days prior to the development of diarrhea are important in differentiating the causes of diarrhea in foals. The potential for peripartum asphyxia, immature gestational age, and sepsis can be assessed through history. Foals with perinatal hypoxic-ischemic injury are at significant risk for gastrointestinal dysfunction, including diarrhea. Premature foals are predisposed to necro-

tizing enterocolitis. Additional information that is pertinent to the workup and support of the diarrheic foal include nursing ability and appetite, mentation and activity level, housing environment, and character and frequency of the diarrhea. Assessment of passive transfer of colostral antibodies is also important, as foals with failure of passive immunity are at increased risk of developing sepsis and possibly infection with pathogenic enteric organisms. On the other hand, foals with high intakes of colostrum and milk may be at increased risk for clostridial enteritis, as it has been hypothesized that colostral trypsin inhibitors may protect clostridial toxins from acid degradation in the stomach. Ingestion of large quantities of milk from heavy lactating mares may provide for additional enteral substrate for proliferation of clostridial organisms. Additional historic information centers on diet. Foals provided milk replacer or a nonequine source milk rather than mare's milk are at increased risk for development of osmotic diarrhea. Foals from poor milkers may be ingesting water or foreign material such as dirt or bedding and are at risk for diarrhea associated with pica.

Some level of epidemiologic data is also very useful in determining the etiology of diarrhea in foals. Information as to whether the foal is part of an outbreak situation (suggesting an infectious, nutritional, or toxic cause) or the sole foal with diarrhea on a farm is useful in directing the diagnostic approach. Hygiene and husbandry practices should be assessed for aiding in education toward minimizing the incidence of diarrhea on farms. Stall versus pasture housing and number of foals per paddock or pasture should also be considered.

Neonatal foals can present with diarrhea at any age between hours and several days of age. Early diarrhea is consistent with hypoxic-ischemic damage or sepsis. Diarrhea in the slightly older foal is indicative of infectious or dietary causes. The neonate with diarrhea should be evaluated for the following: 1) circulatory volume and hydration status, 2) clinical signs consistent with systemic inflammation (e.g. SIRS, sepsis) such as mucosal hemorrhages, congested or hyperemic mucous membranes, injection of vessels, tachycardia, tachypnea, or fever, 3) nutritional status through assessment of body condition or weight, and 4) indicators of concurrent disease such as bacteremia, signs of asphyxial injury, or congenital defects.

Circulatory status should be assessed in the physical examination by close attention to mentation status, capillary refill time, jugular vein fill time, extremity temperature, mucous membrane color, heart rate, and pulse quality. Heart rate can be misleading in the

Table 11.4	Causes of Neonatal Diarrhea			
Bacterial	**Viral**	**Parasitic/Protozoal**	**Environmental**	**Other**
Clostridium perfringens	Rotavirus	*Cryptosporidium*	Pica	Foal heat diarrhea
Clostridium difficile	Coronavirus	*Strongyloides westeri*	Overfeeding	Prematurity (necrotizing enterocolitis)
Salmonella		*Giardia*	Improper mixing of milk replacer	Gastric ulcers
Sepsis		*Eimeria*		Hypoxic-ischemic injury
				Lactose intolerance

neonatal foal, however, as those with hypoxemia, hypothermia, or hypoglycemia can be bradycardic despite significant hypovolemia. Hydration status, reflecting interstitial and intracellular volumes, is indicated by skin turgor, mucous membrane texture, sunken eyes, and corneal quality. The abdomen should be evaluated for distention. Ballottement can indicate ascites or gas distention. The perineum should be assessed for scalding and dermatitis associated with fecal adherence to hair and skin. A cautious digital examination can reveal sand or dirt, rectal impactions, and rectal edema. Body condition scoring can be performed in the neonatal foal, and a subjective evaluation should be performed as a minimum because many diarrheic foals lose substantial amounts of weight (see Chapter 4).[1] Because foals with enterocolitis are at risk for bacterial translocation and subsequent sepsis, they should be evaluated for signs of localized sepsis such as effusive joints or enlarged external umbilical stumps.

PATHOGENESIS

The pathophysiology of diarrhea is multifactorial. Factors resulting in diarrhea from enterocolitis include hypersecretion, osmotic draw, altered motility, altered Starling's forces (as with increased vascular permeability or hydrostatic pressure, or decreased colloid osmotic pressure), maldigestion/malabsorption, and inflammation. Though one mechanism may predominate in some forms of diarrhea, most of them contribute.

Foals with enterocolitis often exhibit signs consistent with abdominal pain. Differential diagnoses that should be considered in foals with acute abdominal disease include strangulating and nonstrangulating obstructions, uroabdomen, and other nongastrointestinal causes of colic, such as liver disease. Foals with impending enterocolitis can be very difficult to differentiate from those with obstructive diseases, because they often exhibit signs of abdominal pain and distention prior to the onset of diarrhea. The presence of

fever and leukopenia are suggestive of enterocolitis, but not specific. Abdominal ultrasonography and radiography can help in differentiation of these conditions.

Causes of diarrhea in neonatal foals include both infectious and noninfectious causes. Noninfectious causes include "foal heat diarrhea," pica, dietary intolerance, gastric ulcer disease, hypoxic-ischemic injury, and necrotizing enterocolitis. Infectious causes include bacterial, viral, parasitic, and protozoal causes (Table 11-4).

Foals with foal heat diarrhea are otherwise bright and nursing well. They do not experience a systemic inflammatory response, and therefore have normal hematologic and vital sign findings.[2,3] The name *foal heat diarrhea* is a misnomer because the diarrhea does not appear to be a result of hormonal changes in the mare.[3] Rather, it is a result of intestinal maturational changes. It usually occurs between seven and 10 days of life and is self-limiting.

Pica results from ingestion of sand, dirt, bedding, or hair.[4] Inflammatory or motility alterations secondary to the presence of foreign material can result in obstructions or impactions as well as diarrhea. Another dietary cause of diarrhea in the foal is dietary intolerance. It occurs when either a foal is lactose-intolerant (secondary to infectious diarrheas such as clostridiosis or rotaviral infection) or is an orphan foal with diarrhea resulting from feeding excessive amounts of milk replacer or milk replacers mixed at higher than 11% total solids.[5] Milk replacers with sucrose or maltose are particularly offensive.[5]

Gastric ulcer disease is associated with diarrhea in some neonatal foals. Clinical signs can be inapparent or include bruxism, ptyalism, dorsal recumbency, diarrhea, or colic (see Case 11-2). Hypoxic-ischemic insult as occurs with peripartum asphyxia can result in gastrointestinal injury, leading to diarrhea. Hypoxic and subsequent reperfusion injury may both contribute to mucosal compromise. Smooth muscle and serosal dysfunction may also result. Energy depletion as occurs secondary to hypoxic-ischemic injury leads to cell membrane pump failure. Subsequent reperfusion injury leads to oxidant injury as well as inflammatory cell activation and "no-reflow" phenomenon.

Necrotizing enterocolitis (NEC) is a state of gastrointestinal necrosis that occurs from mucosal injury, as might occur with asphyxial injury, the presence of enteral nutrition, and bacterial invasion of the GI wall. Ileus, gastric reflux, abdominal distention, intestinal perforations, or diarrhea can result from NEC.[6] Prematurity is a risk factor for development of necrotizing enterocolitis.

Infectious causes of diarrhea often occur in large groups of foals that are housed together; sporadic cases can also occur, particularly with clostridial agents. Viral etiologies include rotavirus and coronavirus. Rotavirus infects and denudes small intestinal microvilli, resulting in maldigestion and malabsorption.[7] It thus interferes with lactase function and sodium-glucose cotransport. Because of relative sparing of crypt epithelium, the virus also results in increased net secretion. Clinical signs vary from mild to severe diarrhea, requiring minimal to intensive therapeutic intervention, respectively. Experimentally, the incubation period is as short as two days.[7] Most affected foals are five to 35 days of age, although younger and older foals can be affected. Older foals (up to 60 days of age) usually have mild diarrhea, and asymptomatic animals can shed the virus.[7,8] Vaccination of gravid mares may reduce the incidence of disease on farms, as well as the severity of clinical signs.[9,10] Phenolic compounds are the optimal disinfectant type used, as rotavirus is resistant to many others. Coronavirus has been associated with diarrhea in foals.[11,12] It infects the small intestine during the first few days of life, with persistence of viral antigen in the crypt cells for three to four days after onset of diarrhea.[11] Complications of coronaviral infections can include coronitis and limb edema associated with inadequate perfusion of the extremities.[11] Other potential viral etiologies of diarrhea include adenovirus and parvovirus, although their exact role in foal diarrhea has not been clearly defined.[13]

The most common bacterial causes of diarrhea include clostridial agents, especially *Clostridium difficile* and *C. perfringens*, and *Salmonella*. The clostridial infections can result in outbreaks or sporadic cases of diarrhea. *C. difficile* is a primary pathogen in neonatal foals and does not require prior antimicrobial administration as a risk factor for development of diarrhea as is usually the case with adult horses.[14,15] The primary virulence factors for pathogenicity include two large exotoxins, toxins A (enterotoxin) and B (cytotoxin). *C. difficile*–associated disease ranges from mild diarrhea to highly fatal, hemorrhagic, or necrotizing diarrhea.[16] It has also been associated with lactose intolerance in foals.[14] It should be noted that toxigenic *Clostridium difficile* can be cultured from the feces of clinically normal foals, just as it can from healthy infants, and it is unknown what circum-

stances or agent-host interactions lead to clinical disease.[17,18]

Clostridium perfringens types A and C have been reported to cause enterocolitis and diarrhea in neonatal foals. As with *C. difficile*, the pathogenicity of *C. perfringens* A and C is dependent upon virulence factors, especially the production of enterotoxins.[19] In a recent epidemiological study, *C. perfringens* was found in 90% of normal three-day-old foals and 64% of normal foals at eight to 12 hours of age. The most common genotype was type A (85%), and *C. perfringens* type C was found in less than 1% of the foals. These results suggest that type A is likely part of the normal microflora of the neonatal foal (and thus the clinical relevance of positive cultures without presence of enterotoxin are questionable), whereas Type C is rarely found in the normal neonatal and has been associated with the clinical signs of watery to hemorrhagic diarrhea, but also includes abdominal distention, colic, and ileus.[20] Therefore, typing of isolates is critical to pursuing positive cultures, because the type of *C. perfringens* varies between clinically normal and affected foals. Foals with *C. perfringens*, type C *infection* can develop rapidly progressive obtundation and colic and may die before the onset of diarrhea. *C. perfringens*–associated diarrhea is associated with a high mortality rate, 54% in one study, and is highly associated with fatal diarrhea in another study.[8,19] Adult horses may serve as reservoirs for spores in the environment.

Salmonellosis is another bacterial form of enterocolitis that can affect the neonatal foal as it can adult horses. Concurrent sepsis is a concern with salmonellae, due to invasiveness and the potential for translocation across the compromised gut barrier. Studies have found an association between isolation of salmonellae from foals with diarrhea and fatality.[8] The severity of the disease, in part, relates to the serotype involved, with group B salmonellae, such as *S. typhimurium*, being among the most pathogenic. Salmonella of other groups can also cause disease, for example, a group C1 *Salmonella ohio* has been reported to cause an outbreak of neonatal salmonellosis.[21] Mares of infected foals may be asymptomatic carriers of Salmonella and the source of the foal's infection. Other bacteria that can cause diarrhea sporadically in the neonate include *Actinobacillus sp.* (in association with bacteremia), enterotoxigenic *E. coli*, *Bacteroides fragilis*, *Clostridium sordelli*, *Aeromonas hydrophila*, and *Streptococcus durans*.[22-27] The significance and pathogenesis of these agents in neonatal foal diarrhea requires further study.

The primary parasitic agent that has been associated with diarrhea in the young foal is *Strongyloides westeri*.[8] It appears that heavy infestations with more than 2000 eggs per gram of feces are required for development of diarrhea, and it is generally not a cause of severe diarrhea.[8] *Strongyloides westeri* is transmitted to foals through suckling milk.

The primary protozoal enteric pathogen of foals is *Cryptosporidium parvum.* It was initially believed that *Cryptosporidium* infections were limited to immunocompromised foals such as Arabians with severe combined immunodeficiency syndrome.[28] More recently, it has been identified as a pathogen of immunocompetent foals as well.[29] The organism invades the microvillus, occupying an intracellular but extracytosolic space. It thus causes villus blunting and maldigestion with a secondary osmotic diarrhea. Most affected foals are five days of age and older, but younger foals can develop disease with high-level exposure. Diarrhea usually lasts between five and 14 days, with recovering animals and asymptomatic older foals and adult horses shedding oocysts. One study identified *Cryptosporidium parvum* causing an outbreak of neonatal diarrhea to be genotypically identical to that associated with bovine diarrhea.[30] However, exposure to cattle was not found to be an important source of infection for foals in another epidemiologic study.[29] Sources of cryptosporidial infection in foals have not been definitively elucidated.[29] Mares, cattle, and municipal water sources have all been suspected as the source of infection in foals, but these remain speculative.[29] Because of the zoonotic risk associated with *Cryptosporidium,* affected foals should be handled carefully with particular attention to good hygiene. The role of other protozoal agents, including *Eimeria leukarti, Trichomonas equi,* and *Giardia sp.,* is poorly understood and requires further study.

A complete blood count from '03 Liquid Assets revealed hyperfibrinogenemia (500 mg/dl) with a normal leukocyte count. A serum biochemical profile was unremarkable except for mild hyperchloremia (105 mEq/liter). Venous blood lactate concentration was mildly increased at 2.1 mmol/liter. Venous blood gas analysis was otherwise unremarkable. Whole-blood immunoglobulin concentration was found to be 400 to 800 mg/dl using a commercial immunoassay (SNAP test: IDEXX Laboratories, Inc., Westbrook, ME). Abdominal ultrasonography revealed multiple distended, fluid-filled small-intestinal loops that were initially hypermotile, and later hypomotile. Thoracic radiography was unremarkable.

Daily fecal cultures for **Salmonella sp.** *were negative. Immunoassays for* **Clostridium difficile** *toxin A were negative, as was fecal culture for* **C. difficile.** *Electron microscopy of feces was negative for viral particles, as was a fecal ELISA for rotavirus. Fecal flotation was negative for nematodes. An immunofluorescent antibody (IFA) assay was positive for large numbers of* **Cryptosporidium** *oocysts. An IFA for* **Giardia sp.** *was negative.*

DIAGNOSTIC TESTS

The clinical pathology of foals with diarrhea can vary depending upon whether there is a concurrent systemic inflammatory response syndrome. The hematologic (CBC) findings can vary from unremarkable to those of hemoconcentration, leukopenia, and hypoproteinemia. A left shift with immature (band, metamyelocytes) neutrophils, with variable toxic cytologic changes, may also be present, reflecting a profound inflammatory response such as sepsis. Hypoproteinemia often reflects protein-losing enteropathy, and hyperfibrinogenemia may be present in the face of inflammatory mediators induced by endotoxemia. Thrombocytopenia occurs when coagulopathies such as disseminated intravascular coagulation are triggered.

As for hematology, serum biochemistry analyses are normal when diarrhea occurs without gastrointestinal inflammation. Enteritis or enterocolitis with subsequent activation of SIRS can lead to organ dysfunction as might occur with severe sepsis. Increases in creatinine and/or BUN and liver enzymes or bilirubin concentrations reflect renal or hepatic dysfunction, respectively. Hypoalbuminemia usually reflects gastrointestinal protein loss. Similarly, hypoglobulinemia may be present, although it may be due to failure of passive transfer of colostral antibodies as well as GI loss. A variety of electrolyte derangements may reflect enteric losses, renal dysfunction, or acid-base derangements and often include hyponatremia, hypochloremia or hyperchloremia, hypokalemia or hyperkalemia, and an increased anion gap. Decreases in total CO_2 concentrations reflect metabolic acidemia. Anion gap may also be increased with hyperlactatemia.

Metabolic acidemia results from both organic and inorganic acidosis. Lactate is the primary organic anion contributing to acidemia. Hyperlactatemia results from a combination of hypoperfusion associated with hypovolemia and hypotension, hypermetabolism, increased glycolysis from inhibition of pyruvate dehydrogenase by inflammatory mediators, enhanced activity of Na-K ATPase due to circulating catecholamines, and reduced hepatic or renal clearance of lactate. Inorganic causes of acidemia in diarrhea cases include hyponatremia or hyperchloremia resulting in a decrease in strong ion difference. The acid-base status is reflected on blood gas analyses as reduced pH and increased base deficit.

As part of intensive management of foals with severe enterocolitis, additional diagnostic monitoring should include indirect blood pressure, urine output measurements, and urinalysis with fractional excretion of electrolytes. Because foals with diarrhea and

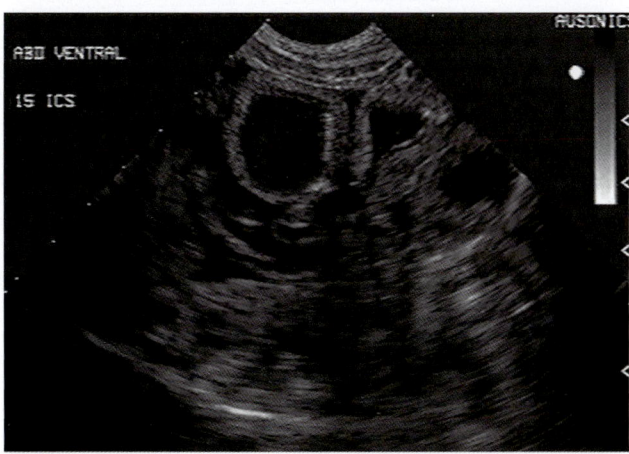

Fig. 11-31 Ultrasound image of dilated small intestine. Note the thickened wall and distended luminal diameter.

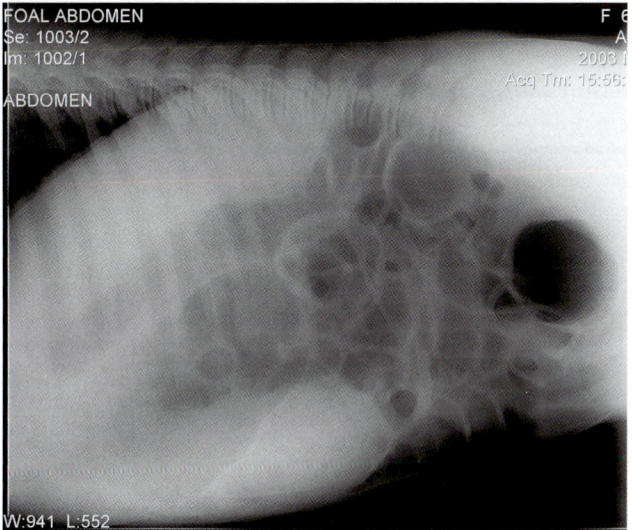

Fig. 11-32 Abdominal radiographs of a foal with diarrhea. Note the distended small and large intestine.

Table 11.5	Specific Diagnostic Tests for Diarrhea
Etiology	**Diagnostic Test**
Rotavirus	Electron microscopy, ELISA
Salmonella	Fecal culture (five samples) or PCR, test mare as well
Clostridium perfringens	Fecal culture with PCR typing, Gram-stain feces, toxin assay
Clostridium difficile	Fecal culture, toxin assay
Cryptosporidium	Immunofluorescence assay, acid-fast stain, flow cytometry
Strongyloides westeri	McMaster fecal flotation method
Lactose intolerance	Lactose tolerance test

pneumatosis intestinalis, or linear gas shadows within the wall of the GI tract, a hallmark of necrotizing enterocolitis. Sand and radiopaque foreign material will also be apparent on abdominal radiographs.

Specific diagnostic evaluation of the neonatal foal with diarrhea includes a number of tests to rule out pathogenic agents (Table 11-5). Fecal samples can be screened for viral particles with electron microscopy. Fecal ELISA and immunoassays are available for rotavirus and coronavirus. Fecal cultures can be performed for *Salmonella sp.* and clostridial organisms. To increase the sensitivity of identifying salmonella shedders, repeated daily cultures should be performed (up to five consecutive samples). Alternatively, PCR techniques are available for salmonellae, although the findings must be interpreted in light of the high-level sensitivity of this test.

Positive cultures for *C. difficile* and *C. perfringens* must be interpreted with caution as nontoxigenic and incidental colonization is possible. The diagnosis of *C. difficile*–associated disease should be coupled to toxin assays. Commercial immunoassays test for toxin A or both toxin A and B. These kits are easy and rapid, however they have variable sensitivities. Stool cytotoxin assays for toxin B are also available and are considered the gold standard for toxin testing, but are time-consuming. PCR techniques for *C. difficile* toxin gene sequences are currently moving from the experimental arena to the clinical setting. Diagnosis of *C. perfringens* enterocolitis is difficult to make. Unfortunately, immunoassays are not available for most toxins, except for enterotoxin. Therefore, cultured isolates must be typed using PCR techniques, such as the multiplex PCR. The diagnosis is made from positive cultures of toxigenic and pathogenic isolates of *C. perfringens* (e.g., type A or C), as well as exclusion of other pathogenic agents. Gram staining of feces can serve as a rapid screen for clostridial overgrowth, however this technique is neither sensitive nor specific (Figure 11-33).

SIRS are at risk for coagulopathies, monitoring should also include clotting times (PT, aPTT) and measurement of fibrin degradation product or D-dimer concentrations. Antithrombin concentrations may be low because of induction of coagulopathies or loss of this small protein through the compromised GI mucosa.

Imaging should be a part of the diagnostic workup of these foals with diarrhea. Abdominal ultrasonography and radiography can aid in differentiating causes of acute abdominal disease. Ultrasound evaluation should include assessment of bowel wall thickness, luminal diameter, and small-intestinal motility (Figures 11-16 and 11-31). Ascites or effusion can also be detected. Radiography can be utilized to assess the degree of gastrointestinal distention (Figures 11-9, 11-12, and 11-32). It can also be utilized to detect

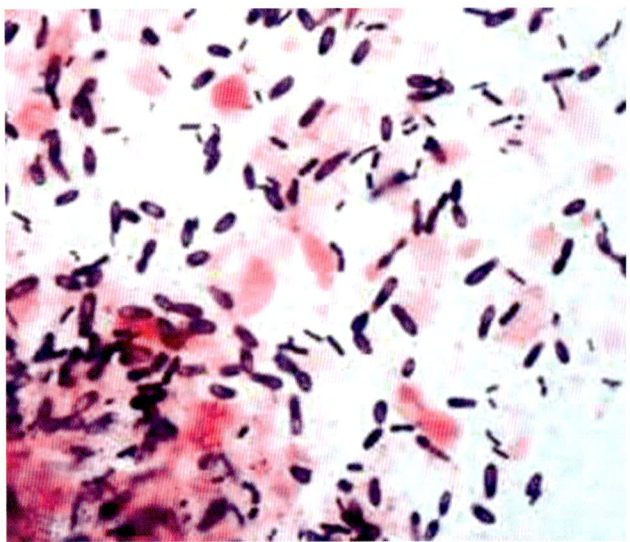

Fig. 11-33 Gram staining of diarrheic feces caused by *Clostridia sp.* may show an increased number of Gram-positive rods.

There are a number of diagnostic tools available for diagnosis of *Cryptosporidium parvum* infection. Immunofluorescence assay (IFA), acid-fast (AF) staining, and flow cytometry have been developed for identification of oocysts.[29] In one study, AF and flow cytometry were determined to be more sensitive than IFA.[29] AF staining was less specific, however. Because of their small size, oocysts are very difficult to visualize microscopically after fecal flotation. Fecal flotation is useful for identifying *Strongyloides westeri* ova, with the McMaster method used for quantification.

If one is concerned that lactose intolerance is playing a role in the continuation of a foal's diarrhea, then the use of a lactose tolerance test may be indicated. After a four-hour fast, the foal is administered lactose (1 g/kg) through a nasogastric tube. Blood samples collected in fluoride oxalate tubes are taken for glucose levels at preadministration, immediately postadministration, and every 30 minutes for three hours. A normal absorption curve would show a doubling of glucose in 60 to 90 minutes. An absence of increase in glucose or a delay in the increase would indicate a problem with lactose digestion and absorption.[31]

Therapy for '03 Liquid Assets was initiated with replacement crystalloid therapy. The foal was rehydrated with Plasma-Lyte 148, and dextrose supplementation was provided through 5% dextrose in water. After rehydration, maintenance fluid requirements were met with Plasma-Lyte 56. Over time the foal developed an inorganic acidosis (hyponatremia, hyperchloremia), which was managed with administration of isotonic sodium bicarbonate. Immunologic and colloid support was provided with a plasma transfusion (2 liters total). With time, the foal developed increasing abdominal distention associated

with ileus. To minimize distention and abdominal discomfort, the foal was kept nothing per os and not allowed to nurse. Nutritional support was provided in the form of parenteral nutrition, consisting of a combination of dextrose, intralipid, and amino acid solutions.

Antimicrobial therapy was instituted as a means of preventing bacterial translocation and bacteremia. Ceftiofur (10 mg/kg, IV, q 12h) and amikacin (21 mg/kg, IV, q 24h) were administered to provide broad-spectrum antimicrobial coverage with potent Gram-negative efficacy. Kaolin pectate and bismuth subsalicylate were utilized intermittently as gastrointestinal protectants.

As the foal's abdominal distention and ileus improved, lactase enzyme (3000 U, PO, q 4h) was provided as enteral feeding was reintroduced and gradually advanced, because of suspected lactose intolerance. As enteral feeding was tolerated, the foal was allowed to nurse the mare for increasing lengths of time and increasing frequency. Intravenous fluid therapy was gradually reduced. The GI motility improved over the next several days as the foal's abdominal distention resolved and fecal character improved. The foal was discharged after eight days of hospitalization.

TREATMENT

The treatment of foals with diarrhea is highly variable, depending upon the severity of clinical signs and physiologic derangements. In general, the management of enterocolitis includes a number of goals. These include hemodynamic, metabolic, and nutritional support; gastrointestinal protectants; antibiotic coverage; and infectious disease control. If a specific agent is identified, then specific therapy for that agent can be instituted.

Hemodynamic disturbances are common among foals with enterocolitis, particularly those with SIRS or sepsis syndrome. Hypoperfusion results from hypovolemia, altered myocardial contractility, inappropriate vasomotor responses, and hypooncotic states associated with hypoalbuminemia. Hemodynamic support occurs primarily in the form of intravenous fluid therapy, consisting of both crystalloids and colloids. A number of crystalloids are appropriate for foals with diarrhea, but because of the tendency for metabolic acidemia, fluids with higher strong ion differences such as Normosol R, Plasma-Lyte 148, or lactated Ringers solution are more ideal than 0.9% saline.[32]

Volume replacement in the neonatal foal should be done with great attention; overzealous administration of crystalloids may potentiate gastrointestinal edema. Monitoring of central venous pressure, urine output, and serial lactate concentration measurements can aid in guiding volume replacement. Colloid therapy is indicated in the hypooncotic and hypovolemic foal. Plasma or synthetic colloid solutions, such as hetastarch, can be used. Plasma has the advantages of providing not only albumin, but also immunoglobulin, antithrombin, clotting factors, and other proteins. If hetastarch is used, platelet counts and clotting times should be monitored, as coagulopathies associated with reduced concentrations of von Willebrand's factor and factor VIII may develop. Once volume replacement has occurred and the central venous pressure (CVP) is at maximum (10 cm H_2O), hypotension should be addressed with inotropes, such as dobutamine (2 to 20 µg/kg/minute, IV CRI). If hypotension and clinical parameters of hypoperfusion persist after initiation of inotropy, then vasopressors should be considered (norepinephrine or vasopressin CRI—see Chapter 7).

Metabolic support occurs in the form of managing acid-base and electrolyte balance. Metabolic acidemia is treated depending upon the cause of acidosis; organic acidoses (lactic acidosis) should be treated with optimizing peripheral oxygen delivery. Inorganic acidoses, as occur with hyponatremia or hyperchloremia associated with electrolyte loss into the GI tract, can be treated by correcting the underlying electrolyte disorder. Sodium bicarbonate is indicated in these situations. Potassium, calcium, and magnesium may need to be supplemented in foals with severe diarrhea. Glucose concentrations should be monitored frequently in the neonatal foal, particularly if the foal is anorexic or receiving parenteral dextrose. Both hypoglycemia and hyperglycemia should be avoided. Recently, tight glucose regulation with insulin has received a great deal of study in human critical care and is associated with improved survival in septic patients (see Chapter 7).[33] In cases with severe diarrhea, ileus and abdominal distention, abdominal discomfort, or suspected osmotic diarrhea, partial or complete withholding of milk should be considered. Parenteral nutritional support is required in these foals (see Chapter 4).

Antimicrobial therapy should be provided in order to minimize the risk for bacterial translocation across the compromised gut barrier. Broad-spectrum coverage, as with a beta lactam and aminoglycoside combination or second- or third-generation cephalosporins, is indicated (see Chapter 5). Gastrointestinal protectants include di-tri-octahedral smectite and activated charcoal, which act as adsorbents. Smectite has been shown to bind clostridial toxins in vitro.[34] However, to the author's knowledge, this product has not been evaluated in neonatal foals and should be used with caution. Other protectants include kaolin/pectin combinations and bismuth subsalicylate.

Nonspecific therapy for diarrhea may include antiulcer medication and probiotics. Sucralfate is also protective, stimulating mucosal blood flow and mucus production because of increased local prostaglandin synthesis. Treatment of gastric ulcers with proton pump inhibitors and/or histamine type 2 receptor antagonists is indicated when ulcers are suspected from clinical signs (bruxism, ptyalism, dorsal recumbency) or documented via gastroscopy (see Case 11-2). Probiotics are often utilized to modulate colonic flora. However, evidence documenting their efficacy in horses is lacking, and their use in neonatal foals prone to bacteremia warrants further study.

If a specific offending agent is identified, then treatment may be more directed. Metronidazole, administered orally or intravenously (10 to 15 mg/kg, q 8 to 12 h), is indicated in clostridiosis cases. The early use of metronidazole in even suspect cases of *C. perfringens* is important because foals can die before the onset of diarrhea. Metronidazole is also the first-line therapeutic for treating *C. difficile* infection in foals, however, cases of metronidazole resistance have been documented.[35,36] In these cases, vancomycin can be used, although it should be restricted to foals in isolation and foals that have severe clinical scores. Unfortunately, bacitracin is uniformly ineffective against equine isolates of *C. difficile*.[36,37] Ivermectin is effective in treating *Strongyloides westeri* infestations.[38] Paromomycin has been suggested as a treatment for *Cryptosporidium* infections, although its efficacy and safety are unproven in foals.[39] Exogenous lactase enzyme (3000 to 6000 U/50 kg foal, PO, q 3 to 6 h) should be provided to foals with rotaviral, cryptosporidial, and streptococcal infections and those with osmotic diarrheas to aid in digestion and prevention of chronic osmotic diarrhea.

Nursing care is very important for the diarrheic neonate. Cleanliness and hygiene are important not only for infectious disease control, but also for preventing secondary complications such as thrombophlebitis in the patient. The foal with diarrhea should be isolated so as to prevent spread of infectious agents. Consideration must be given to efficacy of particular disinfectants for specific agents. Though bleach is effective against most pathogens, rotavirus is best killed with phenolic compounds. *Cryptosporidium* is resistant to most disinfectants. High heat and ultraviolet light may be helpful in eliminating this organism.

Owners should be warned about the potential zoonotic nature of *Salmonella* and *Cryptosporidium*. Frequent handwashing and use of separate clothing when working with sick foals are prerequisites of curtailing the spread of the infection. *Cryptosporidium* can also cause disease through any mucous membrane contact. Protective eyewear and the use of surgical masks may be an important part of disease prevention in caretakers.

OUTCOME

Two follow-up fecal IFA tests on the foal for Cryptosporidium were negative. A source for the Cryptosporidium was not found in this case. The partial failure of passive transfer may have played a role in the pathogenesis of the disease in this case. The owner reported that the foal continued to thrive and grow one month after discharge.

The prognosis for foals with diarrhea is highly variable. Those with diarrhea and no evidence of enterocolitis have a good prognosis, while those with *C. perfringens*, some forms of *C. difficile*, and *Salmonella sp.* infections have a higher mortality rate than those with rotavirus, *Strongyloides*, or *Cryptosporidium* infections.[8]

REFERENCES

1. Paradis, MR: Nutritional support: Enteral and parenteral, *Clin Tech Eq Pract* 1:87, 2003.
2. Masri MD, Merritt AM, Gronwall R et al: Faecal composition in foal heat diarrhea, *Equine Vet J* 18:301, 1986.
3. Johnston RH, Kamstra LD, Kohler PH: Mares' milk composition as related to "foal heat" scours, *J Anim Sci* 31:549, 1970.
4. Ramey DW, Reinertson EL: Sand-induced diarrhea in a foal, *J Am Vet Med Assoc* 185:537, 1984.
5. Buffington CAT, Knight DA, Kohn CW et al: Effect of protein source in liquid formula diets on food intake, physiologic values, and growth of equine neonates, *Am J Vet Res* 53:1941, 1992.
6. Cudd TA, Pauly TH: Necrotizing enterocolitis in two equine neonates, *Compend Cont Educ Pract Vet* 9:88, 1987.
7. Conner ME, Darlington RW: Rotavirus infection in foals, *Am J Vet Res* 41:1699, 1980.
8. Netherwood T, Wood JLN, Townsend HGG et al: Foal diarrhea between 1991 and 1994 in the United Kingdom associated with *Clostridium perfringens*, rotavirus, *Strongyloides westeri*, and *Cryptosporidium spp.*, *Epidemiol Infect* 117:375, 1996.
9. Powell DG, Dwyer RM, Traub-Dargatz JL et al: Field study of the safety, immunogenicity, and efficacy of an inactivated equine rotavirus vaccine, *J Am Vet Med Assoc* 211:193, 1997.
10. Barrandeguy M, Parreno V, Lagos Marmol M et al: Prevention of rotavirus diarrhoea in foals by parenteral vaccination of the mares: Field trial, *Dev Biol Stand* 92:253, 1998.
11. Davis E, Rush BR, Cox J et al: Neonatal enterocolitis associated with coronavirus infection in a foal: A case report, *J Vet Diagn Invest* 12:153, 2000.
12. Guy JS, Breslin JJ, Breuhaus B et al: Characterization of a coronavirus isolated from a diarrheic foal, *J Clin Microbiol* 38:4523, 2000.
13. Corrier DE, Montgomery D, Scutchfield WL: Adenovirus in the intestinal epithelium of a foal with prolonged diarrhea, *Vet Pathol* 19:564, 1982.
14. Weese JS, Parsons DA, Staempfli HR: Association of *Clostridium difficile* with enterocolitis and lactose intolerance in a foal, *J Am Vet Med Assoc* 214:229-232, 1999.
15. Jones RL, Adney WS, Shideler RK: Isolation of *Clostridium difficile* and detection of cytotoxin in the feces of diarrheic foals in the absence of antimicrobial treatment, *J Clin Microbiol* 25:1225, 1987.
16. Jones RL, Adney WS, Alexander AF et al: Hemorrhagic necrotizing enterocolitis associated with *Clostridium difficile* infection in four foals, *J Am Vet Med Assoc* 193:76, 1988.
17. Bolton RP, Tait SK, Dear PR et al: Asymptomatic neonatal colonization by *Clostridium difficile*, *Arch Dis Child* 59:466, 1984.
18. Baverud V, Gustaffson A, Franklin A et al: *Clostridium difficile*: Prevalence in horses and environment, and antimicrobial susceptibility, *Equine Vet J* 35:465, 2003.
19. East LM, Savage CJ, Traub-Dargatz JL et al: Enterocolitis associated with *Clostridium perfringens* infection in neonatal foals: 54 cases (1988-1997), *J Am Vet Med Assoc* 212:751, 1998.
20. Tillotson K, Traub-Dargatz JL, Dickinson CE et al: Population-based study of fecal shedding of *Clostridium perfringens* in broodmares and foals, *J Am Vet Med Assoc* 220:342, 2002.
21. Walker RL, Madigan JE, Hird DW et al: An outbreak of equine neonatal salmonellosis. *J Vet Diagn Invest* 3:223, 1991.
22. Stewart AJ, Hinchcliff KW, Saville WJA et al: *Actinobacillus sp.* bacteremia in foals: Clinical signs and prognosis, *J Vet Int Med* 16:464, 2002.
23. Holland RE, Grimes SD, Walker RD et al: Experimental inoculation of foals and pigs with an enterotoxigenic *E. coli* isolated from a foal, *Vet Microbiol* 52:249, 1996.
24. Holland RE, Sriranganathan N, DuPont L: Isolation of enterotoxigenic *Escherichia coli* from a foal with diarrhea, *J Am Vet Med Assoc* 194:389, 1989.
25. Tzipori S, Hayes J, Sims L et al: *Streptococcus durans*: An unexpected enteropathogen of foals, *J Infect Dis* 150:589, 1984.
26. Hibbs CM, Johnson DR, Reynolds K et al: *Clostridium sordelli* isolated from foals, *Vet Med* 72:256, 1977.
27. Myers LL, Shoop DS, Byars TD: Diarrhea associated with enterotoxigenic *Bacteroides fragilis* in foals, *Am J Vet Res* 48:1565, 1987.
28. Snyder SP, England JJ, McChesney AE: *Cryptosporidium* in immunodeficient Arabian foals, *Vet Pathol* 15:12, 1978.
29. Cole DJ, Cohen ND, Snowden K et al: Prevalence of and risk factors for fecal shedding of *Cryptosporidium parvum* oocysts in horses, *J Am Vet Med Assoc* 213:1296, 1998.
30. Grinberg A, Oliver L, Learmonth JJ et al: Identification of *Cryptosporidium parvum* "cattle" genotype from a severe outbreak of neonatal foal diarrhea, *Vet Rec* 153:628, 2003.
31. Martens RJ, Scrutchfield WL: Foal diarrhea; pathogenesis, etiology and therapy, *Compendium for Continuing Education* 4:175, 1982.
32. Magdesian KG, Madigan JE: Volume replacement in the neonatal ICU: Crystalloids and colloids, *Clin Tech Equine Pract* 2:20, 2003.
33. Van den Berghe, G, Wouters P, Weekers F et al: Intensive insulin therapy in the critically ill patient, *N Engl J Med* 345:1359, 2001.
34. Weese JS, Cote NM, deGrannes RVG: Evaluation of the ability of Di-tri-octahedral smectite to adhere to *Clostridium difficile* toxins and *Clostridium perfringens* enterotoxin in vitro. Proc 48th Annual Convention of the American Association of Equine Practitioners, Orlando 127, 2002.
35. Magdesian KG, Hirsh DC, Jang SS et al: Characterization of *Clostridium difficile* isolates from foals with diarrhea: 28 cases (1993-1997), *J Am Vet Med Assoc* 220:673, 2002.
36. Jang SS, Hansen LM, Breher JE et al: Antimicrobial susceptibilities of equine isolates of *Clostridium difficile* and molecular

characterization of metronidazole-resistant strains, *Clin Infect Dis* 25(S2):S266, 1997.

37. Weese JS, Staempfli HR, Prescott JF: A prospective study of the roles of *Clostridium difficile* and enterotoxigenic *Clostridium perfringens* in equine diarrhoea, *Equine Vet J* 33:403, 2001.

38. Ludwig KG, Craig TM, Bowen JM et al: Efficacy of ivermectin in controlling *Strongyloides westeri* infections in foals, *Am J Vet Res* 44:314, 1983.

39. Byars TD, Divers TJ: Diarrhea in nursing foals. In Orsini JA, Divers TJ, eds: *Manual of equine emergencies*, ed 2, Philadelphia, 2003, WB Saunders.

Case 11-4	Liver Failure in the Foal	Gary Magdesian

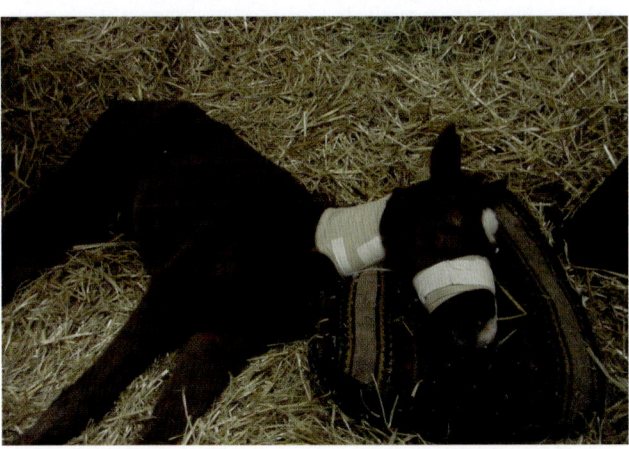

Fig. 11-34 '04 Jaundiced View, a 12-day-old Quarter Horse foal, presented severely depressed with intermittent seizures.

'04 Jaundiced View, a 12-day-old Quarter Horse foal, was presented for depression, intermittent seizures, icterus, and pyrexia (Figure 11-34). The foal had an unremarkable gestational length and parturition history, and had been clinically healthy until the afternoon of presentation. Approximately five hours prior to presentation, she developed acute-onset lethargy and anorexia. The foal's clinical status deteriorated rapidly, leading to seizure activity and pyrexia (104.7°F). The referring DVM administered lactated Ringer's solution, gentamicin, and ampicillin, and referred the foal.

Physical examination revealed the foal to be severely depressed and responsive only to noxious stimuli. The foal exhibited a systemic inflammatory response syndrome, with tachycardia, tachypnea, and pyrexia. Clinical signs compatible with sepsis were found on ophthalmologic exam, including yellow-discolored irides, hyphema, hypopyon, and aqueous flare. The foal was markedly icteric (mucous membranes and sclera) and was in hypovolemic shock as exhibited by prolonged capillary refill time, tachycardia, poor pulse quality, and cold extremities.

HISTORY AND PHYSICAL EXAMINATION

Important historical information for the foal with icterus and altered mentation includes farm epidemiologic data such as the number and percentage of affected foals. The spectrum of clinical signs and course of the disease encountered in outbreak situations are important, as is the age range. Administered supplements or medications should be evaluated for potential hepatotoxicity. For isolated cases, the history leading up to the disease should be investigated. Age of onset is important; for example Tyzzer's disease is limited to foals a few days of age to six weeks of age.[1,2] Management practices, including housing, diet, peripartum history, and additional concurrent disease in the herd, should be considered. Treatment prior to veterinary examination or therapies provided by the referring veterinarian, in the case of specialty practices, should be evaluated.

A detailed physical examination of the foal with liver dysfunction is important not only for elucidating the etiology, but also for management and therapy. With acute hepatic disease, foals may exhibit a systemic inflammatory response syndrome with tachycardia, tachypnea, and/or pyrexia or hypothermia. Hypovolemia and dehydration are common due to lack of nursing, third space losses (diarrhea or ascites), or vascular permeability alterations. Icterus or jaundice is a key finding with liver disease, and mucous membranes, including gingiva, vulvar, and ocular mucous membranes, as well as sclera should be evaluated closely for yellow discoloration (Figure 11-35). Fecal character should be evaluated, as some forms of liver disease can cause diarrhea or changes in fecal color. For example, foals with biliary atresia may have gray feces while those with Tyzzer's disease can exhibit diarrhea.[3-5] Abdominal distention may be present, and abdominal ballottement can be used to reveal ascites or hepatomegaly. Foals with subacute or chronic liver disease may exhibit weight loss or poor growth, which may be apparent as poor body condition. Those with

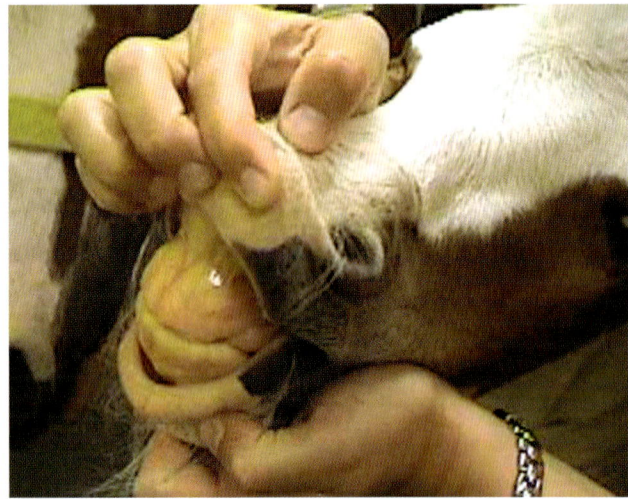

Fig. 11-35 Icteric mucous membranes are a prominent sign in both liver disease and neonatal isoerythrolysis.

acute hepatopathy, such as Tyzzer's disease, have a normal body weight and appear normal until acute onset of signs.[2,6]

The perinatal foal with hepatopathy should be closely evaluated for concurrent signs of hypoxic-ischemic injury, including encephalopathy, enteropathy, and nephropathy. Hepatic dysfunction may occur in these foals as well. Similarly, foals with sepsis can develop hepatitis.

Hepatoencephalopathy is present in many foals with acute liver disease or end-stage liver failure. Signs range from subtle to severe and fulminate. Subtle signs include mild depression and yawning. More obvious signs include central blindness, circling, head pressing, seizures, behavioral changes, and obtundation to coma.

Fundic examinations should be performed in icteric foals because herpes-positive cases often demonstrate dark and red-discolored optic discs and irregularly dilated vessels.[7]

PATHOGENESIS

The pathophysiology of liver disease in the neonatal foal is multifactorial and complex. Because of a large number of etiologies, insult or abnormalities may occur in the form of congenital, genetic, toxic, infectious, and hemodynamic causes.

The differential diagnoses for foals with icterus include fasting hyperbilirubinemia, increased erythrocyte destruction, hepatocellular disease, and cholestatic disorders. Causes of hemolysis include neonatal isoerythrolysis, drug-induced lysis, and increased red blood cell turnover from sepsis or peripartum asphyxial injury. Sepsis may impair bilirubin metabolism

due to the presence of endotoxemia contributing to hyperbilirubinemia.

Liver disease occurs from a number of causes. Infectious causes include bacterial hepatitis secondary to sepsis, and infection with *Actinobacillus equuli* or *Clostridium piliformis*. Bacteremia and sepsis in general can cause hepatic dysfunction by means of inducing hypoperfusion and tissue hypoxia. Inflammatory mediators stimulated by the systemic inflammatory response syndrome (SIRS) will contribute to hepatic damage. Cholangiohepatitis from enteric microbes can result from ileus, enteritis, or ulcerative duodenitis/stricture syndrome. Bacterial hepatopathy may also occur as extension of umbilical vein phlebitis or abscessation. Hepatoencephalopathy was associated with *Rhodococcus equi* infection in one foal. Although not cultured, a liver biopsy suggested a bacterial etiology and the authors speculated that it may have been due to *R. equi* bacteremia or ascending biliary infection.[8]

Tyzzer's disease, caused by *Clostridium piliformis*, formerly known as *Bacillus piliformis*, is an acute and multifocal hepatic necrosis associated with a high mortality rate. Most commonly associated with sporadic cases on farms, outbreaks of disease can also occur. Foals present with a rapidly progressive clinical course including recumbency, hyperthermia or hypothermia, and stupor or coma, icterus, and seizures with marked hypoglycemia and metabolic acidosis.[9] Some foals may be found dead without preceding clinical signs.

Viral hepatitis from equine herpes virus 1 (EHV-1) neonatal infection can occur in association with respiratory distress, neurologic signs, and bone marrow necrosis resulting in leukopenia. Foals are infected in-utero from repeated cell-associated viremia in the dam,[9] so signs are seen immediately at birth. Icterus is a common finding in neonatal herpes infections as a result of multifocal and acute hepatic necrosis. Despite profound necrosis, liver enzymes were not increased in one retrospective report.[10] In the report, herpes-positive foals were more likely to have total white blood cell counts less than 3,000/µl and to be icteric (and hyperbilirubinemic) compared to septic or premature foals. Foals with neonatal herpes infections have a poor prognosis; however, those with milder infections may survive. Treatment with acyclovir can be attempted.[11]

Foals with hypoxic-ischemic injury from peripartum asphyxia most commonly exhibit clinical signs consistent with encephalopathy, nephropathy, or gastroenteropathy, however hepatopathies may also result. Such foals exhibit icterus from biliary stasis and hepatic dysfunction, and have increased concentrations of liver enzymes. Foals with neonatal isoerythrolysis sporadically develop hepatopathies with increases in direct bilirubin concentration in addition to indirect hyperbilirubinemia and increased liver enzymes.[12] Liver disease is suspected to occur as a result of tissue hypoxia, iron overload from hemolysis, or bile stasis caused by the increased amounts of conjugated bilirubin.[12] Another form of liver disease occurs secondary to gastrointestinal disease, primarily strangulating or obstructive lesions and ileus. Endotoxin or bacteria can enter the portal circulation from translocation.

Congenital causes of hepatopathies include portacaval shunts and biliary atresia.[3,13] Portosystemic vascular anomalies include both intrahepatic and extrahepatic shunts.[13-15] Persistent vitelline arteries have been reported in conjunction with intrahepatic portosystemic shunts.[16] Foals with portosystemic shunts have recurrent episodes of blindness, seizures, or altered mentation associated with hepatoencephalopathy. The shunts may not be clinically apparent until affected foals are eating grain or hay. Congenital hepatic fibrosis and cystic bile duct formation is a syndrome suspected to be an autosomal recessive genetic trait of Swiss Freiberger horses.[17] This report included 30 foals that demonstrated jaundice, neurologic signs, colic, and unthriftiness.

Hyperammonemia of Morgan foals and equine glycogen storage disease IV are syndromes suspected to have a genetic basis with some degree of hepatopathy.[18-20] Persistent hyperammonemia in Morgan horses is suspected to be similar to a syndrome of hyperornithinemia, hyperammonemia, and homocitrullinuria (HHH) in humans.[18] These foals exhibit neurologic signs including seizure activity, aimless wandering, yawning, and circling. Supportive care, lactulose, and a low-protein diet resulted in temporary clinical improvement in one of two foals that was treated, however the foal relapsed and was euthanized.[18]

Glycogen-branching enzyme deficiency has been recently attributed to a mutation in the glycogen branching enzyme 1 (GBE 1) gene in Quarter Horses.[20] The syndrome has recently been termed *glycogen storage disease IV* and is believed to be inherited as an autosomal recessive trait, with clinically affected foals being homozygous for the mutation.[19,20] Affected foals are sometimes stillborn, and otherwise exhibit flexural deformities, seizure activity, respiratory or cardiac failure, or recumbency. Leukopenia, hypoglycemia, and high serum CK, AST, and GGT concentrations were common, and all foals died by seven weeks of age.[19] The livers of affected foals contained periodic acid Schiff's (PAS)-positive intracellular inclusions and no GBE activity. An additional consideration for congenital hepatic disease is hepatoblastoma.[21] Polycythemia, hyperbilirubinemia, and increased liver enzymes occur with this liver neoplasm.[21] These foals may survive to weaning or adulthood, but hepatoblastoma has been reported in an aborted fetus and may thus be congenital.[22]

Toxic hepatopathies have been reported in neonatal foals following administration of oral pastes containing ferrous sulfate in the first one to two days of life.[23] Experimental administration of iron to foals confirmed that the hepatotoxicity from the oral paste was indeed due to the contained iron.[23,24] Pathologic changes included liver atrophy, bile duct hyperplasia, lobular necrosis, cholestasis, and periportal fibrosis. Drug-induced hepatopathies can also occur during this time period because of relatively immature hepatic function and increased absorption of macromolecules during colostral IgG absorption.[12] Oral medications should be used with caution in foals less than 24 hours of age because of the potential for increased bioavailability with subsequent hepatotoxicity. Other potential hepatotoxins reported in horses include aflatoxins, pyrrolizidine alkaloids, leukoencephalomalacia, and chlorinated hydrocarbons, although these are considered unlikely in the young foal because of lack of ingestion of feedstuffs by neonates. Steroid hepatopathy has been reported in three- and 10-year-old horses, secondary to intramuscular administration of high doses of triamcinolone acetonide in both cases.[25,26]

A complete blood count from '04 Jaundiced View demonstrated hemoconcentration with a hematocrit of 46%. A mild neutrophilia was present with a toxic left shift (band neutrophils: 500/μl). Hyperfibrinogenemia was also present (600 mg/dl). A venous blood gas revealed metabolic acidemia, with a pH of 7.2 and a base deficit of 12 mEq/liter. Venous blood lactate concentration was high at 8 mmol/liter. Serum biochemistry profile showed marked hypoglycemia (28 mg/dl), and increased liver enzymes (SDH 300 IU/liter, GGT 98 IU/liter, AST 2200 IU/liter). Total, indirect, and direct bilirubin were increased as 9.1, 8.3, and 0.8 mg/dl, respectively. Blood cultures were submitted and subsequently found to be negative. Clotting profiles (PT and aPTT) were within normal limits. Blood ammonia was high at 280 mmol/liter as were bile acid concentrations (50 mg/dl).

Abdominal ultrasonography revealed generalized hepatomegaly with an increased vascular pattern, consistent with a diffuse, acute hepatopathy. Needle biopsies were taken with an automated biopsy instrument. Histopathology showed acute, multifocal, necrotizing hepatitis consistent with Tyzzer's disease. A Warthin-Starry stain (a silver impregnation technique) confirmed the presence of intracellular and filamentous rod-shaped bacteria consistent with **Clostridium piliformis** *(Figure 11-36).*

DIAGNOSTIC TESTS

Clinical pathologic findings in foals with liver disease include increases in concentrations of both hepatocel-

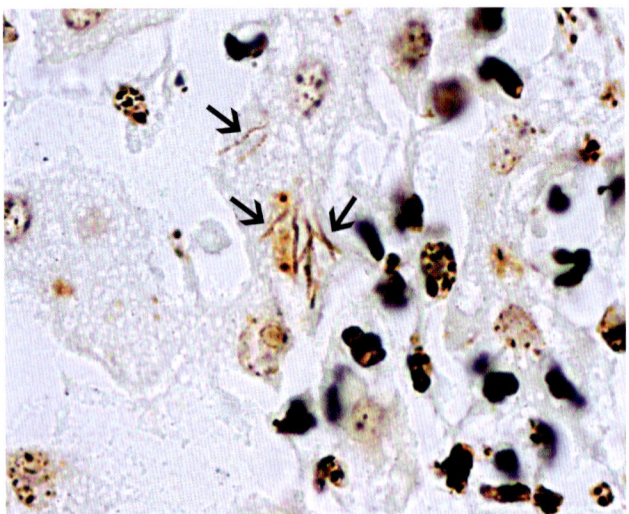

Fig. 11-36 Liver biopsy from a foal with Tyzzer's disease. Note rod-shaped bacteria. Warthin-Starry stain 100×. Courtesy of Dr. Pam Wilkins.

lular and biliary enzymes. Aspartate aminotransferase (AST) and sorbitol dehydrogenase (SDH) are examples of hepatocellular enzymes. AST is not liver-specific, however, having significant components originating from both skeletal and cardiac muscle. SDH is considered to be liver-specific and has a short (two- to three-hour) half-life. Biliary-derived enzymes include γ-glutamyl transferase (GGT) and serum alkaline phosphatase (SAP). GGT is nearly biliary-specific, however pancreatic origins must be considered when concentrations are increased. SAP has isoenzymes from multiple sources, including fast-growing bone in the neonatal foal. It should be noted that serum biochemical indicators of liver status in neonatal foals have some distinct features as compared to adult horses.[27] Serum alkaline phosphatase (152 to 2835 IU/liter), GGT (13 to 39 IU/liter), and SDH (0.2 to 4.8 IU/liter) activities are increased during the first two weeks of life.[27] Serum cholesterol, triglycerides, and total and unconjugated bilirubin concentrations peak during this same neonatal period.

Foals with cholangiohepatitis and infectious hepatopathies usually have increases of both hepatocellular and biliary enzymes. Similarly, those with toxic insults and hypoxic-ischemic disease also have increased liver enzymes. Glycogen-branching enzyme deficiency results in increased GGT concentrations. Those with portacaval shunts often have normal liver enzymes, but liver function tests are abnormal. Foals with herpes hepatopathies also usually have normal enzymes, but increased bilirubin concentrations.

Both indirect-reacting (unconjugated) and direct-reacting (conjugated) bilirubin concentrations increase with liver disease. Cholestatic disease results in increases in both components of bilirubin as well,

while the percentage attributed to direct bilirubin is usually higher than with primary hepatocellular disease, often exceeding 20% to 25% of the total bilirubin concentration. On the other hand, fasting hyperbilirubinemia and that resulting from hemolysis are due exclusively to indirect bilirubin.

Serum bile acid concentrations increase with liver dysfunction, as occurs with portacaval shunts. They represent a good screening test of liver function. Bile acids, such as choleic and chenodeoxycholic acids, are synthesized by the liver from cholesterol, and are excreted into bile after conjugation with amino acids. These conjugated forms form micelles with fat in the intestine and are reabsorbed and recirculated via enterohepatic circulation. Serum concentrations of bile acids increase in the face of hepatocyte damage, biliary stasis, and shunting of portal blood to the systemic circulation as occurs with portosystemic shunts.

Hyperammonemia is often present, also reflecting liver dysfunction. The liver is the primary site of ammonia removal by converting it to urea for renal excretion. Foals with portacaval shunts commonly have high resting ammonia concentrations. Morgan foals with HHH syndrome have very high concentrations of blood ammonia (>200 μmol/liter), while liver enzymes are only mildly to moderately increased and bilirubin is normal to mildly elevated. Proper handling procedures are critical to accurate measurement and interpretation of blood ammonia.[28] Heparinized blood should be used, and the sample should be collected gently (to avoid hemolysis) and kept on ice. The sample should be run within one hour of collection or otherwise spun in order to freeze the plasma at −20° C for subsequent measurement within 48 hours. Blood from aged-matched control foals should be run concurrently.[28]

Additional biochemical indicators of liver function include serum glucose, BUN, albumin, and cholesterol concentrations. Glucose concentrations are variable, and reflect the degree of hepatic necrosis and milk intake. Foals with severe hepatitis or necrosis, such as those with Tyzzer's disease, have profound hypoglycemia. Those with portacaval shunts also commonly exhibit hypoglycemia. As BUN, albumin, and cholesterol are synthesized by the liver, dysfunction is reflected by reduced concentrations of these analytes. However, hypoalbuminemia is uncommon with liver disease, as only 18% and 6% of horses with chronic and acute liver disease had albumin concentrations below the reference value in one report.[29] It has been estimated that greater than 80% of liver mass must be lost for longer than three weeks before hypoalbuminemia develops.[30]

Fractionation of blood amino acids and determination of the branch chain amino acid (BCAA) to aromatic amino acid (AAA) ratio can aid in determining hepatic function. Decreases in the ratio indicate insufficiency, with normal ratios falling between 3.5 and 4.5.[30] Because of liver dysfunction and reduced conversion of blood ammonia to BUN, a decrease in BUN concentration is often observed. It should be noted, however, that BUN concentrations in the normal neonatal foal are lower than those in the adult horse and low concentrations are therefore difficult to interpret in the neonatal liver patient.

Bromsulphalein (BSP) and indocyanine green are dyes that are excreted primarily by hepatic clearance. Clearance and half-life reflect hepatic excretory function and are prolonged in animals with biliary obstruction or hepatocellular failure. It should be noted that alterations in hepatic blood flow alter interpretation of BSP clearance; significant decreases in blood flow as occurs with portosystemic shunts will reduce the delivery of BSP and hence cause an increase in half-life. High bilirubin and low albumin concentrations will result in increased and decreased BSP half-life, respectively. Quantification of serum bile acids has largely replaced the use of BSP clearance as an indicator of hepatic function in horses.[30]

The concentration of triglycerides may increase in foals with liver disease because of reduced hepatic clearance and increased mobilization from adipose tissue associated with a catabolic state. Cholesterol and VLDL concentrations may decrease, however, because of reduced hepatic synthesis. It should again be noted that triglyceride and cholesterol concentrations are higher in healthy neonatal foals compared to adults, and vary with age.[27] In one report, foals had concentrations of 24 to 88 and 30 to 193 mg/dl for triglycerides in <12-hour and in one-day-old foals, respectively. Cholesterol concentrations were 111 to 432 and 110 to 562 in those same age groups.[27]

CBC findings are dependent upon the cause of liver disease. Leukocytosis may be present with cholangiohepatitis. When liver disease is secondary to sepsis or hypoxic-ischemic disease, however, leukopenia with band neutrophils is more common. Hyperfibrinogenemia is usually present with infectious or inflammatory hepatopathies, however fibrinogen may be decreased when coagulopathies such as disseminated intravascular coagulation exist.

Blood cultures should be performed in the neonatal foal with liver disease because of the possibility of sepsis causing hepatitis.

Clotting times may be prolonged with liver failure. Prolongation of prothrombin time (PT) and partial thromboplastin (PTT) occur due to a lack or reduction of synthesis of several clotting factors, including factors II, V, VII, IX, and X. This is an important clinical finding because liver biopsies may have to be delayed in hypocoagulable animals. For similar reasons, plasma antithrombin concentrations may be reduced, leading to coagulopathies such as disseminated intravascular coagulation. In one review, almost half of horses with liver disease had a prolonged PT or PTT.[31] Coagulopathies are common in horses with liver dysfunction due to concurrent systemic inflammatory response syndrome, and fibrin degradation products may be increased and thrombocytopenia may be present.

The acid-base status of foals with liver disease should be evaluated closely through blood gas analysis. With liver dysfunction, acidemia may occur as a result of increased formation and reduced clearance of organic acids such as lactate, pyruvate, and amino acids. Impaired urea synthesis may reduce renal buffering through urine acidification. Serial monitoring of lactate should be included as part of the diagnostic monitoring of the foal with liver disease because lactate clearance may be reduced.

Ultrasonography is a critical component of the diagnostic workup of foals with liver disease. It can be utilized to determine the size of the liver, changes in parenchyma, and dilated bile ducts. With infectious etiologies, such as cholangiohepatitis, hepatitis secondary to sepsis, and Tyzzer's disease, the liver appears subjectively enlarged. Biliary distention is evident in some cases. Evidence of fibrosis (hyperechogenicity) may be present in subacute to chronic cases.

Hepatic scintigraphy will confirm the diagnosis of portacaval shunts. Injection of technetium 99m-labeled sulfur colloid demonstrates alterations in blood flow or the presence of masses. Biliary scans can also be performed looking for biliary obstruction or atresia. Portograms are necessary in cases of portosystemic shunts where surgical correction is contemplated. These are done intraoperatively using radiopaque agents that are injected into a mesenteric vein with subsequent radiography. Simultaneous filling of the portal and azygous veins and caudal vena cava, and lack of intrahepatic filling indicate portacaval shunting.[30]

Histopathology provides the most specific information as to the etiology of liver disease and can aid in diagnostic, prognostic, and therapeutic directions. The safest means of performing liver biopsies is under ultrasonographic guidance and using an automated needle biopsy instrument. It should be pointed out that focal lesions such as neoplasia are easily missed by liver biopsy. Special stains (silver or Warthin-Starry stains) may be helpful in specific diagnoses such as Tyzzer disease. Fine-needle aspirates may also be helpful in the diagnosis of a specific etiology (Figure 11-37).

Culture of liver biopsies is indicated when infectious etiologies are suspected. Cholangiohepatitis is usually associated with Gram-negative enteric aerobes and Gram-negative or Gram-positive anaerobes.

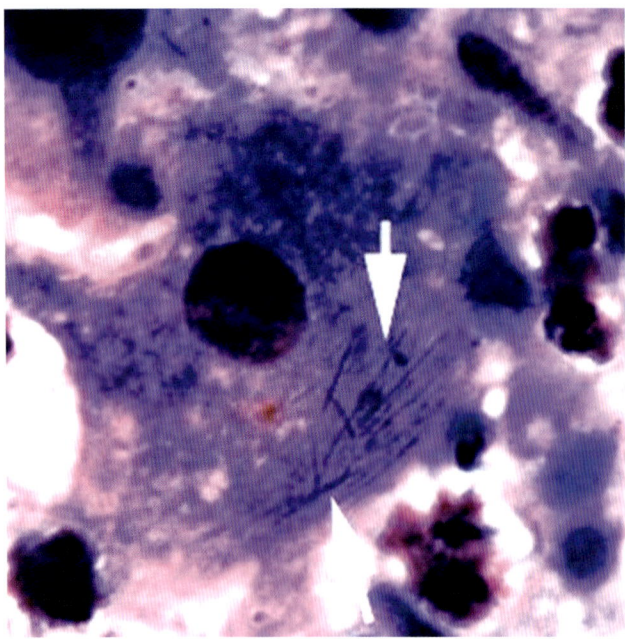

Fig. 11-37 Fine-needle aspirate from the liver of a foal with Tyzzer's disease. Note intracellular rod-shaped bacteria. Courtesy of Dr. Michelle Barton.

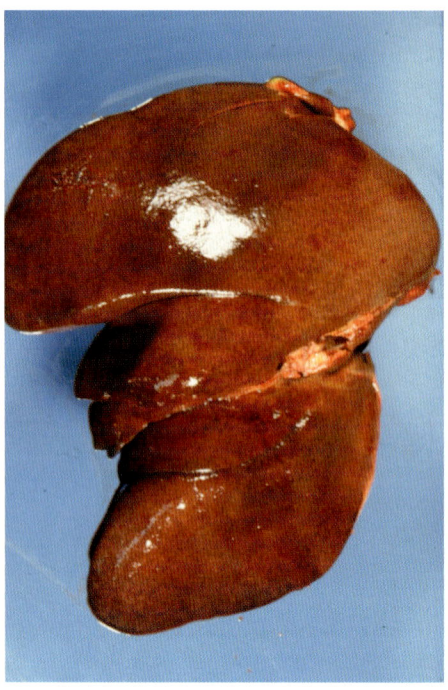

Fig. 11-38 Hepatomegaly is a prominent sign of Tyzzer's disease.

Pathogenesis of and Clinical Findings in Tyzzer's Disease

Foals with Tyzzer's disease develop a peracute to acute multifocal necrotizing hepatitis. Grossly, hepatomegaly is evident. These foals generally have marked increases in AST and SDH concentrations. Other liver enzymes, both hepatocellular and biliary (LDH, SAP, GGT), are also increased, as are both components of bilirubin. Striking hypoglycemia should be a clue to the presence of infection with *Clostridium piliformis*. These foals often have a metabolic acidosis, with hyperlactatemia due to increased production (hypoperfusion, inflammation, catecholamine surges) and reduced hepatic clearance. Complete blood counts often reveal leukopenia with a left shift and cytologic evidence of toxicity, although leukocytosis is present in some cases.[32] Hemoconcentration reflects hypovolemia and dehydration. Hyperfibrinogenemia is common. Physical examination is consistent with septic shock, with petechial hemorrhages and injection being common. Hypovolemic shock is also evident. Mentation is usually depressed, ranging from lethargy to comatose, and icterus is a prominent finding. Clinical signs of hepatoencephalopathy may include depression, weakness, and seizures. Diarrhea is an inconsistent finding. Fever is usually present, although hypothermia from shock may be predominating when initially examined.[32]

Affected foals are often found dead. Serologic testing for recovered or suspected cases can be helpful. Pathology reveals hepatomegaly with rounded margins (Figure 11-38). Histopathologic findings with Tyzzer's disease include multifocal and random necrosis with neutrophilic inflammation (Figure 11-39). Long bacilli are often but not always seen, particularly in hepatocytes at the periphery of necrotic areas. They are best delineated with Warthin-Starry stains (Figure 11-36). An intranuclear location of the microbe has been found using electron microscopy.[33] Myocardial necrosis with Warthin-Starry stained bacilli has also been reported.[32,34] Intestinal necrosis may also be present, and organisms consistent with *C. piliformis* may occasionally be observed in sections of intestine, particularly the large intestine.[36]

Clostridium piliformis is an obligate intracellular spore-forming anaerobe. It is very difficult or nearly impossible to culture in vitro using routine microbiologic methods. Inoculation of embryonated eggs has been one means of trying to assess antimicrobial susceptibility. Penicillin, tetracycline, erythromycin, and streptomycin appear to be effective in vitro, while sulfonamides and chloramphenicol do not.[37] Treatment with dextrose, volume replacement, and sodium bicarbonate can result in temporary improvement of mentation, however most foals are reported to die.

The exact pathophysiology of infection is unknown but is believed to be oral with subsequent distribution to the liver. Ingestion of spores from feces shed by

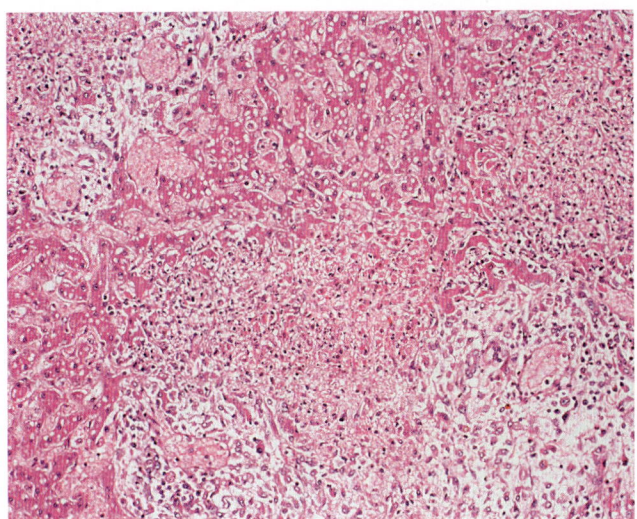

Fig. 11-39 Histopathology of a foal liver with Clostridium piliformis, Tyzzer's disease. Hematoxylin and eosin stain 10×.

subclinical carriers may play a role in development of disease, and the disease has been experimentally reproduced.[35] It has also been suspected that rabbit and rodent populations could serve as reservoirs of infection.[33] Most reported cases have been sporadic, however a number of cases have been noted on particular premises.[38] Preventive measures are unknown, however efforts should be directed at environmental hygiene on affected farms, including the use of 0.3% sodium hypochlorite to eliminate spores from barns housing affected foals.[39]

Risk factors for *Clostridium piliforme* infection in foals include foaling season, farm residency and age of mare. In one study, foals born between March 13 and April 13 were 7.2 times as likely to develop infection as those born at any other time of the foaling season.[38] Foals of nonresident visiting mares were 3.4 times as likely to develop the disease as were foals born to mares that were permanent residents of the farm. Foals born to young mares were 2.9 times as likely to develop Tyzzer's disease as those born to mares ≥6 years of age.[38]

Oxygen insufflation was administered (10 liters/ minute) because of the foal's moribund state. The foal was administered Plasma-Lyte 148 and dextrose supplementation at 2% to provide 4 to 8 mg/kg/minute. The foal was administered a total of 3 liters over two hours. Once hypovolemia was corrected, the foal was administered Plasma-Lyte 56 with potassium supplementation (q 40 mEq/liter) at a maintenance rate of 4 ml/kg/hour. Parenteral nutrition (PN) was administered for nutritional support. B complex vitamins were added. Antimicrobials were continued, using a combination of ampicillin (22 mg/kg IV, q 8 h) and gentamicin (6.6 mg/kg IV, q 24 h). Seizure activity was controlled with phenobarbital.

Lactulose was administered (0.1 ml/kg PO, q 8 h). Sucralfate was provided for gastric ulcer prophylaxis (20 mg/kg PO, q 8 h).

TREATMENT

Treatment of liver disease is largely supportive, with specific therapies available for certain diseases. Foals with acute hepatopathies often present in hypovolemic crises. A combination of crystalloids and colloids is indicated in volume replacement. Ideal crystalloids for liver disease include those containing acetate and/or gluconate instead of lactate, such as Plasma-Lyte 148 or Normosol-R (Abbott Laboratories, Abbott Park, IL). The liver is the primary site of lactate clearance, whereas muscle and renal metabolize acetate and gluconate is utilized by most tissues. Though accumulation of lactate from LRS does not lead to lactic acidosis (the cation associated with lactate in LRS is sodium as opposed to hydrogen ion), lactate is depressive to the myocardium; therefore iatrogenic increases in lactate concentration should be avoided. Foals with septic shock, such as those with Tyzzer's disease, should be treated with aggressive fluid therapy. Boluses of 10 to 20 ml/kg of isotonic replacement crystalloids or 3 to 5 ml/kg of colloids should be administered over 20 to 30 minutes until the hypovolemic crisis is improved or fails to improve with further volume.

If hypotension persists despite volume resuscitation, inotropes and pressors are indicated. If systemic blood pressure does not normalize in the face of a maximum or high CVP (>10 cm H_2O), dobutamine should be administered as a β-agonist inotrope (2 to 20 μg/kg/ minute). Lastly, vasopressors should be administered. Norepinephrine (0.1 to 3 μg/kg/minute) or vasopressin (0.25 to 1 mU/kg/minute) can be used in an attempt to normalize blood pressure and perfusion (see Chapter 7). Oxygen insufflation (5 to 10 liters/ minute) should be provided to foals with central depression, hypoventilation, or concurrent respiratory tract disease.

Because hepatic biotransformation and elimination of drugs is reduced, medications metabolized by the liver should be used judiciously and dosage alterations should be considered.

Antimicrobial therapy is indicated in cases of bacterial cholangiohepatitis or hepatitis. Broad-spectrum antimicrobials should be administered to foals with cholangiohepatitis. A combination of beta lactam, such as penicillin or ampicillin, and aminoglycoside, such as amikacin or gentamicin, is a reasonable initial choice. Ceftiofur is also a good choice, and potentiated sulfonamides can be used for long-term therapy. Foals with Tyzzer's disease may be treated with any of a number of antimicrobials as the agent appears very susceptible to penicillin, gentamicin, tetracycline, and metronidazole.

Plasma transfusions (20 to 40 ml/kg) can be beneficial to foals with liver disease. Plasma provides additional colloid support, albumin and immunoglobulin replacement, and provision of antithrombin or clotting factors for foals with coagulopathies.

Dextrose supplementation in polyionic nonlactated fluids should be provided. Potassium chloride should be supplemented even if potassium concentrations are normal because it aids in renal excretion of ammonia. Neomycin (4 to 8 mg/kg PO, once) or metronidazole (low doses because of reduced hepatic metabolism (10 mg/kg PO q 12h) may be administered to reduce enteric bacterial production of ammonia. Alternatively, lactulose can be used and is preferred by the author (0.1 to 0.25 ml/kg PO q 6 to 8h).[28] Lactulose is a synthetic disaccharide that bypasses the small intestine. Fermentation in the colon results in increased nitrogen incorporation into the enteric flora, with less available for absorption. Lactulose also reduces the pH of ingesta, resulting in inhibition of ammonia generation and increased ionization of ammonia with ion trapping within the GI lumen.

For severe neurologic signs, mannitol (0.25 to 1.0 g/kg) may be administered if increased intracranial pressure is suspected. Sodium bicarbonate should not be administered unless a significant inorganic acidosis is present; rapid correction of acidemia can increase the concentration of ionized ammonia and exacerbate clinical signs. Benzodiazepines, such as diazepam, should be avoided in foals with hepatic insufficiency as they can potentiate clinical signs of hepatic encephalopathy by enhancing the effects of GABA. Seizures should be controlled with phenobarbital or pentobarbital. Flumazenil (0.5 to 1.0 mg/kg slowly IV), a benzodiazepine antagonist, can be tried in foals with clinical signs of hepatic encephalopathy that are unresponsive to other therapeutics.

Nutritional support of foals with hepatic disease is vital to a successful outcome. Parenteral nutrition should be administered to foals with fulminate hepatitis or liver dysfunction, including those with Tyzzer's disease. Formulations for patients with hepatic failure should be utilized. Protein requirements should be met but not exceeded in order to avoid contributing to hyperammonemia. Formulations with increased branch chain amino acids (valine, isoleucine, leucine) and decreased aromatic amino acids (phenylalanine, tryptophan, tyrosine, methionine) are being evaluated for use in human liver patients. Vitamin K_1 should be administered in foals with long-term liver disease. Since the liver is the primary source of vitamin C synthesis and storage of vitamins A, D, and riboflavin, a multivitamin should be provided to foals with chronic liver disease. B vitamins should be administered diluted in fluids. Vitamin E can be supplemented as an antioxidant.

Foals with portacaval shunts should be stabilized for hepatic encephalopathy, and then surgical correction can be attempted after diagnostic venography to localize the shunt.[13]

Gastric ulcer prophylaxis is indicated in select cases, particularly those with hypovolemic or hypotensive shock. Sucralfate is advantageous in that it does not undergo hepatic biotransformation. For treating ulcers, famotidine or ranitidine should be utilized, because unlike cimetidine, they are excreted primarily in the kidneys and do not inhibit hepatic metabolism of other drugs.

To everyone's surprise, '04 Jaundiced View made gradual clinical improvement over the next 24 hours. After 48 hours, her mentation improved to the point of ambulation and normal nursing behavior. The liver enzyme bilirubin and bile acid concentrations gradually decreased. The filly was discharged after 10 days with a continued course of antimicrobials for an additional week. This was a very unusual outcome for a foal with Tyzzer's disease, which is uniformly fatal.

OUTCOME

The outcome in Tyzzer's disease is generally grave. There are currently no reports of survival in documented (definitively diagnosed) cases. Some cases will improve temporarily with volume replacement and administration of dextrose and sodium bicarbonate. However, there are three reported cases and a few anecdotal reports of survival in presumptive cases of *Clostridium piliforme* infection.[38,40] Early therapy with antimicrobials and aggressive intensive care including parenteral nutrition appear to be key to a successful outcome.[40]

REFERENCES

1. Brown CM, Ainsworth DM, Personett LA et al: Serum biochemical and haematological findings in two foals with focal bacterial hepatitis (Tyzzer's disease), *Equine Vet J* 15:375, 1983.

2. Turk MAM, Gallina AM, Perryman LE: *Bacillus piliformis* infection (Tyzzer's disease) in foals in northwestern United States: A retrospective study of 21 cases, *J Am Vet Med Assoc* 178:279, 1981.

3. Bastianello SS, Nesbit JW: The pathology of a case of biliary atresia in a foal, *J S Afr Vet Assoc* 57:117, 1986.
4. St. Denis KA, Waddell-Parks N, Belanger M: Tyzzer's disease in an 11-day-old foal, *Can Vet J* 41:491, 2000.
5. Copland MD, Robartson CW, Fry J et al: Tyzzer's disease in a foal, *Austr Vet J* 61:302, 1984.
6. Paradis, MR: Nutritional support: Enteral and parenteral, *Clin Tech Equine Pract* 1:87, 2003.
7. Golenz MR, Madigan JE, Zinkl J: A comparison of the clinical, clinicopathological, and bone marrow characteristics of foals with equine herpes and neonatal septicemia. Proceedings of the Thirteenth ACVIM Forum 585, 1995.
8. Freestone JF, Shoemaker S, McClure JJ: Pulmonary abscessation, hepatoencephalopathy and IgM deficiency associated with *Rhodococcus equi* in a foal, *Aust Vet J* 66: 343, 1989.
9. Hess-Dudan F: Four possible causes of hepatic failure and/or icterus in the newborn foal, *Equine Vet Educ* 6:310, 1994.
10. Perkins G, Ainsworth DM, Erb HN et al: Clinical, haematological and biochemical findings in foals with neonatal equine herpesvirus-1 infection compared with septic and premature foals, *Equine Vet J* 31:422, 1999.
11. Murray MJ, del Piero F, Jeffrey SC et al: Neonatal equine herpesvirus type 1 infection on a Thoroughbred breeding farm, *J Vet Int Med* 12:36, 1998.
12. Divers TJ, Perkins G: Urinary and hepatic disorders in neonatal foals, *Clin Tech Equine Pract* 1:67, 2003.
13. Fortier LA, Fubini S, Flanders JA et al: The diagnosis and surgical correction of congenital portosystemic vascular anomalies in two calves and two foals, *Vet Surg* 25: 154, 1996.
14. Hillyer MH, Holt PE, Barr FJ et al: Clinical signs and radiographic diagnosis of a portosystemic shunt in a foal, *Vet Rec* 132:457, 1993.
15. Bounanno AM, Carlson GP, Kantrowitz B: Clinical and diagnostic features of portosystemic shunt in a foal, *J Am Vet Med Assoc* 192:387, 1988.
16. De Bosschere H, Simoens P, Ducatelle R et al: Persistent vitelline arteries in a foal, *Equine Vet J* 31:542, 1999.
17. Haechler S, Van den Ingh TSGAM, Rogivue C et al: Congenital hepatic fibrosis and cystic bile duct formation in Swiss Freiberger horses, *Vet Pathol* 37:669, 2000.
18. McConnico RS, Duckett WM, Wood PA: Persistent hyperammonemia in two related Morgan weanlings, *J Vet Int Med* 11:264, 1997.
19. Valberg SJ, Ward TL, Rush BM et al: Glycogen branching enzyme deficiency in Quarter Horse foals, *J Vet Int Med* 15:572, 2001.
20. Ward TL, Valberg SJ, Adelson DL et al: Glycogen branching enzyme (GBE1) mutation causing equine glycogen storage disease IV, *Mamm Genome* 15:570, 2004.
21. Cantile C, Arispici M, Abramo F et al: Hepatoblastoma in a foal, *Equine Vet J* 33:214, 2001.
22. Neu, SM: Hepatoblastoma in an equine fetus, *J Vet Diagn Invest* 5:634, 1993.
23. Mullaney TP, Brown CM: Iron toxicity in neonatal foals, *Equine Vet J* 20:119, 1988.
24. Swerczek TW, Ward Crowe M: Hepatotoxicosis in neonatal foals (letter), *J Am Vet Med Assoc* 183:388, 1983.
25. Cohen ND, Carter GK: Steroid hepatopathy in a horse with glucocorticoid-induced hyperadrenocorticism, *J Am Vet Med Assoc* 200:1682, 1992.
26. Ryu S, Kim B, Lee C et al: Glucocorticoid-induced laminitis with hepatopathy in a Thoroughbred filly, *J Vet Sci* 5:271, 2004.
27. Bauer JE, Asquith RL, Kivipelto J: Serum biochemical indicators of liver function in neonatal foals, *Am J Vet Res* 50:2037, 1989.
28. Divers TJ: Liver failure and hemolytic anemia. In Orsini JA, Divers TJ, eds: Manual of equine emergencies, ed 2, Philadelphia, 2003, WB Saunders.
29. Parraga ME, Carlson GP, Thurmond M: Serum protein concentrations in horses with severe liver disease: A retrospective study and review of the literature, *J Vet Int Med* 9: 154, 1995.
30. Barton MH: Disorders of the liver. In Reed SM, Bayly WM, Sellon DC, eds: *Equine internal medicine*, ed 2, St Louis, 2004, WB Saunders.
31. McGorum B, Murphy D, Love S et al: Clinicopathological features of equine primary hepatic disease: A review of 50 cases, *Vet Rec* 145:134, 1999.
32. Humber KA, Sweeney RW, Saik JE et al: Clinical and clinicopathologic findings in two foals infected with *Bacillus piliformis*, *J Am Vet Med Assoc* 193:1425, 1988.
33. Pulley LT, Shively JN: Tyzzer's disease in a foal, *Vet Pathol* 11:203, 1974.
34. Carrigan MJ, Pedrana RG, McKibbin AW: Tyzzer's disease in foals, *Aus Vet J* 61:199, 1984.
35. Swerczek TW: Multifocal hepatic necrosis and hepatitis in foals caused by *Bacillus piliformis*, *Vet Annu* 17:130, 1977.
36. Harrington DD: Naturally-occurring Tyzzer's disease (*Bacillus piliformis* infection) in horse foals, *Vet Rec* 96:59, 1975.
37. Ganaway JR, Allen AM, Moore TD: Tyzzer's disease, *Am J Pathol* 64:717, 1971.
38. Fosgate GT, Hird DW, Read DH et al: Risk factors for *Clostridium piliforme* infection in foals, *J Am Vet Med Assoc* 220:785, 2002.
39. St. Denis KA, Waddell-Parks N, Belanger M: Tyzzer's disease in an 11-day-old foal, *Can Vet J* 41:491, 2000.
40. Peek SF, Byars TD, Rueve E: Neonatal hepatic failure in a Thoroughbred foal: Successful treatment of a case of presumptive Tyzzer's disease, *Equine Vet Educ* 6:307, 1994.

Umbilical and Urinary Disorders

| Case 12-1 | Umbilical Infection/Patent Urachus | Rose Nolen-Walston |

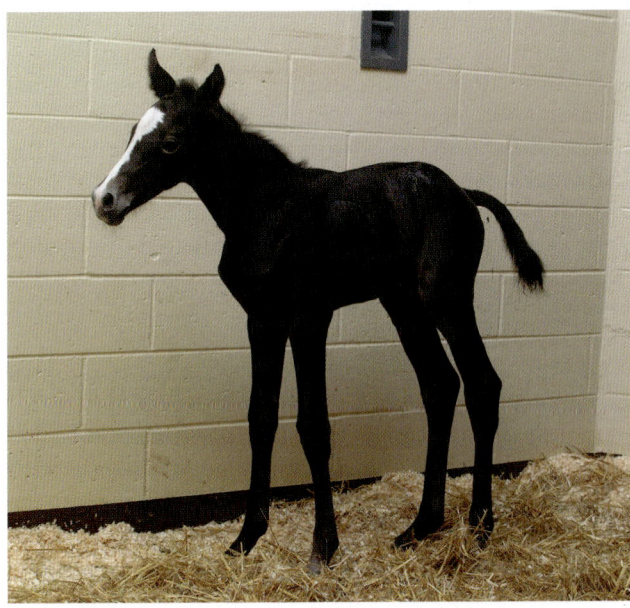

Fig. 12-1 Mutiny, a nine-day-old Hanoverian foal, presented for diarrhea and was screened for umbilical infection.

Mutiny, a 59 kg Hanoverian colt, presented with his dam at nine days of age for evaluation of mild diarrhea and mild lethargy (Figure 12-1). On physical examination, the foal was found to be bright and alert, and auscultation of the thorax and abdomen revealed no murmurs, arrhythmias, or adventitial lung sounds. The heart rate and respiratory rates were normal, but the foal had a rectal temperature of 103.2° F. His mucous membranes were moist but slightly injected, and the capillary refill time was less than two seconds. The foal's tail was wet, and the hindquarters were stained with watery manure. No heat or effusion was noted in any palpable joint, but the umbilical stump was wet and subjectively thickened.

The owner reported that Mutiny was born after a mild dystocia that was easily corrected by the referring veterinarian after approximately 20 minutes of manipulation. At birth, the foal took several hours to stand. He nursed poorly overnight, although he seemed much improved by morning. The umbilicus was dipped in a 7% iodine solution once the foal had stood and nursed. The following day, the veterinarian found the foal's IgG to be low at 400 mg/dl, and administered 1 liter of hyperimmune plasma intravenously. Since that time, the foal had been apparently healthy until the previous day when the diarrhea and decreased activity were noted.

HISTORY AND PRESENTATION

There is no published data that describes the prevalence of umbilical disease in foals; however, in neonates with failure of passive transfer or frank infection, omphalitis is a common comorbidity. The external signs of omphalitis include a thickened umbilical stump, perinavel edema, purulent drainage, and/or patent urachus (Figure 12-2). However, umbilical infection is frequently not apparent on physical examination, but only found via additional imaging when a clinical suspicion arises. Studies performed at two large referral centers found that approximately 50% of foals with evidence of ongoing infectious processes demonstrated ultrasonographic evidence of omphalitis or omphalophlebitis.[1,2] An additional data set shows that 25% of septic foals had an umbilical infection, as did 50% of foals with septic arthritis or osteomyelitis.[3] Because of this, the majority of foals treated within the hospital setting for omphalitis,

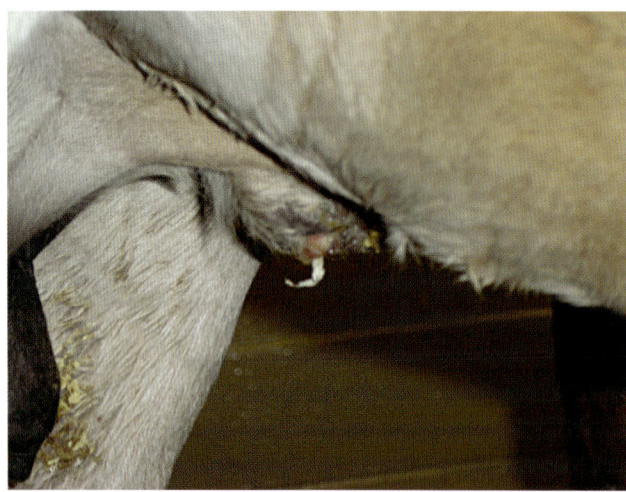

Fig. 12-2 Often umbilical infections have no external clinical signs but the presence of perinaval edema. Purulent drainage from the umbilicus may be present in some cases.

omphalophlebitis, or urachitis were presented for other complaints. The important diagnosis of umbilical infection can often be delayed for days if foals at high risk are not evaluated in a timely manner.

Although umbilical infections have been documented in horses up to 16 months of age,[4] more than 95% of cases are patients under eight weeks old and are associated with organisms that are common isolated in septicemic foals.[5] The majority of equids mentioned in the literature are horse foals, although the condition has also been described in a Grevy's zebra.[6] The urachus is the most commonly involved structure,[5,7,8] either patent, infected, or both. The vascular remnants are also commonly involved, showing extraluminal and intraluminal inflammation or abscessation, as well as involvement of the surrounding tissues.

. PATHOGENESIS

The umbilicus consists of the two umbilical arteries, the umbilical vein, and the urachus, all of which are enclosed in an umbilical sheath. In equine practice, commonly encountered disturbances of the umbilical remnant include omphalitis/omphalophlebitis, patent urachus, liver abscess, and umbilical hernia. There is no single pathogenesis for umbilical infection, but two studies look at risk factors.[1,2] In both studies, criteria for sonographic evaluation of the umbilicus included grossly abnormal navel as described above, fever of unknown origin, leukopenia or leukocytosis, hyperfibrinogenemia, septic arthritis/osteomyelitis, body wall abscesses, positive blood culture, positive sepsis score, diarrhea, or pneumonia. These studies found that approximately half of the cases that fulfilled one

or more of these criteria demonstrated umbilical pathology sonographically.

Postnatal treatment of the umbilicus has also been examined as a risk factor for omphalitis. Although dipping with 7% iodine or 1% povidone is traditional, a study comparing different bactericidal solutions found 0.5% chlorhexidine superior in decreasing the number of bacteria colonizing the stump, as well as minimizing chemical irritation of the tissues.[9] In the case of 7% iodine, local tissue necrosis after treatment may be sufficient to provide an ideal culture medium for bacteria, actually increasing the likelihood of infection.

Much folklore also exists regarding the correct technique for severing the umbilical cord after birth. It is generally accepted that allowing the cord to break spontaneously when the mare rises is ideal, but contrary to popular belief, the cord can be severed immediately after parturition with no appreciable effect on the foal's blood volume.[10] The cord is narrowest at about 5 cm from the foal's body wall, and it is at this area that the cord usually separates. The umbilical arteries retract approximately 6 cm within the abdominal cavity after rupture of the cord.[11] If the cord must be manually separated, providing steady traction on the cord distal to the narrowing while supporting the foal's abdomen at the umbilicus most closely resembles the natural event. Sharp transaction of the cord with clamp or ligature placement prevents retraction of the umbilical structures, and may explain why this procedure has been anecdotally associated with a greater number of complications.

Of the umbilical structures, the urachus is most commonly affected when omphalitis is diagnosed.[7,8] Patent urachus is can be diagnosed by palpation (consistently wet umbilical remnant), visually (seeing "two streams" of urine during micturition from both the urethra and the umbilicus), or sonographically. Most of the literature suggests that patent urachus is usually associated with umbilical infection,[7,12] although more recent data questions that assertion.[5] It has also been hypothesized that excessive abdominal pressure from foal handling or lifting can contribute to the development of urachal patency.[13] Congenital patent urachus, where urine is seen from the umbilicus from the first urination, is generally considered to respond well to conservative therapy such as cauterization. Patent urachus occurring after the first few days of life or secondary to umbilical infection is generally more refractory to medical management,[8] although several authors describe considerable success with nonsurgical treatment.[1]

A diagnostic plan was devised for Mutiny. A complete blood count revealed a neutrophilic leukocytosis of 17,000 WBC/μl, and a fibrinogen of 500 mg/dl. The chemistry panel was unremarkable, and no evidence of dehydration or hypoperfusion was noted. Fecal samples were submitted for analysis for common foal diarrheic pathogens, and an ultrasound examination of the umbilical structures was performed. The umbilical stump was wider than normal (31 mm diameter) with significant edema, and the urachal wall was thickened with fluid and areas of gas shadowing within the lumen. The right umbilical artery was 25 mm in diameter, with a small amount (2 mm) of heterogeneous material in the lumen cranial to the bladder. The left umbilical artery and umbilical vein showed no abnormalities along its entire length.

DIAGNOSTIC TESTING

As most patients with omphalitis do not have umbilical abnormalities as a presenting complaint, the first aspect of diagnosis includes early clinical suspicion. An absence of palpable abnormalities in no way rules out omphalitis and should not be considered a reason to delay further diagnostic testing. Foals under eight weeks of age who have a history of failure of passive transfer or evidence of infectious or inflammatory disease should be considered for ultrasonographic screening. Evaluation of umbilical structures, both normal and abnormal, is well-described[1,5,14,15] and within the capabilities of many equine veterinarians in general practice with some ultrasound experience and appropriate equipment.

A 7.5 mHz transducer is used for the evaluation, and the foal can be evaluated in lateral recumbency or standing (Figure 12-3). A linear transrectal or tendon probe is acceptable. The abdomen is prepared by closely clipping a 4-cm strip along the ventral midline from the xiphoid to the umbilical stump, and a 5-by-5-cm area caudal to the stump (to the udder or prepuce), and cleaning the skin thoroughly. A full evaluation is made of each structure, in short- and long-axis, looking for enlargement from wall thickening or luminal dilation, as well as the presence of abscesses, gas shadows, or fluid accumulation. The umbilical stump is scanned first, and is usually less than 18 mm in diameter at 24 hours of age, decreasing to less than 15 mm at seven days of age (Figure 12-4, Table 12-1). The vein is then followed cranially and very superficially on midline until it terminates within the hepatic parenchyma, where it will eventually become the falciform ligament (Figure 12-5). It should be less than 10 mm in diameter at 24 hours of age, and reduced to less than 7 mm by seven days of age. There should be no areas of thickened wall, or heterogeneous fluid within the lumen (a small amount of anechoic fluid in the lumen for one to two weeks is usually normal), and the liver around the vein should be examined for the presence of abscesses. The arteries course caudally on either side of the urinary bladder, and mature into the round ligaments of the bladder. As the arteries are scanned caudally, deeper settings may

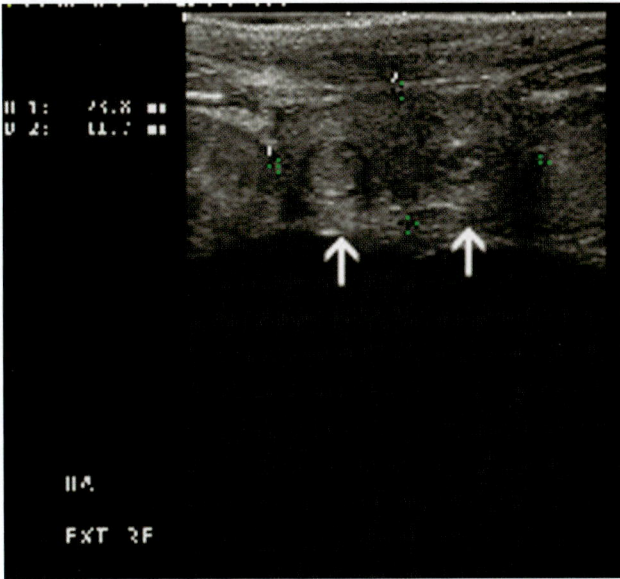

Fig. 12-4 Ultrasound image of the umbilical stump of a normal foal. Note the presence of the two arteries *(a)*. Courtesy of Dr. Kate Chope.

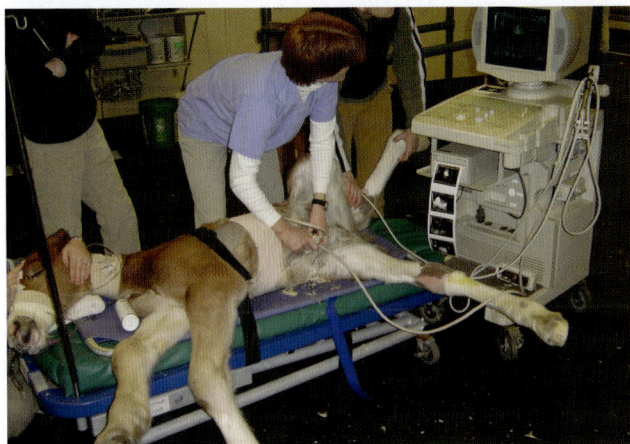

Fig. 12-3 Ultrasound evaluation can be performed in the standing or recumbent foal using a 7.5 mHz ultrasonic probe on the ventral midline of the foal cranial and caudal to and including the umbilical stump.

Table 12.1	Ultrasound Measurement of the Normal Umbilical Structure of the One-Day-Old and Seven-Day-Old Foal	
	One Day of Age	**Seven Days of Age**
Umbilical stump	<18 mm	<15 mm
Umbilical vein	<10 mm	<7 mm
Umbilical artery	<13 mm	<10 mm

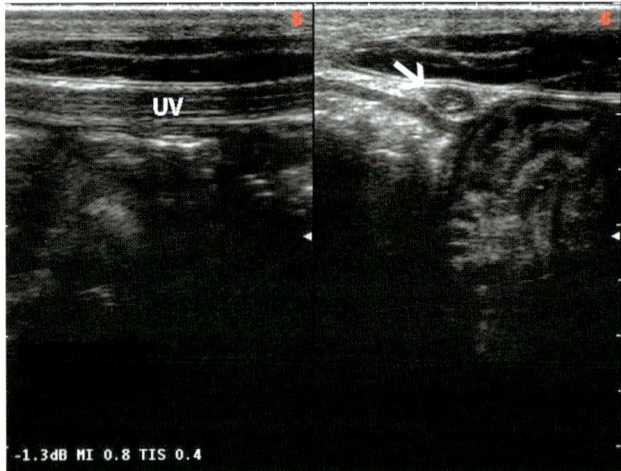

Fig. 12-5 Ultrasound image of the umbilical vein of a normal foal. The vein is found superficial on midline and heads cranially from the umbilical stump until it enters the liver. Note the longitudinal *(left)* and cross-sectional *(right)* views of the vein. Image courtesy of Dr. Kate Chope.

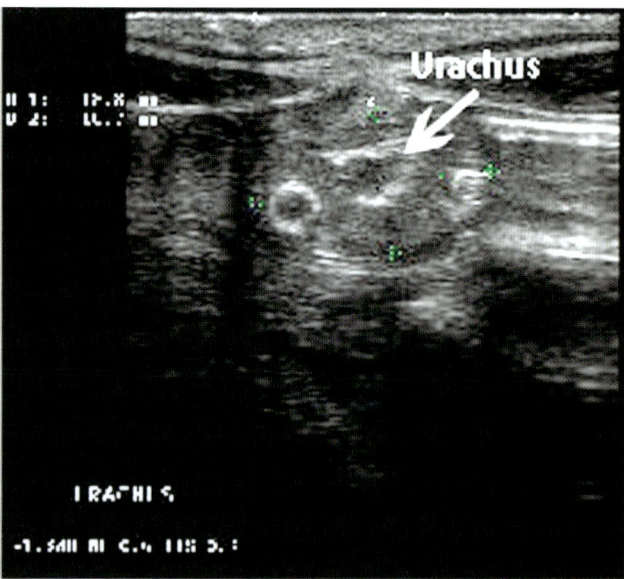

Fig. 12-7 Ultrasound image of an abnormal umbilical stump. Though normal in size, there is fluid in the area of urachus *(u)*. Image courtesy of Dr. Kate Chope.

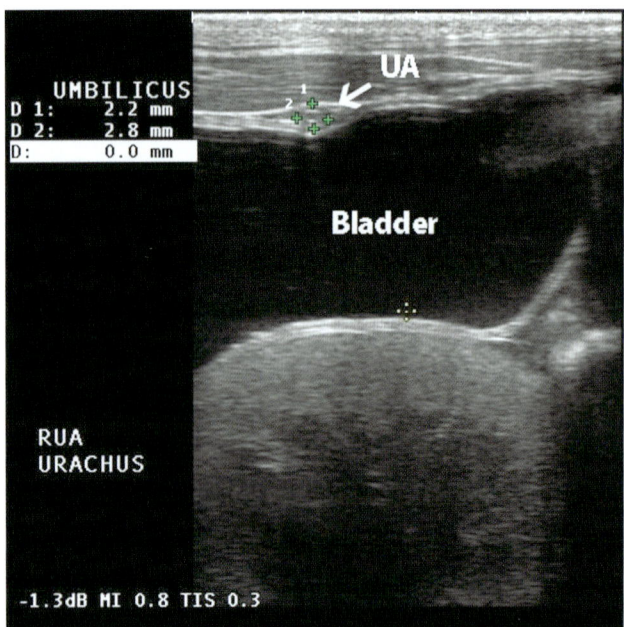

Fig. 12-6 Ultrasound image of the umbilical artery *(ua)* of a normal foal in relationship to the bladder. The umbilical arteries diverge at the apex of the bladder to eventually the round ligaments of the bladder in the adult. Image courtesy of Dr. Kate Chope.

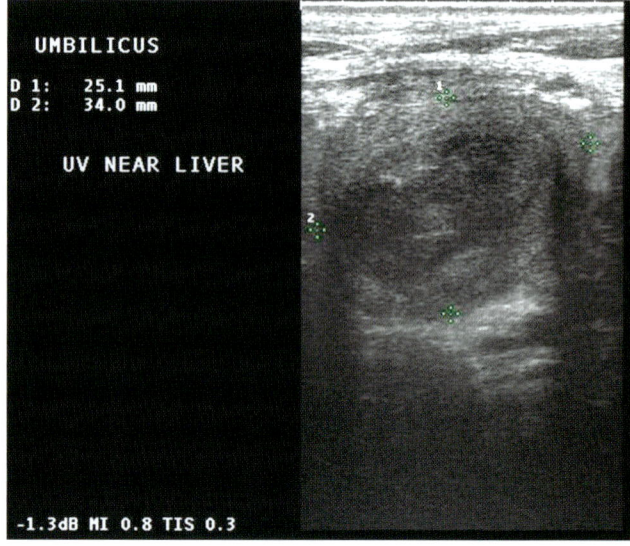

Fig. 12-8 Ultrasound image of an enlarged umbilical vein prior to entering the liver. Image courtesy of Dr. Kate Chope.

need to be used. The arteries may contain echoic clot material, but it should not be inhomogeneous or contain gas shadows. Generally slightly larger than the umbilical vein, the arteries have a diameter of less than 13 mm at 24 hours of age, and less than 10 mm at seven days of age (Figure 12-6, Table 12-1).[15]

Ultrasonographic abnormalities of umbilical structures that can be evident in foals with omphalitis/ omphalophlebitis include enlargement of the vessels beyond the normal limits, asymmetry of arteries with enlargement, abscessation of stump or single vessel, gas shadowing indicative of an anaerobic infection, edema of structures, and hematoma formation (Figures 12-7 and 12-8). The urachus is scanned both longitudinally and in cross-section, although patency is often most apparent in the former view. Longitudinally, a small "beak" at the bladder by the umbilical remnant can be normal in younger foals, but any evidence of urine extending through the urachus at the

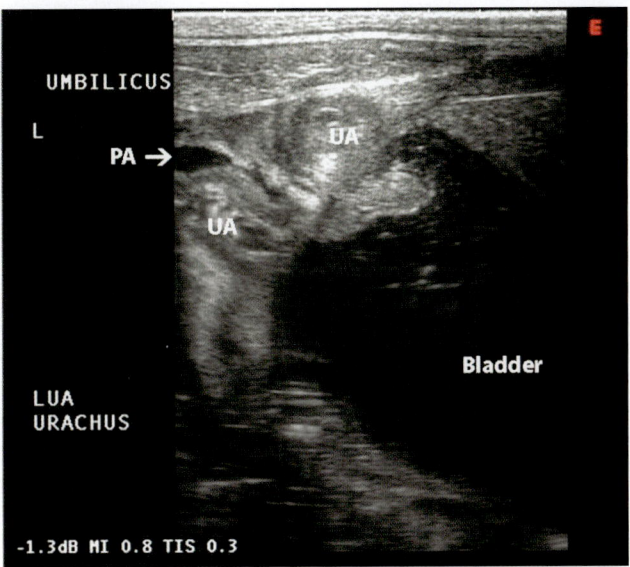

Fig. 12-9 Ultrasound image of the neck of the bladder of a foal. Note the umbilical arteries *(a)* and the evidence of patent urachus *(pa)*.

umbilical stump should be considered evidence of patency (Figure 12-9). The urachus is also evaluated for thickened walls and gas, and when imaged with the arteries, is found to have a composite diameter of less than 25 mm. The bladder should also be evaluated, and found to be oval with anechoic or slightly speckled urine.

As there were no obvious abscesses or large areas of purulent accumulation, the foal was treated with amikacin, ampicillin, and oral metronidazole. Topical procaine penicillin G (PPG) was used on the umbilical stump and distal urachal orifice to promote closure of the patent urachus. The enteric pathogen screen was diagnostic for rotavirus, Mutiny was monitored closely for signs of dehydration, acid-base abnormalities, and electrolyte balance. After 24 hours, the foal's temperature normalized at 101.1° F, and a repeat CBC performed three days after admission showed that the WBC count had decreased to 13,000 cells/μl.

By the fifth day of hospitalization, the foal was producing formed manure. An ultrasound examination was repeated on day seven, and showed that the urachal wall was much less thickened, although gas shadows remained in the urachal remnant at the tip of the umbilicus. This was suspected to be secondary to introduction of room air during the topical PPG treatment. The right umbilical artery still was larger than the reference range, but the intraluminal material was only apparent for a length of 2 cm close to the umbilicus.

TREATMENT

Traditional treatment for infection of the umbilical structures has included complete resection of the umbilical remnant by celiotomy.[16] More recently, Fischer described a laparoscopic-assisted resection of umbilical structures to minimize soft-tissue swelling, edema, and associated morbidity and discomfort.[17] Large venous abscesses are sometimes too large for full excision, but have been treated successfully with a one-stage marsupialization procedure.[18] This condition may carry a worse long-term prognosis due to an apparently greater risk for adhesions.[5] In recent years, there has been increasing interest in treating umbilical infections medically. In one study of approximately 75 foals with umbilical abnormalities, 75% were treated with medical management alone. After three to seven days, the majority of foals showed ultrasonographic improvement, although in some cases an alteration in antibiotic change was necessary before improvement was noted. The majority of foals were treated for two or more weeks before full resolution was achieved.[1]

Foals that should be referred to surgery include those with substantial abscessation or venous involvement that extends as far as the liver.[1] Other suggested criteria for surgical treatment include extremely large umbilical structures, the presence of multiple infected structures (especially infected joints, which suggests the presence of a septic focus), or ultrasonographic evidence of purulent material.[5] Patients that are potentially going to receive surgical resection should receive one to four days of parenteral antibiotics prior to celiotomy in an attempt to minimize abdominal contamination. Considerable variation exists among centers in the proportion of cases that are treated surgically versus medically. Although one might assume that medical therapy would be a good option for owners with financial constraints, this is not necessarily the case. In one hospital, otherwise healthy foals treated with antibiotics only for umbilical remnant infections did not show a significant decrease in cost when compared to surgery.[2]

Antibiotic therapy for omphalitis generally precedes the acquisition of culture and sensitivity results, and selection is therefore empirical. Mixed infections are likely, and common isolates include Gram-negative bacteria (such as *E. coli*, *Klebsiella*, and *Enterococcus*), Gram-positive organisms (especially β-hemolytic *Streptococcus*), and anaerobes (including *Bacteroides* and *Clostridium*).[5,19] A broad-spectrum coverage that includes the aerobic spectrum is appropriate, typically a β lactam antibiotic, such as penicillin, and an aminoglycoside, such as amikacin. Although penicillin drugs have good anaerobic coverage, many strains of *Bacteroides* are resistant to it. In cases in which gas shadows are observed sonographically, additional anaerobic coverage with metronidazole is probably warranted.[1]

For congenital patent urachus and many milder cases of patent urachus secondary to omphalitis, local therapy (chemical cautery with silver nitrate, topical procaine penicillin G,[8] and thermocautery)[20] is often curative, but caution must be used not to place anything further than 1 cm into the stump. Treatments that cause necrosis may also predispose to further bacterial infection.[21]

The urachus remained patent for nine days, and no umbilical moisture or urine flow was noted after that day. On day 14, a repeat ultrasound of the umbilical structures showed a resolution of urachal inflammation, and no evidence of patency could be visualized. The right umbilical artery was still thicker than the left, but both were within the reference range for diameter and no luminal contents were apparent. Mutiny was discharged on the fifteenth day of hospitalization, and no medical sequelae were described on follow-up one month later.

PROGNOSIS

An early study reports a guarded prognosis with a survival rate of 66.6% in foals treated surgically and 42.9% treated with antibiotic therapy alone (Figure 12-10).[8] Advances in therapeutic techniques have improved

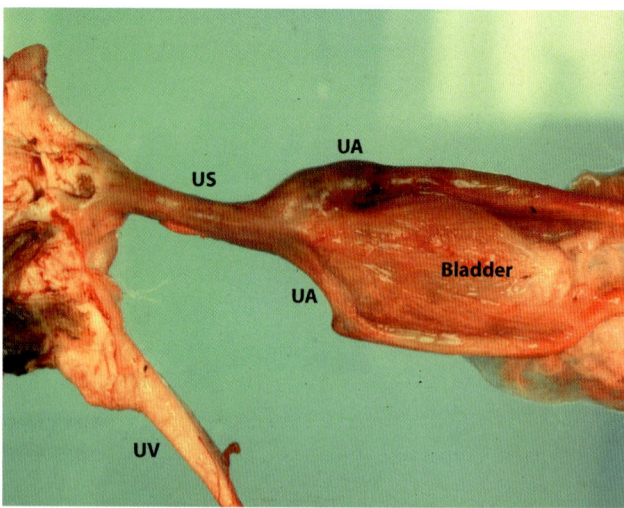

Fig. 12-10 Postmortem example of asymmetry of the umbilical arteries on a foal with omphalophlebitis.

the overall survival rates to 87%. Nonsurvivors died of causes unrelated to the umbilical infection.[15] Severe concurrent disease such as sepsis or multiple joint arthritis, as well as the presence of hepatic abscessation, are suggestive of a poorer outcome.[5]

As the owner walked the mare and foal to the trailer, she thanked the clinician for all her work. "Mutiny sure turned out to be a fitting name for the colt," she commented. The attending veterinarian asked her what she meant. "Well," said the owner, "Mutiny—that's a really bad naval problem, isn't it?"

REFERENCES

1. Reimer JM: Ultrasonography of umbilical remnant infections in foals, Proceedings 39th Ann Convention AAEP, 247, 1993.
2. White SL, Huff T: Retrospective study of surgical vs. medical management of umbilical remnant infections in neonates, Dorothy R. Havemeyer Neonatal Septicemia Workshop, Boston, 48, 1998.
3. Paradis MR: Update on Septicemia. In Vaala W, ed: *Veterinary Clinics of North America: Equine Practice,* Philadelphia, 1994, WB Saunders.
4. Collatos C, Reef VB, Richardson DW: Umbilical cord remnant abscess in a yearling colt, *J Am Vet Med Assoc* 195:9, 1252, 1989.
5. Reef VB, Collatos C, Spencer PA et al: Clinical, ultrasonographic, and surgical findings in foals with umbilical remnant infections, *J Am Vet Med Assoc* 1:195(1):69, 1989.
6. Ndung'u FK, Ndegwa MW, Maar TWJ: Patent urachus with subsequent joint infection in a free-living Grevy's zebra foal, *J Wildl Dis* 39:1, 244, 2003.
7. Adams SB, Fessler JF: Umbilical cord remnant infections in foals: 16 cases (1975-1985), *J Am Vet Med Assoc* 1:190(3):316, 1987.
8. Adams, R: Urachal and umbilical disease. In *Equine clinical neonatology,* Philadelphia, 1990, Lea & Febiger.
9. Lavan RP, Madigan JE, Walker R et al: Effect of disinfectant treatments on bacterial flora of the umbilicus of neonatal foals, Proceedings 40th Ann Convention AAEP 37, 1994.
10. Doarn RT, Threlfall WR, Kline R: Umbilical blood flow and the effects of premature severance in the neonatal horse, *Theriogenology* 28:789, 1987.
11. Whitewell KE: Morphology and pathology of the equine umbilical cord, *J Reprod Fertil Suppl* 23:599, 1975.
12. Turner TA, Fessler JF, Ewert KM: Patent urachus in foals, *Equine Pract* 4:24, 1982.
13. Madigan JE, House JK: Patent urachus, omphalitis, and other umbilical abnormalities. In Smith BP, ed: *Large animal internal medicine,* ed 3, 2002, Mosby.
14. Reef VB, Collatos C: Ultrasonography of umbilical structures in clinically normal foals, *Am J Vet Res* 49:2143, 1988.
15. Lavan RP, Craychee T, Madigan JE: Practical method of umbilical ultrasonographic examination of one-week old foals: The procedure and the interpretation of age-correlated size ranges of umbilical structures, *J Equine Vet Sci* 17:96, 1997.
16. Trent AM, Smith DF: Surgical management of umbilical masses with associated umbilical cord remnant infections in calves, *J Am Vet Med Assoc* 185:1531, 1984.
17. Fischer AT Jr: Laparoscopically assisted resection of umbilical structures in foals, *J Am Vet Med Assoc* 214:1813, 1999.
18. Edwards RB III, Fubini SL: A one-stage marsupialization procedure for management of infected umbilical vein remnants in calves and foals, *Vet Surg* 24:32, 1995.

19. Vaala WE, Clark ES, Orsini JA: Omphalophlebitis and osteomyelitis associated with *Klebsiella* septicemia in a premature foal, *J Am Vet Med Assoc* 193:1273, 1988.

20. Kumaran D, Bhuvanakumar CK: Thermocautery as a treatment for pervious urachus—a clinical study, *Centaur (Mylapore)* 10:43, 1993.

21. Madigan JE, Lavan R: Umbilical disorders—new aspects of pathogenesis and preliminary considerations of methods of umbilical cord treatment regimens. Equine anaesthesia, abdominal surgery and medicine of the foal: In Proceedings of Fourteenth Bain-Fallon Memorial Lectures, Sydney, Australia, *Aust Equine Vet Assoc* 237, 1992.

Case 12-2	Rupture of the Urinary Bladder	Pamela A. Wilkins and Bettina Dunkel

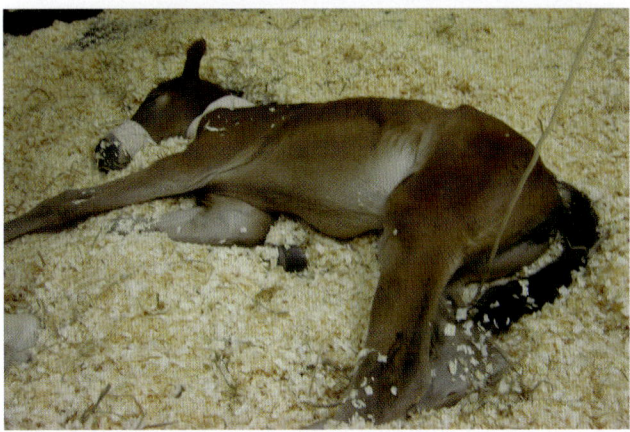

Fig. 12-11 '04 Unzipped at presentation to the neonatal intensive care unit.

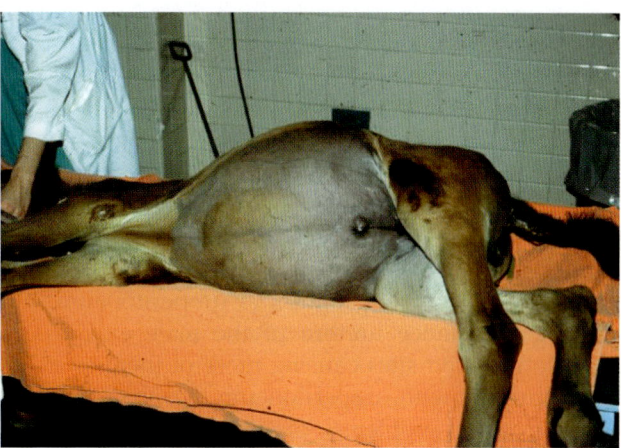

Fig. 12-12 Foal with uroperitoneum anesthetized in lateral recumbency. Note severe abdominal distention. In this case, the external umbilical remnant is also fluid-distended. Image courtesy of Dr. Dean Richardson.

'04 Unzipped, a six-day-old Thoroughbred filly, presented to the NICU at 12:45 PM on April 17, 2004, with a primary complaint of progressive abdominal distention, inability to urinate, depression, and anorexia (Figure 12-11). Historically both the gestation and parturition had been unremarkable. The referring veterinarian had performed an abdominal ultrasound examination and suspected uroperitoneum secondary to a bladder defect.

At presentation, the foal was bright and ambulating but did not suckle from the dam. She weighed 55.45 kg. The foal was tachycardic (108 beats/minute), tachypneic (42 breaths/minute) with increased respiratory effort and nostril flare, and afebrile (101.7° F) on physical examination. Her abdomen was large and tautly distended (Figure 12-12). Mucous membranes were light pink with a capillary refill time of approximately two seconds. Jugular refill was sluggish. On auscultation, the foal's lungs were harsh bilaterally with decreased lung field size bilaterally; the foal had a normal sinus rhythm with no evidence of murmurs. Distal peripheral arteries were difficult to palpate, and distal limbs, particularly the hindlimbs, were cool. She was judged to be mildly (5%) dehydrated. The foal postured to urinate, but the urination attempt was not productive.

HISTORY AND PHYSICAL EXAMINATION

Uroperitoneum has been recognized as a syndrome in foals for over 50 years.[1,2] Traditionally, it has been thought to present most frequently in the 24- to 36-hour-old male foal during the postparturient period.[2-4] However, in 18 foals presenting to New Bolton Center with a primary complaint of uroperitoneum between 1989 and 2004, the average age at presentation was 9.4 days (range 2 to 42 days), with 12 foals presenting between two and seven days of age. There were 17 additional foals that developed, or were diagnosed with, uroperitoneum after being hospitalized for other problems during the same time period. In this group, the mean age of diagnosis was 6.6 days (range 2 to 31 days), with 14 cases diagnosed at seven days of age or less. Once foals presenting at more than 21 days of age were removed, the average age at diagnosis was 6.2 days and was not different between foals presenting for uroperitoneum and foals developing uroperitoneum in the hospital.[5]

Previous reports had a proportionately larger affected male than female population.[2-6] A more recent report suggested that such extreme sex bias may have been an artifact of small case numbers in the early reports.[7] In our study population, the ratio of males to females was approximately 2 to 1; however, within the population hospitalized first for other problems, there was no difference in numbers of colts and fillies. For both groups of foals combined, 40% of all foals (70% of foals where the birth was known to be observed) had been born following dystocia, induction of parturition, or Caesarian section, suggesting that adverse periparturient events are associated with uroperitoneum. A history of dystocia was significant in foals developing uroperitoneum in the hospital.[5] Although speculative, we might suggest that injury to the urinary tract (traumatic, hypoxic, or septic) underlies most cases of uroperitoneum in foals.

In our study population, dystocia was common, providing opportunity for both physical trauma and hypoxia. Documented infection was present in 63% of the foals. For foals presenting with a complaint of uroperitoneum, it is possible that fillies suffering less-severe injury do not progress to uroperitoneum, but the high-resistance urethra of the male exacerbates stress on injured sites causing more of them to eventually present with uroperitoneum. For foals presenting for other problems, the injury appears to be similarly severe for fillies and colts, or perhaps persistent lateral recumbency contributes to eventual development of uroperitoneum. Congenital bladder wall defects are not reported in other species, with the large majority of neonatal urinary ascites cases in humans attributed to iatrogenic trauma or posterior urethra valves in males.[8]

Clinical signs associated with uroperitoneum in the neonatal foal typically include straining to urinate, dribbling urine, and a "stretched-out" stance. Weakness, tachycardia, tachypnea, and failure to suckle well are also commonly present. A distended abdomen may be observed, and a fluid wave may be felt on ballottement of the abdomen. Abdominal distention is significantly more common in foals presenting with a complaint of uroperitoneum than in foals developing uroperitoneum in the hospital.[5] Occasionally urine will accumulate in the scrotum and should not be confused with hernia (Figure 12-13). Urachal tears occurring near or outside the body wall may present with significant ventral abdominal "edema," which is actually subcutaneous urine accumulation, with or without increased peritoneal fluid volume. Foals developing uroperitoneum while hospitalized for other problems are likely to have early signs of decreased urination frequency and urine volume and excessive weight gain. Foals may also show signs of sepsis, including

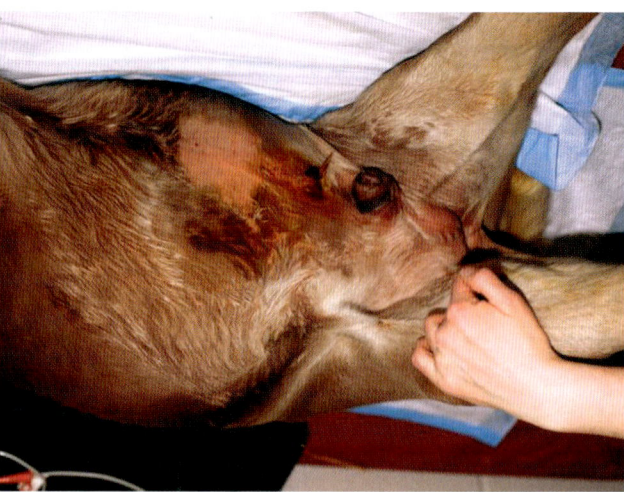

Fig. 12-13 Scrotal and preputial edema present in a male foal presenting with uroperitoneum. Image courtesy of Dr. Joanne Hardy.

fever, injected mucus membranes, diarrhea, and disease of other body systems.

PATHOGENESIS

It has been hypothesized that colts were more at risk due to their long, narrow high-resistance urethra that was less likely to allow bladder emptying, resulting in rupture of a full bladder during parturition when high pressures were applied focally or circumferentially around the bladder.[1] Rupture or disruption of any structure of the urinary tract can occur. The dorsal wall of the bladder has been reported to be a frequent disruption site, with the ventral wall less likely to be involved.[4] The urachus appears to be the next most commonly affected structure. A few cases of ureteral and urethral defects have been reported.[4,6] Sepsis does not appear to favor one site over the others.[7]

The pathophysiology of uroperitoneum is not yet fully understood. It was once thought that high pressures exerted on a full bladder during parturition was the main cause. Full bladder and obstruction due to umbilical cord torsion or trauma at parturition, strenuous exercise, and external trauma have been reported as causes.[9] However, there are anecdotal reports of fetuses with very enlarged bladders observed *in utero* that do not experience bladder rupture during delivery (Figures 12-14 and 12-15, FT Bain and JE Palmer, personal communication, 2005). A few reports describe possible congenital bladder wall defects, proposed due to the smooth and noninflamed edges of the tissue present at the time of surgical correction.[7,10,11] Sepsis as a factor leading to urinary tract rupture and

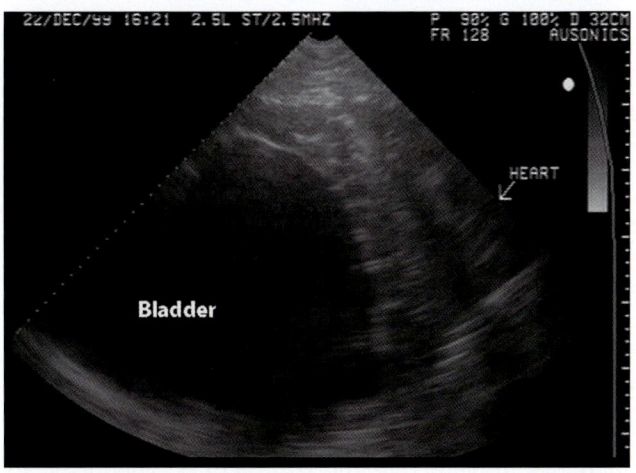

Fig. 12-14 Enlarged bladder seen during transabdominal ultrasonographic fetal evaluation. Image courtesy of Dr. Fairfield Bain.

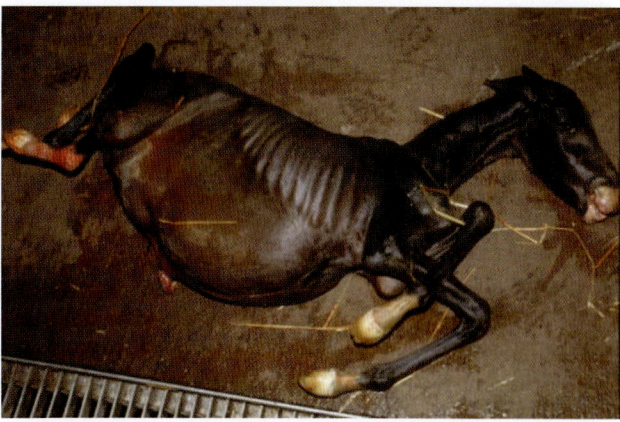

Fig. 12-15 Fetus aborted from pregnancy examined in 12-14. Note large abdomen, all due to bladder distention. The enlarged bladder was secondary to umbilical cord torsion resulting in urachal obstruction. The bladder did not rupture during delivery. Image courtesy of Dr. Fairfield Bain.

Table 12.2	Sequential Arterial Blood Gas and Clinical Chemistry Results for '04 Unzipped					
	Hospitalization Day					
Parameter	Admission	Anesthesia Day 1	Post-Op Day 1	Post-Op Day 2	Post-Op Day 3	Post-Op Day 4[‡]
pH	7.438	7.347	7.463	7.458	—	—
PaO_2 (mm Hg)	51.7*	214.8**	61.4***	70.3***	—	—
$PaCO_2$ (mm Hg)	40.5	62.6	37.9	39.6	—	—
SBE (mmol/liter)	+3.9	+6.2	+4.1	+4.9	—	—
Lactate (mmol/liter)	3.6	0.9	1.8	0.4	—	—
Sodium (mEq/liter)	117	123.1	123.2	128.5	131	129
Chloride (mEq/liter)	81	86	89	93	97	95
Potassium (mEq/liter)	4.45	4.38	4.40	4.55	3.81	4.21
Plasma creatinine (mg/dl)	3.39	—	—	2.38	1.73	1.85
Peritoneal creatinine (mg/dl)	9.78	—	—	—	—	5.06
BUN (mg/dl)	17	19	14	15	—	—

*INO_2 at 15 liters/minute.
**100% O_2.
***Room air.
[†]Recurrent uroperitoneum diagnosed.

uroperitoneum has received more attention in the literature recently, and is a particular problem in foals hospitalized for other problems, as its course is less obvious and more insidious.[7] A history of dystocia is a significant risk factor for the development of uroperitoneum in foals hospitalized for other primary problems.[5]

The foal was in obvious respiratory distress at arrival, and intranasal oxygen insufflation (INO_2) was immediately instituted at 15 liters/minute. An arterial blood gas (ABG) obtained from the left metatarsal artery on nasal O_2 revealed significant hypoxemia (temperature corrected PaO_2 51.7 mm Hg) (Table 12-2). Additional ABG abnormalities included desaturation of Hb (SaO_2 85.4%) and *hyperlactatemia (lactate 3.6 mmol/liter). Temperature-corrected $PaCO_2$ was 40.5 mm Hg (lower than usually seen in this age foal at this clinic), which suggested hyperventilation.*

CARDIOPULMONARY COMPLICATIONS

The foal in this report presented in respiratory distress, and oxygen insufflation at a large flow rate was immediately initiated. An arterial blood gas obtained after inspired nasal O_2 was initiated revealed significant hypoxemia without hypercapnia. The marked

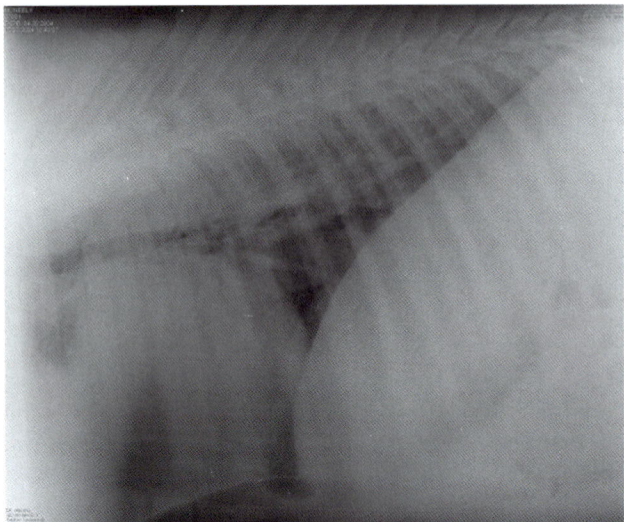

Fig. 12-16 Lateral thoracic radiograph of a foal with increased abdominal fluid. Note the diffuse interstitial pattern, particularly evident dorsally. Also note the pronounced rounded shape of the diaphragm with cranioventral separation of the diaphragm halves.

abdominal distention was a likely contributor to respiratory distress by interfering with normal chest wall, diaphragmatic, and lung expansion, essentially creating a form of restrictive pulmonary disease in the foal (Figure 12-16). '04 Unzipped was suffering from intra-abdominal hypertension (IAH), which can progress to abdominal compartment syndrome (ACS) secondary to significant interperitoneal fluid accumulation.[12]

Increased intra-abdominal pressure, the root cause of abdominal compartment syndrome, has a direct effect on pulmonary function.[12] Pulmonary compliance suffers with resultant progressive reduction in total lung capacity, functional residual capacity, and residual volume—all contributing to significant ventilation-perfusion relationship aberrations.[13] Pulmonary vascular resistance increases as a result of reduced alveolar oxygen tension and increased intrathoracic pressures. Ultimately, pulmonary organ dysfunction is manifest by hypoxia and hypercapnia.

Decompression of the abdominal cavity results in nearly immediate reversal of respiratory failure, although some degree of atelectasis may persist.[13] As yet, unpublished data from a retrospective study of foals with uroperitoneum at New Bolton Center revealed that at least 20% of foals with uroperitoneum had clinically important hypoxemia at the time uroperitoneum was recognized. This was more common in foals presenting with uroperitoneum (27%) than in foals developing uroperitoneum after hospitalization.[5] Ventilation-perfusion relationship abnormalities and mechanical restriction resulting in hypoxemic respiratory failure secondary to IAH were the most likely pulmonary sources of the respiratory distress present in '04 Unzipped at admission.[14-17]

Increased intra-abdominal pressure is also consistently correlated with reduction in cardiac output.[12] Reduction in cardiac output is a result of decreased cardiac venous return from direct compression of the caudal vena cava and portal vein. Increased intrathoracic pressure also results in reduced cranial vena cava flow, further decreasing venous return to the heart. Increased intrathoracic pressure causes cardiac compression (thoracic tamponade) and reduction in end-diastolic volume. Increased systemic vascular resistance results from the combined effect of arteriolar vasoconstriction and increased intra-abdominal pressure. These derangements result in reduced stroke volume that is only partly compensated for by increases in heart rate and contractility. The tachycardia commonly observed in foals with clinically important uroperitoneum is likely due to this mechanism, at least in part. The Starling curve is thus shifted down and to the right, and cardiac output progressively decreases with increasing intra-abdominal pressure.[12,14,18,19] These derangements are exacerbated by concomitant hypovolemia.[20] Although not determined in this case, increased intrapleural pressure resulting from transmitted intra-abdominal forces can increase measured hemodynamic parameters including central venous pressure and pulmonary artery wedge pressure. Significant hemodynamic changes have been demonstrated with intra-abdominal pressures above 20 mm Hg (~27 cmH$_2$O).[12,18] Poor cardiac output is also a potential contributor to hypoxemia.[14,15]

An intravenous catheter was placed in the left jugular vein of the foal, and blood was withdrawn and submitted for blood culture and routine clinical chemistry and hematology testing. Identified abnormalities included hyponatremia (Na 117 mEq/liter), hypochloremia (Cl 81 mEq/liter), hyperglycemia (glucose 226 mg/dl), increased plasma creatinine concentration (3.39 mg/dl), leukocytosis (total WBC count 19, 800 cells/μl), neutrophilia (18,612 cells/μl), lymphopenia (990 cells/μl), and hyperfibrinogemia (705 mg/dl). The potassium concentration was 4.45 mEq/liter. The calculated effective osmolality was decreased at 248 mOsm/liter. Plasma IgG concentration was >800 mg/dl.

Abdominal ultrasonography revealed a fluid-filled abdomen. The fluid was hypoechoic and was also observed surrounding the kidneys. A defect was seen in the dorsal wall of the bladder (Figures 12-17 and 12-18), and the urachus appeared to be fluid-filled. No pleural fluid was seen in either side of the thorax. Abdominocentesis was performed, and the fluid appeared to be clear. Creatinine concentration of the peritoneal fluid was 9.6 mg/dl and the peritoneal fluid to plasma creatinine ratio was 2.83. A Foley catheter was placed transabdominally (Figure 12-19), and the intra-abdominal pressure was measured in lateral recumbency as 31 cm H$_2$O

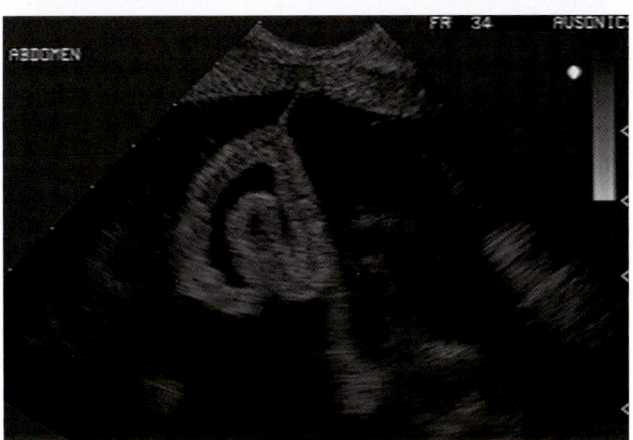

Fig. 12-17 Cross-sectional view of '04 Unzipped's bladder with dorsal wall defect. Note the inverted U-shape of the bladder.

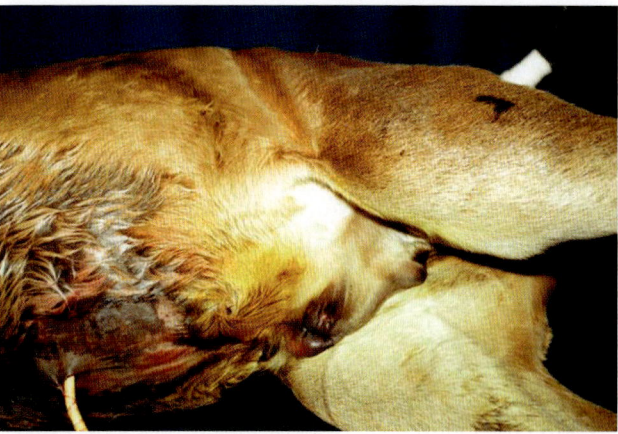

Fig. 12-19 A Foley catheter is placed in the ventral abdomen of a male foal to measure intra-abdominal pressure and aid in drainage of urine from the peritoneal space. Note the scrotal and preputial edema present. Image courtesy of Dr. Joanne Hardy.

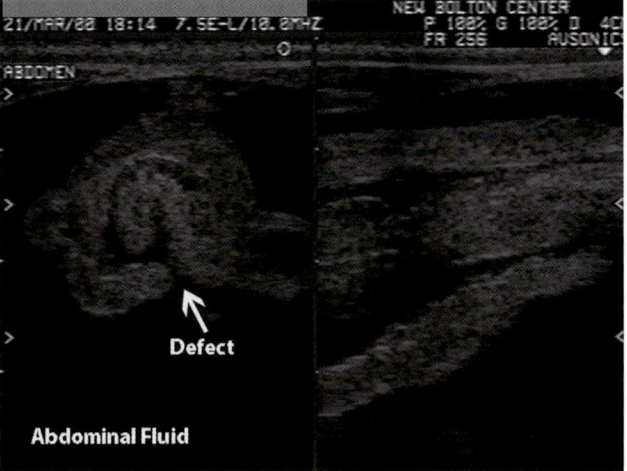

Fig. 12-18 A defect in dorsal bladder wall is clearly visible (arrow) In a transverse image of '04 Unzipped's bladder. Note the large amount of free abdominal fluid.

(~23 mm Hg) with the zero point at the pubic symphysis. The urinary catheter was left in place to aid in draining urine from the abdomen. A diagnosis of uroperitoneum secondary to dorsal bladder wall defect complicated by intra-abdominal hypertension was made, and the foal was prepared for surgical exploration. Intravenous fluids were administered as 0.9% NaCl with 5% added dextrose at 120 ml/hour, and ceftiofur sodium (10 mg/kg IV over 20 minutes) was administered as perioperative antimicrobial therapy. Anesthesia induction occurred less than two hours after presentation.

DIAGNOSIS

Laboratory findings are variable, depending upon the duration of the uroperitoneum as well as the presence and severity of sepsis and diet. Classic findings include hyperkalemia, hyponatremia, and hypochloremia arising from equilibration of urine electrolytes and water with blood across the peritoneal membrane.[3-6] The usual foal diet of milk, which is high in potassium and free water and low in sodium, promotes the electrolyte abnormalities. Foal urine is also low in sodium and chloride and high in potassium, therefore accumulation of urine into the abdomen allows diffusion of a low sodium, low-chloride, and high potassium fluid into the system thus diluting sodium and chloride and elevating potassium. Foals that develop uroperitoneum while receiving sodium-containing intravenous fluids may not have electrolyte imbalances due to correction of electrolyte derangements, although hyperkalemia may be apparent if milk is provided.

Increased serum creatinine concentration is often present while blood urea nitrogen concentrations are occasionally, but not consistently, increased.[3,4,6] Metabolic and/or lactic acidosis and hypoxemia may be part of the clinical picture. Some patients also have serum hypo-osmolality. Foals should be tested for failure of passive transfer. In an unpublished retrospective study of foals with uroperitoneum, 32% had plasma IgG concentrations less than 800 mg/dl at admission.[5]

One of the most sensitive laboratory tests for uroperitoneum is the peritoneal-to-serum creatinine ratio. A ratio ≥2 to 1 is considered diagnostic of uroperitoneum. This ratio was 2.83 in '04 Unzipped. Peritoneal fluid should be collected and tested for creatinine concentration, as well as for cytology, culture, and sensitivity. It is important that the clinician be aware of the techniques used in the laboratory to measure peritoneal fluid creatinine concentration. Although it has been reported by others that peritoneal creatinine concentration is larger in foals with urachal lesions, this has not been the case in our experience.[5,7] In '04 Unzipped's case, the peritoneal fluid creatinine concentration was first reported as 4.3 mg/dl. The high clinical suspicion of uroperitoneum resulted in re-evaluation by the laboratory at the clinician's prompting, and uncovered a dilution error. Other laboratory errors that may occur include evaluation of the peritoneal fluid sample as a urine sample, which in our laboratory falsely increases creatinine concentration by as much as 6 mg/dl, resulting in foals with peritoneal effusions due to other problems having, perhaps unnecessary, abdominal exploration.

Cytologic evaluation of peritoneal fluid is necessary to identify concurrent peritonitis or other gastrointestinal compromise.[21-23] An electrocardiogram may be performed on initial evaluation of a foal with suspected uroperitoneum as hyperkalemia can result in bradycardia, increased duration of the QRS complex, shortened QT interval, increased P-wave duration, prolonged P-R interval, or AV conduction disturbances. As '04 Unzipped had a normal potassium concentration, tachycardia, and a normal sinus rhythm, an ECG was not performed in this case. Other possible cardiac sequelae to hyperkalemia include cardiac arrest, third-degree A-V block, ventricular premature contractions, and ventricular fibrillation.[6,10]

Ultrasonography has become the tool of choice in the diagnosis of uroperitoneum and is a useful tool available to the practitioner. Imaging of free peritoneal fluid can be readily accomplished, and large tears within the bladder, and sometimes urachus, are readily seen. In a fluid-filled abdomen, the empty bladder with a large defect will collapse on itself and often have a U-shape (Figures 12-17 and 12-18). Six of eight foals in one study had urinary tract lesions identified sonographically, and all 31 foals in a second study underwent sonographic evaluation with significant correlation between ultrasonographic findings and location of the lesion at surgery.[4,7]

Additional diagnostics that have potential utility include instillation of new methylene blue dye within the bladder.[22,23] Abdominocentesis following a brief waiting period (15 to 30 minutes) should allow visualization of a color change of peritoneal fluid if the defect is within the bladder and/or urachus. Radiopaque material can be used for a similar purpose, with abdominal radiographs obtained after the material is injected into and has distended the bladder.[22,23] If ureteral lesions are suspected or if no evidence of disruption of the bladder or urachus can be uncovered, an intravenous pyelogram can be attempted.[22,23] Radiographs obtained in foals using this technique are frequently less than ideal for diagnosis, at least in the author's experience, and may be related to the larger intravascular volume of the foal compared to the adult, resulting in relative underdosing of the dye.

TREATMENT

Initial treatment is aimed at stabilizing the patient, correcting electrolyte and acid-base abnormalities, and providing fluid volume replacement. 0.9% or 0.45% saline should be used until laboratory data are available. Potassium concentration >5.5 mEq/liter can be life-threatening. Hyperkalemia can be managed by peritoneal drainage to decrease whole-body potassium stores. This can be performed with teat cannulas, Foley catheters, large-gauge (16 ga or 14 ga) intravenous catheters, or human peritoneal dialysis catheters (Figure 12-19).

Fluid replacement should at least equal the amount of fluid removed from the abdomen to prevent acute hypotension due to expansion of previously collapsed capillary beds. Abdominal drainage will also help ventilation by decreasing pressure on the diaphragm. One caution with peritoneal drainage is the possibility of omental eventration, via the hole made through the abdominal wall, once large-bore drainage devices have been removed. To prevent this problem, many clinicians will leave drainage devices in place until the time of surgery or suture the defect closed at the time of removal.

Intravenous calcium gluconate, glucose, sodium bicarbonate, and insulin can be used to decrease potassium concentration. These maneuvers do not correct the whole-body potassium overload, however, and hyperkalemia can reappear until the urine is removed from the abdomen. Hyponatremia should be slowly corrected.

Because of the real possibility of concurrent sepsis, blood cultures should be obtained prior to administration of preoperative antimicrobials. Broad-spectrum coverage, penicillin and amikacin or ceftiofur sodium, is recommended until culture results become available. Therapeutic drug monitoring should be performed if aminoglycoside therapy is used. However, the peak value may be depressed due to the increased volume of distribution represented by the volume of urine in the abdomen, so dose adjustment based on a low peak should not be made until a new peak is obtained after surgical correction of the uroperitoneum. Foals with failure of passive transfer should be treated with adequate volumes of intravenous plasma.

Once the metabolic abnormalities have been addressed, surgical management can be considered. Medical management using an indwelling Foley catheter has been described.[24] Preoperative medical stabilization reduces the anesthetic risk. Safer inhalant

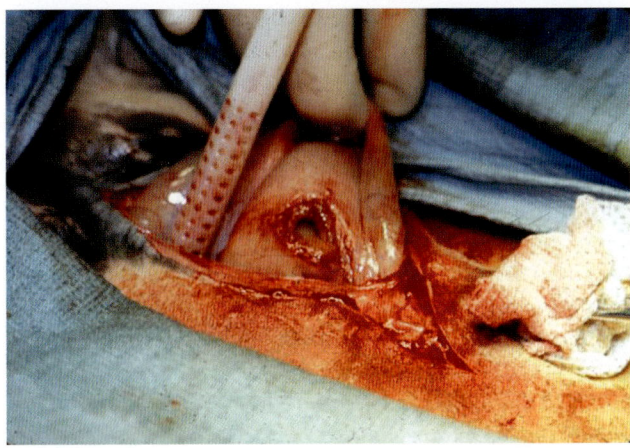

Fig. 12-20 Defect in the bladder of a foal. This is a ventral defect seen in a different foal than '04 Unzipped. Image courtesy of Dr. Dean Richardson.

agents, such as isoflurane, have also decreased risk. It is usual for the internal umbilical remnant to be removed at the time of surgery. Consideration should be given to culture of any removed umbilical remnant, and the peritoneal cavity, and the remnant should be submitted for histopathologic evaluation. In '04 Unzipped's case, the decision was made to go straight to surgery based upon the normal potassium concentration and the degree of respiratory compromise. As INO_2 failed to resolve the severe hypoxemia, it was desirable to relieve the IAH rapidly.

Surgical repair of '04 Unzipped's bladder tear was unremarkable. Approximately 4 liters of peritoneal fluid was suctioned from the abdominal incision. The surgeons identified a 1.5cm tear in the dorsal apex (Figure 12-20). The apex of the bladder was removed and the cystotomy was closed in two layers (Lembert followed by Cushing) using 3-0 vicryl. One liter of carboxymethyl cellulose (CMC) was instilled in the abdomen prior to closure. The remaining internal and external umbilical remnant was removed, and the abdominal incision was routinely closed. The urachus and umbilicus were cultured and appeared grossly normal. The cultures were eventually reported as positive. The foal experienced no anesthetic problems and was maintained on 0.9% saline with 5% dextrose throughout the procedure at 120 ml/hour. The foal's weight on return to the NICU from surgery was 52.3kg for a weight loss of 3.2kg; ~6% of her body weight at admission), corresponding to the approximate net fluid loss from her abdomen at surgery.

SURGICAL AND ANESTHETIC CONCERNS

When IAH and/or ACS are present, abdominal decompression may precipitate adverse physiologic and metabolic events that should be anticipated. Although '04 Unzipped did not receive positive pressure ventilation, large airway pressures are frequently required for mechanical ventilation in these patients; when combined with the return to more normal negative pleural pressures and acutely increased cardiac output following abdominal decompression, there is risk for the development of "re-expansion" pulmonary edema.[25]

Re-expansion pulmonary edema is probably related to increased pulmonary vascular permeability, secondary to hypoxic damage to capillary endothelium, and mechanical damage to blood vessels from overstretching during the process of re-expansion. Additionally, there may be an acute change in transmural pulmonary vascular pressures. Clinical signs can present from seconds to hours after the injury. Both acute lung injury (ALI) and acute respiratory distress syndrome (ARDS) have been recognized as significant complications of abdominal compartment syndrome, and ALI has been reported in foals with uroperitoneum.[16,21,26]

"Washout" of accumulated intra-abdominal products of anaerobic metabolism may result in a bolus of acid and potassium systemically delivered to the heart. This may contribute to adverse cardiac events such as dysrhythmia or asystole. Foals with significant preexisting electrolyte derangements (hyponatremia, hypochloremia, and hyperkalemia) may be at greater risk for these types of cardiac complications. Anticipating, recognizing, and treating these effects is of critical importance.[12,13,27]

In early reports of uroperitoneum, cardiac dysrhythmias were common associated with anesthesia and were generally attributed to hyperkalemia. The use of isoflurane, in place of halothane, and perioperative management aimed at correcting hyperkalemia prior to induction of anesthesia, has minimized these complications. Only 4 of 25 foals undergoing anesthesia for correction of uroperitoneum experienced dysrhythmia in one recent report; only 2 of 4 had increased potassium concentrations.[5] This compared favorably to 9 of 18 foals experiencing dysrhythmia or other anesthetic complications in one early report.[6]

In '04 Unzipped's case, positive pressure ventilation was not used. There was some evidence of increased dead space ventilation as the arterial $PaCO_2$ was 61.4 mm Hg one hour following induction of anesthesia at a time when the end-tidal CO_2 ($ETCO_2$) was 46 mm Hg (Table 12-2). The foal was receiving 100% oxygen, and her PaO_2 was only 215 mm Hg, resulting in a PaO_2/FiO_2 ratio of 215, consistent with ALI. Her lactate concentration had decreased to 0.9 mmol/liter. At this time, approximately three hours after presentation, her electrolyte concentrations were Na 123 mEq/liter, Cl

86 mEq/liter, and K 4.28 mEq/liter. She remained hyperglycemic.

On return to her stall '04 Unzipped was tachycardic (210 beats per minute) and tachypneic (60 breaths per minute) while receiving 10 liters/minute inspired nasal O_2. Once the foal had been allowed some time to recover, an arterial blood gas was obtained without intranasal O_2 and revealed persistent modest hypoxemia (62 mm Hg; see Table 12-2) in lateral recumbency. Intranasal O_2 was continued at 3 liters/minute. Fluid therapy was altered to bolus therapy every four to six hours as 0.9% NaCl without dextrose. The foal was assisted to her feet and allowed to suckle from the dam as desired. Intramuscular butorphanol (2 to 4 mg) was administered for postoperative pain relief as needed, and oral phenazopyridine treatment was initiated to relieve urinary tract discomfort.

'04 Unzipped recovered fairly uneventfully from surgery but remained oxygen dependent for the next 48 hours. It was noted that the foal had progressive abdominal distention and her respiratory rate remained increased. She was noted to urinate frequently and produce a normal stream and apparently normal volume, but her weight gain was more rapid than anticipated. The foal would episodically tail-flag and posture to urinate without urine production. Her appetite was somewhat capricious. The foal's hyperglycemia and electrolyte abnormalities resolved. Her plasma creatinine concentration decreased to 1.73 mg/dl.

Despite normalizing creatinine concentration and apparent normal urine volume, the foal's increasing abdominal distention led to clinical suspicion of continued urine leak. A repeat abdominal ultrasound examination revealed accumulation of hypoechoic fluid within the peritoneal space. No defect was seen in the urinary bladder during this examination. Abdominocentesis was performed, and the creatinine concentration of the peritoneal fluid was 5.63 mg/dl, confirming reoccurrence of uroperitoneum. Approximately 2 liters of fluid was drained from the abdomen. Re-exploration of the abdomen was offered, but the owners declined. A urinary catheter was placed and secured with sutures to relieve tension on the bladder, and the foal was observed closely. Fluid was drained from the abdomen once daily over the next two days and was discontinued when ultrasonography revealed minimal to no fluid accumulation. Drainage was simplified because the omentum had been removed at the previous surgery. Antimicrobial therapy was changed to oral trimethoprim sulfa, and fluid boluses were discontinued. Intranasal O_2 was also discontinued as the PaO_2 in lateral recumbency was acceptable (see Table 12-2). The foal was discharged six days after admission with the indwelling urinary catheter still sutured in place. The catheter was removed at home 10 days after it was placed, and '04 Unzipped continued to recover uneventfully.

OUTCOME

Many of these foals are persistently oxygen dependent for several days following surgical correction, and serial arterial blood gas analyses should be performed before intranasal oxygen supplementation is discontinued. Thoracic radiographs may be indicated and may reveal diffuse, patchy interstitial and alveolar patterns. Sepsis, persistent hypoxemia, pneumonia, peritonitis, and acute respiratory distress syndrome all complicate the management of uroperitoneum. Recurrence of the urinary tract rupture can occur. Many clinicians leave the urinary catheter in place for several days following surgical correction to prevent pressure on the repair and hopefully circumvent the complication of small leak experienced by this foal.

Prognosis is closely associated with concurrent illness, especially septicemia. Uncomplicated uroperitoneum from a defect in the bladder has a good prognosis. If the location of the lesion is other than the bladder, the prognosis is not as favorable.[6] Foals with septicemia have a much poorer prognosis.[5-7]

REFERENCES

1. Bain AM: Disease of foals, Aust Vet 30:9, 1954.
2. Du Plessis JL: Rupture of the bladder in the newborn foal and its surgical correction, J S Afr Vet Assoc 29:261, 1958.
3. Behr MJ, Hackett RP, Bentinick-Smith J et al: Metabolic abnormalities associated with rupture of the urinary bladder in neonatal foals, J Am Vet Med Assoc 178:263, 1981.
4. Adams R, Koterba AM, Cudd TC et al: Exploratory celiotomy for suspected urinary tract disruption in neonatal foals: A review of 18 cases, Equine Vet J 20:13, 1988.
5. Dunkel BD, Palmer JE, Boston RC et al: Uroperitoneum in 32 foals (1987-2004), In publication, 2005.
6. Richardson DW, Kohn CW: Uroperitoneum in the foal, J Am Vet Med Assoc 182:267, 1983.
7. Kablack KA, Embertson RM, Bernard WV et al: Uroperitoneum in the hospitalized equine neonate: Retrospective study of 31 cases, 1988-1997, Equine Vet J 32:505, 2000.
8. Checkley AM, Sabharwal AJ, MacKinlay GA et al: Urinary ascites in infancy: Varied etiologies, Pediatr Surg Int 19:443, 2003.
9. Pascoe RR: Repair of a defect in the bladder of a foal, Aust Vet J 47:343, 1971.
10. Hackett RP: Rupture of the urinary bladder in neonatal foals, Comp Cont Ed 6:S488, 1984.
11. Wellington JKM: Bladder defects in newborn foals (letter), Aust Vet J 48:426, 1972.
12. Bailey J, Shapiro MJ: Abdominal Compartment Syndrome, Crit Care 4:23, 2000.

13. Kron IL, Hartman PK, Nolan SP: The measurement of intra-abdominal pressure as a criterion for abdominal re-exploration, *Ann Surg* 199:28, 1984.

14. Wilkins PA: Lower respiratory problems of neonates. In Parente EJ, ed: *Equine respiratory disease, Vet Clin N Amer Eq Pract* 19:19, 2003.

15. Wilkins PA: Acute respiratory failure: Diagnosis, monitoring techniques and therapeutics, *Clin Tech Equine Pract* 2:56, 2003.

16. Wong DM, Leger LC, Scarratt WK et al: Uroperitoneum and pleural effusion in an American Paint Filly, *Equine Vet Educ* 16:290, 2004.

17. Wilkins PA: Respiratory distress in foals with uroperitoneum: Possible mechanisms, *Equine Vet Educ* 16:293, 2004.

18. Barnes GE, Laine GA, Giam PY et al: Cardiovascular responses to elevation of intra-abdominal hydrostatic pressure, *Am J Physiol* 248:R208, 1985.

19. Ridings PC, Bloomfield GL, Blocher CR et al: Cardiopulmonary effects of raised intra-abdominal pressure before and after intravascular volume expansion, *J Trauma* 39:1071, 1995.

20. Baggot MG: Abdominal blow-out: A concept, *Curr Res Anesth Analg* 30:295, 1951.

21. Hyman S, Wilkins PA, Palmer JE et al: Uroperitoneum associated with *Clostridium perfringens* urachitis in two neonatal foals, *J Vet Intern Med* 16:489, 2002.

22. Hyman SS: Uroperitoneum in the equine neonate. In Wilkins PA, ed: *Recent advances in equine neonatal care,* Ithaca: International Veterinary Information Service (www.ivis.org), Document No. A0415.1101, 2001.

23. Hardy J: Uroabdomen in foals, *Equine Vet Educ* 10:21, 1998.

24. Lavoie JP, Harnagel SH: Nonsurgical management of ruptured urinary bladder in a critically ill foal, *J Am Vet Med Assoc* 192:1577, 1988.

25. Ozlu O, Kilic A, Cengizlier R: Bilateral re-expansion pulmonary edema in a child: A reminder, *Acta Anaesthesiol Scand* 44:884, 2000.

26. Offner PJ, de Souza AL, Moore EE et al: Avoidance of abdominal compartment syndrome in damage-control laparotomy after trauma, *Arch Surg* 136:676, 2001.

27. Eddy V, Nunn C, Morris JA: Abdominal compartment syndrome, *Surg Clin North Am* 77:801, 1997.

13 Cardiac Disorders

| Case 13-1 | Foal with Congenital Cardiac Defect | Katherine Chope |

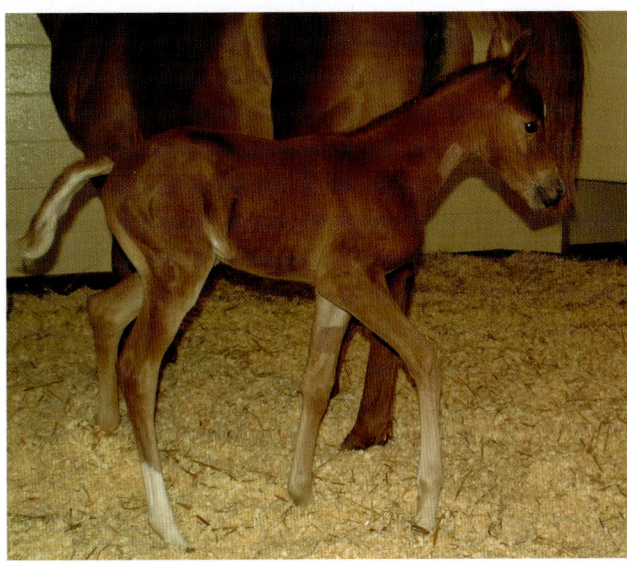

Fig. 13-1 '01 Dear John at two days of age when the murmur was first discovered.

'01 Dear John, a 21-day-old Arabian filly presented for evaluation of a loud heart murmur audible on both sides of the chest, and a palpable precordial thrill. '01 Dear John's birth 21 days prior to admission to a maiden mare was uncomplicated, and the foal stood and nursed within two hours of birth. Her IgG level was >800 mg/dl. The foal was active and similar in size to other foals of the same age on the farm. The murmur had been detected on routine neonatal examination, and when it persisted at three weeks of age, she was sent to a referral facility for evaluation (Figure 13-1).

Upon presentation to the hospital, '01 Dear John was bright, alert, responsive, and active. Her temperature was 100.5°F, her heart rate 90 to 100 beats per minute in a normal sinus rhythm, and her respiratory rate was 40 to 50 breaths per minute. Her mucous membranes were pale pink, moist, and demonstrated a normal capillary refill time. Peripheral pulses were strong and jugular refill was normal on the filly. Auscultation of her heart revealed a grade 6/6 harsh, band-shaped pansystolic murmur with the point of maximal intensity over the tricuspid valve region, and a grade 5/6, coarse, crescendo-decrescendo pansystolic murmur with the point of maximal intensity over the pulmonic valve region and radiating caudally. Auscultation of her lungs was unremarkable.

HISTORY AND PHYSICAL EXAMINATION

Cardiac murmurs are very common in neonatal foals. The majority are not pathologic in origin. Nonpathologic causes of murmurs detected in the neonatal period include murmurs caused by the normal transition from fetal circulation and systolic physiologic flow murmurs. Pathologic causes of murmurs are less common and include persistent elements of fetal circulation that remain patent beyond normally expected dates of closure, congenital cardiac defects, and rarely an acquired valvular insufficiency or bacterial endocarditis.

In a study of Thoroughbred foals, 90% of foals had continuous machinery murmurs present for the first 15 minutes of life, most likely due to persistent flow through the ductus arteriosus.[1] Waxing and waning murmurs, associated with flow through the closing ductus arteriosus, can be heard for the first three to four days of life. In a study of 10 pony foals, Livesey and colleagues found that systolic murmurs were present in all foals during the first three days of life, and persisted in six foals on day 35 and two foals up to day 49.[2] In the same study, turbulent flow through the ductus was identified via echocardiography in a number of foals up to day 49 (seven weeks). The relationship between detection of a systolic murmur and detection of flow in the ductus was described as inconsistent, suggesting that some flow in the ductus may be present in the absence of a detectable murmur, and that a proportion of the systolic murmurs were purely physiologic in origin.[1] Arrhythmias are also common in the first few minutes of life of the newborn foal, but typically disappear shortly thereafter. They are likely due to high vagal tone and hypoxia at birth.[3]

Physiologic murmurs may be detected in foals that present for any variety of reasons. Typical findings on auscultation of a physiologic murmur are a grade 3/6 or less holosystolic, crescendo, crescendo-decrescendo or band-shaped murmur with the point of maximal intensity over the pulmonic to aortic valve area. Physiologic murmurs also may change in grade with changes in heart rate. Physiologic murmurs have been described as being up to a grade 4/6, however, this may be due to variations in the murmur grading system, rather than interpretation of a murmur with a palpable thrill being nonpathologic.[4] Physiologic murmurs typically are not right-sided systolic or diastolic. The presence of a grade 4/6 or above holosystolic or pansystolic murmur, bilateral murmurs, multiple systolic murmurs, a diastolic murmur or a continuous murmur, which persist beyond 96 hours of age, is indicative of a pathologic, not physiologic process. Similarly, grade 3 to 4/6 (or lower) systolic murmurs should be investigated if the clinical presentation suggests cardiac disease or any uncertainty exists regarding their origin.

The initial cardiac evaluation of a neonatal foal should include careful auscultation of both sides of the heart over all valve areas. This is ideally accomplished in an area with a minimum of background noise, with the foal relatively still and the front leg on the side of the examiner extended slightly forward. The pulmonic, aortic, and mitral valve regions are located in the left third, fourth, and fifth intercostal spaces, respectively. The tricuspid valve region is located in the right third to fourth intercostal space. Murmurs, if identified, should be characterized according to grade, timing, location or point of maximal intensity, shape or pitch, character, and radiation. Murmurs are graded on a scale of 1 to 5 or 1 to 6, depending upon clinician's training and preference. In a six-grade system, grade 1 murmurs are audible only after careful auscultation for several minutes and only over one valve area, grade 2 murmurs are slightly louder, readily audible when the stethoscope is placed over the point of maximal intensity, and grade 3 murmurs are easily audible immediately upon auscultation and may

radiate over more than one valve area. Murmurs of grade 4 or above by definition have a palpable thrill. Grade 6 murmurs are audible with the stethoscope removed slightly off of the chest wall. Timing is defined as pansystolic (obliterating one or both heart sounds); holosystolic (between the heart sounds); early, mid, or late systolic; or holodiastolic. Shape or pitch refers to whether the murmur increases (crescendo) in pitch, decreases in pitch (decrescendo), increases then decreases (crescendo-decrescendo), or does not change in pitch (band-shaped). The modifiers describing quality of sound are not universally agreed upon but are most frequently *soft and blowing, coarse, harsh, musical, honking,* or *machinery.* Harsh or machinery murmurs are generally associated with a pathologic process. The palm of the hand should be laid flat over the region of the cardiac silhouette on both sides to palpate for a thrill (vibration).

The remainder of the cardiac exam should include evaluation of mucous membranes, capillary refill time, jugular refill, presence or absence of jugular pulse, arterial pulse quality, and auscultation of the lungs. The size and activity level of the foal should be appropriate, baring unrelated disease processes, and the foal should not demonstrate signs of exercise intolerance. Signs of cardiac disease include jugular pulses or distension, bounding pulses, pleural effusion, ascites, dependant edema, severe exercise intolerance, collapse, and cyanosis. Clinical signs that can occur in cardiac disease but are less specific include tachycardia, tachypnea, and weak thready pulses. Bounding pulses reflect an especially large difference in pressure between systole and diastole such as occurs in a patent ductus arteriosus. They may also be appreciated in aortic regurgitation or an aorta-cardiac fistula, although this is unlikely in a neonate.

Cyanosis is rare in the horse. Central cyanosis (detectable in mucous membranes) is most commonly due to severe respiratory disease, resulting in hypoxia, or congenital cardiac or circulatory conditions causing right-to-left shunting of blood, thereby bypassing oxygenation in the lungs (Figure 13-2). Central cyanosis is generally not detectable until PaO_2 is below 40 mm Hg, below the 60 mm Hg level defined for hypoxia. Evaluation of the response of the PaO_2 to nasal insufflation with 100% oxygen, if available, can help indicate whether the cyanosis is due to a right-to-left shunt. A PaO_2 of less than 100 mg Hg after nasal insufflation with 100% oxygen is strongly suggestive of a right-to-left shunt.[5]

The clinical presentation of neonatal foals with a ventricular septal defect (VSD) ranges from normal to debilitated based on the size, location, and number of defects, and the presence of any additional cardiac abnormalities. Small defects may have no gross clinical manifestations, and the defect may go unnoticed

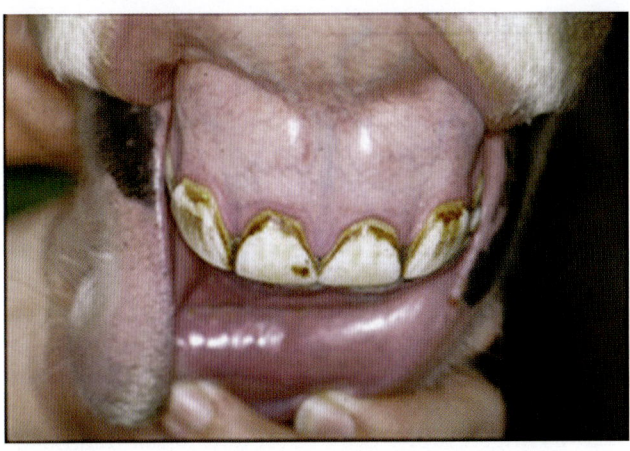

Fig. 13-2 Foal with cyanotic mucous membranes. Photo courtesy of Dr. Michelle Barton.

PATHOGENESIS

Physiologic flow murmurs are murmurs of left ventricular ejection, due to nonlaminar flow in the great vessels, as in adult horses. Echocardiographic examinations of foals with murmurs that are consistent with normal physiologic flow murmurs have indicated that there is often no other echocardiographically detectable cause for the murmur, such as valvular regurgitations, shunts, or ductal flow.[1] Murmurs due to flow in patent remnants of fetal circulation (ductus arteriosus or foramen ovale) can also be normal in the neonate, if not detected beyond the normal time window for closure.

In utero, the fetus receives oxygen via the placental blood flow and the fetal lungs are bypassed, in essence a right-to-left shunt. Fetal circulation bypasses the lungs via the ductus arteriosus, which forms a communication between the pulmonary artery and aorta, and the foramen ovale, which forms a communication between the right and left atria. At birth, decreases in pulmonary resistance and increases in oxygen content associated with inflation of the lung stimulate physiologic closure of the ductus and the foramen ovale. Anatomic closure follows.[1,8,9] Physiologic closure of the ductus typically occurs within 24 to 72 hours. Thus, continuous or systolic murmurs within that time frame are considered nonpathologic. Occasionally, systolic flow persists in the ductus for up to several weeks post-birth. This may be a normal variation or secondary to disease processes that result in sustained elevation in right-sided pressures or hypoxia (pneumonia, pulmonary hypertension, dysmaturity/immaturity, maladaptive foal syndrome, or other pulmonary disease). However, systolic murmurs associated with ductal flow should not persist beyond seven weeks of age. Functional closure of the foramen ovale has been suggested to be associated with elevation of left atrial pressures secondary to ductal closure, as well as changes in oxygen tension. Anatomic closure of the foramen ovale occurs during the first few weeks of life.[1,9]

The true incidence of congenital cardiac abnormalities in the horse is unknown although relatively rare overall.[6,10] In an evaluation of approximately 2500 foals, fetuses, and horses presenting for necropsy over four years, Rooney and Franks found four congenital cardiac anomalies.[11] Cardiac defects accounted for 3.6% of the abnormalities in a survey of congenitally abnormal fetuses and foals. Marr reports detecting congenital abnormalities in 3.4% of 380 horses presenting for cardiac evaluation.[1,12] VSDs are recognized as the most common type of congenital cardiac abnormality in the horse, as in cattle and llamas.[1,4,6,23,24] However, a variety of congenital and complex congenital cardiac defects have been described in foals including atrial septal defect, patent ductus arteriosus,

until the horse reaches training age or beyond. Typical findings on auscultation of an isolated VSD are a grade 3/6 or higher, harsh, band-shaped pansystolic murmur with the point of maximal intensity over the right third to fourth intercostal space (tricuspid valve region) and a grade lower crescendo-decrescendo ejection-type murmur, with the point of maximal intensity over the pulmonic valve region. The right-sided murmur represents flow through the septal defect, and the left-sided murmur represents the relative pulmonic stenosis that occurs secondary to the right ventricular volume overload created by the defect (i.e., more blood than normal flowing through a normal pulmonic valve). A left-sided murmur that is louder than the right-sided murmur suggests that the septal defect is located in the right ventricular outflow portion of the septum or that other abnormalities exist.[6,7] Diastolic murmurs may also exist in conjunction with the typical systolic murmurs of a septal defect and are usually due to prolapse of an aortic leaflet into the defect, and resulting aortic regurgitation.

The clinical presentation of foals with other types of congenital cardiac diseases can also vary widely, ranging from normal to recumbent, hypoxic, or cyanotic depending upon the type and severity of the lesion. Typically, however, foals with complex congenital cardiac disease are severely debilitated.[1,4,6] Most foals with congenital cardiac disease demonstrate grade 3/6 or higher holosystolic or pansystolic murmurs. Care should be taken to not equate the loudness or grade of the murmur with the severity of the suspected disease process, as complex congenital abnormalities may have murmurs that are a lower grade than those of a VSD. Likewise, the absence of a detectable murmur should not rule out congenital cardiac disease in cases when it would otherwise be suspected.

VSD with pulmonic stenosis, tetralogy of Fallot, endocardial cushion defect, tricuspid atresia, truncus arteriosus, pseudotruncus arteriosus, transposition of the great vessels, and double outlet right ventricle, among others.[1,4,6,10,13-26] Other congenital defects, such as an anomalous origin of the right coronary artery, have been echocardiographically detected in the adult horse and are unlikely to be of clinical significance in the neonate.[27]

Congenital cardiac abnormalities represent either persistent remnants of fetal circulation after birth (patent ductus arteriosus or patent foramen ovale) or failure of a step or steps during embryologic development of the heart. Membranous VSDs are a result of failure of fusion of the muscular septum with the endocardial cushion during early fetal development, and right ventricular outflow septal defects are a result of abnormal development of the bulbus cordis.[4] Defects may also occur in the muscular portion of the septum. VSDs may be present as part of more complex congenital cardiac disease.

The cause of VSD is unknown although evidence suggests it is a heritable defect in cattle and dogs.[28] Certain breeds of horse, including Standardbreds, Arabians, American Miniatures, and Welsh Mountain ponies, appear to have an increased incidence of congenital cardiac disease.[1,4,29,30] Using horses with VSDs or other congenital cardiac abnormality for breeding purposes is not recommended. Genetic defects, maternal infection, nutrition, and hypoxia have been implicated in small animals and suggested as a cause in large animals.[12,19,31,32] Exposure to teratogens in early gestation could potentially play a role in causing abnormal cardiac development in utero, but little evidence exists in this regard.

The initial workup on '01 Dear John was composed of an echocardiographic examination using real-time two-dimensional imaging (B-mode), M-mode, color, pulsed, and continuous-wave Doppler studies. Standard B-mode imaging revealed the presence of a 1.3 to 0.17 cm (long-axis view) by 3 to 3.2 cm (short-axis view) defect in the membranous portion of the interventricular septum. Color-flow Doppler demonstrated a jet of regurgitant bloodflow from left to right across the defect in the interventricular septum. Pulsed-wave Doppler confirmed a left-to-right high-velocity shunt, and continuous-wave Doppler revealed the shunt velocity to be 4.2 to 4.5 ml/ second. Mild left ventricular and left atrial enlargement was present, and a mild volume overload pattern was present on M-mode examination. No other cardiac abnormalities or valvular regurgitations were identified. '01 Dear John was in sinus rhythm throughout the examination. As she was otherwise clinically healthy, no further diagnostic tests were performed.

DIAGNOSTIC TESTS

The diagnostic test of choice for evaluation of a murmur or suspected cardiac disease is an echocardiographic examination using B-mode (two-dimensional real-time) ultrasound, M-mode ultrasound, pulsed and/or continuous-wave Doppler, and color-flow Doppler examination.[1,4,6,19,29,31-34] Thoracic radiographs may be useful in suggesting gross cardiac enlargement and vascular changes, but are nonspecific. Likewise, electrocardiographic changes are nonspecific in the equine. Rarely, more invasive techniques such as angiography may be of additional diagnostic benefit. However, they are generally performed when indicated following an initial echocardiographic examination, are limited by the animal's size (less than 300 pounds), and are generally performed at referral centers.

Echocardiography alone can be used to diagnose most fetal congenital abnormalities or acquired pathologies. Echocardiographic examination provides both structural and functional information. Measurements obtained during the echocardiogram may also help determine prognosis and, in applicable cases, treatment success. Additional techniques, such as a bubble or contrast study, may be used in conjunction with the echocardiographic exam to help confirm an intracardiac shunt.

Echocardiographic examination is noninvasive and can be performed with practice in the foal with many commercially available ultrasound machines. The examination is most easily performed with the foal standing; however, if necessary, diagnostic quality images can also often be obtained with the foal in lateral or sternal recumbency. A phased array, sector, or small footprint curvilinear probe should be used. A mid-range frequency (5.0 MHz) transducer and a depth setting of 12 to 20 cm should suffice for most neonatal foals. The majority of the echocardiographic examination should be performed from the right fourth intercostal space (right parasternal view), switching to the left parasternal windows only after the basic views and measurements have been obtained. It is often necessary to extend the right forelimb, particularly in recumbent or sternal foals, in order to obtain diagnostic images from the right fourth intercostal space (Figure 13-3).[6]

Three standard long-axis or sagittal views (right ventricular outflow, left ventricular outflow, and four-chamber), three standard short-axis or transverse views (level of aortic valve, level of mitral valve, and level of left ventricle), and three standard M-mode views (through aortic valve, mitral valve, and left ventricle just below the mitral valve) should be obtained (Figures 13-4 to 13-12). Care should be taken to

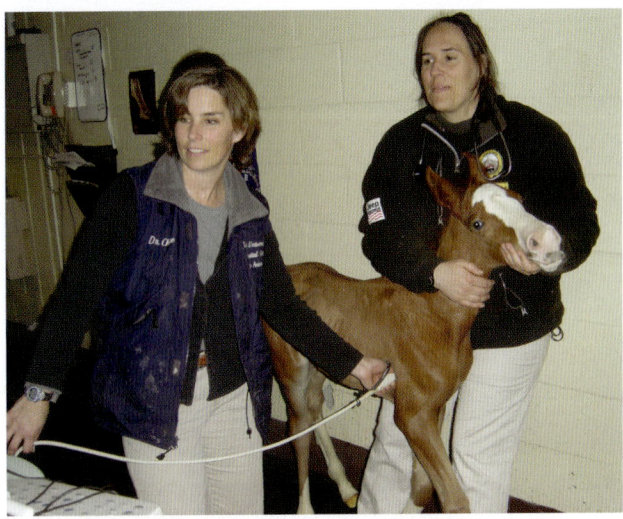

Fig. 13-3 Extension of the right forelimb allows for ultrasound imaging from the right fourth intercostal space.

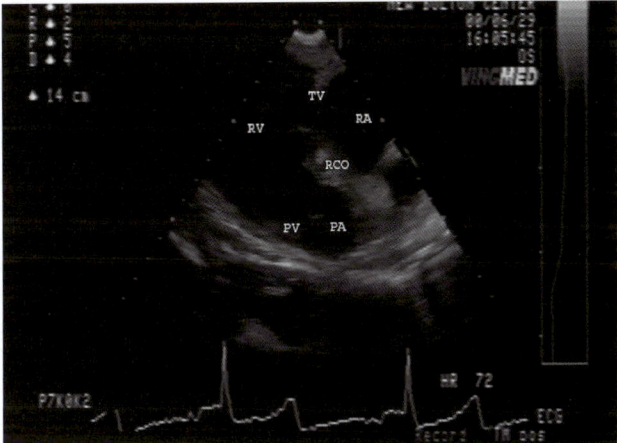

Fig. 13-4 Long-axis view of the right ventricular outflow tract of a one-month-old Warmblood foal. Taken from the right cardiac window, displayed depth 14 cm. *RA,* right atrium; *TV,* tricuspid valve; *RV,* right ventricle; *PV,* pulmonic valve; *PA,* main pulmonary artery; *RCO,* right coronary artery. Image courtesy of New Bolton Center, University of Pennsylvania School of Veterinary Medicine.

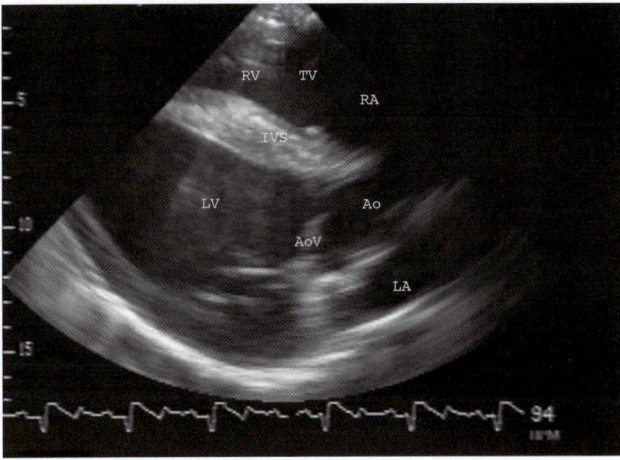

Fig. 13-5 Long-axis view of the left ventricular outflow tract of a two-week-old Thoroughbred cross foal. Taken from the right cardiac window, displayed depth 18 cm. *RA,* right atrium; *TV,* tricuspid valve; *RV,* right ventricle; *LV,* left ventricle; *AoV,* aortic valve; *Ao,* aorta; *LA,* left atrium (portion of); *IVS,* interventricular septum. Image courtesy of New Bolton Center, University of Pennsylvania School of Veterinary Medicine.

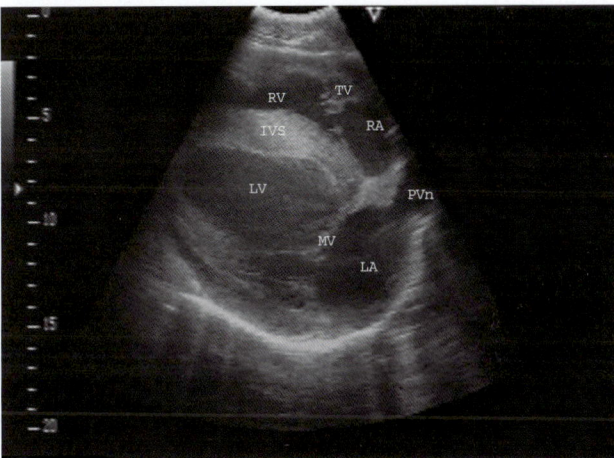

Fig. 13-6 Long-axis four-chamber view of a two-week-old Thoroughbred cross foal. Taken from the right cardiac window, displayed depth 20 cm. *RA,* right atrium; *TV,* tricuspid valve; *RV,* right ventricle; *LV,* left ventricle; *MV,* mitral valve; *LA,* left atrium; *PVn,* pulmonary vein; *IVS,* interventricular septum. Image courtesy of New Bolton Center, University of Pennsylvania School of Veterinary Medicine.

identify each cardiac chamber and valve, and ensure that they present a normal appearance and relationship to one another. Some normal "drop out" or hypoechoic regions can occur in the middle of the atrial septum (region of foramen ovale) in the long-axis views and the proximal portion of the interventricular septum in the four-chamber long-axis view, so any suspicious region should be evaluated in two planes. In neonatal foals, the "flaps" of the foramen ovale can be rather easily imaged on 2-D normally, and should not be mistaken for a defect. Patency should be confirmed with Doppler examination. The region between the pulmonary artery and aorta in the right outflow view

should be examined for evidence of a patent ductus, although frequently the ductus is very difficult to image in the standard B-mode image.

Pulsed-wave and/or color Doppler, if available, should be applied across the atrioventricular (tricuspid and mitral) and semilunar (pulmonic and aortic) valves, the interventricular septum, interatrial septum, and in cases of suspected persistent ductus arteriosus, the main pulmonary artery. Pulsed and/or color Doppler should be applied across the atrial side of the

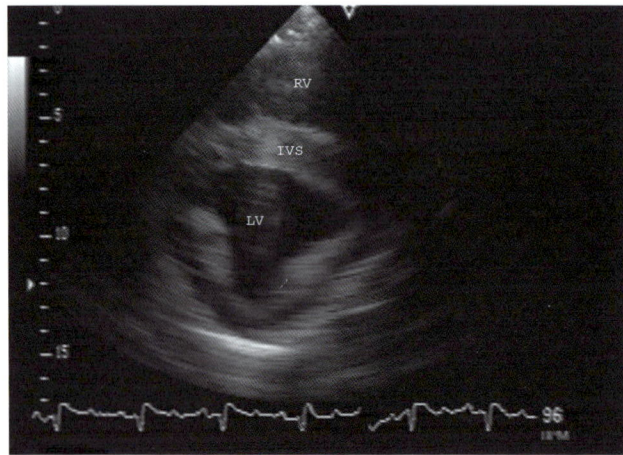

Fig. 13-7 Short-axis view of left ventricle of a two-week-old Thoroughbred cross foal. Taken from the right cardiac window, displayed depth 20 cm. *LV,* left ventricle; *IVS,* interventricular septum; *RV,* right ventricle. Image courtesy of New Bolton Center, University of Pennsylvania School of Veterinary Medicine.

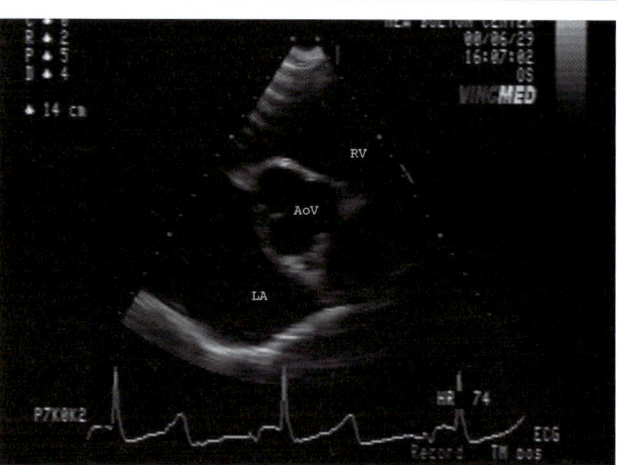

Fig. 13-9 Short-axis view of aortic valve of four-week-old Warmblood foal. Taken from the right cardiac window, displayed depth 14 cm. *AoV,* aortic valve; *LA,* left atrium; *RV,* right ventricle. Image courtesy of New Bolton Center, University of Pennsylvania School of Veterinary Medicine.

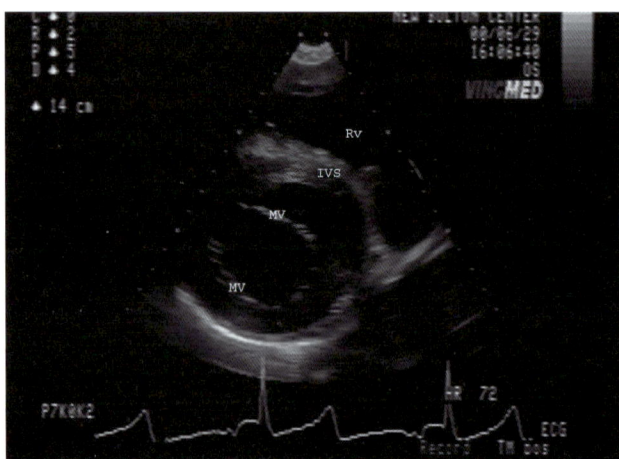

Fig. 13-8 Short-axis view of mitral valve in the open position of a four-week-old Warmblood foal. Taken from the right cardiac window, displayed depth 14 cm. *MV,* mitral valve; *IVS,* interventricular septum; *RV,* right ventricle. Image courtesy of New Bolton Center, University of Pennsylvania School of Veterinary Medicine.

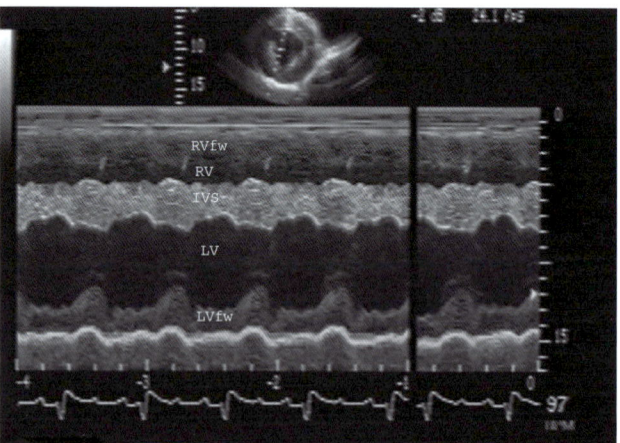

Fig. 13-10 Two-dimensional short-axis view of left ventricle with M-mode cursor and M-mode echocardiogram of left ventricle of a four-week-old Warmblood foal. Taken from the right cardiac window, displayed depth 17 cm. *RVfw,* right ventricular free wall; *RV,* right ventricular chamber; *IVS,* interventricular septum; *LV,* left ventricular chamber; *LVfw,* left ventricular free wall. Image courtesy of New Bolton Center, University of Pennsylvania School of Veterinary Medicine.

atrioventricular valves (looking for backflow during systole) and the ventricular side of the semilunar valves (looking for backflow during diastole). Pulsed Doppler is used to precisely map the location of any abnormal or regurgitant flow. Color flow is used similarly, and when available, is often a more simply applied survey tool. In most standard color maps, red and blue represent normal flow toward and away from the transducer; disturbed or high-velocity flows are coded in the green or light color range. Continuous-wave Doppler can be used to quantify the velocity of any high-velocity flow identified by pulsed-wave or color Doppler.

If a shunt is suspected, contrast echocardiography can also be used as a diagnostic aid, if the Doppler findings are unclear. It is performed using a commercially available contrast agent or agitating several milliliters of saline, removing any large air bubbles, and injecting it into the jugular vein while the suspect region is being evaluated sonographically. The air-laden solution will appear echodense or strongly reflective in contrast to normal blood. These small air

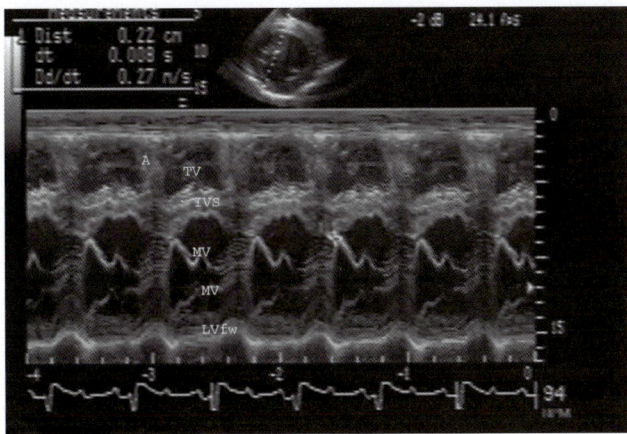

Fig. 13-11 Two-dimensional short-axis view of mitral valve with M-mode cursor and M-mode echocardiogram of mitral valve of a two-week-old Thoroughbred cross foal. Taken from the right cardiac window, displayed depth 17 cm. *TV*, tricuspid valve; *IVS*, interventricular septum; *MV*, mitral valve; *LVfw*, left ventricular free wall; *A*, artifact created by lung field extending into imaging window. Image courtesy of New Bolton Center, University of Pennsylvania School of Veterinary Medicine.

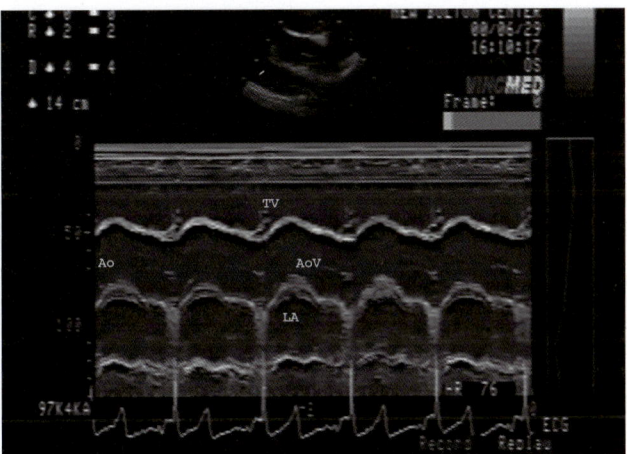

Fig. 13-12 Two-dimensional short-axis view of aortic valve with M-mode cursor and M-mode aortic valve of a four-week-old Warmblood foal. Taken from the right cardiac window, displayed depth 14 cm. *TV*, tricuspid valve; *Ao*, aorta; *AoV*, aortic valve; *LA*, left atrium. Image courtesy of New Bolton Center, University of Pennsylvania School of Veterinary Medicine.

bubbles do not pass through the pulmonary microcirculation, and thus should only be seen on the right side of the heart. A positive contrast jet means bright echoes are seen in a normally dark region (right-to-left shunt), whereas a negative contrast jet means anechoic fluid (unaltered blood) is entering the region of echoes (left-to-right shunt).

Once a thorough examination has been performed from the right parasternal window, the examination may be continued from the left third, fourth, and fifth intercostal spaces in order to obtain a left atrial diam-

eter, evaluate the pulmonary artery and aorta, particularly if a patent ductus arteriosus is suspected, and interrogate the mitral valve with pulsed- and/or color Doppler.

Few published normals for cardiac size in the equine neonate exist. In a study of sixteen normal pony and Thoroughbred foals (average body weight 64.67 kg) by Stewart and colleagues, average left ventricular end diastolic M-mode measurements at 14 days of age were 6.91 +/− .51 cm, right ventricular end diastolic measurements were 2.55 +/− .86 cm, and aortic root measurements were 3.75 +/− .26 cm.[35] Generally, the right ventricular chamber size should be less than half that of the left ventricular chamber size. Due to the nature of fetal circulation, however, the right ventricular free wall is thicker relative to the left ventricular free wall at birth and in the first few weeks of life than it is in the adult.[35]

A physiologic flow murmur should result in no detectable abnormalities on the echocardiogram. A patent ductus arteriosus can be difficult to identify in a two-dimensional view, but may appear as a hypoechoic tubular structure between the aorta and pulmonary artery, best seen from the right parasternal view. Volume overload of the pulmonary artery, left atrium, left ventricle, and aorta may be present. Continuous or disturbed flow should be detected on pulsed-wave Doppler of the main pulmonary artery. A patent foramen ovale appears as anechoic region in the central portion of the atrial septum (secundum region), although caution should be used, as anatomically closed foramen ovale are often still visible echocardiographically even in adult horses. Doppler or contrast findings should be used to confirm patency.

Echocardiographically, abnormal valves may appear thickened, irregular, or lacking in normal valve motion. Vegetative lesions appear as hypoechoic clumps on the valve surface. Valvular regurgitation appears as turbulent or aliased flow during the appropriate phase of the cardiac cycle for that valve.

A careful, thorough, and methodical echocardiographic examination is essential to making an accurate diagnosis of congenital cardiac disease. A variety of potential cardiac abnormalities exists, and normally readily identifiable structures may be almost unrecognizable. As always, in addition to the standard long- and short-axis views, the heart should be carefully scanned from base to apex in both planes. Care should be taken to identify that each of the typically visualized cardiac chambers and vessels are accounted for and that no unidentifiable structures are visible. Chambers and vessels should present a normal appearance and relationship to one another. Structures that are not readily identifiable should be methodically followed to determine relationships and communications with structures that can be identified.

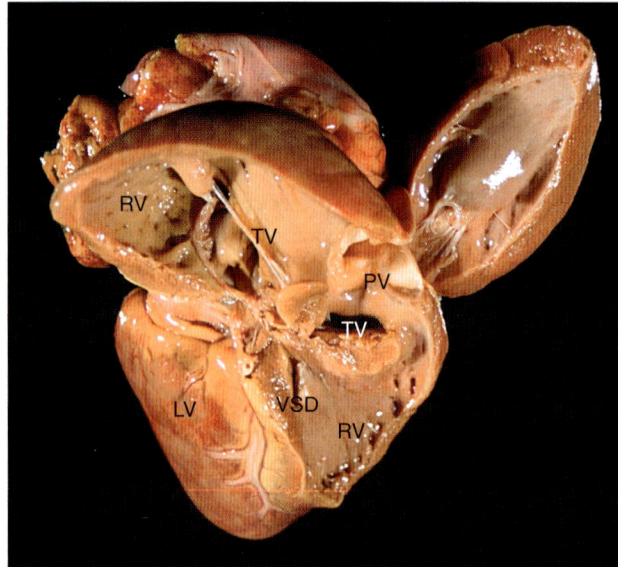

Fig. 13-13 Pathology specimen of American Miniature Horse heart with a ventricular septal defect and right ventricular hypertrophy. *RV*, right ventricle; *LV*, left ventricle; *VSD*, ventricular septal defect; *TV*, tricuspid valve; *PV*, pulmonic valve. Image courtesy of Dr. Fabio Del Piero, Diplomate ACVP, University of Pennsylvania.

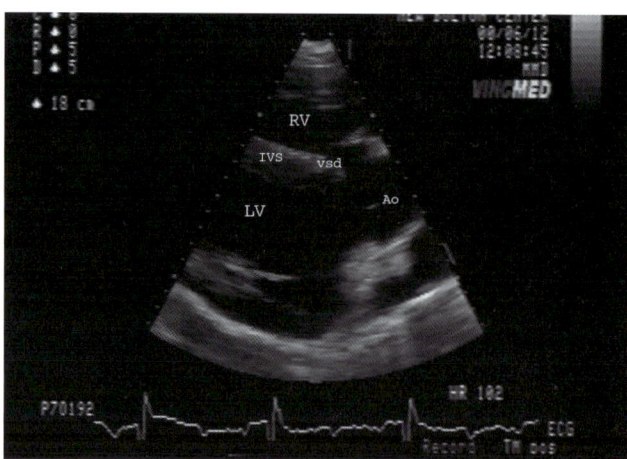

Fig. 13-14 Long-axis view of left ventricular outflow tract of an eight-week-old Tennessee Walker foal with a membranous ventricular septal defect. Taken from the right cardiac window, displayed depth 18 cm. *RV*, right ventricle; *LV*, left ventricle; *IVS*, interventricular septum; *VSD*, ventricular septal defect; *AO*, aorta. Image courtesy of New Bolton Center, University of Pennsylvania School of Veterinary Medicine.

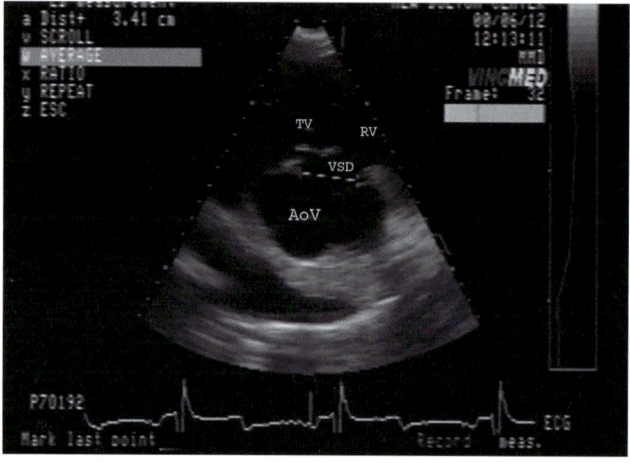

Fig. 13-15 Short-axis view just below level of aortic valve of a membranous ventricular septal defect in an eight-week old Tennessee Walker foal. Dotted lines indicate 2-D measurement. Taken from the right cardiac window, displayed depth 18 cm. *RV*, right ventricle; *TV*, tricuspid valve; *VSD*, ventricular septal defect; *AoV*, aortic valve. Image courtesy of New Bolton Center, University of Pennsylvania School of Veterinary Medicine.

VSDs are most commonly located in the membranous portion of the interventricular septum[1,4,6,29] (Figure 13-13). They may also present in the right ventricular outflow portion of the septum or the muscular septum where they can be more difficult to detect on 2-D images. When in the right ventricular outflow portion (subpulmonic), they are reported to be easier to identify in a short-axis view. Muscular or apical muscular defects are often best seen in an extreme caudal or apical four-chamber long-axis view. In 2-D imaging, septal defects appear as anechoic region or absence of echoes within the otherwise echoic septum. Care should be taken however, not to confuse the normal hypoechoic region of drop out that is seen in the basilar portion of the septum in the four-chamber long-axis view. Defects should be confirmed in two planes (long- and short-axis views), and long- and short-axis measurements should be obtained (Figures 13-14 to 13-16). Due to normal drop out at the edges of a septal defect, overestimation of the size of the defect is more likely than underestimation of size.[6]

Color-flow Doppler applied over the region of the septal defect demonstrates aliased flow colors (blue-green, orange-yellow-red) across the region of the defect and extending into the right ventricle (Figure 13-17). Pulsed-flow Doppler should be applied in the absence of color flow or in addition to color flow. Pulsed-flow Doppler applied from the right side of the septum will reveal an aliased systolic signal towards the transducer, if the typical left-to-right shunt is present. Continuous-wave Doppler of a VSD demonstrates a high-velocity systolic envelope directed toward the right side of the chest in left-to-right shunts. Continuous-wave Doppler should be used to measure the peak velocity of flow through the shunt, which provides important information about the hemodynamics of the shunt and is of prognostic value (Figure 13-18). Peak shunt velocities of greater than 4 m/second through the defect indicate that the VSD is restrictive and of less hemodynamic significance.

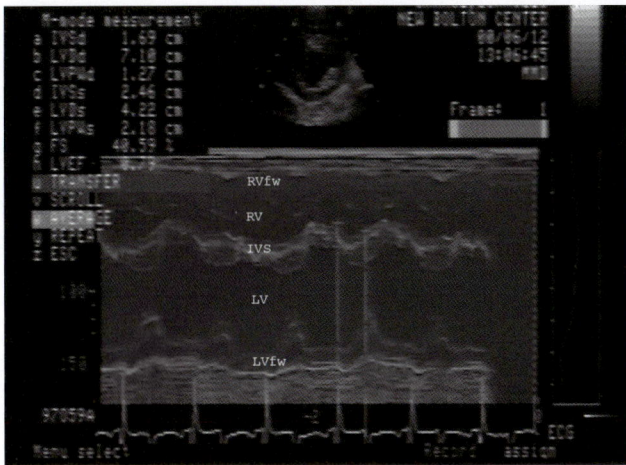

Fig. 13-16 M-mode echocardiogram of left ventricle of an eight-week-old Tennessee Walker foal with a ventricular septal defect. Volume overload pattern present, demonstrated by movement of the interventricular septum toward the right side in diastole. Image courtesy of New Bolton Center, University of Pennsylvania School of Veterinary Medicine.

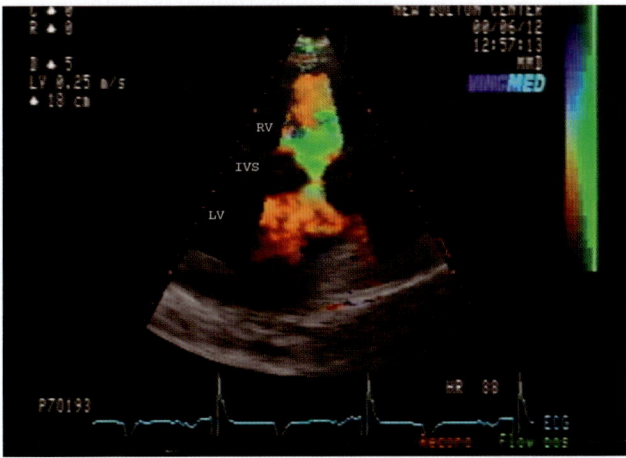

Fig. 13-17 Color-flow Doppler interrogation of a membranous ventricular septal defect in the left ventricular long-axis view. Taken from the right cardiac window, displayed depth 18 cm. *RV,* right ventricle; *IVS,* interventricular septum; *LV,* left ventricle; Green color indicates high-velocity turbulent flow extending from left to right ventricle across ventricular septal defect (left-to right-shunt); red and blue colors represent normal flow. Image courtesy of New Bolton Center, University of Pennsylvania School of Veterinary Medicine.

Rarely, right-to-left or bidirectional shunts are identified. These are typically associated with very large defects, muscular defects, significant right outflow obstruction, or end-stage disease and a worse prognosis. Examination of the defect with contrast echocardiography should reveal a negative contrast jet in the right ventricle in left-to-right shunts, and a positive contrast jet in right-to-left shunts.

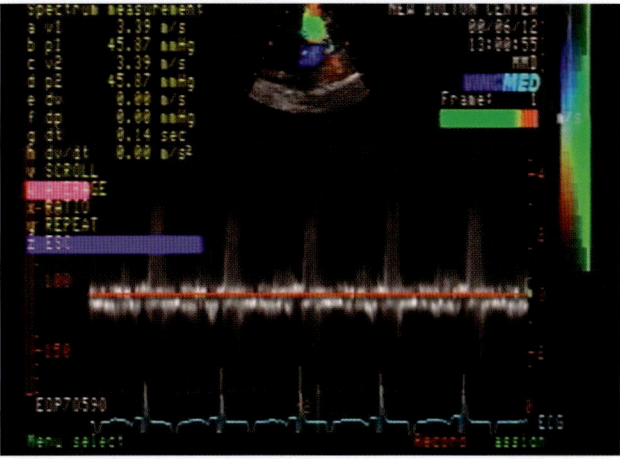

Fig. 13-18 Continuous-wave (CW) Doppler interrogation of right ventricle in the region of ventricular septal defect in an eight-week-old Tennessee Walker foal. Taken from the right cardiac window in left ventricular long-axis view, with cursor placed through region of turbulent flow identified by Color-flow Doppler in Figure 13-17. A high velocity (3.39m/second) shunt is identified traveling toward the transducer from the left to the right side of the heart *(shunt flow appears as echoic peak above the baseline).* Image courtesy of New Bolton Center, University of Pennsylvania School of Veterinary Medicine.

As most other congenital defects of the horse are even rarer, and can be quite complex, in-depth discussion of echocardiographic findings is reserved for a cardiology text, and only basic findings in a few conditions are summarized. A VSD may also present with a hypoplastic pulmonary artery, and a hypoplastic pulmonary artery as an isolated finding is very rare in horses. Atrial septal defects, rare in isolation, appear as a region of drop out visible in two planes in the atrial septum. They can be located in the primum portion near the ventricular septum, the secundum portion in the region of the foramen ovale, or more basilar, in the sinus venosus. They are described as having a characteristic "T" sign, a bright echo imaged perpendicular to the defect.[6] Flow should be documentable across the defect. In tetralogy of Fallot, a perimembranous VSD with a large, overriding aorta should be clearly evident. The pulmonary valve or pulmonary artery is hypoplastic, and the right ventricular free wall is hypertrophied.

Persistent truncus arteriosus occurs when the truncus arteriosus, the precursor of the aorta and pulmonary artery, fails to divide.[4] It appears echocardiographically as a single large vessel overriding a large VSD with no detectable pulmonary artery arising from the right ventricle. It may be seen in a variety of anatomic conformations arising from the aorta. In pseudotruncus, the pulmonary artery is present although atretic, and may be difficult to identify. Identification of the two great vessels arising in parallel, rather than being oriented perpendicular to one another, is abnormal and indicates severe malformation. This can be seen in transposition of the great vessels, and double outlet right ventricle, both of which often have other defects (VSD, ASD, PDA) of necessity for any survival outside the womb.

Tricuspid atresia occurs when the tricuspid valve is poorly formed or imperforate. Echocardiographically the valve appears as a thick band of echoes. The right ventricle is very small, the right atrium is large, and an atrial septal defect and VSD are present. Defects of the endocardial cushion or absence of the atrioventricular canal occurs when there is a large primum atrial septal defect (near the ventricle), a large VSD, and abnormalities of both the tricuspid and mitral valves. The valves may appear cleft.

No treatment options were available for '01 Dear John. She was discharged with instructions to allow her the normal access to turn out as the other foals. She was to be carefully monitored, however, for signs of reduced exercise tolerance, elevated respiratory or heart rate at rest, lethargy, coughing, or nasal discharge. Repeat echocardiographic examination was to be sought should any of these symptoms occur. Echocardiographic re-evaluation in one year was recommended to re-evaluate her cardiac function and ensure that no new valvular regurgitations develop.

TREATMENT

Currently, no published reports exist of surgical repair of a VSD or other congenital cardiac defect in a foal. Foals with small VSDs may not need medical intervention to live a comfortable life. The potential exists to apply some of the current transvascular techniques currently being developed and used in small animals and humans for repair of an appropriate defect in a small foal. An "umbrella" or "clamshell"-type device could potentially be used to seal a single, small VSD that is located far enough from the aortic valve to prevent interference. Coils have been used to stimulate closure of patent ductus arteriosus in large dogs, and could be used in theory in small foals; however success is also dependant upon the anatomic shape of the ductus.

Complete cardiopulmonary bypass to patch a VSD or correct a tetralogy of Fallot is theoretically possible in a small foal but is clearly highly invasive and would require early identification and decision for surgery in a foal small enough and of personal or commercial value to warrant the procedure. This type of procedure would need to be performed in a referral center with a veterinarian experienced in cardiopulmonary bypass surgery in other species. However, the decision to repair a congenital defect entails ethical considerations, and the animal should not be used for breeding purposes.

Medical therapy may help stabilize foals that are decompensating or have concurrent complicating pulmonary disease; however, it should be viewed as a short-term solution. Foals demonstrating clinical and/or echocardiographic evidence of heart failure due to a persistent fetal remnant, congenital abnormality, or acquired disease can be treated medically in order to stabilize them prior to further evaluation or intervention. Furosemide (1 to 2 mg/kg prn SQ, IM, or IV, longer term .5 to 2 mg/kg PO), a loop diuretic, can be used for treatment of pulmonary edema.[36] Digoxin (.011 to .0175 mg/kg PO bid or .0022 mg/kg IV bid maintenance dose) is a cardiac glycoside and positive inotrope that can be used to improve myocardial function.[6,36] Digoxin should not be used in animals that may be dehydrated or have compromised renal function (or the dose should be reduced and serum digoxin levels followed). Serum potassium levels should be obtained, as hypokalemia may potentiate the toxic effects of digoxin.[37] Foals receiving digoxin should have their serum peak (one to two hours after oral administration) and trough (prior to next dose) concentrations monitored until a stable therapeutic level is reached. The therapeutic range of digoxin is 1 to 2 ng/ml.[36,37] Serum concentrations of digoxin, and serum creatinine levels should be periodically re-evaluated while undergoing treatment. Additionally, the foal should be monitored for signs of dehydration or digoxin toxicity, which include anorexia, depression, colic, or cardiac arrhythmias. Anecdotally, foals with congenital defects resulting in volume overload have been stabilized with short-term medical therapy, after which time they have been able to thrive and grow successfully without further medical or surgical intervention.[38]

Identification of an infectious process such as valvular bacterial endocarditis would warrant long-term treatment with an appropriate (based on blood culture) intravenous, bactericidal antibiotic. Serial echocardiographic examinations are recommended to monitor response to treatment. Echocardiographic confirmation of resolution of the lesions (significant decrease in size, increase in echogenicity, and a smoother appearance of the lesion) is necessary prior to discontinuation of antibiotic therapy and should be repeated within one to two weeks after discontinuation of antibiotic therapy to confirm no recrudescence of infection.

In foals with more severe isolated congenital cardiac disease or complex cardiac disease, treatment may transiently prolong life but is not indicated beyond the period required for accurate diagnosis.

In the absence of the development of further significant cardiac disease, '01 Dear John's prognosis for life is good, and she should be able to be ridden at lower levels of athletic work, including pleasure and low-level showing. It is unlikely that she will be able to compete successfully in more rigorous athletic disciplines. She should be re-evaluated prior to breaking to ride, and yearly thereafter to ensure that no new developments have occurred and that she remains safe to ride as a pleasure/low-level show horse. She should not be used for breeding, as her defect may be heritable, and the increased circulatory volume of late gestation may be detrimental to her condition.

OUTCOME

Murmurs due to physiologic flow in the equine neonate typically do not persist beyond several months of age. As the murmurs do not represent a pathologic state, the presence of a physiologic or functional-flow murmur in the neonatal period should not affect a foal's life expectancy or place any restrictions on his intended use or athletic performance. Likewise, transient murmurs due to patent remnants of the fetal circulation that then undergo normal closure do not alter performance or life expectancy.

The prognosis for life and use with an isolated VSD depends upon the size, location, and number of defects and the shunt velocity through the defects, as well as the presence of any concomitant valvular disease. Single membranous defects less than 2.5 cm in either axis with a shunt velocity of greater than 4 m/second are compatible with a normal life expectancy and successful use at most disciplines.[4,6,29] Horses with small VSDs have been reported to race successfully (Standardbreds).[29] Horses with VSDs between 2.5 and 3.5 cm and shunt velocities from 3 to 4 m/second typically do not have normal exercise tolerance, but may be able to be pleasure horses or perform at lower-level disciplines.[1,6,29] Horses with septal defects greater then 3.5 cm or shunt velocities lower than 3 m/second have a shortened life expectancy and are likely to develop congestive heart failure.[6,29] Additionally, using the ratio of the size of the septal defect to the aortic root may be useful in smaller horses, ponies, and potentially foals.[1,7] Septal defects that are less than one third the diameter of the aortic root have been suggested to be restrictive and carry a better prognosis.[1,7]

The presence of prolapse of an aortic cusp and resultant aortic regurgitation may shorten life and performance expectancy. Horses with muscular defects or multiple defects generally have a worse prognosis for performance and life than those with a membranous or perimembranous VSD. Although reported in a very small number of cats, dogs, and people, spontaneous closure of a VSD has not been described in the horse.

Horses with a small patent ductus arteriosus may be able to survive into adulthood, and reports exist of horses being used successfully for light riding. In milder forms of some of the complex congenital diseases (such as tetralogy of Fallot), horses that do not exhibit undue poor growth and are not asked to work at a young age may occasionally go undiagnosed until young adulthood. Overall, however, horses with complex congenital cardiac disease have a grave prognosis.

Patent foramen ovale is rare as an isolated finding and would normally result in left-to-right shunting (in cases of normal right-sided pressures) and eventual development of chamber enlargement. Clinical manifestations would depend upon the size of the defect and the presence of other congenital abnormalities. In complex cardiac disease, the shunting associated with a patent ductus arteriosus and/or patent foramen may be essential for life.

The prognosis for foals with acquired valvular disease varies on an individual basis depending upon the valve affected, severity of regurgitation, and cause. Typically, mitral insufficiency is the least well tolerated. In a report of three foals with acquired mitral valvular regurgitation, one of which was idiopathic and another secondary to bacterial endocarditis, all three developed congestive heart failure and were euthanized.[39] It is likely that even less severely affected foals having valvular disease would result in gradual volume overload and potentially cardiac failure over time. In neonatal foals in which valvular disease is identified, echocardiographic evaluation in several months and periodically thereafter is recommended.

The prognosis for acquired valvular disease due to bacterial endocarditis will again be influenced by the valve affected, severity of lesion, and response to antimicrobial therapy. Provided antibiotic therapy is successful in eliminating infection, the foal is still at risk for the subsequent development of more severe regurgitation due to long-term changes in valvular anatomy and stiffness.

REFERENCES

1. Marr CM: Cardiac murmurs: Congenital heart disease. In Marr CM, ed: *Cardiology of the horse*, London, 1999, WB Saunders.
2. Livesey LC, Marr CM, Freeman S et al: Auscultatory and two dimensional spectral, M mode and colour Doppler echocardiographic findings in pony foals from birth to seven weeks of age, *J Vet Intern Med* 12:255, 1998.
3. Yamoto K, Yasuda J, Too K: Arrhythmias in newborn foals, *Equine Vet J* 23:169, 1992.

4. Patteson MW: *Equine cardiology,* ed 1, Oxford, 1996, Blackwell Science.

5. Wilson WD, Lofstedt J: Alterations in respiratory function. In Smith BP, ed: *Large animal internal medicine,* ed 3, St Louis, 2002, Mosby.

6. Reef VB: Cardiovascular ultrasonography. In Reef VB: *Equine diagnostic ultrasound,* Philadelphia, 1998, WB Saunders.

7. Bonagura JD, Blissitt KJ: Echocardiography, *Equine Vet J* Suppl 19:5, 1995.

8. Machida N, Yasuda J, Too K et al: A morphological study on the obliteration processes of the ductus arteriosus in the horse, *Equine Vet J* 20:249, 1988.

9. Macdonald AA, Fowden AL, Silver M et al: The foramen ovale of the foetal and neonatal foal, *Equine Vet J* 20:255, 1988.

10. Reef VB: Echocardiographic findings in horses with congenital cardiac disease, *Compendium on Continuing Education* 13:09, 1991.

11. Rooney JR, Franks WG: Congenital cardiac anomalies in the horse, *Vet Path* 1:454, 1964.

12. Crowe MW, Swerczek TW: Equine congenital defects, *Am J Vet Res* 46:353, 1984.

13. Reef VB: Cardiovascular disease in the equine neonate, *Vet Clin North Am* 1:117, 1985.

14. Gehlen H, Bubeck K, Stadler P: Valvular pulmonic stenosis with normal aortic root and intact ventricular and atrial septa in an Arabian horse, *Equine Vet Educ* 13:286, 2001.

15. Critchley KL: An interventricular septal defect, pulmonary stenosis and a bicuspid pulmonary valve in a Welsh pony foal, *Equine Vet J* 8:176, 1976.

16. Vitums A, Bayly WM: Pulmonary atresia with dextroposition of the aorta and ventricular septal defect in three Arabian foals, *Vet Pathol* 19:160, 1982.

17. Reef VB, Mann PC, Orsini P: Echocardiographic detection of tricuspid atresia in two foals, *J Am Vet Med Assoc* 191:225, 1987.

18. Wilson RB, Haffner JC: Right atrioventricular atresia and ventricular septal defect in a foal, *Cornell Vet* 77:187, 1987.

19. Stephen JO, Abbott J, Middleton DM et al: Persistent truncus arteriosus in a Bakshir Curly foal, *Equine Vet Educ* 12:251, 2000.

20. McClure JJ, Gaber CE, Watters JW et al: Complete transposition of the great arteries with ventricular septal defect and pulmonary stenosis in a Thoroughbred foal, *Equine Vet J* 377, 1983.

21. Vitmus A, Grant BD, Stone EC et al: Transposition of the aorta and atresia of the pulmonary trunk in a horse, *Cornell Vet* 63:41, 1973.

22. Vitmus A: Origin of the aorta and pulmonary trunk from the right ventricle in a horse. *Path Vet* 7:482, 1970.

23. Chaffin MK, Miller MW, Morris EL: Double outlet right ventricle and other associated congenital cardiac anomalies in an American Miniature Horse foal, *Equine Vet J* 24: 402, 1992.

24. Peppas GP, Canfield PJ, Hartley WJ et al: Multiple congenital cardiac anomalies and idiopathic thoracic aortitis in a horse, *Vet Rec* 14, 1996.

25. Bayly WM, Reed SM, Leathers CW et al: Multiple congenital heart anomalies in five Arabian foals, *J Am Vet Med Assoc* 181:684, 1982.

26. Seco Diaz O, Desrochers A, Hoffman V et al: Total anomalous pulmonary venous connection in a foal, *Vet Radiol Ultrasound* 46:83, 2005.

27. Karlstam E, Ho SY, Agren et al: Anomalous aortic origin of the left coronary artery in a horse, *Equine Vet J* 31:350, 1999.

28. Reef VB, McGuirk SM: Diseases of the cardiovascular system. In Smith BP, ed: *Large animal internal medicine,* ed 3, St Louis, 2002, Mosby.

29. Reef VB: Evaluation of ventricular septal defects in horses using two dimensional and Doppler echocardiography, *Equine Vet J* Suppl 19:86, 1995.

30. Del Piero F: Personal communication, 2004.

31. McGuirk SM, Shaftoe S, Lunn DP: Diseases of the cardiovascular system. In Smith BP, ed: *Large animal internal medicine,* St Louis, 1990, Mosby.

32. Bonagura JG, Darke, PG: Congenital heart disease. In Ettinger SJ, Feldman EC eds: *Textbook of veterinary internal medicine,* ed 4, Philadelphia, 1995, WB Saunders.

33. Pipers FS, Reef VB, Wilson J: Echocardiographic detection of ventricular septal defects in large animals, *J Am Vet Med Assoc* 187:810, 1985.

34. Boon JA: *Manual of veterinary echocardiography,* Baltimore, 1998, Williams and Wilkins.

35. Stewart JH, Rose JA, Barko AM: Echocardiography in foals from birth to three months old, *Equine Vet J* 16:332, 1984.

36. Plumb DC: *Veterinary drug handbook,* ed 4, Ames, 2002, Iowa State Press.

37. Reef VB: Arrhythmias. In Marr CM, ed: *Cardiology of the horse,* London, 1999, WB Saunders.

38. Leblanc M: personal communication at 2004 Havenmeyer Foundation Equine Neonatology Conference, Talloires, France.

39. Reef VB: Mitral valvular insufficiency associated with ruptured chordae tendinae in three foals, *J Am Vet Med Assoc* 191:329, 1987.

40. Lombard CW, Scarratt WK, Buergelt CD: Ventricular septal defects in the horse, *J Am Vet Med Assoc* 183:562, 1983.

41. Glazier DB, Farelly BT, O'Connor J: Ventricular septal defect in a seven year old gelding, *J Am Vet Med Assoc* 161:49, 1975.

42. Kvart C, Carlsten J, Jeffcott B et al: Diagnostic value of contrast echocardiography in the horse, *Equine Vet J* 17:357, 1985.

43. Bonagura JD, Pipers FS: Diagnosis of cardiac lesions by contrast echocardiography, *J Am Vet Med Assoc* 182:396, 1983.

44. Blissett KJ, Bonagura, JD: Colour flow Doppler echocardiography in normal horses, *Equine Vet J* Suppl 19:47, 1995.

45. Critchley KL: The importance of blood gas measurement in the diagnosis of an interventricular septal defect in a horse: A case report, *Equine Vet J* 8:128, 1976.

46. Cottrill CM, O'Connor WN, Cudd T et al: Persistence of foetal circulatory pathways in a newborn foal, *Equine Vet J* 19:252, 1987.

47. Machida N, Yasuda K, Too K: A morphometric study of foetal and newborn cardiac growth in the horse, *Equine Vet J* 20: 261, 1988.

48. Lombard CW, Evans M, Martin L et al: Blood pressure, electrocardiogram and echocardiogram measurements in the growing pony foal, *Equine Vet J* 16: 342, 1984.

14 Ophthalmologic Disorders

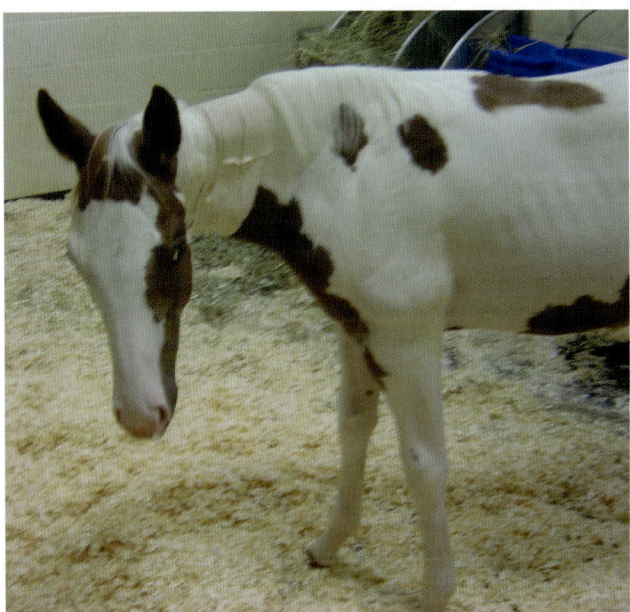

Fig. 14-1 '04 FortyLashes, a five-day-old Paint foal colt, presented with ocular discomfort.

'04 FortyLashes, a five-day-old Paint foal colt, presented for evaluation of ocular discomfort of the right eye (OD), evident as tearing and squinting that developed two days after birth (Figure 14-1). The referring veterinarian had made a diagnosis of lower-lid entropion OD. Upon closer examination of the eyes, a lens opacity in the left eye (OS) was also evident. The otherwise healthy foal was referred to the hospital for cataract evaluation and further management of the eyelid condition after treatment with an ophthalmic broad-spectrum antibiotic three times daily had failed to improve the clinical signs of OD.

Ocular disorders in neonates have been reported to represent 5% of all equine ocular disorders and may be categorized as congenital, inherited, or acquired.[1-4] While congenital disorders (present at the time of birth) may be genetically based, they also may develop secondary to various insults in utero, including infection, nutritional deficiencies or excesses, drugs, toxins, trauma, ionizing radiation, and other unknown or idiopathic factors. Ocular examination of the equine neonate should be performed in the immediate newborn period and at any follow-up visits as part of the routine physical exam. This approach ensures early detection and, if treatable, proper management of ocular conditions that may otherwise result in life-long visual impairment. It will also help to optimize breeding programs since patients affected by inherited ocular disease may be excluded from breeding, therefore limiting economic losses.

The ophthalmic evaluation of the newborn foal is similar to that for an adult horse with the exception of systemic and local anesthesia, which usually is not necessary in these young patients. It is recommended to keep the foal and mare close together to allow for speedy examination of the neonate. Technical support is required to keep the foal's head steady for the ocular exam and to restrain the mare, if necessary. The ocular exam should take place in bright and dim light conditions.

THE NORMAL EQUINE NEONATAL EYE

Foals are born with their eyes open. The pupils are initially round to oval in shape and become more horizontal at three to five days postpartum with a lighter-colored iris than adult horses. A reliable menace response is absent until two weeks of age and can therefore not be used as assessment of vision in the immediate postnatal period.[5] While the pupillary light reflex (PLR) is present at the time of birth, it may be sluggish in a highly excited foal due to a high sympathetic tone. Therefore, optimal testing for PLRs should take place in a quiet and relaxed environment; a bright focal illuminator (e.g. Finoff illuminator) should be used to evaluate for PLRs in bright and dim light.

Neonatal foals also show a lower tear secretion than adults, which may be accompanied by decreased corneal sensitivity and lagophthalmos in sick foals.[6-8] A mild ventro-medial deviation of the eyes can be seen in foals less than one month old. Iris color in most foals is brown, but variations known as "Heterochromia iridis" may be seen in color-dilute foals or those carrying color-dilute genes (e.g., Palomino, Appaloosa, Paint).[4] Heterochromia iridis refers to a lack of iridal stromal pigment and clinically manifests itself as a combination of white and blue iris color with brown corpora nigra ("wall eye") or white iris with brown corpora nigra ("china eye").

Lens suture lines ("Y-sutures") are commonly observed in newborn foals and are, unlike cataracts, insignificant without impact on vision.[1,2] Persistent hyaloid artery remnants are another frequent finding in equine neonates, especially in premature foals.[4,9] They result from a failure of part or all of the hyaloid artery to regress and can be appreciated as a fine gray-white linear opacity (in some cases containing blood) spanning from the optic disc to the posterior lens capsule. Regression of these remnants usually occurs at three to four months of age. Attachment of these remnants to the posterior lens capsule may result in focal posterior capsular and subcapsular cataracts that are nonprogressive and often not associated with visual impairment.

Normal variations in the appearance of the retina may occur and may be misinterpreted as congenital fundic lesions that are uncommonly found in equine neonates. The tapetum in foals resembles that of adult horses with tapetal coloration related to coat color. Color combinations of green-blue or green-yellow are common, with small dots uniformly distributed throughout the tapetum, representing the end-on views of choroidal capillaries or "Stars of Winslow." Color-dilute foals have a yellow tapetum with red Stars of Winslow. The non-tapetum is usually of a dark-brown color. A "red" fundus is found in albinotic or subalbinotic horses due to an absence of pigmentation in the retinal pigment epithelium that results in exposure of choroidal vasculature against a pale scleral background. The pink-orange optic nerve in foals is rather round compared to the elliptically shaped disc seen in adult horses and is located in the inferotemporal region of the non-tapetum.

On presentation, an ocular examination was performed on '04 FortyLashes unsedated. The findings were as follows: severe lacrimation, blepharospasm with moderate to severe lower-lid entropion OD, absent menace response, but positive direct and consensual PLRs in both eyes (OU). A fluorescein stain uptake was absent in both eyes indicating an intact cornea. A 10% incipient central axial cataract OS was seen. Application of topical proparacaine OD resulted in mild temporary improvement of the entropion and increased comfort level of the patient. The diagnosis was moderate congenital lower-lid entropion OD resulting in secondary corneal irritation and congenital incipient cataract OS.

CONGENITAL OPHTHALMIC ABNORMALITIES

Several congenital ophthalmic abnormalities have been noted in the newborn foal. They can involve all parts of the eye, including the eyelids, the lens, the globe, and the retina.

Inversion of the upper and especially lower eyelids is the most common congenital lid abnormality in foals and may occur on a primary basis or secondary to microphthalmia or lid trauma. Sick or premature foals are predisposed to develop entropion due to dehydration, a negative energy balance, or malnutrition, which all lead to mild enophthalmos and secondary inversion of the lids due to lack of support by the globe.[1,10,11]

Clinical signs of entropion include blepharospasm, increased lacrimation, conjunctivitis, and/or corneal ulceration. The pain from continuous corneal irritation results in a dominant spastic component of the lid inversion which, in a vicious cycle, exacerbates the underlying anatomic entropion. Application of a topical anesthetic (Proparacaine®) allows short-term pain relief and estimation of the spastic component of the entropion. Corneal surface anesthesia occurs after 10 to 30 seconds and may last for 15 to 20 minutes. Because of their short duration and epithelial toxicity, frequent application of topical anesthetics for long-term pain relief is not only impractical but can also result in severe corneal damage.

Reports of delayed or incomplete lid opening in foals have been rare.[12] Manual opening by applying minimal digital pressure and traction may be attempted, and if unsuccessful, surgical opening of the palpebral fissure should be performed under heavy sedation or general anesthesia.[13] The eyelids are prepared using a diluted (1:10 to 1:50) povidone-iodine solution. After at least three scrubs, the area is rinsed with 0.9% sterile saline (alcohol should be avoided since it can severely damage corneal and conjunctival epithelia). The line of separation between the lids is cut using a scissor blade in sliding motion. Great care must

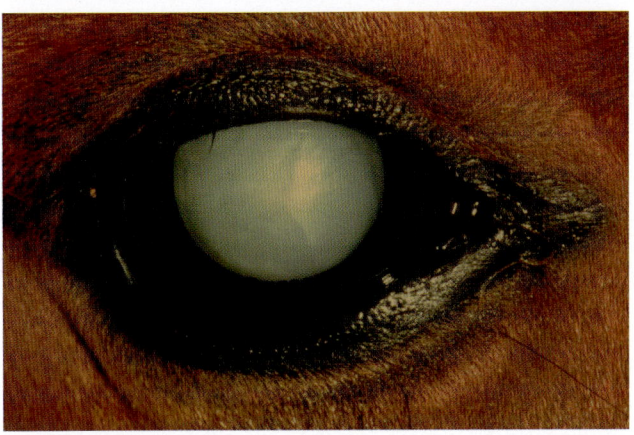

Fig. 14-2 Mature cataract in a foal.

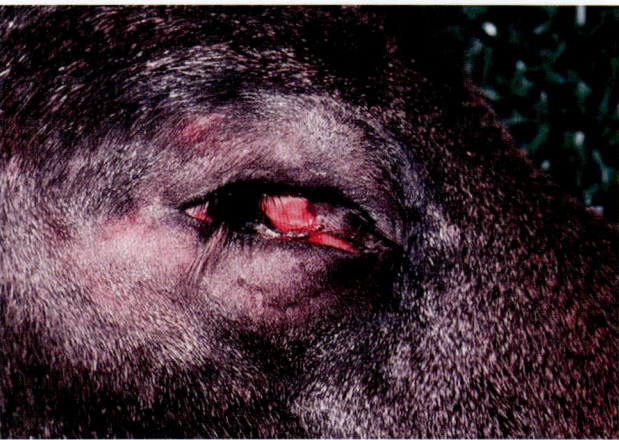

Fig. 14-3 Rudimentary ocular tissue can be seen in this foal with severe microphthalmia.

be taken to avoid injury to the cornea. Postoperative treatment includes application of a topical broad-spectrum antibiotic four to six times daily for 10 days, or longer if necessary.

Congenital cataracts are commonly found in foals and have been reported to represent up to 35.3% of all congenital ocular lesions.[1,3,4] Etiologic factors include heritability, uveitis, trauma, and nutritional deficiencies.[1,11] Since genetic factors may contribute to congenital cataracts, affected patients should not be used for breeding.

Congenital cataracts may occur unilaterally or bilaterally and may range from smaller cataracts associated with persistent hyaloid artery remnants to nuclear to mature cataracts (Figure 14-2). Inherited cataracts have been reported in Belgians (associated with aniridia), Quarter Horses, Thoroughbreds, and Morgans.[4,10,14,15] Congenital cataracts in Morgans appear as finely reticulated spherical nuclear translucencies that occur in a symmetrical fashion in both eyes without impairing sight. Cataracts and lens luxations are also frequent findings in Rocky Mountain Horses affected by anterior segment dysgenesis.[16]

Congenital lens subluxation or lens luxation can also be seen in the neonatal foal. It can occur as a single lesion or as part of multiple ocular anomalies and occurs secondary to a defect in lens zonule formation.[17] Cardinal signs of lens dislocation include vitreous prolapse (white vitreal strands prolapsing through pupil), presence of an aphacic crescent (edge of displaced lens and ciliary zonules remnants appreciated through pupil), phacodonesis (lens tremor seen with globe movement), iridonesis (tremulousness of iris), and asymmetry in anterior chamber depth.

Microphthalmos is a congenitally small globe and can be found sporadically in all breeds of horses, especially Thoroughbreds.[1,18] It can occur unilaterally or bilaterally with different degrees of severity. *Pure microphthalmos* describes a small but functional globe. *Complicated microphthalmos* refers to a small globe

affected by other ocular defects, including cataracts and retinal dysplasia. Foals with only subtle microphthalmia usually suffer from marked visual impairment despite an only small reduction in globe size. The diagnosis can be facilitated by comparing the ocular dimensions of the affected eye with the contralateral eye (in case of unilateral disease) or with the eyes of healthy, age-matched control foals. Caliper measurements of the dorsoventral and horizontal corneal diameters are useful. Globe diameter can be determined via ocular ultrasound (B-scan). The degree of third-eyelid protrusion is directly related to the degree of microphthalmos.

In severely affected patients, no lid opening may be found and anophthalmos may be suspected. However, closer inspection of the eyes will show rudimentary ocular tissue (Figure 14-3). In these patients, enucleation is strongly recommended to prevent future ocular complications such as chronic conjunctivitis and corneal irritation from entropion. The enucleation procedure should include placement of an orbital implant (especially in young patients) to prevent malformation of the growing skull, since globe development dictates development of the bony orbit. If a foal is suffering from complete blindness due to bilateral severe microphthalmia, euthanasia should be considered for humane reasons.

Multiple ocular anomalies have been seen in the neonatal foal. These congenital abnormalities may include corneal lesions, microcornea, megalocornea, dermoids, persistent papillary membranes, aniridia, iridal hypoplasia, anterior segment dysgenesis, enlarged corpora nigra, iridal colobomata, lens luxation, cataracts, retinal dysplasia, and retinal detachment.[1,3,4,15,16,19,20] Any breed may be affected with lesions occurring in either one or both eyes. Affected eyes are often blind in cases of multiple anomalies and should be enucleated in cases of unilateral disease.

Congenital buphthalmia (globe enlargement) is often associated with multiple ocular abnormalities and chronic glaucoma.[21,22] Treatment consists of enucleation for pain relief and prevention of complications such as exposure keratitis from subsequent inability to fully close the eyelids over the enlarged globe.

Congenital strabismus (hyperopia) and dorsomedial strabismus, a deviation of the eye from its physiological position, have been reported in Appaloosa foals and may be associated in this breed with congenital stationary night blindness.[23,24] This strabismus becomes more evident when the foal tries to focus on an object or when it is placed in an unfamiliar environment. Corrective surgery consisting of ocular rectus muscle transposition may result in improvement of clinical vision and behavior. While congenital strabismus is rarely found in foals, it has been reported in mules with an incidence of 1 in 200.[25]

Glaucoma refers to an increase in intraocular pressure that is no longer compatible with normal physiologic function of the eye. Congenital glaucoma in foals of various breeds has been described and was attributable in these patients to abnormal differentiation of the iridocorneal angle (goniodysgenesis).[4,22,26,27] While glaucoma in adult equine patients is often secondary to underlying uveitis, it has not been reported in equine neonates. Accurate diagnosis of glaucoma requires applanation tonometry using a tonopen. The mean intraocular pressure in horses has been reported to range from 16.5 to 32.5 mm Hg with a mean of 24.5 mm Hg. A thorough ocular examination should rule out presence of other ocular abnormalities before medical or surgical treatment recommendations are made. Clinical signs depend upon the stage of glaucoma and include moderate buphthalmia, conjunctival injection unresponsive mydriasis, iris atrophy, corneal edema and/or striae, lens luxation or subluxation, retinal atrophy, optic nerve cupping, and blindness.

Treatment goals for glaucoma are to preserve sight for as long as possible and to minimize pain. Medical management includes decreasing aqueous humor production via topical β-blockers (i.e. Timoptic, twice daily) or topical carbonicanhydrase inhibitors such as dorzolamide (Trusopt q 8 hours); a combined product is also commercially available (Cosopt, twice daily). While some ophthalmologists advocate use of a topical miotic such as 1% pilocarpine solution twice or three times daily or 4% pilocarpine gel once daily to increase aqueous humor outflow, others recommend use of topical 1% atropine once or twice daily in selected cases. Topical ocular miotics such as pilocarpine may lead to painful spasms of the iris and ciliary body musculature as well as breakdown of the blood aqueous barrier and should therefore not be administered in horses affected by uveitis. Systemic nonsteroidal anti-inflammatory drugs (NSAIDS) also have their place in the treatment of glaucoma patients to address the mild uveitic component often seen with glaucoma and for pain relief.

The owner should be informed that medical management of equine glaucoma is often ineffective in controlling intraocular pressure, and early surgery is usually recommended to preserve sight. Surgery may include laser cyclophotocoagulation of the iris ciliary body or high-flow gonioimplants to increase aqueous outflow in these foals. An irreversibly blind, medically unresponsive, glaucomatous eye should be enucleated for pain relief.

Congenital retinal diseases include retinal dysplasia, chorioretinitis, optic nerve hypoplasia, optic nerve colobomas, and night blindness. Retinal dysplasia is anomalous retinal differentiation with proliferation of one or more of its constituent elements. Histologic characteristics are folding of the sensory retina and formation of retinal "rosettes" that are composed of one or more layers of neuroblasts surrounding a central lumen. The condition is congenital and suspected secondary to infectious, traumatic, and toxic insults occurring during fetal development.[1,4,28] It is usually bilateral and nonprogressive, and vision depends upon severity of the lesion and presence of other ocular anomalies. Ophthalmoscopic findings include single or multiple focal dots or linear streaks as well as geographic lesions.

Fetal exposure during late gestation to various infectious agents (especially in mares with active respiratory disease) may result in congenital chorioretinitis.[29] Clinically, gray or grayish-white indistinct circular lesion in the non-tapetal fundus indicate active chorioretinitis. Healed lesions appear as chorioretinal scars or "bullet-hole" lesions in the non-tapetum. They are characterized as sharply demarcated circular depigmented lesion with a darkly pigmented center. Unless the scars are numerous (>20) or the horse appears to have visual difficulties, they are considered insignificant.[10]

Optic nerve hypoplasia is a congenital condition referring to a smaller than normal optic disc due to a failure of retinal ganglion cells to develop. Fundic examination shows a pale, small optic disc and either attenuated or completely absent retinal vasculature. One or both eyes may be affected, and other ocular abnormalities may be present.[10] Affected patients show abnormal PLRs but may still have some vision, depending upon the severity of the condition.

Optic nerve colobomas are congenital malformations of the optic nerve head and peripapillary area. They appear as excavations of the optic disc, and their size is directly related to the severity of visual impairment.[30]

Equine night blindness (nyctalopia) is a nonprogressive congenital condition that has been described in

Appaloosas, Quarter horses, Thoroughbreds, Paso Finos, and Standardbreds.[10,24] In Appaloosas, the condition is thought to be inherited as a recessive or sex-linked recessive trait with the defect on the X-chromosome. A defect in neural transmission between the photoreceptor layers and bipolar cells has been proposed as pathogenesis. The degree of visual impairment differs considerably among affected patients. Mildly affected patients may only show clinical signs (i.e. behavioral uneasiness, more injury-prone) at reduced light levels or at night. With more severe disease, patients become increasingly more apprehensive during daylight hours and may react unpredictably in a darkened environment. Affected horses seek light and may try to move closer to a light source such as a window or hallway. Unusual head carriage or "star-gazing" in an attempt to focus on objects in their environment as well as bilateral dorso-medial strabismus in more severely affected patients may also be noticed. A maze test in dim and bright light conditions can be helpful in establishing the diagnosis. Ophthalmoscopic findings are usually normal. While history, behavior, and clinical exam findings may be suggestive of nyctalopia, the final diagnosis requires electroretinography (ERG). The ERG of nyctalopic horses is characteristically "negative" or a-wave dominated with simple negative potentials without a normal scotopic b-wave.[31]

Congenital abnormalities of the nasolacrimal duct system mainly involve atresia of the nasal puncta, and less commonly atresia of the eyelid puncta or naso-lacrimal duct agenesis.[1,4] Clinical signs are often not seen until the foal is a couple months old and initially consist of unilateral or bilateral ocular discharge accompanied by conjunctivitis. Chronicity of the condition often leads to dacryocystitis with copious mucopurulent ocular discharge and facial dermatitis from tear drainage. The diagnosis usually is confirmed by the fluorescein dye test. For this test, fluorescein dye is applied to the eye and expected to appear in the ipsilateral nostril within five minutes. If the dye is absent, the distal puncta should be closely examined for their presence. They should be located in the ventral meatus of the nasal cavity 5 to 8 cm caudal to the external nares. If present, the nasolacrimal duct should be flushed to establish patency of the duct, which may be occluded. If absent, a stiff polyethylene tubing is passed through the upper or lower-lid punctum into the proximal lacrimal duct and flushed with saline.

In foals, heavy sedation or general anesthesia is indicated for this procedure. A bulging of the nasal mucosa overlying the imperforate nasal puncta may be seen, or the catheter tip may be gently palpated through the mucosa indicating the distal end of the nasolacrimal duct. A mucosal incision is made over the expected location of the distal punctum, and the tubing is pulled through this newly created distal opening. The tubing may be sutured to the facial skin and should be left in place for at least three weeks to allow for epithelialization of the new duct and puncta. Topical antibiotic solution is applied to the eye four times daily until removal of the tubing. Systemic flunixine megulamine is recommended for five days to minimize any possible soft-tissue swelling and discomfort associated with this procedure; systemic broad-spectrum antibiotics are indicated in cases of dacryocystitis.

Contrast radiography (dacryocystorhinography) may be used to localize the site of obstruction. The nasolacrimal duct is cannulated, and 2 to 5 ml of radiopaque contrast material (ethiodized poppy seed oil or propyliodone oil) is injected. Subsequent lateral and dorsoventral or oblique radiographic views are taken. Surgery to treat nasolacrimal duct atresia usually involves surgical creation of a fistula for tear drainage directly into the nose—conjunctivorhinostomy with drainage into the caudal nasal cavity or conjunctival-maxillary sinusotomy with drainage into the maxillary sinus.[22]

'04 FortyLashes was hospitalized, and an eyelid-tacking procedure for temporary eversion of the lower-right eyelid was performed under heavy sedation. Postoperative treatment included application of a one-inch strip of a topical ophthalmic broad-spectrum antibiotic ointment four times daily in the right eye for 10 days and intravenous flunixine meglumine (0.5 mg/kg) twice daily for two days.

'04 FortyLashes was discharged two days after the procedure and rechecked by the referring veterinarian two days later. The referring veterinarian reported excellent improvement in comfort level. The sutures were removed 12 days after the procedure without recurrence of entropion.

A recheck appointment in two months was scheduled to monitor for progression of the cataract OS. Cataract surgery was recommended in case progression of the cataract was noticed.

TREATMENT FOR ENTROPION

While mild cases of entropion may respond to contact lens placement and frequent manual eversion of the affected lid, most patients require "eyelid tacking" with temporary sutures to maintain the eyelid margins in a more normal position for 10 to 20 days. Under heavy sedation and after multiple applications of a local anesthetic (i.e. Proparacaine®), three "soft" 4.0 nonabsorbable (silk or nylon) single vertical mattress sutures are placed in the affected eyelid (Figure 14-4). Correct suture placement is imperative with the first

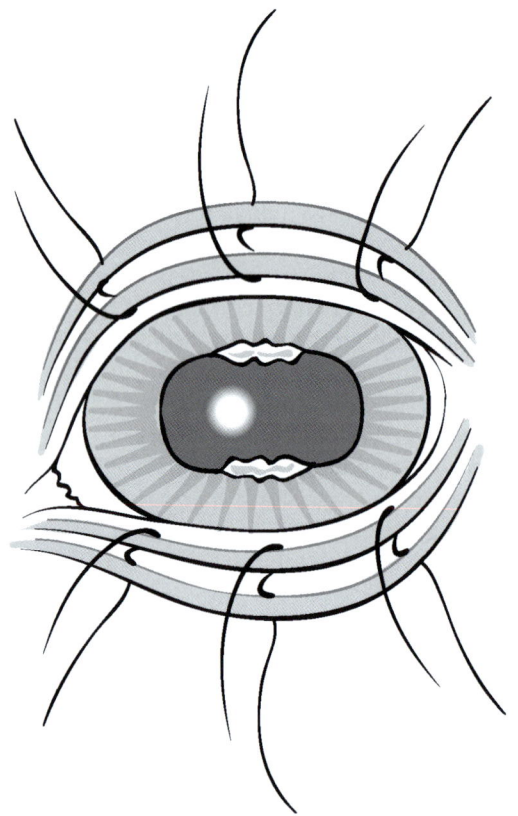

Fig. 14-4 Treatment for temporary correction of entropion involves the placement of vertical mattress sutures in the affected lid. This may be either the lower or upper lid.

bite entering the lid tissue partial thickness 2 to 3 mm from the lid margin, and the second bite entering about 1 cm away from the lid; both bites are approximately 5 mm long. The suture close to the cornea is cut short, whereas the other end is left long for easier removal later on. In most patients, this procedure will help avoid surgical correction later in life by buying the patient enough time until normal growth has led to more developed retrobulbar tissue. Additional medical treatment includes a topical broad-spectrum antibiotic ointment four times daily, and if corneal damage is present, topical 1% atropine ophthalmic ointment or drops once to twice daily to maintain cycloplegia. In case of contact lens placement, topical solution rather than ointment should be used.

Stainless-steel skin staples or blood vessel clips should not be utilized for this procedure since inappropriate placement can lead to painful abscessation of eyelid tissue, and dislodged staples or clips carry a high risk of causing severe corneal injuries. Subcutaneous injections of saline, lidocaine, or procaine peni-

cillin may be complicated by granuloma and abscess formation and should therefore be discouraged.

Permanent entropion surgery should be reserved for older foals with unresponsive entropion.[33] These patients should be referred for surgery to a specialist since the delicate equine eyelid tissue is at a high risk to respond with hematoma formation and secondary cicatrical entropion or ectropion when inadequately handled.

On re-evaluation of '04 FortyLashes at three months of age, the cataract in the left eye had grown significantly and was now involving about 40% of the lens. The foal appeared to have some visual impairment on that side. The right eye did not show any signs of cataract development. Ocular ultrasound and an electroretinogram were performed on OS and found to be normal besides the lenticular opacity. Cataract surgery for OS was recommended and performed. Recovery was uneventful.

TREATMENT FOR CATARACTS

Cataract surgery should be recommended if the foal shows signs of visual impairment from the cataract.[10,34-37] Preoperative workup should include ocular ultrasound and ERG to evaluate integrity of intraocular structures and retinal function. Foals should be screened for subclinical infections since systemic illness may predispose these patients to postoperative endophthalmitis, which may result in loss of the eye. Active uveitis should be treated preoperatively until resolution of clinical signs to optimize the result of surgery. Owner compliance as well as a friendly personality in the patient itself is crucial for the final success of surgery, which is dependent upon postoperative medical care.

The success rate of cataract surgery is estimated at 80%. Foals under six months of age seem to have the highest success rate. This may be attributable to the only mild postoperative uveitis they experience. Early return of sight in these young patients has been shown to be crucial for proper development of the central visual pathways. Phacoemulsification of the lens via ultrasonic fragmentation of the lens and subsequent aspiration of the emulsified lens has been proven to be the most useful technique in the horse. Artificial intraocular lenses for equine patients are currently unavailable. While aphacic foals should be severely farsighted, they seem to have functionally normal vision after surgery.

Case 14-2   Foal with Corneal Ulceration   Isabel Jurk

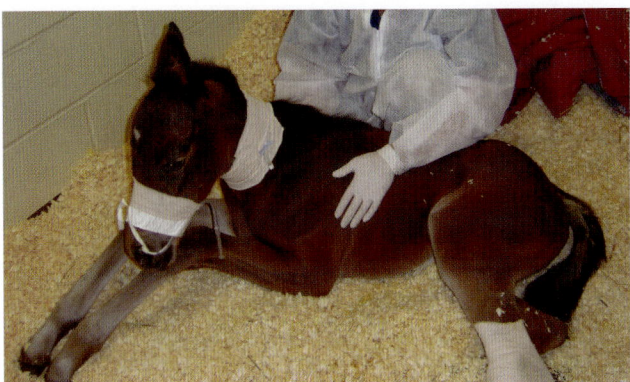

Fig. 14-5 '05 Misty presented with signs of mild peripartum asphyxia. Recumbent foals are at high risk for the development of corneal ulcers.

'05 Misty, a six-hour-old Thoroughbred colt, was hospitalized for intensive care after a complicated birth (Figure 14-5). Delivery was delayed due to malpositioning of one of his forelimbs. On initial physical examination, '05 Misty was recumbent and mildly depressed. He was tube fed 1 liter of good colostrum and placed on broad-spectrum antibiotics and intravenous fluid support. His bloodwork was within normal limits. The working diagnosis for his overall condition was mild peripartum asphyxia and hypoxic encephalopathy (see Chapter 10).

'05 Misty's initial ocular evaluation revealed conjunctival and retinal hemorrhages in both eyes (OU). Because of his recumbency, both eyes were prophylactically stained on a daily basis to rule out secondary corneal ulceration. Two days after initial presentation, the foal was standing and nursing from his dam, but a superficial corneal stain uptake was evident in his left eye (OS). Clinical ophthalmic exam findings at that time included mild conjunctival hemorrhages OU; mild photophobia and lacrimation OS; absent menace response with sluggish direct PLRs OU; mild central corneal edema in palpebral fissure with superficial, elliptically shaped area of fluorescein stain uptake; mild miosis with only mild 1+ aqueous flare; and focal areas of retinal hemorrhages OU (Figure 14-6).

Ophthalmic Diagnosis: Superficial corneal ulcer OS with mild secondary uveitis. Conjunctival and retinal hemorrhages OU.

PATHOGENESIS

Conjunctival hemorrhages can occur secondary to blunt trauma and chest compression during foaling

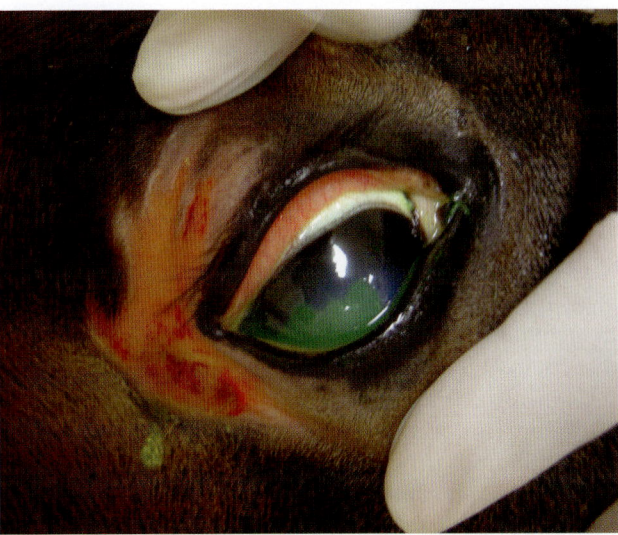

Fig. 14-6 A superficial corneal ulcer takes up fluorescein stain.

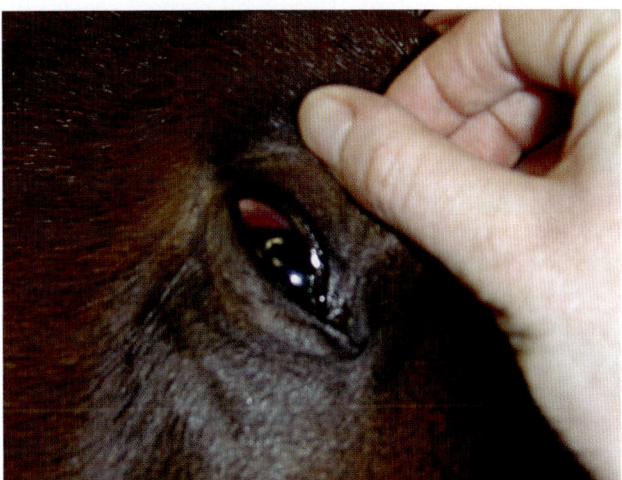

Fig. 14-7 Conjunctival hemorrhages are often seen in foals that have experienced dystocia.

(Figure 14-7).[38] Usually located dorsally or dorsonasally and extending into the limbus, they resolve within 10 days without requiring treatment. They do not cause any short-term or long-term effect on vision. Differentials include subconjunctival or scleral petechiation and hemorrhage seen with coagulation disorders or associated with neonatal maladjustment syndrome in newborn foals.

Retinal hemorrhages often present an incidental finding in equine neonates. A recent survey of neonatal Thoroughbred foals found retinal hemorrhages in 27 of 167 (16%) newborn foals; four eyes were additionally affected by papilledema.[39] The hemorrhages were typically located in the tapetal fundus and ranged from small punctuate-type lesions to splashlike hemorrhages. Often both eyes were affected. A direct correlation between the incidence of retinal hemorrhages and foal size/dystocias has been suggested. A larger than average foal may suffer from increased thoracic pressure and elevated intracranial pressure during parturition. This may explain why larger male foals are predominantly affected compared to the significantly lower incidence in premature neonates. Also, asphyxic episodes during foaling as well as individual variations in blood supply and vascular fragility may play a role in the pathogenesis of retinal hemorrhages. Retinal hemorrhages in foals may also be seen with trauma, chorioretinitis, retinal detachment, clotting disorders, neoplasia, and other disorders.[10]

Corneal ulceration in neonatal foals is not uncommon and can occur due to various factors, including lagophthalmos, low tear production, struggling, lying in a bedded stall, and entropion. Sick foals are at high risk of developing corneal lesions, which in part may be due to a significantly lower corneal sensitivity compared to healthy foals, predisposing these patients to sustain corneal trauma. Decreased corneal sensitivity also may explain in part lack of clinical signs in these patients. Therefore, sick foals should be monitored daily for presence of corneal lesions.

Because of this decreased corneal sensitivity, neonates may only show subtle clinical signs (e.g., mild photophobia, epiphora, blepharospasm) that may not correlate with the seriousness of their condition and often can be overlooked. Rapid melting of the cornea may follow once the cornea becomes infected. The location of the ulcer may give valuable clues about possible underlying causes such as entropion, distichia, and trichiasis from long eyelashes, which have to be corrected before proper wound healing can be expected. The diagnosis of corneal ulceration is made via positive fluorescein stain uptake in the cornea. If a corneal ulcer is evident before dye application (a descemetocele has to be ruled out!), corneal scrapings for aerobic and fungal cultures as well as for immediate cytology and Gram staining for antibiotic selection may be helpful. A topical anesthetic must be applied before corneal scraping can be performed, using a Kamura spatula or the back of a #15 Bard-Parker blade. Ideally, immediate referral to a specialist without further diagnostic workup is indicated in cases of deep corneal ulceration ($>\frac{1}{2}$ stromal thickness) or melting corneal ulcers.

Treatment with topical ophthalmic bacitracin-neomycin-polymyxin B ointment (one-inch strip four times daily), once daily 1% atropine ointment ($\frac{1}{2}$-inch strip) OS, and artificial tear ointment OU (one-inch strip four times daily) was initiated in '05 Misty. A small face-mask was placed to protect the eye from further insult. After 48 hours without dramatic improvement but also no deterioration, the cornea OS was anesthetized with topical proparacaine and a corneal scraping was performed, which revealed unremarkable cytology. A soft contact lens was placed, and the foal was switched to topical Ciloxan® drops (two drops four times daily), topical I-drops® (two drops four times daily), and topical atropine drops (two drops once daily). The eye medications were given 5 to 10 minutes apart with the I-drops given last. Systemic treatment was initiated with intravenous flunixine meglumine (0.5 mg/kg) twice daily for two days, then once daily for three days. Systemic antibiotics were continued throughout this time.

The patient's comfort level and the appearance of the eye improved rapidly. A 3-mm area of central superficial stain uptake was present after removal of the contact lens five days later. The patient was continued on the same treatment regimen, and the ulcer resolved after another four days. At that time, all medications were discontinued. All hemorrhages resolved within 10 days, and no other short- or long-term ocular complications were noted

TREATMENT

Initial medical treatment of a superficial ulcer includes application of a topical ophthalmic broad-spectrum antibiotic ointment (e.g., bacitracin-neomycin-polymyxin B) four times daily. Topical gentamicin should not be used in cases of noninfectious persistent corneal ulcers since it can slow down corneal wound healing.[10] If no improvement is noted within 24 to 48 hours, one should reassess the original diagnosis and try to identify an underlying cause.

In cases of progressive or deeper ulceration, frequent topical treatment (at least 6 to 8 times daily) is required. Agents used to treat gentamicin-resistant Pseudomonas infection include topical Ciloxan (0.3% ciprofloxacin, Alcon Labs, Fort Worth, TX), amikacin (10 mg/ml) and polymyxin B (0.25% IV solution). Fortified cefazolin (50 mg/ml), chloramphenicol, bacitracin, and carbenicillin (0.4% or 4 to 8 mg/ml) are effective against beta-hemolytic *Streptococcus*.[40,41] Topical natamycin, miconazole, itraconazole, fluconazole, and ketoconazole have been used successfully in equine patients with fungal keratitis.[28,42] Antifungal agents may be commercially available for ophthalmic use (e.g. natamycin) or should be compounded. In general, one should refrain from using antifungal vaginal cream for treatment of fungal keratitis since its high alcohol content makes it unsuitable for ocular use.

Soft contact lenses may be placed in the eye to aid in epithelial adhesion in superficial corneal ulcers and allow for a longer contact time with the topical antibiotic. While ointments in general provide a longer contact time than drops, the author recommends using solution instead once a contact lens has been placed. In uncooperative patients, placement of a subpalpebral lavage system may greatly facilitate administration of topical medication. Depending upon the size of the foal, facemasks are helpful in protecting the eye from irritation from bedding, especially in recumbent foals. Facemasks with plastic eye cups should not be used since severe ocular injury can result from breaking of the material, and the increasing humidity underneath the cups may predispose patients to fungal keratitis. The author prefers either Cashel® fly masks or Guardian masks® for this purpose.

With severe corneal infection, frequent topical medication every two hours may be required to achieve optimal results. If this type of intensive care cannot be provided, referral to an equine clinic should be considered. Infected corneal ulcers or ulcers with extensive stromal involvement can be complicated by rapid corneal "melting" (keratomalazia) that can result in corneal perforation within 24 hours. Clinically, corneal liquefaction becomes evident as grayish, gelatinous appearance of the cornea that may "bulge" forward or form gelatinous tissue "oozing" from the cornea. Mediators of this stromal collagenolysis are mainly metalloproteinases and serine proteinases derived from tear film and corneal cells, leucocytes, and microbes.[43] Immediate hourly treatment with a specific proteinase inhibitor for ophthalmic use or combinations of them should be initiated, including N-acetylcysteine (a 20% IV preparation can be diluted down with artificial tears to a 5% solution), 0.05% disodium or potassium ethylene diamine tetraacetate (EDTA), heparin (1000 IU/ml), tetracycline antibiotics, or preferably, autogenous serum. When using the latter, care should be taken to prepare fresh serum every 24 to 48 hours and to keep it refrigerated at all times. Systemic antimicrobial treatment should also be considered for patients with infected corneal ulcers; systemic antifungal treatment is a must in patients with suspected deep fungal keratitis.

In equine patients, severe painful uveitis is frequently encountered as sequela of corneal disease.[10] Evident clinically by photophobia, a difficulty to keep the pupil dilated, and a greenish-yellowish aqueous flare in foals, uveitis should be treated with topical 1% atropine and systemic NSAIDS. Atropine sulfate is effective in minimizing pain from cilicary muscle spasm (cycloplegic), stabilizing the blood aqueous barrier and reducing the risk of posterior synechia formation.[40,44] It also has been shown to reduce intestinal motility in equine patients who should be closely monitored for signs of colic. In foals, the author recommends using a ½-inch strip of 1% atropine ointment once or twice daily for a few days or until effect. Alternatively, 1% tropicamide may be used two to three times daily. However, tropicamide is mainly a mydriatic and not so much a cycloplegic agent, and therefore is limited to treatment of mild uveitis. Systemic NSAIDS will provide pain relief from the anterior uveitis as well as help stabilize the blood aqueous barrier.[40,45] Flunixin meglumine (0.5 mg/kg twice daily, IV, IM, or PO) may be used in foals. Since side effects of systemic NSAIDS include gastroduodenal ulceration, concomitant use of oral ranitidine (6.6 mg/kg orally, q 8 h) or sucralfate (20 mg/kg orally, q 8 h) is highly recommended for gastric ulcer prophylaxis.[10]

While use of topical NSAIDS such as flurbiprofen has been advocated to help treat anterior uveitis secondary to corneal ulceration, it can also predispose patients to bacterial and fungal keratitis as well as keratomalazia and should only be considered in cases with the most severe and otherwise medically uncontrollable uveitis.[46,47] Corticosteroids are contraindicated in treatment of corneal ulceration or even after healing of an ulcer to treat corneal scarring or corneal vascularization since they may exacerbate possible residual fungal keratitis.[48] Heavy artificial tear preparations (e.g., 0.5 to 1% Celluvisc [Allergan, Irvine, CA] drops or I-drops) should be considered in patients with possible underlying tear film abnormalities.

As soon as progressive corneal ulceration despite aggressive medical treatment becomes evident, surgical keratectomy with placement of a conjunctival flap should be recommended to halt progression of disease and prevent corneal rupture. The benefits of this procedure by far outweigh any concerns about corneal scarring associated with this surgery, since healing of a deep corneal ulcer will result unavoidably in scar formation. However, in order to minimize scarring via preparation of a very thin flap tissue and to optimize the outcome of surgery, this procedure should only be performed by a trained specialist.

Once the cornea has perforated from an infected corneal ulcer, painful panophthalmitis of the globe ensues and makes these patients poor candidates for any other surgery besides enucleation for pain relief.

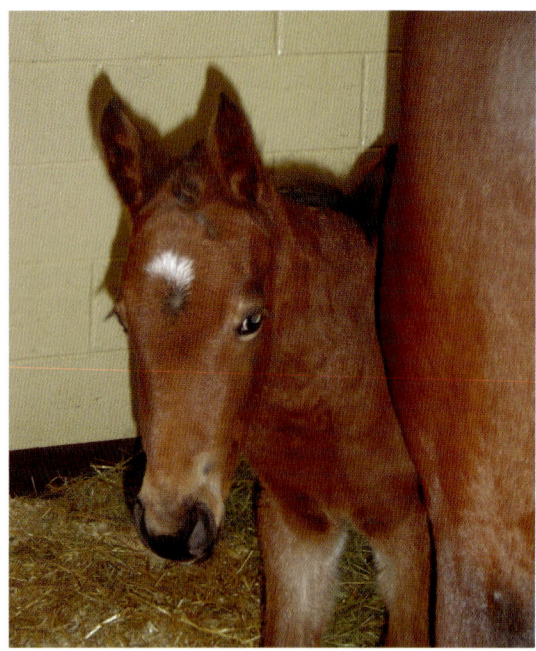

Fig. 14-8 '05 MrMagoo presented with signs of disseminated infection—fever, septic arthritis, and bilateral uveitis.

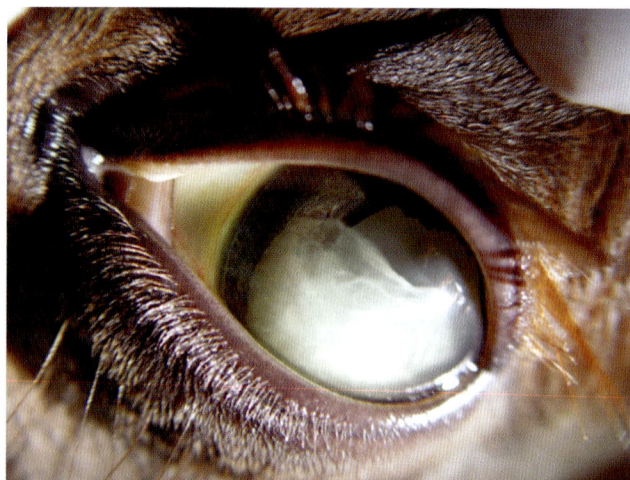

Fig. 14-9 Fibrin clot present in the anterior chamber at presentation.

'05 MrMagoo, a Thoroughbred colt, had a normal birth and was standing and nursing by two hours of age (Figure 14-8). Unfortunately, the owner did not realize that because the mare had leaked colostrum for four days preceding the birth that the foal was at risk for septicemia. The veterinarian was called to examine the foal at 18 hours of age for a normal foal check. The foal was bright and alert but perhaps a little quieter than to be expected. Immediately recognizing the possibility of failure of passive transfer, the veterinarian administered 1 liter of intravenous plasma.

At three days of age, '05 MrMagoo was hospitalized for intensive care after developing a high fever (103°F), left hock joint effusion, and bilateral uveitis. A neutrophilia and a high fibrinogen were present on his initial CBC. Blood and joint fluid cultures were submitted. The joint fluid had an increased WBC count and elevated protein indicating septic arthritis. His IgG levels were low at 400 mg/dl. The working diagnosis was partial failure of passive transfer with septicemia and septic arthritis.

'05 MrMagoo's ocular evaluation revealed lacrimation, moderate conjunctival injection, moderate-severe miosis and a 2+ aqueous flare in both eyes (OU). A large fibrin clot was present in the anterior chamber in both eyes, overlying the pupils and preventing visualization of structures in the posterior segment (Figure 14-9). The intraocular pressure was low at 7 mm Hg OU. Otherwise,

there was no corneal fluorescein stain uptake noted in either eye, and a positive dazzle response was present OU. In order to better evaluate the intraocular structures, an ocular ultrasound was performed, which was normal with the exception of the intracameral fibrin. The diagnosis was severe bilateral uveitis, suspected secondary to septicemia.

Systemic illness in neonatal foals frequently results in either immune-mediated or endotoxic uveitis or in uveitis secondary to ocular invasion of an infectious organism. Organisms implicated in the pathogenesis of neonatal uveitis are similar to those associated with neonatal septicemia. These include *Rhodococcus equi*, *Streptococcus sp.*, *Salmonella sp.*, *E. coli*, *Actinobacillus equuili*, adenovirus, and equine viral arteritis.[10]

Early clinical signs of uveitis include photophobia, lacrimation and blepharospasm, conjunctival hyperemia, aqueous flare, and miosis. Since untreated uveitis in foals may quickly lead to severe corneal edema, hypopyon (fibrin accumulation in the anterior chamber), hyphema, posterior synechia, and cataract formation, a thorough workup and early aggressive medical treatment are imperative to avert sight- and globe-threatening sequela of severe uveitis.

Systemic treatment with broad-spectrum antibiotics (amikacin and ampicillin) was initiated in '05 MrMagoo's. The affected hock was lavaged with 1 liter of sterile saline, and intra-articular amikacin was administered (see Chapter 6, Case 6-2). Another liter of intravenous plasma was administered to increase IgG levels.

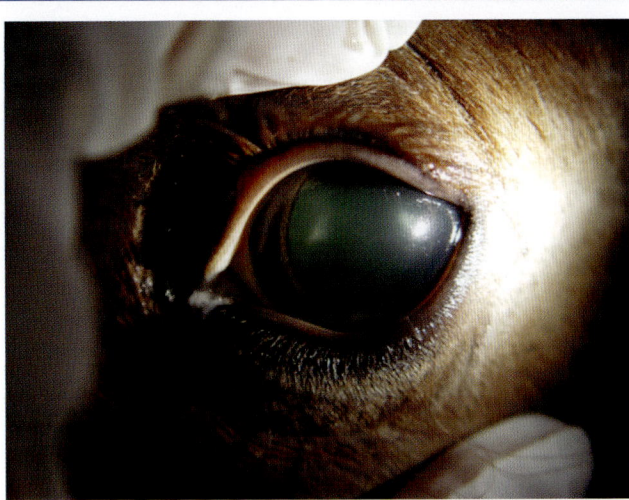

Fig. 14-10 Appearance of eye three hours postinjection of tissue-plasminogen activator.

Ocular treatment involved topical Neopolydex (Qualitest Pharmaceuticals, Inc., Huntsville, AL) ointment (½-inch strip q 4 hrs) OU as well as topical atropine, twice daily, OU. At the same time of the joint lavage, a bilateral intracameral tissue plasminogen activator (TPA) injection was performed, which resulted in resolution of the fibrin clots within three hours (Figure 14-10).

'05 MrMagoo's ocular treatment was continued with Neopolydex ointment in a tapering dose (q 6 hours OU for four days, q 8 hours for four days, q 12 hours for four days, once daily for four days) as well as atropine (once daily for 5 days, then discontinue). Flunixine meglumine was administered at .5 mg/kg once daily for four days.

TREATMENT

Since topical corticosteroids (e.g., 0.2% dexamethasone, 1% prednisolone acetate) are the preferred treatment for anterior uveitis, a corneal fluorescein dye test should be applied first to rule out presence of a corneal ulcer.[49] It should be noted that topical hydrocortisone is ineffective in treating anterior uveitis due to its poor corneal penetration. The severity of the uveitis dictates frequency of topical steroid use, which may range from q 6 hours to q 2 hours. Treatment also typically includes use of a topical mydriatic/cycloplegic, topical and systemic NSAIDS, as well as a broad-spectrum topical antibiotic (i.e. chloramphenicol, ofloxacin) and systemic antibiotics.

A topical antibiotic-corticosteroid preparation (e.g. NeoPolyDex) may be considered to improve owner compliance and minimize patient handling. If concerns about side effects of topical atropine (i.e., colic) prevent more frequent administration of the drug, combination with 2.5% to 10% phenylephrine may be used to optimize pupillary dilation.

Intracameral injection of TPA as enzymatic therapy to aid fibrinolysis should be considered in patients with large fibrin accumulation or a large blood clot in the anterior chamber.[10,50] It should be ideally used within three to 10 days after fibrin formation. If used too early or in cases of active bleeding, TPA may result in severe intraocular bleeding, which ultimately may lead to loss of the eye. The procedure is routinely performed under general anesthesia or heavy sedation combined with local and topical anesthesia. The eye is surgically prepared with topical 1% Betadine solution or 1:50 povidone-iodine solution. An intracameral injection along the limbus with a 27-gauge needle of 50 to 150 μg of TPA per eye is performed while the globe is stabilized with a pair of small forceps (e.g. Bishop-Harmon). Great care must be taken to avoid injury of the iris, especially the corpora nigra, and lens. As the needle is being retracted, the needle tract exit should be grasped with the forceps and held off for a few seconds to allow for rapid sealing. This prevents a "backward-splashing" of TPA underneath the conjunctival tissue. Because of the high risk of complications (i.e. recurrent hemorrhage, corneal/iris/lens perforation, immediate postoperative changes in intraocular pressure), this procedure should be performed by a trained specialist.

Depending upon the underlying cause, prognosis for an uveitic eye may range from good to guarded, and the owner should be made aware of the seriousness of this condition early on, including the possibility of future recurrent uveitis episodes (equine recurrent uveitis or ERU) in the affected eye.

'05 MrMagoo's uveitis resolved within five days of treatment, and both eyes continued to appear comfortable. The septic hock was lavaged twice more on an every-other-day schedule. Systemic antibiotics were continued for a total of two weeks when all signs of infection were resolved. The foal was discharged from the hospital on day 14.

REFERENCES

1. Roberts SM: Congenital ocular anomalies, *Vet Clin North Am Equine Pract* 8:459, 1992.
2. Latimer CA, Wyman M, Hamilton J: An ophthalmic survey of the neonatal horse, *Equine Vet J Suppl* 2:9, 1983.
3. Priester WA: Congenital ocular defects in cattle, horses, cats, and dogs, *J Am Vet Med Assoc* 160:1504, 1972.
4. Gelatt KN: Congenital and acquired ophthalmic diseases in the foal, *Anim Eye Res* 1:15, 1993.

5. Enzerink E: Short communication: The menace response and pupillary light reflex in neonatal foals, *Equine Vet J* 30:546, 1998.

6. Clark CK, Brooks DE, Lester GD: Corneal sensitivity and tear production in hospitalized neonatal foals, *Proc Am Coll Vet Ophthalmol* 134, 1996.

7. Brooks DE, Clark CK, Lester GD: Cochet Bonnet aesthesiometer-determined corneal sensitivity in neonatal foals and adult horses, *Vet Ophthalmol* 3:133, 2000.

8. Adams R, Mayhew IG: Neurological examination of newborn foals, *Equine Vet J* 16:306, 1984.

9. Munroe G: Study of the hyaloid apparatus in the neonatal Thoroughbred foal, *Vet Rec* 146:579, 2000.

10. Brooks DE: Equine ophthalmology. In Gelatt KN, ed: *Veterinary ophthalmology,* Philadelphia, 1999, Lippincott Williams & Wilkins.

11. Whitley DR: Neonatal equine ophthalmology. In Koterba AM, Drummond WH, Kosch PC, eds: *Equine clinical neonatology,* Philadelphia, 1990, Lea & Febiger.

12. Fox LM, Thurmon JC: Bilateral ankyloblepharon congenital, *Vet Med* 64:237, 1969.

13. Turner AG: Ocular conditions of neonatal foals, *Vet Clin North Am* 20:429, 2004.

14. Beech J, Aguirre G, Gross S: Congenital nuclear cataracts in the Morgan horse, *J Am Vet Med Assoc* 184:1363, 1984.

15. Joyce JR, Martin JE, Storts RW et al.: Iridial hypoplasia (aniridia) accompanied by limbic dermoids and cataracts in a group of related Quarterhorses, *Equine Vet J Suppl* 10:26, 1990.

16. Ramsey DT, Ewart SL, Render JA et al.: Congenital ocular abnormalities of Rocky Mountain Horses, *Vet Ophthalmol* 2:47, 1999.

17. Matthews AG, Handscombe MC: Bilateral cataract formation and subluxation of the lenses in a foal: A case report, *Equine Vet J Suppl* 2:23, 1983.

18. Dziezyc J, Kern TJ, Wolf ED: Microphthalmia in a foal, *Equine Vet J Suppl* 2:15, 1983.

19. Mosier DA, Engelman RW, Confer AW: Bilateral multiple congenital ocular defects in Quarterhorse foals, *Equine Vet J Suppl* 2:18, 1983.

20. Ueda Y: Aniridia in a Thoroughbred horse, *Equine Vet J Suppl* 10:29, 1990.

21. Gelatt KN: Glaucoma and lens luxation in a foal, *Vet Med Small Anim Clin* 261, 1973.

22. Barnett KC, Cottrell BD: Buphthalmos in a Thoroughbred foal, *Equine Vet J* 20:132, 1988.

23. Gelatt KN, McClure JR: Congenital strabismus and its correction in two Appaloosa horses, *Florida Agric Experim Stat J* Series No. 1364:240.

24. Rebhuhn WC, Loew ER, Riis RC: Clinical manifestation of night blindness in the appaloosa horse, *Comp Cont Educ Vet Suppl* 6:103, 1984.

25. Munroe G: Congenital ocular disease, In Robinson NE, ed: *Current therapy in equine medicine,* ed 4, Philadelphia, 1997, WB Saunders.

26. Wilcock BP, Brooks DE, Latimer CA: Glaucoma in horses, *Vet Pathol* 28:74, 1991.

27. Halenda RM, Grahn BH, Sorden SD et al: Congenital equine glaucoma: Clinical and light microscopic findings in two cases, *Vet Comp Ophthalmol* 7:105, 1997.

28. Lavach JD: *Large animal ophthalmology,* St Louis, 1990, CV Mosby.

29. Rebhuhn WC: Retinal and optic nerve diseases, *Vet Clin North Am* 8:587, 1992.

30. Matthews AG, Crispin SM, Parker J: The equine fundus II: Normal anatomical variants and colobomata, *Equine Vet J Suppl* 10:50, 1990.

31. Witzel DA, Smith EL, Wilson RD et al: Congenital stationary night blindness: An animal model, *Invest Ophthalmol Vis Sci* 17:188, 1978.

32. Gelatt KN, Gelatt JP: Surgery of nasolacrimal apparatus and tear systems, In Gelatt KN, Gelatt JP, eds: *Small animal ophthalmic surgery. Practical techniques for the veterinarian,* Boston, 2001, Butterworth-Heineman.

33. Molleda JM, Martin E, Novales M et al: Congenital bilateral entropion of the upper eyelid in a pony, *Equine Pract* 19:8, 1997.

34. Gelatt KN, Myers VS, McClure JR: Aspiration of congenital and soft cataracts in foals and young horses, *J Am Vet Med Assoc* 165:611, 1974.

35. Dziezyc J, Millichamp NJ, Keller CB: Use of phacofragmentation for cataract removal in horses: 12 cases (1985-1989), *J Am Vet Med Assoc* 198:1774, 1991.

36. Dziezyc J: Management of cataracts in horses, *Equine Comp* 1640, 1993.

37. Millichamp NJ, Dziezyc J: Cataract phacofragmentation in the horse, *Vet Ophthalmol* 3:157, 2000.

38. Munroe G: Subconjunctival hemorrhages in neonatal Thoroughbred foals, *Vet Rec* 144: 278, 1999.

39. Munroe G: Survey of retinal haemorrhages in neonatal Thoroughbred foals, *Vet Rec* 146: 95, 2000.

40. Regnier A: Antimicrobial, anti-inflammatory agents, and antiglaucoma drugs, In Gelatt KN, ed: *Veterinary ophthalmology,* Philadelphia, 1999, Lippincott Williams & Wilkins.

41. Kern TJ: Antibacterial agents for ocular therapeutics, *North Am Vet Clin Small Anim Pract* 34:7655, 2004.

42. Ford MM: Antifungals and their use in veterinary ophthalmology, *North Am Vet Clin Small Anim Pract* 34:669, 2004.

43. Brooks DE, Ollivier FJ. Matrix metalloproteinase inhibition in corneal ulceration, *North Am Vet Clin Small Anim Pract* 34:611, 2004.

44. Klaus G, Constantinescu GM: Nonhypotensive autonomic agents in veterinary ophthalmology, *North Am Vet Clin Small Anim Pract* 34:777, 2004.

45. Giulana E: Nonsteroidal anti-inflammatory drugs in veterinary ophthalmology, *North Am Vet Clin Small Anim Pract* 34:707, 2004.

46. Reviglio VE, Rana TS, Li QJ: Effects of topical nonsteroidal anti-inflammatory drugs on the expression of matrix metalloproteinases in the cornea, *J Cataract Refract Surg* 29:989, 2003.

47. Moreira H, McDonnell PJ, Fasano AP: Treatment of experimental Pseudomonas keratitis with cyclo-oxygenase and lipoxygenase inhibitors, *Ophthalmol* 98:1693, 1991.

48. O'Day DM, Ray WA, Robinson R et al.: Efficacy of antifungal agents in the cornea. II. Influence of corticosteroids, *Invest Ophthalmol Vis Sci* 25:331, 1984.

49. Holmberg BJ, Maggs DJ: The use of corticosteroids to treat ocular inflammation, *North Am Vet Clin Small Anim Pract* 34:693, 2004.

50. Wilkie DA, Gemensky-Metzler AJ: Agents for intraocular surgery, *North Am Vet Clin Small Anim Pract* 34:801, 2004.

Index

Page numbers followed by f indicate figures; t, tables; b, boxes.

A

Abdominal adhesions, ultrasonography of, 201, 201f
Abdominal compartment syndrome (ACS), 240, 243
Abdominal distension, 194, 214, 221, 238, 240
Abdominal examination, of foal, 124, 194
Abdominal pain. See Colic
Abdominocentesis
  in foals, 195–196
  in peripartum mares, 24
Abortion, late-term, causes of, 16
Abscesses, intra-abdominal, 84, 210
Acetylcysteine
  ophthalmic preparation, 267
  retention enemas, for colic, 205, 206
  for septic pneumonia, 109
α-1-acid-glycoprotein, in acute phase immune
    response, 79
Acidified milk replacer, 59
ACS (abdominal compartment syndrome), 240, 243
ACTH (adrenocorticotropic hormone), for advancing
    fetal maturity, 18
Actinobacillus equuli, 84, 89, 94, 222
Acute lung injury (ALI), 105, 106, 144
Acute phase immune response, 79
Acute respiratory distress syndrome (ARDS), 105,
    106
Adrenergic agonists. See Inopressor therapy; *specific
    drugs*
Adrenocorticotropic hormone (ACTH), for advancing
    fetal maturity, 18
Agalactia, treatment of, 73
Airway patency, maintenance of, 109
Albumin, blood, 9
Albuterol inhalants, for septic pneumonia, 109
ALI (acute lung injury), 105, 106, 144
Alkaline phosphatase, 9
Allanto-chorion. See Chorioallantois
Alloimmune disorders, 46–47. See also Immune-
    mediated thrombocytopenia; Neonatal
    Isoerythrolysis
Alpha-tocopherol. See Vitamin E
Altrenogest, 17

Alveolar hypoventilation, etiology of, 102
Alveolar–arterial oxygen gradient, 103–104
Alveoli
  Laplace relationship in, 138, 138f
  surfactant function in, 139
Amikacin, 90, 91t, 108, 117
Amino acids, blood, fractionation of, 224–225
Amino acid solutions, in parenteral nutrition, 66–67,
    66t
Aminoglycosides. See also *specific drugs*
  for septic arthritis/osteomyelitis, 117
  for septic pneumonia, 108
  for septicemia, 90
Aminophylline, for septic pneumonia, 109
Ammonia, blood, in hepatopathy, 223, 224
Amnion, 5, 19
Ampicillin, 90, 91t, 117
Amyloid, serum, 9, 79
Analgesics, 196t, 205. See also *specific drugs*
Anemia, isoerythrolysis and, 40, 42
Anesthesia, uroperitoneum and, 243
Angular limb deformities. See Limb deformities,
    angular
Anorexia, in high-risk mares, 18
Antibiotic therapy. See also *specific drugs*
  for aspiration pneumonia, 154
  for cholangiohepatitis, 227
  for neurologic disease, 186–187
  for omphalitis, 235–236
  for placentitis, 16, 17t
  for septic arthritis/osteomyelitis, 117
  for septic meningitis, 187
  for septic pneumonia, 108
  for septicemia, 90–92, 90t, 91t, 131–132
Antibodies, maternal. See also IgG;
    Immunoglobulins
  antiplatelet, in immune-mediated
    thrombocytopenia, 46, 47
  anti–red blood cell, in isoerythrolysis, 41–42, 44b,
    45
  half-life of, 33
Anti-endotoxin plasma, 92

Anti-inflammatory drugs. *See* Corticosteroids; Nonsteroidal anti-inflammatory agents
Anti-inflammatory response syndromes, 80
Antiplatelet antibodies, in immune-mediated thrombocytopenia, 46, 47
Anti–red blood cell antibodies, in isoerythrolysis, 41–42, 44b, 45
APGAR scoring system, 26, 27t
Apnea, after foaling, 27
Arabian foals, congenital neurologic disorders in, 183
ARDS (acute respiratory distress syndrome), 105, 106
Arterial blood gas analysis. *See* Blood gas analysis
Arthritis, septic, 112–119
    diagnostic testing for, 115–116, 115f
    history and physical examination, 112–113, 112–113f
    pathogenesis of, 112–113f, 113–114
    prognosis for, 118–119, 119f
    treatment of, 116–118, 117–118f
Arthrocentesis, 88, 114, 115
Arthroscopy, for septic arthritis, 118
Arytenoid chondritis, 150, 152, 155
Ascorbic acid, as neuroprotectant, 187, 188t
Aspartate amino transferase (AST), 9, 224
Asphyxia
    and encephalopathy, 181–182, 185–189
    during foaling. *See* Neonatal asphyxia
    systemic effects of, 182
Aspiration pneumonia. *See* Pneumonia, aspiration
AST (aspartate amino transferase), 9, 224
Ataxia, spinal, 181
Athletic performance
    cardiac defects and, 257
    neonatal pneumonia and, 110
    septic arthritis and, 119, 119f
Atlantooccipital spinal tap, 184
Atresia coli, 199f, 203
Atrial septal defects, 255
Atropine, for cardiovascular resuscitation, 28
Azithromycin, 91t

B
Bacillus piliformis. *See* *Clostridium piliformis*
Bacitracin, 219
Bacteria, blood cultures for, 85–86, 115–116, 225
Bacterial infection. *See also specific diseases, e.g.,* Salmonellosis
    and diarrhea, 214t, 215, 217, 217t
    and endotoxemia, 77
    and hepatopathy, 222
    and meningitis. *See* Meningitis, bacterial
    and placentitis, 16
    and pneumonia, 100
    and septicemia, 89–90, 89t, 90t
Bandages
    for decubital ulcers, 188, 188f
    for limb deformities, 161–162, 170, 172
Barium enema, 198–199, 199f
Behavior, neonatal, 3f, 4f, 5–7. *See also* Suckling behavior
Behavioral problems, in hand-raised orphan foals, 59
Bile acids, 9, 224
Bilirubin, 9, 133, 224
Biopsy
    bone marrow, 48
    liver, 224f, 225
Birth resuscitation of foals, 26–29
Bladder, urinary. *See* Urinary bladder
Blood clotting disorders. *See* Coagulopathies
Blood cultures, 85–86, 115–116, 225
Blood donors, 42–43
Blood gas analysis, 101–104, 102t, 103f
    in critically ill foals, 124, 133
    in detection of hypoxemia, 137
    in pulmonary prematurity, 141–142
Blood pressure
    fetal/neonatal transition and, 123
    measurement of, noninvasive, 122–123, 123f
Blood transfusions, 42–43, 124
Blood urea nitrogen, 9–10, 133
Body condition scoring, 54–55, 54–55f, 54t
Body wall tears, 22–26, 23f
Body weight, at birth, 54
Bone development, angular limb deformities and, 167
Bone diaphysis, angular limb deformities and, 174
Bone marrow aspirate/biopsy, 48
Borborygmi, in colic, 194
Bottle feeding, 58
Bovine colostrum, 36–37
Bovine hemoglobin (Oxyglobin), for isoerythrolysis, 42
Bradycardia
    fetal, 15
    paradoxical, with hypoperfusion, 124, 214
    perinatal, 27
Bromsulphalein (BSP) clearance, 225
Bronchodilators, for septic pneumonia, 109
Broodmare. *See* Mare
BSP (bromsulphalein) clearance, 225
Bucket feeding of orphan foals, 58–59, 58f
Buphthalmia, congenital, 262
Buscopan, 196t
Butorphanol, for colic pain, 196t
N-Butylscopolammonium bromide, 196t

C
Caffeine, for respiratory stimulation, 186, 188, 188t
Calcium
    in mammary secretions, and prediction of foaling, 1–2

maternal dietary deficiency of, and fetal development, 52–53
Candidiasis, and oral ulcers, 49f
Capnography, 107–108
Carbon dioxide. *See also* Hypercapnia
    end-tidal, 107–108, 143, 144
    partial pressure of
        estimation of, 107–108
        in respiratory disease, 102
Cardiac arrhythmias. *See also* Bradycardia; Tachycardia
    in critically ill foals, 123–124
    perinatal, 248
Cardiac auscultation, 7, 123–124, 248
Cardiac disorders, 247–257. *See also specific disorders and defects*
    congenital, 123, 249–250
    diagnostic testing for. *See* Echocardiography
    history and physical examination, 247–249, 249f
    pathogenesis of, 249–250
    treatment and prognosis for, 256–257
Cardiac murmurs
    in critically ill foals, 123
    grading of, 248
    pathologic, 247–248, 249
    physiologic, 248, 249, 257
Cardiac shunting, 103, 109, 110f, 248
Cardiac valves
    acquired disease of, 257
    congenital disorders of, 250, 256
    echocardiography of, 250–251, 252–253f, 253, 256
Cardiopulmonary complications, of uroperitoneum, 239–240, 240f, 243
Cardiovascular resuscitation, 28–29
Cardiovascular system
    evaluation of, 7, 122–123, 213–214
    in transition to extrauterine life, 3
Carpus
    angular deformities of
        diagnosis of, 168, 168f, 169f
        history and physical examination, 165–166, 165–166f
        prognosis for, 175–176
        treatment of, 170, 172–174
    cuboidal bones of, incomplete ossification of, 166, 171f, 174
    hyperextension of, 159, 160, 164
    hyperflexion of, 157f, 158, 158f, 161–162, 164
CARS (anti-inflammatory response syndrome, compensatory), 80
Castor oil, for colic, 205
Casts, for limb deformities, 162, 172
Cataracts, 261, 261f, 264
Catheters, intravenous, for parenteral nutrition, 67, 71
Cefotaxime, 91t, 187

Ceftazidime, 91t, 187
Celiotomy, exploratory, in colic, 202, 205–206
Cephalosporins
    for septic arthritis/osteomyelitis, 117
    for septic meningitis, 187
    for septic pneumonia, 108
    for septicemia, 90, 91t
Cephalothin, 91t, 117
Cerebellar abiotrophy, 183
Cerebral edema, treatment of, 187
Cerebrospinal fluid analysis, 184–185
Cervical star, 19
Chest, examination of, 7
Chest wall
    in respiratory function, 137–138, 137f
    rib fractures, 7, 28, 29f
Chloramphenicol, 91t, 187
Cholangiohepatitis, 222, 227
Chondroitin sulfate, for septic arthritis, 118
Chorioallantois, 5. *See also* Hydrops allantois; Placenta
Chorioretinitis, congenital, 262
Cimetidine, for gastric ulceration, 211, 211t
Circulatory status evaluation, 7, 122–123, 213–214
Clarithromycin, 91t
Cleft palate, 150, 151, 151f, 155
Clenbuterol, for placentitis, 17
Clinical pathology. *See* Hematology; Serum chemistry panel
Clostridial enteritis, 213, 215
    diagnostic testing for, 217, 217t, 218f
    treatment and prognosis for, 219, 220
Clostridium difficile, 215, 217, 217t, 219, 220
Clostridium perfringens, 215, 217, 217t, 219, 220
Clostridium piliformis, 226. *See also* Tyzzer's disease
Clotting disorders. *See* Coagulopathies
Cluster differentiation antigen 14, 77–78
Coagulation system
    acute phase immune response and, 79
    diagnostic testing of, 88–89
Coagulopathies
    diarrhea and, 217
    hepatopathy and, 225
    septicemia and, 85, 89, 93
Colic, 191–206
    abdominocentesis in, 195–196
    analgesics/sedatives for, 196t, 205
    clinical signs of, 192–195, 194f
    diagnostic approach to, 191–192, 193t
    diagnostic clinical pathology in, 195–196, 196f
    diagnostic imaging in, 195f, 197–201, 197–201f, 205f
    differential diagnosis of, 192, 193t, 202–204, 203f
    isoerythrolysis and, 40
    in prepartum mare, 22–23
    prognosis for, 206
    treatment of, 196t, 204–206

Colitis. *See also* Enterocolitis
  and colic, 192, 193t
  ultrasonography of, 199–200
Colloids, for critically ill foals, 125
Coloboma, 262
Colon. *See* Large intestine
Colostrometer, 36, 37f
Colostrum
  absorption of, 31–32, 33. *See also* Failure of passive
    transfer (FPT)
  anti–RBC antibody testing of, 44b, 45
  constituents of, 33
  evaluation of quality of, 32, 36, 37f
  feeding of, 36–37
  in immunocompetence of foal, 31, 33
  mammary production of, 1–2
Colostrum banks, 36
Colostrum substitutes, 36–37
Common digital extensor tendon rupture, 159,
    160f
Compensatory anti-inflammatory response
    syndrome (CARS), 80
Complement system, in acute phase immune
    response, 79
Complete blood count. *See* Hematology
Computed tomography (CT)
  in neurologic disease, 185, 185f
  in septic arthritis/osteomyelitis, 114f, 116
  in septic pneumonia, 105, 106f
Congenital disorders
  bladder wall defects, 238
  cardiac, 123, 249–250
  cleft palate, 150, 151, 151f, 155
  of gastrointestinal tract, 193t, 202–203
  limb deformities. *See* Limb deformities
  and liver failure, 223
  neurologic disorders, 183–184, 189
  ocular, 259, 260–263, 261f
  patent urachus, 232, 236
Conjunctival hemorrhages, 265, 265f
Contact lenses, 266–267
Continuous positive airway pressure (CPAP), 145
Coombs' test, for isoerythrolysis, 42
Coprophagy, 6, 53, 53f
Corneal ulcers, 265–267, 265f
  seizures and, 188–189
Coronavirus, and diarrhea, 214t, 215, 217t
Corticosteroids
  adverse effects of, 49
  for cerebral edema, 187
  for endotoxemia, 92–93
  for immune-mediated thrombocytopenia, 48, 49
Cortisol, fetal levels of, 1, 143
Cow's milk, 57t, 63
CPAP (continuous positive airway pressure), 145
Cranial nerves, examination of, 180

C-reactive protein, in acute phase immune response,
    79
Creatine kinase, 9
Creatinine
  blood levels of, 9
    fetal distress and, 132
    in uroperitoneum, 241
  peritoneal fluid/serum ratio, 196, 241–242
Creep feeding, 57, 59
Critically ill foals, 121–133
  clinical examination of, 121–124
  dextrose therapy for, 128–130
  fluid therapy for, 124–125, 125f, 130–131
  inopressor therapy for, 125–128, 127t
  laboratory evaluation of, 132–133
  oxygen supplementation for, 124, 124f
  recognition of, 121–122
Cryptosporidiosis, 216, 217t, 218, 219, 220
Crystalloids, for critically ill foals, 125
C-section, and pulmonary prematurity, 136
CT. *See* Computed tomography (CT)
Cuboidal bones, of carpus/tarsus
  incomplete ossification of, 166, 169, 170f, 171–172f,
    174
  normal ossification of, 167
Cultures
  blood, 85–86, 115–116, 225
  fecal, 217
  liver biopsy, 225
  synovial fluid, 116
Cyanosis
  cardiac disorders and, 248
  hypoxemia and, 100, 100f, 137
Cytokines
  in acute phase immune response, 79
  in lung maturation, 141

D
Dalteparin, for coagulopathy, 93
Dam. *See* Mare
Dead space–tidal volume ratio, 108
Dead space ventilation, 102–103
Decubital ulcers, 112, 112f, 118, 188, 188f
Defecation, stance for, 191f, 193
Dehydration, in neonates, 125
Deoxycholic acid, 53
Depression, neurologic disease and, 180
Dermatitis, in immune-mediated thrombocytopenia,
    46, 47
Detomidine, for colic pain, 196t
Dexamethasone
  for cerebral edema, 187
  for immune-mediated thrombocytopenia, 48
Dextrose therapy
  for critically ill foals, 128–130
  for high-risk mares, 18

for hypoglycemia, 61
for liver disease, 228
in parenteral nutrition, 66t
Diaphragmatic hernias, and colic, 192, 204
Diaphysis of long bones, angular limb deformities
and, 174
Diarrhea, 213–220
and colic, 194
diagnostic testing for, 216–218, 217f, 217t, 218f
history and physical examination, 213–214
milk replacer and, 59, 214
pathogenesis of, 214–216, 214t
prognosis for, 220
and sodium loss, 131
treatment of, 218–219
Diazepam
for sedation, 196t
for seizures, 186, 188t
DIC (disseminated intravascular coagulation), 80, 84f,
85
Diet. See also Nutrition
calcium deficient, 52–53
iodine deficient, 53
and milk composition, 52–53
selenium/vitamin E deficient, 153
Digit, hyperextension of, 159, 160, 160f, 163–164,
163f
Digital extensor tendon, common, rupture of, 159,
160f
Digoxin, 256
Dimethyl sulfoxide (DMSO), for cerebral edema, 187,
188t
Dioctyl sodium sulfosuccinate (DSS), 205
Dipalmitoylphosphatidylcholine, 139–140, 141
Disseminated intravascular coagulation (DIC), 80,
84f, 85
Distal interphalangeal joint, flexural deformities of,
158, 159f, 160, 162, 163, 164
DMSO (dimethyl sulfoxide), for cerebral edema, 187,
188t
Dobutamine, for hypovolemic shock, 126, 127t
Domperidone, for agalactia, 73
Donors
blood, 42–43
plasma, 34–35
Dopamine, for hypovolemic shock, 126–127, 127t
Doxapram, for cardiovascular resuscitation, 29
Doxycycline, 91t
DSS (dioctyl sodium sulfosuccinate), 205
Ductus arteriosus
and cardiac murmurs, 247–248
closure of, 249
patent, 253, 257
Duodenal ulcers, 210, 212
Dysmaturity, 19, 20t, 136, 166. See also Intrauterine
growth restriction (IUGR)

Dysphagia, 150–153
and aspiration pneumonia, 148–150, 154,
156
clinical signs of, 149, 149f
diagnostic testing for, 150–153, 151f, 152f
differential diagnosis of, 149t, 150
nutritional myodegeneration and, 153,
155
Dyspnea, 100
Dystocia, uroperitoneum and, 238, 239

E
Ears, petechiae of, 47f, 81f, 82
Ecchymoses, 46, 47f, 48
Echocardiography, 250–256. See also specific specific
cardiac defects
abnormal findings, 253–256, 254–255f
contrast technique, 252–253
examination procedure, 250–253, 251f
normal images, 251–253f
Electrocardiogram, fetal, 15, 16f
Electrolytes. See also specific electrolytes
derangements of, 216, 241
fluid therapy and, 130–131
Encephalopathy
hepatic, 222, 228
neonatal, 181–182, 185–189
Endocarditis, 83–84
Endoscopy. See also Gastroscopy
in colic, 201
in dysphagia, 151–152, 151f, 152f
of joints, 118
Endotoxemia, 61, 92
Endotoxins
assays for, 86
effects of, 78
in septicemia, 77–78
End-tidal carbon dioxide, 107–108, 143, 144
Enemas
barium, 198–199, 199f
for meconium retention, 205, 206
Energy requirements, calculation of, 65–66
Enrofloxacin, 91t
Enteral nutrition, 62–65, 70–71, 71f. See also
Nutritional support
Enteritis. See also Clostridial enteritis; Enterocolitis
and colic, 192, 193t
radiography of, 197, 197f, 198f
ultrasonography of, 199–200, 199f, 200f
Enterocolitis. See also Colitis
and diarrhea, 213, 214–216
necrotizing, 71, 193t, 198, 215, 217
Entropion, 260, 263–264, 264f
Enzyme-linked immunosorbent assay for FPT
testing, 33–34, 34f
Epilepsy, benign pediatric, 183, 189

Epinephrine
  for cardiovascular resuscitation, 28
  for hypovolemic shock, 127, 127t
  and lactate levels, 132
Epiphyseal (E-type) joint lesions, 113, 113f
Equine herpes virus 1, and hepatitis, 222
Erythromycin, 91t
Escherichia coli, and septicemia, 89, 90
Esophageal dysfunction, and dysphagia, 149, 152
Esophagitis, reflux, 209, 209f, 210
Esophagoscopy, 209, 209f
Esophagotomy tube placement, 154
Extremities, temperature of, in evaluation of ill foal, 122
Eye, 259–269. See also Ophthalmologic disorders; specific ocular structures
  anatomy and physiology of, 259–260
  congenital disorders of, 259, 260–263, 261f
  fundic abnormalities, hepatitis and, 222
  as secondary infection site, 83, 84f
Eyelid abnormalities, 260–261, 263–264, 264f

F
Failure of passive transfer (FPT), 31–49
  diagnosis of, 33–34, 34f
  history and physical examination, 31–32
  in neonatal encephalopathy, 181, 186
  pathogenesis of, 32–33
  prevalence of, 9, 9f
  prevention of, 36–38
  and respiratory infection, 100
  and susceptibility to infection, 79
  treatment of, 34–36, 35f
Famotidine, for gastric ulceration, 211, 211t
Fecal analysis, in diarrhea, 217–218
Fecaliths, 203, 203f
Feces, normal appearance, 54
Feeding. See Diet; Nutrition
Feeding methods, for orphan foals, 58–59, 58f
Feeding tubes, nasogastric, 64, 70, 154
Fescue toxicity, 20, 32
Fetlocks. See Metacarpophalangeal joint; Metatarsophalangeal joint
Fetus
  abortion of, 16
  development of, and maternal diet, 52–53
  electrocardiogram of, 15, 16f
  hormone levels in, 1
  in initiation of labor, 1
  placentitis-associated maturation problems, 19–20, 20t
  transition to extrauterine life in, 3, 123, 128
  ultrasonography of, 15, 15f, 15t
Fever, sepsis and, 82
Fibrinogen, 9, 86, 132
Fibrinolytic indexes, in neonates vs. adults, 88–89

Fibrinolytic system, in acute phase immune response, 79
Flexural limb deformities. See Limb deformities, flexural
Flow cytometric analysis, 48
Fluconazole, 91t
Fluid requirements, maintenance, 67
Fluid therapy
  for critically ill foals, 124–125, 125f, 130–131
  for diarrhea, 218–219
  for liver disease, 227
  potassium supplementation in, 131
  sodium levels and, 130–131
Flumazenil, 228
Flunixin meglumine
  for colic pain, 196t
  for endotoxemia, 93
  for placentitis, 16–17
Foal heat diarrhea, 214
Foaling environment, preparation and disinfection of, 36, 76–77
Foals
  birth resuscitation of, 26–29
  clinical examination of, 6–7, 6t
  clinical pathology, normal values, 7–10, 8t
  critical illness and. See Critically ill foals
  nutritional requirements of, 51–53, 61
  postpartum behavior of, 3f, 4f, 5–7
  progestagen levels in, 1, 2f
  rejection of, by dam, 6
  signs of infection in, 82
  transition to extrauterine life in, 3, 123, 128
Foramen ovale
  closure of, 3, 249
  patent, 253, 257
FPT. See Failure of passive transfer (FPT)
Fractures, rib, 7, 28, 29f
FRC. See Functional residual capacity (FRC)
Functional residual capacity (FRC), 106, 107, 107f, 137–138, 138f, 144
Fungi, and pneumonia, 101
Furosemide, for pulmonary edema, 256

G
Gait analysis, 180
Gastric emptying, delayed, 197, 199f, 209–210
Gastric ulcers, 208–212
  and colic, 192, 193t
  diagnostic testing for, 199, 201, 209–210, 209f
  and diarrhea, 214
  history and physical examination, 208–209, 208f
  pathophysiology of, 210
  prophylaxis for, 93
  treatment and prognosis for, 211–212, 211t, 219
Gastrointestinal reflux, 194–195

Gastrointestinal tract. *See also specific organs, e.g.,*
  Small intestine
  bacterial defense systems in, 78
  congenital disorders of, 193t, 202–203
  development of, 53, 62
  diagnostic imaging of, 197–201, 197–201f
  inflammatory disease of. *See also* Colitis; Enteritis;
    Enterocolitis
    and colic, 193t, 194
    radiography, 197, 198f
    ultrasonography, 199–200, 200f
  obstruction of
    and colic, 192, 193t, 202, 203–204
    radiography, 197, 197f, 198f, 199f
    ultrasonography, 200, 200f
  as route of infection, 76, 82, 82f
Gastroscopy, 201, 209, 209f
Genitourinary tract, bacterial defense systems in,
  78
Gentamicin, 16, 91t, 117
Gestation, hormone levels in, 1
Gestation length
  and prematurity, 136
  prolonged, 19–20
  variability of, 146
GGT (γ-glutamyl transferase), in hepatopathy, 224
Glaucoma, 262
Globe, congenital disorders of, 261, 261f, 262
Glucogenesis, 128
Glucoregulatory response in neonates, 61
Glucosamine, for septic arthritis, 118
Glucose, blood. *See also* Hyperglycemia;
    Hypoglycemia
  hepatopathy and, 224, 226
  monitoring of, 70f, 219
  parenteral nutrition and, 61, 72
  prematurity and, 143
  regulation of, in neonates, 128
  sepsis and, 86
Glucose intolerance, 61, 129
Glucose metabolism, fetal/neonatal transition and,
  128
Glucose therapy. *See* Dextrose therapy
γ-Glutamyl transferase (GGT), in hepatopathy,
  224
Glutaraldehyde coagulation
  for colostrum evaluation, 36
  for FPT testing, 33–34
Glycogen storage disease IV, 223
Goat's milk, 57t, 63
Goats, nurse, 56t, 57, 57f
Goiter, neonatal, 53
Gram-negative bacteria
  blood cultures for, 86
  and endotoxemia, 77
  and septicemia, 89–90, 89t, 90t

Gram-positive bacteria, and septicemia, 89t, 90, 90t
Growth rate, monitoring of, 10

H
Hand-raised orphan foals, behavioral problems in, 59
Head trauma, and neurologic disease, 182, 185
Heart
  arrhythmias of. *See* Cardiac arrhythmias
  auscultation of, 7, 123–124, 248
  disorders of. *See* Cardiac disorders
  echocardiography of. *See* Echocardiography
  valves of. *See* Cardiac valves
  vasopressin and, 127
Heart murmurs. *See* Cardiac murmurs
Heart rate. *See also* Bradycardia; Tachycardia
  of fetus, 15
  of neonate, 6, 6t
Hematology
  in hepatopathy, 225
  normal values, 8, 8t
  in sepsis, 85t, 86–87, 87t, 101
  in septic arthritis, 115
Hemicircumferential transection of periosteum, 173
Hemoglobinemia, isoerythrolysis and, 40
Hemoglobinuria, isoerythrolysis and, 40, 40f
Hemolysis. *See* Neonatal isoerythrolysis
Hemorrhage, reproductive tract, 22, 25, 25f
Hemostatic indexes, in neonates vs. adults, 88–89
Heparin, for coagulopathy, 93
Hepatic abscesses, 84
Hepatic failure. *See* Liver failure
Hepatoencephalopathy, 222, 228
Hepatotoxicity, 221, 223
Hernias
  and colic, 192, 204
  of ventral body wall, in dam, 24–25, 26f, 29
Herpes virus, equine, and hepatitis, 222
Heterochromia iridis, 260
High-risk pregnancy
  and birth resuscitation of foals, 26–29
  body wall tears and, 22–26
  painful prepartum disorders and, 22
  placentitis. *See* Placentitis
  twin pregnancies, 15, 23, 26
Hippomane, 18
Holliday-Segar formula for maintenance fluids, 130
Hoof trimming, for angular limb deformities, 170
Hormones
  in initiation of labor, 1
  in neonates, 1, 2f
Hyaline membrane disease, 138, 139, 140f
Hyaluronan, 115
Hyaluronate sodium, for septic arthritis, 118
Hyaluronic acid, for septic arthritis, 118
Hydranencephaly, 183–184, 184f
Hydration, evaluation of, 125, 214

Hydrocephalus, internal, 183, 183f
Hydrops allantois, 22, 23, 23f, 24, 25f, 26
Hyperammonemia, hepatopathy and, 223, 224
Hyperbilirubinemia, 133, 224
Hypercapnia
    etiology of, 102
    in neonatal encephalopathy, 182
    treatment of, 186
Hypercreatinemia, 132, 241
Hyperemia, sepsis and, 82, 83f
Hyperfibrinogenemia, 86, 132
Hyperglycemia
    causes of, 129
    parenteral nutrition and, 61, 72
    treatment of, 72, 129–130
Hyperkalemia, in uroperitoneum, 241, 242, 243
Hyperlactic acidemia
    in dam, 24
    in neonates, 10, 132–133
Hypernatremia, in critically ill foals, 130–131
Hyperopia, 262
Hypertension
    intra-abdominal, 240, 243
    pulmonary, 142
Hypoglycemia
    glucogenesis and, 128
    in hepatopathy, 224, 226
    in premature foals, 143
    sepsis and, 86
    treatment of, 60, 128–130
Hypokalemia, fluid therapy and, 131
Hyponatremia, 128, 131
Hypoperfusion
    and blood pressure, 123
    in critically ill foals, 124–125
Hypopyon, 268–269, 268f
Hypothermia, 82, 128
Hypovolemic shock
    recognition of, 122–124
    treatment of, 124–128, 127t
Hypoxemia
    and brain injury, 181
    detection of, 137
    signs of, 100, 100f
    uroperitoneum and, 239–240
Hypoxia
    fetal, bradycardia as indication of, 15
    response to, in fetus and neonate, 27
Hypoxic encephalopathy. See Neonatal
    encephalopathy (NE)

I

Icterus. See Jaundice
IgG. See also Immunoglobulins
    colostral, absorption of, 31–32, 33. See also Failure
        of passive transfer (FPT)

lypholyzed equine preparations, 37
Ileus, functional, and colic, 192, 193t, 204
Imipenem, 91t
Immune disorders, 31–49
    failure of passive transfer. See Failure of passive
        transfer (FPT)
    immune-mediated thrombocytopenia, 46–49, 47f
    isoerythrolysis. See Neonatal isoerythrolysis
Immune system
    acute phase response of, 79
    at birth, 31
    innate, as septicemia defense, 76, 77–79
Immune-mediated thrombocytopenia, 46–49, 47f
Immunocompetency
    colostrum and, 31, 33, 79
    factors affecting, 80b
Immunoglobulins. See also Antibodies; IgG
    in colostrum, 31–32, 33
    in innate immune system functioning, 79
Indocyanine green clearance, 225
Infection. See also Bacterial infection; Parasitic
        infection; Viral infection
    defenses against, 77–79
    factors associated with increased risk of, 80b
    pathogenesis of, 76–77
    prevalence of, 75–76
    primary site of, 81–82, 82f
    secondary sites of, 82–84, 84f
Inflammation, and pulmonary development, 141
Inflammatory response syndromes, 80
Inguinal hernias, and colic, 192, 204
Inopressor therapy
    in critically ill foals, 125–128, 127t
    "rule of 6" for, 126
Insulin
    administration of, 129–130
    for hyperglycemia, 72, 129–130
Insulin response, in premature foals, 143
Interphalangeal joints
    distal, hyperflexion of, 158, 159f, 160, 162, 163,
        164
    hyperextension of, 159, 160, 160f, 163–164, 163f
Intestines. See Large intestine; Small intestine
Intra-abdominal hypertension, 240, 243
Intra-articular antibiotics, for septic arthritis, 117
Intranasal oxygen administration, 109, 109f, 124, 124f,
        144
Intrauterine growth restriction (IUGR), 19–20, 20t
Intravascular hemolysis. See Neonatal isoerythrolysis
Intravenous catheters, for parenteral nutrition, 67, 71
Intussusception, 192, 193t, 200, 200f, 204
Iodine, maternal dietary deficiency of, and fetal
        development, 53
Iris, 260
Isoerythrolysis. See Neonatal isoerythrolysis
Isoxsuprine, for placentitis, 17

IUGR (intrauterine growth restriction), 19–20, 20t
Ivermectin, for strongyloidosis, 219

J

Jaundice
   differential diagnosis of, 222
   isoerythrolysis and, 40, 40f
   liver failure and, 221, 222f
Jaundiced foal agglutination (JFA) test, 44b, 45
Joint lavage, for septic arthritis, 116, 117–118, 118f
Joints. *See also specific joints*
   abnormal, diagnostic testing for, 88
   blood supply to, 113
   deformities of. *See* Limb deformities
   infection of. *See* Arthritis, septic
   periarticular ligament laxity, 166, 170, 174
   as secondary infection site, 83, 84f

K

Kernicterus, 41
Kidney. *See also* Nephropathy
   abscesses of, 84
   functional assessment of, 9–10, 124, 132

L

Labor. *See* Parturition
Lactase, 53, 219
Lactate, blood
   in dam, 24
   in neonates, 10, 132–133
Lactation
   inadequate milk production, 53–54
   maintenance of, in non-nursing mare, 72, 73
   milk volume, normal, 52
   onset of, 1–2
   premature, causes of, 13, 16
Lactose intolerance, 214, 217t, 219
Lactose intolerance test, 218
Lactulose, for hepatopathy, 228
Lameness, causes of, 113
Laplace relationship, 138, 138f
Large intestine
   atresia of, 199f, 203
   inflammatory disease of. *See* Colitis
   obstruction of
      lethal white syndrome and, 202–203
      meconium impaction and, 202, 205, 206
      radiography in, 197, 198–199, 198f, 199f
Laryngeal paralysis, 150, 150f, 152, 155
Lavender foal syndrome, 183, 189
Lens
   anatomy of, 260
   congenital cataracts, 261, 261f, 264
   luxations of, 261
Lethal white syndrome, 192, 202–203, 203f

Leukocytes, 8, 8t. *See also* Lymphocytes; Neutrophils; Platelets
Ligament laxity, periarticular, 166, 170, 174
Limb deformities
   angular, 165–176
      acquired, 167
      diagnostic testing for, 168–170, 168–171f
      history and physical examination, 165–167
      pathogenesis of, 167
      prognosis for, 175–176, 175f
      treatment of, 170–174, 171–172f
   flexural, 157–164
      diagnostic testing for, 160–161
      history and physical examination, 157–159, 157–160f
      pathogenesis of, 159–160
      prognosis for, 164
      treatment of, 161–164, 163f
Limbs, normal angular deviation, at birth, 167, 168
Lipid emulsions, in parenteral nutrition, 66t
Lipid intolerance in neonates, 61
Lipopolysaccharide-binding protein, 77
Liver abscesses, 84
Liver failure, 221–228
   diagnostic testing for, 9, 223–225, 224f, 226f
   history and physical examination, 221–222, 222f
   pathogenesis of, 222–223
   prognosis for, 228
   treatment of, 227–228
   Tyzzer's disease and, 222, 224f, 226–227, 226–227f, 228
Lumbosacral spinal tap, 184
Lungs. *See also* Pneumonia; *entries at* Pulmonary
   acute injury to, 105, 106, 144
   auscultation of, 7
   maturation of, 136, 141
   postpartum adaptations of, 3
   prematurity of. *See* Pulmonary prematurity/immaturity
   radiographs of, 104–105, 104–105f
   surfactant deficiency in, 139–140
Lymphocytes, 8, 101
Lymphopenia, 8, 101
Lyphomune, 37

M

Magnesium sulfate, as neuroprotectant, 187, 188t
Magnetic resonance imaging (MRI), in neurologic disease, 185
Malnutrition, detection and etiology of, 54–55, 55t
Maltase, 53
Mammary development, 1–2, 13, 16. *See also* Lactation
Mannitol, for cerebral edema, 187, 188t

Mare
  bond with foal, 6, 27, 73
  as infection source for foal, 76–77
  rejection of foal by, 6
MARS (mixed anti-inflammatory response
      syndrome), 80, 85
Maternal antibodies, 33, 41–42, 45, 46–47
Maternal stress, and pulmonary maturation, 136
Maturity
  abnormalities of, at birth, 19–20, 20t. *See also*
      Dysmaturity; Prematurity
  assessment of, 7, 136–137
Mean corpuscular volume, 8, 8t
Mean platelet volume, 48
Mechanical ventilation, 109, 143, 144–145
Meconium
  aspiration of, 101, 149, 153–154
  impaction of
      and colic, 191, 192, 193t, 202
      diagnosis of, 195f, 197, 198f, 200–201, 201f
      prognosis for, 206
      treatment of, 204–205
  passage of, 6, 54
Melena, isoerythrolysis and, 40, 41f
Meningitis, bacterial
  diagnostic testing for, 184–185
  prognosis for, 189
  and seizures, 182
  septicemia and, 83, 84f
  treatment of, 187
Metabolic acidosis, 133, 216, 219
Metabolic status
  assessment of, 124
  and lactate levels, 132
  and maintenance fluid therapy, 130
Metacarpophalangeal joint
  angular deformities of, 168–169, 169f, 173, 175–176
  flexural deformities of, 158–159, 158f, 159f, 162, 164
Metatarsophalangeal joint, angular deformities of,
      168–169, 169f, 173, 175–176
Metoclopramide, for gastric ulceration, 211–212, 211t
Metronidazole, 91t, 219
Microbes, recognition of and defenses against, 77–79
Microphthalmos, 261, 261f
Midazolam, for seizures, 186
Milk
  aspiration of, and pneumonia, 148–150, 154, 156.
      See also Dysphagia
  constituents of, 52, 57t
  dietary influences on composition of, 52–53
  regurgitation of, 149, 149f
  volume produced, normal, 52
Milk of magnesia, for colic, 205
Milk pellets, 59
Milk replacers, 56t, 57–58, 57t, 63
  and diarrhea, 59, 214

Mineral oil, for colic, 205
Mixed anti-inflammatory response syndrome
      (MARS), 80, 85
MODS (multiple organ dysfunction syndrome), 80,
      88
MRI (magnetic resonance imaging), in neurologic
      disease, 185
Mucolytic agents, for septic pneumonia, 109
Mucous membranes
  as defense against infection, 78
  immune-mediated thrombocytopenia and, 46, 47f
  isoerythrolysis and, 40, 40f
  normal, 7
Mule foals
  immune-mediated thrombocytopenia in, 46
  isoerythrolysis and, 41
Multiparous mares, and isoerythrolysis, 40
Multiple organ dysfunction syndrome (MODS), 80,
      88
Musculoskeletal system
  evaluation of, 10, 10f
  infection of. *See* Arthritis, septic
  limb deformities. *See* Limb deformities
Muzzle, for foal, 45f
Myocardial damage, and cardiac arrhythmias, 124

N
Naloxone, as neuroprotectant, 187, 188t
Narcolepsy, 183, 189
Nasal flare, as sign of respiratory distress, 137
Nasogastric feeding tubes, 64, 70, 154
Nasogastric intubation, for colic, 194–195
Nasolacrimal duct obstruction, 263
NE (neonatal encephalopathy), 181–182, 185–189
Neck trauma, and neurologic disease, 182, 185
Necrotizing enterocolitis, 71, 193t, 198, 215, 217
Neonatal asphyxia. *See also* Neonatal encephalopathy
      (NE)
  and diarrhea, 214–215
  etiology of, 27
  and liver failure, 222
  systemic effects of, 182
Neonatal encephalopathy (NE), 181–182, 185–189
Neonatal goiter, 53
Neonatal isoerythrolysis, 39–45
  diagnostic testing for, 42
  and hepatitis, 222–223
  history and physical examination, 40–41, 40–41f
  with immune-mediated thrombocytopenia, 47
  pathogenesis of, 41–42
  prevention of, 43–45, 44b, 45f
  treatment of, 42–43
Neonatal maladjustment syndrome. *See* Neonatal
      encephalopathy (NE)
Neonatal respiratory distress syndrome (NRDS), 139,
      140f

Nephropathy
  isoerythrolysis and, 40, 41f
  oxytetracycline and, 162
  and sodium loss, 131
Nervous system
  autonomic, failure of, 124
  as secondary infection site, 83
Neurologic dysfunction, 179–189
  diagnostic testing for, 184–186, 185f
  differential diagnosis of, 181–184
  isoerythrolysis and, 41
  physical examination in. *See* Neurologic
    examination
  prognosis for, 189
  treatment of, 186–189, 188t
Neurologic examination, 7, 124, 179–181
Neutropenia
  with alloimmune thrombocytopenia, 49
  in neonates, 8
  sepsis and, 86–87, 101
  septic arthritis and, 115
Neutrophilia, sepsis and, 101
Neutrophils. *See also* Neutropenia; Neutrophilia
  in neonates, 8, 101
  in sepsis, 86–87, 88f
Night blindness, equine, 262–263
NMD (nutritional myodegeneration), 153, 155
Nonsteroidal anti-inflammatory agents. *See also*
  specific drugs
  for endotoxemia, 93
  for placentitis, 16–17, 17t
Norepinephrine, for hypovolemic shock, 127,
  127t
Nostrils, milk in, dysphagia and, 149, 149f
NRDS (neonatal respiratory distress syndrome), 139,
  140f
Nuclear scintigraphy, for lung function testing, 107
Nurse goats, 56t, 57, 57f
Nurse mares, 56–57, 56t
Nursing behavior. *See* Suckling behavior
Nutrition. *See also* Diet
  in fetal development, 52–53, 153
  of foal
    determining adequacy of, 53–54, 54–55f, 54t
    normal requirements, 51–53, 61
    orphans, 56–59, 56t, 57t
    requirements in premature/unfed/sick foals, 61
  of mare, 52–53, 153
Nutritional myodegeneration (NMD), 153, 155
Nutritional support, 60–73. *See also* Enteral nutrition;
  Parenteral nutrition
  complications of, 61, 70–73
  delivery route selection for, 62–64
  emergencies in, 60–61
  in hepatopathy, 228
  monitoring of, 69–70, 70f, 70t
  plan for, 62
  requirements of neonatal foals, 61

O
Occipitoatlantoaxial malformations, 183
Ocular disorders. *See* Ophthalmologic disorders
Omeprazole, for gastric ulceration, 211, 211t
Omphalitis, 231–236
  diagnostic testing for, 233–235, 233t, 233–235f
  history and physical examination, 231–232, 232f
  pathogenesis of, 232
  and septic arthritis/osteomyelitis, 116
  treatment and prognosis for, 235–236, 236f
Omphalophlebitis, 77, 81–82, 82f
Ophthalmic medications, 266–267, 269
Ophthalmologic disorders, 259–269. *See also specific*
  disorders
  congenital, 259, 260–263, 261f
  corneal ulceration, 265–267, 265f
  hypopyon, 268–269, 268f
Optic nerve disorders, congenital, 262
Oral ulcers/erosions, 47f, 49f
Orphan foals, 56–59, 56t, 57t
Osteomyelitis, types of, by location, 113. *See also*
  Arthritis, septic
Overfeeding, 61, 71
Oxygen, decreased. *See* Hypoxia
Oxygen gradient, alveolar–arterial, 103–104
Oxygen, partial pressure of. *See also* Hypoxemia
  in neonates, 3, 3t
  in respiratory disease, 100
Oxygen supplementation
  for critically ill foals, 124, 124f
  for placentitis, 17
  for pulmonary prematurity, 144
  for septic pneumonia, 109, 109f
  for septicemia, 93
Oxyglobin, for isoerythrolysis, 42
Oxytetracycline, 91t, 162
Oxytocin, for milk let-down, 73

P
Packed cell volume, normal values, 8, 8t
Paint horses, and lethal white syndrome, 192,
  202–203
Parasitic infection, and diarrhea, 214t, 215–216, 218,
  219, 220
Parenteral nutrition, 64–69. *See also* Nutritional
  support
  complications of, 71–72
  discontinuance of, 72
  formulation and preparation of diet, 65–67, 65b,
    66t, 68–69b
  indications for, 62
  initiation of, 67–68
  monitoring of, 69–70, 70f, 70t

Parenteral nutrition bag, 70f
Paromomycin, for cryptosporidiosis, 219
Parturition
    hormonal signaling of, 1–2
    impending, signs of, 1
    induction of
        and pulmonary prematurity, 136, 146
        timing of, 146
    normal, 2
    prediction of, from mammary gland secretions,
        1–2
    stages of, 3–4, 4f
Patent ductus arteriosus, 253, 257
Patent foramen ovale, 253, 257
Patent urachus, 232, 236
Pathogen-associated molecular patterns, 77
Pathogen-specific DNA assays, 86, 116
Pattern-recognition receptors, 77–78
PEEP (positive end expiratory pressure), 143, 145
Penicillin, 91t
    for placentitis, 16
    for septic arthritis/osteomyelitis, 117
    for septic pneumonia, 108
    for septicemia, 90
Pentazocine, for colic pain, 196t
Pentoxifylline, for placentitis, 17
Percutaneous ultrasonography. See Transabdominal
        ultrasonography
Perfusion
    blood pressure as indicator of, 123
    in critically ill foals, 124–125
Periarticular ligament laxity, 166, 170, 174
Periosteal stripping, 173
Peritoneal drainage, 241f, 242
Peritoneal fluid analysis, 196, 196f, 241–242
Persistent truncus arteriosus, 255
Petechiae
    differential diagnosis of, 48
    in immune-mediated thrombocytopenia, 46, 47f
    sepsis and, 48, 81f, 82
Phalangeal joints. See Interphalangeal joints
Pharyngeal cysts, 150, 151, 152f, 155
Phenobarbital, for seizures, 186, 188t
Physeal growth, angular limb deformities and, 167
Physeal (P-type) joint lesions, 113, 114f, 119, 119f
Physical examination
    critically ill foals, 121–124
    neurologic examination, 7, 124, 179–181
    normal foals, 6–7, 6t
Pica, and diarrhea, 214
Pinnae, petechiae of, 47f, 81f, 82
Placenta
    inspection of, 5, 5f
        in hydrops allantois, 24, 25f
        in placentitis, 18–19, 18f
    premature separation of, 181

Placentitis, 13–20
    diagnostic testing for, 14–15, 14–16f
    fetal effects of, 19–20, 20t
    history and physical examination, 13–14, 13f
    and isoerythrolysis, 41, 42
    and lung maturation, 141
    and neonatal encephalopathy, 181
    pathogenesis of, 16
    placental appearance in, 18–19, 18f
    treatment of, 16–18, 17t
Plasma
    anti-endotoxin, 92
    oral administration, for FPT, 37–38
Plasma donors, 34–35
Plasma transfusions
    for critically ill foals, 125, 132
    for failure of passive transfer, 34–36, 35f
    for immune-mediated thrombocytopenia, 49
    for liver disease, 228
Platelet factor 3 test, 48
Platelets, 8
    antibodies against, in immune-mediated
        thrombocytopenia, 46, 47
    decreased numbers of. See Thrombocytopenia
Pneumatosis intestinalis, 198, 217
Pneumocytes, surfactant production by, 139, 139f
Pneumonia
    aspiration, 101, 148–156
        diagnostic testing for, 150–153, 151f
        dysphagia and, 148–150, 154, 156. See also
            Dysphagia
        prognosis for, 156
        treatment of, 153–155, 155f
    septic, 99–110
        diagnostic testing for, 101–106, 102t, 103–106f
        history and physical examination, 99–100, 100f
        lung function testing in, 106–108, 107f
        pathogenesis of, 100–101
        pathophysiology of, 106
        prognosis for, 110
        treatment of, 108–110, 109f, 110f
Pneumoperitoneum, 197–198, 205f
Polymyxin B, for endotoxemia, 92
Portosystemic shunts, 223, 224, 225, 228
Positive end expiratory pressure (PEEP), 143, 145
Postmaturity, 19–20, 20t
Postpartum causes of malnutrition, 54, 55t
Potassium, blood
    fluid therapy and, 131
    in uroperitoneum, 241, 242, 243
Potassium supplementation, in fluid therapy, 131
Pregnancy
    high-risk. See High-risk pregnancy
    normal, 1–2, 1f
Premature foals
    and incomplete ossification of cuboidal bones, 166

lung surfactant in, 140
nutritional requirements of, 61
physiology of, 143
Prematurity, 19–20. *See also* Pulmonary prematurity/immaturity
definition of, 19, 136
endogenous vs. exogenous causes of, 136
indications of, 20t, 136–137
Prepartum causes of malnutrition, 54, 55t
Prepartum period
disorders of
body wall tears, 22–26
and colic-like symptoms, 22
placentitis. *See* Placentitis
normal, 1–2, 1f
Prepubic tendon rupture, 23, 24–25
Pressure sores, 112, 112f, 118, 188, 188f
Primary pulmonary hypertension, 142
Probiotics, for diarrhea, 219
Progestagens
in fetal maturation and initiation of labor, 1
newborn levels of, 1, 2f
Progesterone, for placentitis, 17
Prolonged gestation, 19–20
Protein, blood, 9
Protein C, for septicemia, 93
Protein requirements, calculation of, 66–67, 66t
Proteinuria, 10
Protozoal infection, and diarrhea, 214t, 216, 218, 219, 220
Ptyalism, 208f
Pulmonary artery, hypoplastic, 255
Pulmonary complications, of uroperitoneum, 239–240, 240f, 243
Pulmonary edema, 256
Pulmonary function testing, 106–108, 107f
Pulmonary gas exchange, 102–103
Pulmonary hypertension, primary, 142
Pulmonary maturation, 136, 141
Pulmonary prematurity/immaturity, 135–147
diagnostic testing for, 141–142
history and physical examination, 136–137
induction of parturition and, 136, 146
inflammation and, 141
pathogenesis of, 137–138, 137f, 138f
primary pulmonary hypertension and, 142
radiography in, 141f, 142f
surfactant and, 138–140
treatment and prognosis for, 143–146
Pulmonary shunting, 103, 109, 110f
Pulse oximetry, 101
Pulse quality, evaluation of, 122, 248
Pyloric outflow obstruction, diagnosis of, 197, 199f, 209–210

R
Radiography
in angular limb deformity, 168–170, 168–172f
in colic, 197–199, 197–199f, 205f, 209–210
contrast, of gastrointestinal tract, 198–199, 199f, 209–210
in diarrhea, 198f, 217, 217f
in dysphagia, 152, 153f
in pneumonia, 104–105, 104–105f, 151f, 152
in pulmonary prematurity/immaturity, 141f, 142f
in septic arthritis/osteomyelitis, 113–114f, 116
Radionucleotide bone imaging, in septic arthritis/osteomyelitis, 116
Ranitidine, for gastric ulceration, 211, 211t
RDS. *See* Respiratory distress syndrome (RDS)
Recombinant granulocyte colony-s factor, 48, 49
Rectal examination, in pregnant mare, 23–24
Rectal ultrasonography, in placentitis, 14, 14f
Rectus abdominus rupture, 23
Recumbency
critical illness and, 122
and decubital ulcers, 112, 112f, 118, 188, 188f
Red blood cell antibodies, 41–42, 44b, 45
Red blood cell antigens (factors), in isoerythrolysis, 41–42, 43
Red blood cell count, 8, 8t
Red blood cell typing, 43
Refractometry, for colostrum evaluation, 36, 37f
Regional limb perfusion, for septic arthritis/osteomyelitis, 116, 117, 117f
Regumate. *See* Altrenogest
Regurgitation of milk, 149, 149f
Rejection of foal, 6
Renal abscesses, 84
Renal function, assessment of, 9–10, 124, 132
Renal sodium wasting, 131
Reperfusion injury, 181, 187, 214
Reproductive tract. *See also* Uterus
hemorrhage of, 22, 25, 25f
Respiratory distress
signs of, 100, 137
uroperitoneum and, 239
Respiratory distress syndrome (RDS)
acute, 105, 106
mechanical ventilation in, 145
neonatal, 139, 140f
Respiratory patterns, abnormal, neurologic disorders and, 181–182, 188
Respiratory rate, of neonates, 6, 6t
Respiratory resuscitation, 27–28, 28f
Respiratory system. *See also* Lungs
bacterial defense systems in, 78
diagnostic sampling of, 106
evaluation of, 124
infection of. *See* Pneumonia
physical examination of, 137

physiology of, 137–139, 137f, 138f
prematurity of. *See also* Pulmonary prematurity/
    immaturity
as route of infection, 82, 100
in transition to extrauterine life, 3
vulnerability of, 99, 100
Resuscitation, at birth, 26–29
Retina
    abnormalities of, hepatitis and, 222
    anatomy of, 260
    congenital disorders of, 262
    hemorrhages of, 265–266
    inflammation of. *See* Uveitis
Rhodococcus pneumonia, and athletic function, 110
Rib fractures, 7, 28, 29f
Rifampin, 91t
Rotavirus, 214t, 215, 217t, 220
"rule of 6" for inopressor therapy, 126

S
SAA (serum amyloid A), 9, 79
Salmonellosis, 215, 217, 219, 220
SAP (serum alkaline phosphatase), in hepatopathy,
    224
Scintigraphy, of liver, 225
Scrotal edema, uroperitoneum and, 238, 238f
Sedatives, for colic, 196t
Seizures
    clinical presentation of, 180
    diagnostic testing for, 184–186, 185f
    differential diagnosis of, 181–184
    hepatopathy and, 222, 228
    prognosis for, 189
    treatment of, 186–189, 188f, 188t
Selenium, and nutritional myodegeneration, 153, 155
Sepsis. *See also* Septicemia
    and bacterial meningitis, 182
    and colic, 192, 194
    ecchymoses and petechia in, 48, 81f, 82
    and hyperglycemia, 72
    and icterus, 222
Sepsis scoring system, 86–88, 87t
Septic arthritis. *See* Arthritis, septic
Septic meningitis. *See* Meningitis, bacterial
Septic pneumonia. *See* Pneumonia, septic
Septic shock, 84–85, 88
Septicemia, 75–95. *See also* Sepsis
    clinical signs and physical examination, 81–85,
        81–84f
    definition of, 76
    diagnosis of, 85–89, 85t, 87t, 88f, 132–133
    mortality from, 76, 88
    pathogenesis of, 76–80, 80b
    pathogens in, 89–90, 89t, 90t
    prevalence of, 75–76
    prognosis for, 94

treatment of, 89–94, 93f
    antibiotic therapy in, 90–92, 91t, 131–132
    dextrose/insulin therapy in, 129
Seramune, 37
Serum alkaline phosphatase (SAP), in hepatopathy,
    224
Serum amyloid A (SAA), 9, 79
Serum chemistry panel
    in hepatopathy, 223–225
    normal values, 8t, 9–10
    in sepsis, 85t, 87, 87t
SGA (small for gestational age). *See* Intrauterine
    growth restriction (IUGR)
Shock
    hypovolemic
        recognition of, 122–124
        treatment of, 124–128, 127t
    septic, 84–85, 88
Shoeing, corrective
    for angular limb deformities, 170
    for flexural limb deformities, 163–164, 163f
Single radial immunodiffusion, for FPT testing, 34
SIRS. *See* Systemic inflammatory response syndrome
    (SIRS)
Skin, as defense against infection, 78
Skin lesions, in immune-mediated thrombocytopenia,
    46, 47
Small for gestational age (SGA). *See* Intrauterine
    growth restriction (IUGR)
Small intestine
    development of, 53
    inflammatory disease of. *See* Enteritis
    obstruction/strangulation of, 192, 193t, 203–204
        diagnostic imaging, 197, 197f, 200, 200f
Snap test for IgG, 33, 34f
Sodium, blood, 128, 130–131
Sodium requirements, 130–131
Soft palate, dorsal displacement of, 150, 152, 152f,
    153f, 155
Sorbitol dehydrogenase, in hepatopathy, 224
Spinal ataxia, 181
Spinal nerves, examination of, 180
Spinal tap, procedure for, 184
Splenic abscesses, 84
Splints, for limb deformities, 161–162, 170, 172
Standardbreds, blood types in, 43
Stomach
    acid secretion in, 210
    delayed emptying of, 197, 199f, 210
    mucosal defenses in, 210
    ulcers of. *See* Gastric ulcers
Strabismus, congenital, 262
Streptococcus spp., and septicemia, 89
Stridor
    causes of, 149, 149t
    tracheotomy for, 154–155, 155f

Strongyloidosis, 215–216, 217t, 218, 219, 220
Suckling behavior
    critical illness and, 121, 122
    inadequate milk production and, 53–54
    neurologic disease and, 180
    normal, 3f, 5, 6, 51–52, 52t
Sucralfate, 211, 211t, 219
Sugar refractometer, for colostrum evaluation, 36, 37f
Sulfonamides. See Trimethoprim-sulfonamides
Sulpiride, for agalactia, 73
Surfactant, 138–140
    composition and functions of, 138–139
    deficiency of, 139–140
    production of, 3, 139, 139f, 140, 143
    for treatment pulmonary prematurity, 144, 145
Surgical intervention
    for angular limb deformities, 173, 174
    for colic, 202, 205–206
    for flexural limb deformities, 162–163
    for omphalitis, 235
    for uroperitoneum, 243
Synovial fluid analysis, 115–116, 115f
Synovial (S-type) joint infections, 113
Systemic inflammatory response syndrome (SIRS)
    diagnostic testing and, 88
    diarrhea and, 216, 217
    and hepatitis, 222
    septicemia and, 80, 84–85, 84f

T
Tachycardia
    abdominal pain and, 194
    fetal, 15
Tail, for blood pressure measurement, 123, 123f
Tarsal bone (T-type) osteomyelitis, 113
Tarsus
    angular deformities of, 169, 170f, 174
    cuboidal bones, incomplete ossification of, 166, 169, 170f, 171–172f, 174
Team approach, to critically ill foal, 121, 122
Tear secretion, 260
Temperature
    core to extremity gradient, in critically ill foals, 122
    normal, of neonates, 6t, 7
Tendon contracture/laxity. See Limb deformities, flexural
Tetralogy of Fallot, 255
Theophylline, for septic pneumonia, 109
Thermoregulation in foals, 7
Thiamine, as neuroprotectant, 187, 188t
Thrombocytopenia
    differential diagnosis of, 8, 48
    immune-mediated, 46–49, 47f
Ticarcillin, 91t
Tissue plasminogen activator, intraocular injection of, 269, 269f

Tocolytic agents, for placentitis, 17, 17t
Tocopherol. See Vitamin E
Toll-like receptors, 77, 78
Toxicity, hepatic, 221, 223
Tracheotomy, 154–155, 155f
Transabdominal ultrasonography
    in mares with abdominal pain, 24, 25, 25f, 26f
    in placentitis, 14–15, 14f, 15t
Transfusion reactions, 35
Transfusions
    blood, 42–43, 124
    plasma
        in critically ill foals, 125, 132
        for failure of passive transfer, 34–36, 35f
        for immune-mediated thrombocytopenia, 49
        in liver disease, 228
Transphyseal bridging, 173, 174
Trauma
    and angular limb deformities, 167
    and neurologic disease, 182, 185, 189
Tricuspid atresia, 256
Triglycerides, blood, in hepatopathy, 225
Trimethoprim-sulfonamides, 91t
    for placentitis, 16
    for septic arthritis/osteomyelitis, 117
    for septic meningitis, 187
Truncus arteriosus, persistent, 255
Twin pregnancies, 15, 23, 26
Tyzzer's disease, 222, 224f, 226–227, 226–227f, 228

U
Udder enlargement. See Mammary development
Ultrasonography
    in colic, 195f, 199–201, 199–201f
    in diarrhea, 200f, 217, 217f
    of heart. See Echocardiography
    in hepatopathy, 225
    in mares with abdominal pain, 24, 25, 25f, 26f
    in placentitis, 14–15, 14f, 15t
    in septic pneumonia, 105
    for umbilicus inspection, 233–235, 233–235f, 233t
    in uroperitoneum, 241f, 242
Umbilical cord, 5, 18, 232
Umbilical hernias, and colic, 192, 204
Umbilicus
    anatomy of, 232
    infection of. See Omphalitis
    postnatal care of, 5, 77, 232
Underfeeding, consequences of, 61
Urachus
    infection of, 232
    patent, 232, 236
    rupture of, 238, 242. See also Uroperitoneum
    ultrasonography of, 234–235, 234–235f
Urea nitrogen, blood, 9–10, 133

Urinary bladder, rupture of. *See also* Uroperitoneum
  diagnosis of, 241f, 242
  pathogenesis of, 22, 238–239
  surgical repair of, 242–243, 243f
Urinary sodium loss, 131
Urinary tract, bacterial defense systems in, 78
Urination, 6, 54, 193, 194f
Urine, normal volume of, 54
Uroperitoneum, 237–244
  cardiopulmonary complications of, 239–240, 240f, 243
  and colic, 192, 193t
  diagnosis of, 196, 201, 241–242, 241f
  history and physical examination, 237–238, 237f, 238f
  pathogenesis of, 238–239, 239f
  prognosis for, 244
  treatment of, 242–244, 243f
Uterus
  tears of, 22
  torsion of, 22, 24
Uveitis, 83, 84f, 267, 268–269, 268f

V
Vaginal discharge, 16
Vancomycin, for clostridial enteritis, 219
Vasopressin
  for cardiovascular resuscitation, 28
  for hypovolemic shock, 127–128, 127t
  pharmacology of, 127–128
Ventilation, assisted, at birth, 27–28. *See also* Mechanical ventilation
Ventricular septal defect (VSD)
  clinical presentation of, 248–249
  echocardiography of, 254–255, 254–255f

pathogenesis of, 250
  treatment and prognosis for, 256, 257
Viral infection. *See also specific viruses*
  and diarrhea, 214t, 215, 217t, 220
  and liver failure, 222
  and placentitis, 16
  and pneumonia, 100–101
  and thrombocytopenia, 48
Vitamin B complex, in parenteral nutrition, 67
Vitamin C, as neuroprotectant, 187, 188t
Vitamin E
  deficiency of, and nutritional myodegeneration, 153
  as neuroprotectant, 187, 188t
  for nutritional myodegeneration, 155
  for placentitis, 17–18
VSD. *See* Ventricular septal defect (VSD)

W
Warming, external, in hypovolemic shock, 128
Water losses, and maintenance fluid therapy, 130
Weakness, critical illness and, 121, 122
Weight gain, normal, 54
Weight, monitoring of, 10, 10f
White blood cell count, normal values, 8, 8t
White muscle disease. *See* Nutritional myodegeneration (NMD)

X
Xylazine, for colic pain, 196t

Z
Zinc sulfate coagulation for FPT testing, 33
Zoonotic diseases, 219

Table 5-5   Commonly Used Antimicrobials for Treatment of Equine Neonatal Septicemia

Drug	Dose	Route	Interval	Comments
Amikacin	21 mg/kg[80] 25 mg/kg[81,82]	IV	Once daily	Trough levels should be <2 µg/ml; potentially nephrotoxic; efficacy is based on C_{max} : MIC > $10^{54,82}$
(Na) Ampicillin	22 mg/kg*	IV	6 hours	Prediction of efficacy is based on AUC_{0-24} : MIC
Azithromycin	10 mg/kg[83]	PO	q 24 hours; q 48 hours after 5 days	Prediction of efficacy is based on AUC_{0-24} : MIC
Ceftazidime	50 mg/kg	IV	6 hours slow over 15 minutes	Prediction of efficacy is based on T > MIC†
Cefotaxime	40 mg/kg[84]	IV	4–6 hours	Higher or more frequent dosing may be needed for meningitis; prediction of efficacy is based on T > MIC†
Ceftiofur	5 mg/kg[85] 10 mg/kg[86]	IV IV	12 hours 6 hours, over 30 minutes	Prediction of efficacy is based on T > MIC†
Ceftriaxone	25 mg/kg[87]	IV	q 12 hour	Third generation; prediction of efficacy is based on T > MIC†
Cephalothin	10–20 mg/kg*	IV	6 hours	First generation; prediction of efficacy is based on T > MIC†
Cefazolin	8–16 mg/kg[15]	IV	6–8 hours	First generation; prediction of efficacy is based on T > MIC†
Chloramphenicol palmitate	50 mg/kg[88]	PO	6–8 hours	Potential for aplastic anemia in humans
Cefuroxine axetil	30 mg/kg/day[86]	PO	Divided BID or TID	Second generation; prediction of efficacy is based on T > MIC†
(Na) Cefuroxine	50–100 mg/kg/day[86] 200–240 mg/kg/day	IV IV	Divided TID Divided TID	Second generation; Higher dose for meningitis; prediction of efficacy is based on T > MIC†
Cefpodoxime proxetil	10 mg/kg	PO	8–12 hours	Third generation; prediction of efficacy is based on T > MIC†
Doxycycline	10 mg/kg*	PO	12 hours	
Clarithromycin	7.5 mg/kg[89]	PO	12 hours	
Enrofloxacin	5–10 mg/kg[81]	PO or IV	24 hours	Potential for arthropathy; prediction of efficacy is based on C_{max} : MIC > 10
Erythromycin stearate	25 mg/kg[90] 37.5 mg/kg	PO PO	8 hours 12 hours	Prediction of efficacy is based on T > MIC†
Erythromycin lactobionate	5 mg/kg	IV	6 hours	
Fluconazole	4 mg/kg[56]	PO	Once daily	
Gentamicin sulfate	6.6 mg/kg 10–16 mg/kg if <7 days old[86]	IV	Once daily	Trough levels should be <2 µg/ml; potentially nephrotoxic; prediction of efficacy is based on C_{max} : MIC > 10
Imipenem	10 mg/kg†	IV	6 hours	
Metronidazole	10–15 mg/kg*	PO	6–12 hours	
Oxytetracycline	5–10 mg/kg*	IV	12 hours	
(K or Na) Penicillin	22,000 IU/kg[91]	IV	6 hours	Prediction of efficacy is based on T > MIC†
Rifampin	5–10 mg/kg[92]	PO	12 hours	
Ticarcillin or Ticarcillin/ clavulanic acid	50 mg/kg[93]	IV	6 hour	
Timethoprim sulfa	20–30 mg/kg*	PO	12 hours	

*Dose established in adult horses
†Dose established in humans
†T > MIC = plasma concentration of the drug should be one to five times the MIC for 40% to 100% of the time between dosing intervals